ALZHEIMER DISEASE
THERAPEUTIC STRATEGIES

Advances in Alzheimer Disease Therapy

Series Editors:
Ezio Giacobini
Robert Becker

This series periodically brings up-to-date advances in basic and clinical sciences that are relevant to understanding the etiology, pathogenesis, diagnosis, and treatment of Alzheimer disease. Experts from the various fields relevant to understanding Alzheimer disease report their new research findings and discuss the newest developments in possible Alzheimer disease therapies.

Books in the Series

Cholinergic Basis for Alzheimer Therapy
Edited by Robert Becker and Ezio Giacobini
ISBN 0-8176-3566-1

Alzheimer Disease: Therapeutic Strategies
Edited by Ezio Giacobini and Robert Becker
ISBN 0-8176-3757-5

ALZHEIMER DISEASE
THERAPEUTIC STRATEGIES

Ezio Giacobini
Robert Becker

Editors

with the editorial assistance of
Diana L. Smith *&* **Joyce M. Barton**

Birkhäuser

Ezio Giacobini
Chairman of Pharmacology
Southern Illinois University
School of Medicine
P.O. Box 19230
Springfield, IL 62794-9230
USA

Robert E. Becker
Chairman of Psychiatry
Southern Illinois University
School of Medicine
P.O. Box 19230
Springfield, IL 62794-9230
USA

Library of Congress Cataloging-in-Publication Data

Alzheimer disease: therapeutic strategies / Ezio Giacobini, Robert
    Becker, editors, with the editorial assistance of Diana L. Smith and
    Joyce M. Barton.
        p.   cm. — (Advances in Alzheimer disease therapy)
    Includes bibliographical references and index.
    ISBN 978-1-4615-8151-2   ISBN 978-1-4615-8149-9 (eBook)
    DOI 10.1007/978-1-4615-8149-9
        1. Alzheimer's disease—Chemotherapy. 2. Alzheimer's disease—
    Pathophysiology. 3. Alzheimer's disease—Treatment.
    I. Giacobini, Ezio. II. Becker, Robert E. III. Series.
        [DNLM: 1. Alzheimer's Disease—therapy. WM 220 A4755 1994]
    RC523.A39757 1994
    616.8'31—dc20
    DNLM/DLC
        for Library of Congress   94-34494
                                                               CIP

Printed on acid-free paper.

Birkhäuser

©1994 Birkhäuser Boston
Softcover reprint of the hardcover 1st edition 1994

ISBN 978-1-4615-8151-2

Camera-ready text prepared by the editors using WordPerfect 6.0 on an IBM PS2

9 8 7 6 5 4 3 2 1

CONTENTS

Introductions

Part I. Neuropathologic and Genetic Basis of AD Treatment

Part II. Therapeutical Strategies to Arrest Production and Processing of Amyloid

Part III. The Cholinergic System of Human Brain

Part IV. Cholinesterase Inhibitors in AD Treatment

Part V. Nicotinic Agonists as Drugs for AD Treatment

Part VI. Muscarinic Agonists: Preclinical and Clinical Approaches

Part VII. Drugs to Enhance Acetylcholine Synthesis and Release

Part XI. Antioxidant, Protective, and Anti-Inflammatory Agents in AD Therapy

Part XII. Treatment of Behavioral and Gait Disturbances

Part XV. Clinical Testing of Efficacy of New Drugs in AD

Part XVI. Socio-Economic Aspects in the
Treatment of Alzheimer's Disease

Part XVII.   Alzheimer Disease Treatment: The Future

INTRODUCTIONS

Alzheimer Disease: Therapeutic Strategies
edited by E. Giacobini and R. Becker.
© 1994 Birkhäuser Boston

DEVELOPMENT OF DRUGS FOR ALZHEIMER THERAPY: A DECADE OF PROGRESS

Ezio Giacobini and Robert Becker

Departments of Pharmacology and Psychiatry, Southern Illinois University School of Medicine, P.O. Box 19230, Springfield, IL 62794-9230

We have reached the third publication of the series on Advances in Alzheimer Therapy (Giacobini and Becker, 1988; Becker and Giacobini, 1991), therefore, some comparisons seem both useful and appropriate. In the seven years (1988-1994) since our first volume (Giacobini and Becker, 1988) we have identified approximately 100 compounds proposed for use in Alzheimer disease (AD) therapy. We have found reference to over 300 studies conducted in humans. These studies have involved a total of about 3,000 patients.

A brief retrospective of AD therapeutical approaches represented by these different compounds tells us something about the course of drug development and the potential of the various therapeutic approaches as a future treatment of AD, the most common degenerative disease of the central nervous system.

The Drugs That Made it Through (the Reviews)
An overview of the compounds that were discussed in our three volumes (Giacobini and Becker, 1988; Becker and Giacobini, 1991; Giacobini and Becker, 1994) gives some indication of persisting interests, successful trends, approaches with marginal benefits and strategies that have already begun to be abandoned. There has been disappointment with the cholinergic approaches and the major thrust of basic research has turned to the cellular and molecular biology of AD. From the number of papers and the results presented in this volume, it appears that the only group of drugs which has successfully survived through the three meetings are the cholinesterase inhibitors (ChEI).

As seen in Table I, the number of ChEI reported and discussed increased from 7 in 1988 to 13 in 1994. Their representation in clinical trials (mainly Phase II) tripled during the same period of time.

In spite of this positive trend, the number of registered and approved drugs is still limited to one single compound (tacrine, THA, tetrahydroaminoacridine) which was registered in the USA in September, 1993 as the first drug with an indication for AD. THA will soon be registered also in European countries such as France and Italy.

	Number of Compounds Reported	In Clinical Trials	Registered in USA, Europe or Japan
Springfield I (1988)	7	4	0
Springfield II (1991)	9	9	0
Springfield III (1994)	13	13	1 (THA, 1993, USA)

TABLE I.   Cholinesterase Inhibitors in AD Therapy (1988-1994).   Number of compounds reported in our publications.

As seen by the data presented here, the tacrine experience continues to contribute to our knowledge of ChEI effect and helps to improve methodology of clinical trials. The most recent and comprehensive study of tacrine efficacy described here (Knapp et al., this publication) focuses on higher dosages (120-160 mg). A rise in dosage and a corresponding increase in cholinesterase (ChE) inhibition also augmented percentage of responders to 40% as well as quality of response. In addition, perhaps most importantly, cognitive abilities of most patients may have declined at a lower rate than expected. The successful experience with tacrine has been confirmed in more than 2,000 patients in placebo-controlled, double-blind parallel trials. This clearly indicates the possibility of improving efficacy with new (second and third generation) ChEIs (Table II). Cholinergic therapy, strengthened by these clinical results has demonstrated its rationality but not yet its limits in AD treatment. The benefits observed in AD patients treated with tacrine provide strong support for other cholinomimetic approaches such as muscarinic and nicotinic agonists. It also suggests that drugs which are capable of raising acetylcholine (ACh) levels in cortex or stimulating specific cholinergic receptor subtypes should produce some improvement in AD symptoms.

Other hypotheses related to the cholinergic system and based on other pathogenic mechanisms should also be explored as alternative therapies. Among them, nerve growth factor (NGF) administration, continues to be of interest in spite of limited experience (a total of three patients in Sweden) and severe side effects (weight loss, confusion and pain). In conclusion, tacrine represents the first but very important step toward an effective therapy. Although the benefits of tacrine are limited qualitatively and quantitatively, they are above the expectations of our first publication (Giacobini and Becker, 1988).

1. Pseudo-reversible or irreversible inhibitor.

2. Selective AChE inhibitor, possibly G_4 isoform selective.

3. Produces long-lasting 40-60% steady state AChE inhibition in brain (12-24 hrs/dose).

4. Doubles ACh concentration in affected brain areas.

5. Has low toxicity at <u>80-90%</u> AChE (RBC) inhibition.

TABLE II.   Characteristics of a New ChEI

How Many ChEI Can Survive?
Presently, at least 15 ChEI are being actively studied preclinically and clinically around the world.   This large number of ChEI which are still alive and well represent the strongest support in favor of the "hypothesis of cholinergic therapy" launched more than 10 years ago. The results presented at this meeting clearly indicate that 3-4 of these compounds either do not show significant advantages in comparison to tacrine, or are even inferior as far as clinical efficacy or less suitable for severity and number of side effects. The reasons for such failure might be multiple: difficulties for the compound to reach sufficiently high acetylcholinesterase (AChE) inhibition in brain; too low ACh increase produced; numerous peripheral side effects or "new" side effects such as bone marrow toxicity. Limited penetration of the compound through the blood brain barrier (BBB) and lack of specificity for AChE are also limitations. To us the data indicate that close to 50% of the ChEI presented in 1994 either will not be seriously considered at our next meeting (1996) or will be abandoned completely by drug companies.

Muscarinic Agonists: A New Life?
Within the area of the hypothesis of cholinergic therapy, the use of muscarinic agonists seemed to be dwindling up to very recently, because of failures in clinical trials for at least five compounds (arecoline, bethanechol, oxotremorine, pilocarpine and RS86) between 1981 and 1991. Now, it seems likely that a new series of compounds, a second generation of muscarinic agonists, with higher selectivity for M_1-M_3 receptors is already in the clinic, heralded by AF-102B and xanomeline.

The Drugs that Never Made It

As expected, this last decade, a period of intense experimental trials witnesses already several victims (drugs) or doubtful successes. Unfortunately, entire classes of compounds are not pursued any longer by the industry because of lack of efficacy. Many of them never made their way out of Europe or Japan or reached registration in the USA. The most important representative of this group are the so-called nootropic drugs (see Voronina et al. and Pepeu et al., this publication). Numerous clinical trials failed to demonstrate clear efficacy of these drugs lowering the expectation of clinicians and drug companies as well as the interest of the FDA. Other probable or possible candidates for extinction are so-called cholinergic function-enhancers such as choline, phosphatidylcholine, L-acetylcarnitine and L-alpha-glycerophosphorylcholine. A series of negative or non-convincing clinical results has made the development of these drugs not totally unlikely but doubtful.

Other cholinomimetics, the acetylcholine releasers and modulators such as aminopyridines, phosphatidylserine and linopyridine, have not demonstrated (yet) convincing efficacy in AD patients. Other less interesting drugs or potential victims are antigalanin-agents, neuropeptides such as THR and somatostatin and hormone precursors such as dihydroepiandosterone (DHEA). Growth factors such as NGF, and gangliosides are still under discussion. However, the very limited number of cases treated so far (3 for NGF and 5 for GM_1) does not allow us to draw any conclusion, not even preliminarily. Other growth factors (FGF, BDNF and CGF) seem to be less likely candidates in AD therapy.

The Unfulfilled Promises

This publication (Giacobini and Becker, 1994) has devoted a substantial number of chapters to fields other than cholinomimetic drugs and the next one in 1996 will probably continue to present new areas of research and novel directions.

The strong emphasis of basic research studies *in vitro* and the elegant hypotheses put forward to stimulate the design of new strategies has obviously not yet paid off in terms of producing new compounds ready for clinical studies. Among the yet unfulfilled promises are three major categories of drugs such as Ca^{++} uptake blockers, antioxidant compounds and drugs to prevent synthesis, or to decrease deposition and slow down processing of β-amyloid. Among Ca^{++} uptake blockers only nimodipine is in clinical trial. The use of Ca^{++} antagonists based on the "glutamate hypothesis of neurotoxicity" is still debatable. It is a matter of speculation whether the treatment should be with glutamate agonists (glutamate itself or glycine) or partial agonists such as cycloserine would be more indicated. Others suggest that quite oppositely, treatment with glutamatergic antagonists to suppress the presumed neurotoxic effects would be useful, particularly in the initial stages of AD. Among drugs with antioxidant properties, only deprenyl, a MAO-B inhibitor, is being tested. The latest field of research based on apolipoproteins is still too young to be evaluated. However, we should not be discouraged but continue to accumulate new evidence and knowledge in these three areas. The lesson is that excellent basic hypotheses can not always be translated into clinical successes.

The Winner Is ...
Significant advances have been made in the understanding of the etiology, particularly genetics, pathogenesis and cellular biology of AD since our first publication (Giacobini and Becker, 1988). Although β-amyloid, tau protein, oxidative damage, apoptotic cell death and other pathogeneses are still central foci for consideration of therapeutical approaches, no drugs or even drug precursors have been presented which could presage a breakthrough. Meanwhile, considerable clinical experience and new basic knowledge have been gained in the field of cholinomimetic therapy. Cholinesterase inhibitors, particularly, are the only class of drugs with proven efficacy in AD patients which are being tested in various phases (I to III) of clinical study. As pointed out in several chapters of this book, the latest ChEI candidates (second and third generation) for therapy have been developed following rational pharmacological and chemical lines. The most desirable characteristics for an efficacious ChEI are summarized in Table II. The emphasis is on reaching high enough ChE inhibition in CNS to at least double ACh concentration. This is an achievable goal and one or several of the compounds presently tested might already satisfy these criteria. X-ray crystallography of ChEI-AChE complexes can show residues crucial for ligand binding. A detailed description of the active site of the enzyme as presented in this publication by Silman et al. makes it possible to use a structure-based drug design of inhibitors with even higher selectivity and specificity.

Clinical Trials, Still a Problem
As underlined in the chapter of Thal in this publication, there are still several problems inherent to the conduct of clinical trials. Outcome measures have been recently refined and improved. Standardized tests have been introduced so that data from different trials can be compared among several countries. Instruments of cognitive changes have improved and current trials use a few but specific end-points. As pointed out by Zec et al. in this publication, the low error score seen with our brief screening tests [Mini-Mental State Exam (MMSE) and Alzheimer Disease Assessment Scale (ADAS)] in very early AD patients makes it difficult to detect improvement in cognitive functioning as a result of drug efficacy. This is a major concern since it is early in the course of AD that treatment might have its maximal effect. At the same time, and because of the improvements, the requirements for approval of a drug for an antidementia claim have become more stringent. New studies will be more lengthy with an increased duration from 30 weeks to at least 52 weeks. It is felt that long-term studies of up to one year or more are indispensable in order to detect unequivocal changes in rate of decline. They will probably be requested by

	TACRINE * Point Diff./6 mo (40-160 mg/day)	1996 COMPOUND Point Diff./year	IDEAL COMPOUND Point Diff./year
Measures			
1. MMSE	+3-4	+6-8	+6-8
2. ADAS - Cog	+2-4	+4-8	+4-8
3. GDS	+	+ +	+ +
4. CIBI or CGIC	+	+ +	+ +
5. IADL	+	+ +	+ +
Dose Response (plasma levels)	significant for for 1, 2, 3, 4 and 5	highly significant for 1, 2, 3, 4 and 5	highly significant for 1, 2, 3, 4 and 5
Side Effects at Therapeutic Doses			
Hepatotoxicity	+ + +	0	0
Hematology	+	0	0
Cholinergic	+ +	0	0
Other Improvements			
Percent of patients tolerating drug	40	95-100	100
Reduction in care giver burden	+	+ +	+ + +
Slowing or arresting disease progression	0	0	+ + +
Cost/patient/year	$3,500-4,000	$1,500	$1,500
Access of AD population to drug	limited	improved	unlimited
Estimated number of AD patients treated with drug	250,000	1,000,000	10,000,000

TABLE III. Results from 30-52 week, 500 patients, double-blind, placebo controlled, parallel-group study, 4 doses (4 groups). * CIBI = Clinician Interview-Based Impression of Change; ADAS = Alzheimer Disease Assessment Scale; CGIC = Clinical Global Impression of Change; MMSE = Mini-Mental State Examination; IADL = Instructional Activities of Daily Living; GDS = Global Deterioration Scale; + = significant improvement; + + highly significant improvement or less deterioration.
* Results for tacrine from Knapp et al. (this publication).

regulatory authorities. Effects on decline will have to be studied to differentiate symptomatic suppression of disease expression from pathogenic alteration of disease progression. Finally, the pharmaco-economic evaluation of a compound will become central to clinical studies. Cost/benefit analysis based on evaluations of 30-52 week long treatment will be made. Given these premises, a conservative profile of a new compound to be successfully developed within the next 2-5 years emerges and the characteristics of an ideal compound can be identified (Table III). Based upon the favorable reports about ChEI in this volume, it appears possible to us that significant improvement will be made in cholinomimetic therapy already in the next 2-3 years. If our hypothesis (Giacobini and Becker, 1988; Becker and Giacobini, 1991) that the beneficial effect from ChE inhibition is limited by the appearance of side effects is correct, then significant improvements in multiple areas should be within reach. We have described these improvements in Table III. Improvements in efficacy, safety, accessibility and cost are all achievable for a compound with an improved safety profile. Articles in this volume describe a number of potential candidates with these characteristics.

Although there are still relatively very few complete clinical trials of ChEI, results to date indicate that lost cognitive function and the accompanying functional disabilities will not be restored by drug therapy. This is understandable in view of the loss of cells and synapses found in persons with clinically evident AD (DeKosky, this publication). Our probable inability to replace lost brain function reinforces the importance of early diagnosis (Becker and Giacobini, 1990) and the need for pharmacotherapy that will slow or arrest the progressive deterioration that is characteristic of AD. Presently, there is little evidence that cholinomimetic therapy will affect the disease course significantly. In Table III we have indicated that an ideal ChEI would have this property. The interference of side effects may have prevented the study of this particular aspect of the therapy. The availability of the new compound(s) we have mentioned above will allow this study. It is probable we will be able to evaluate the potential for ChEI therapy aimed at disease decline within the next 3-5 years. The next meeting in 1996 will demonstrate whether we were realistic in setting these basic goals or not and whether ChEIs may have any effect on disease progression.

REFERENCES

Becker R and Giacobini E (editors) (1990): *Alzheimer Disease: Current Research in Early Diagnosis*. New York: Taylor and Francis.

Becker R and Giacobini E (editors) (1991): *Cholinergic Basis for Alzheimer Therapy*. Boston: Birkhauser.

Giacobini E and Becker R (editors) (1988): *Current Research in Alzheimer Therapy*. New York: Taylor and Francis.

Alzheimer Disease: Therapeutic Strategies
edited by E. Giacobini and R. Becker.
© 1994 Birkhäuser Boston

EPIDEMIOLOGY OF AD: IMPACT ON THE TREATMENT

Luigi Amaducci and Laura Fratiglioni
Department of Neurological and Psychiatric Sciences, University of Florence, Florence, Italy

INTRODUCTION

The principal aims of the epidemiologic research are to understand the natural history of the diseases, and to discover strategies to positively modify such a natural history. This implies that the epidemiological research may be conducted at two different levels: explanatory or scientific, versus pragmatic or action-oriented (Kleinbaum et al., 1982). Great contribution to the treatment of diseases can derive from both levels.

In the case of a chronic and invalidating disease as Alzheimer's disease (AD), the main contributions can be summarized in the following three points:

1. Epidemiological studies have shown the relevance of AD for the public health and the medical science. One of the consequences is the allocation of resources in all fields of the research, especially in studies aimed at discovering possible therapies.
2. Population surveys have stressed the need of precise and accurate diagnostic criteria for AD, sometimes giving the opportunity and data to assess the diagnostic validity. The implication of such studies for the clinical trials is obvious.
3. Studies on the natural history of AD have already shown different possible levels of therapeutic intervention, and suggested useful guidelines for the study design of future clinical trials.

RELEVANCE OF AD

The 1-2% AD prevalence in people aged 65-74 years, 4% in people aged 75-84 years, and 10% in subjects aged over 85, clearly show and quantify the public health importance of AD (for a review and references, see Fratiglioni, 1993). Moreover, a time trend study of incidence from Rochester, Minnesota, indicates a tendency towards increasing rates in the oldest age groups in the last two quinquina (Kolmen et al., 1993). This trend, if confirmed, will have big consequences in the health care organization.

The frequency of the disease together with the unprecedented increase in the developed countries of the elderly persons, with the proportion of the very old doubling within one generation, causes formidable costs, both financial or psychosocial. The great part of the economical costs is due to the care of the patients. A Swedish study carried out in Stockholm found that most of the subjects (84%) with questionable-mild dementia live in their own homes, while most of the moderate-severe cases (77%) are in institutions (Fratiglioni et al., 1994). Differently from physically handicapped, a subject affected even by mild form of dementia, needs constant domiciliarity assistance and continuous surveillance. On the other hand, institutional cases who suffer from severe disease request higher amount and specialized type of staff effort. As was shown in surveys in the United States, Australia, New Zealand, and Sweden, 40-50% of all demented subjects are in institutions. Lower figures were reported in Italy from a rural area and from Germany (for references see Fratiglioni et al., 1994).

Growing insight into the psychological and social stresses associated with the family caregivers in the home setting has indicated the true breadth of the devastation caused by this disease. In a controlled, population-based study on caregiver burden, Grafström et al. (1992) found that caregivers of demented persons living at home experience a very stressful situation and as a consequence they had an increased use of psychotropic drugs. The institutionalization of the demented relative does not relieve the closest relative from the subjective feeling of stress.

The scientific relevance of AD is based on many intellectually stimulating aspects, first of all the dilemma of AD as disease entity. The descriptive epidemiological data have been taken as support to the hypothesis that AD is not differentiated from "normal aging" (Brayne and Calloway, 1988). In community samples there is a continuous distribution of at least some of the manifest variables associated with AD. Thus, the changes in brain function found in normal aging, benign forgetfulness, and AD can be seen as a continuum, which may reflect a single underlying process. This implies the concept of AD as an accelerated, but physiological, aging process. In other words if we will be able to live until 120 years, shall we all develop AD? This dilemma is still debated (Berg, 1985; Hofman et al., 1988). Prevalence data from the very old ages have not yet given a clear evidence supporting one of the two hypothesis. In the Swedish study, the Kungsholmen Project, where a substantial number of subjects were aged over 90 (8.6% of the study population) the prevalence figures increased even in the most advanced ages (Fratiglioni et al., 1991), although uncertainty remains for ages over 90 due to the instability of the prevalence figure (large confidence interval).

VALIDITY OF AD DIAGNOSIS

Even if the conceptual definition of AD as a disease is problematic, assuming that AD is a disorder that is revealed when a threshold is reached, some operational criteria can be defined. As there are no biological markers of the disease, clinical diagnostic criteria, such as the DSM III-r (APA, 1987), the NINCDS-ADRDA (McKhann et al., 1984), and the ICD-10 (WHO, 1987) are the most frequently used. They include both criteria for diagnosis of dementia and of AD.

The precision of the AD diagnosis has been studied in a few investigations as agreement among different clinicians. The results showed values of Kappa index around 0,60 (for a review see Fratiglioni, 1993).

From a population survey, possibilities of improvement of the reliability for the DSM III-r criteria for dementia diagnosis have been suggested, simply adding some specifications and a category of questionable dementia (Fratiglioni et al., 1992).

Finally, as a part of a cross-sectional project on the prevalence of dementia, the interobserver agreement was studied when the three main diagnostic systems were used (Baldereschi et al., 1994). This study showed that clinicians from different cultures and medical traditions can use the DSM III-r as well as the ICD-10 criteria in a reliable way (Kappa=0.67 and 0.69). For the AD diagnosis the Kappa values suggested the need to merge the two categories, probable and possible AD, to improve the reliability.

The validity of the clinical diagnostic criteria of AD has been investigated mostly in terms of positive predictive value. Few studies have been carried out on the sensitivity and specificity, and there has been none in the general population. On the basis of the available information, the use of codified criteria appears more accurate than the clinical judgement. The NINCDS-ADRDA seems less specific than the DSM III-r criteria. On average, when both diagnostic criteria are considered, the sensitivity was 0.82 and the specificity 0.65 (for a review and references, see Fratiglioni, 1993). These data are essential in the study of the efficacy of a treatment, where a high specificity is the goal of the diagnostic procedure.

NATURAL HISTORY OF AD: LEVELS OF INTERVENTION

As said in the introduction, one of the basic aims of the epidemiological research is to understand the natural history of disease. In general, the natural history of the disease can be described by three sequential processes (induction, promotion and expression) that correspond to three alternative strategies of treatment. Kleinbaum et al. (1982) call these strategies prevention. The primary prevention aims at preventing and postponing the first new occurrences of the disease, which implies the detection of risk factors and their climation or treatment. The secondary prevention is aimed at decreasing the duration of the disease and/or prolonging life. This implies the detection of markers of early phases and the availability of treatment able to stop or slow the disease process. The tertiary prevention is aimed at making the disease outcome less severe. The knowledge of the course of the disease and the detection of efficacious treatments are necessary.

Presently, primary prevention of AD is more an aim for the future than a practical possibility. Our knowledge of the risk factors of the disease is still limited and the only universally accepted risk factors (aging and genetic alterations) are not yet preventable. However, many possible risk factors (such as head trauma, thyroid disease, depression and low education), and some of the putative risk factors (maternal advanced age, non-smoking, aluminum exposure, diet, alcohol, occupational toxins), if definitely confirmed, can be prevented or controlled (for a view of risk factors of AD, see Fratiglioni, 1993).

Secondary prevention deals with the problem of the early diagnosis and with the detection of valid predictive tests. At the moment, such instruments are lacking, as well as treatments.

The efficacy of a treatment in the tertiary prevention is based on the results of controlled, randomized, double blind clinical trials. In the next paragraph we will discuss how further data about the course of the disease may help the planning of such clinical trials.

NATURAL HISTORY OF AD: GUIDELINES FOR THE DESIGN OF CLINICAL TRIALS

The discrepancy among study results and the frequent failure in the detection of a positive effect of a treatment of AD can both be due to methodological shortcomings.

First, reliable measures of progression are essential in clinical trials. Recently, the concept of reliability of a measure has been applied to its change over time (van Belle et al., 1990). The authors used the Mini-Mental State Examination (MMSE) and the Blessed and Tomlinson Dementia Rating scale (DRS), and found that the reliability of these estimates of change were primarily dependent upon the length of time between observations, more than upon the number of observations. The authors concluded that changes in cognitive status as measured by the MMSE and DRS scale have a reasonable reliability if the time interval between the observations is more than one year. The same conclusions are reached by Morris et al. (1993) analyzing longitudinal data from the CERAD study. They suggested the inclusion of other clinical scales in the evaluation protocol.

Second, prognostic variables such as age at onset, patient age, language dysfunction, extrapyramidal signs, psychosis, and dementia severity, although they have not yet been definitely confirmed, need to be controlled in clinical trials.

Third, there is agreement among the researchers and the clinicians on the fact that AD is characterized by heterogeneity. Clinical data as age at onset, symptoms, and pathological findings suggest the possibility of a clinical heterogeneity, as well as progression and survival data seem to show a functional heterogeneity (Ritchie and Touchon, 1992). Finally, findings from etiopathogenetic research indicate an heterogeneity also in the etiology and pathophysiology. Examples are the identification of genetic defects only in few families, and the presence of a familiar aggregation in many cases, but not in all (for review and references, see Fratiglioni, 1993); and the association between apolipoprotein E allele epsilon4, and some cases of AD. Despite all these data, there is still debate if this heterogeneity corresponds to different subtypes (Jorm, 1985; Ritchie and Touchon 1992). Although no definite conclusions have been reached, it seems necessary to begin to take these aspects into account in the design of clinical trials.

Finally, the course of the disease in the general population, and in the placebo group (Knopman and Gracon, 1994) need further investigation in order to understand which is the minimum duration of a treatment needed to detect the effect of an efficacious drug or other medical interventions.

REFERENCES

American Psychiatric Association (APA) (1987): Diagnostic and Statistical Manual of Mental Disorders, 3rd Ed, revised (DSM III-r). Washington DC: American Psychiatric Association, pp. 97-163.

Baldereschi M, Amato MP, Nencini P, Pracucci G, Lippi A, Amaducci L et al. (1994): Cross-national interrater agreement on the clinical diagnostic criteria for dementia. *Neurology* 44:239-242.

Berg L (1985): Does Alzheimer's disease represent an exaggeration of normal aging? *Arch Neurol* 42:737-739.

Brayne C and Calloway P (1988): Normal ageing, impaired cognitive function, and senile dementia of the Alzheimer's type: a continuum. *Lancet* i:1265-1267.

Fratiglioni L (1993): Epidemiology of Alzheimer's disease. Issues of etiology and validity. *Acta Neurol Scand* 87(Suppl. 145):1-70.

Fratiglioni L, Forsell Y, Agucro Torres H and Winblad B (1994): Severity of dementia and institutionalization in the elderly: Prevalence data from an urban area in Sweden. *Neuroepidemiology* (In Press).

Fratiglioni L, Grut M, Forsell Y, Grafström M, Holmen K, Eriksson K, Viitanen M, Bäckman L, Ahlbom A and Winblad B (1991): Prevalence of Alzheimer's disease and other dementias in an elderly urban population: Relationship with age, sex and education. *Neurology* 41:1886-1892.

Fratiglioni L, Grut M, Forsell Y, Viitanen M and Winblad B (1992): Clinical diagnosis of Alzheimer's disease and other dementias in a population survey. Agreement and causes of disagreement in applying DSM III-r criteria. *Arch Neurol* 49:227-32.

Grafström M, Fratiglioni L, Sandman P-O and Winblad B (1992): Health and social consequences for relatives of demented and non-demented elderly. A population-based study. *J Clin Epidemiol* 45:861-870.

Hofman A, van Duijn CM and Rocca WA (1988): Is Alzheimer's disease distinct from normal ageing? *Lancet* i:226-227.

Jorm AF (1985): Subtypes of Alzheimer's disease - A conceptual analysis and critical review. *Psychol Med* 15:543-553.

Kleinbaum DG, Kupper LL and Morgenstern H (1982): Epidemiologic research. Principles and quantitative methods. Belmont, California: *Lifetime Learning Publication*.

Knopman D and Gracon S (1994): Observations on the short-term "natural history" of probable Alzheimer's disease in a controlled clinical trial. *Neurology* 44:260-265.

Kolmen E, Beard CM, O'Brien PC, Offord MS and Kurland LT (1993): Is the incidence of dementing illness changing? A 25-year time trend study in Rochester, Minnesota (1960-1984). *Neurology* 43:1887-1892.

McKhann G, Drachman D, Folstein M, Katzman R, Price D and Stadlan M (1984): Clinical diagnosis of Alzheimer's disease: Report of the NINCDS-ADRDA Work Group under the auspices of Department of Health and Human Services Task Force on Alzheimer's Disease. *Neurology* 34:939-44.

Morris JC, Edland S, Clark C, Galasko D, Koss E, Mohs R, van Belle G, Fillenbaum G and Heyman A (1993): The Consortium to Establish a Registry for Alzheimer's Disease (CERAD). Part IV. Rates of cognitive change in the longitudinal assessment of probable Alzheimer's disease. *Neurology* 43:2457-2465.

Ritchie K and Touchon J (1992): Heterogeneity in senile dementia of the Alzheimer type: Individual differences, progressive deterioration or clinical subtypes? *J Clin Epidemiol* 45:1391-1398.

van Belle G, Uhlmann RF, Hughes JP and Larson EB (1990): Reliability of estimates of changes in mental status test performance in senile dementia of the Alzheimer type. *J Clin Epidemiol* 43:589-595.

World Health Organization (WHO) (1987): ICD-10 draft of Chapter V: Categories F00-F99, mental and behavioral disorders (including disorders of psychological development): Diagnostic criteria for research (WHO/MNH/MEP/87.1,REV 4), Geneva: World Health Organization, Division of Mental Health.

PART I
NEUROPATHOLOGIC AND GENETIC BASIS OF AD TREATMENT

Alzheimer Disease: Therapeutic Strategies
edited by E. Giacobini and R. Becker.
© 1994 Birkhäuser Boston

NEUROPATHOLOGICAL BASES OF ALZHEIMER DISEASE, IMPLICATIONS FOR TREATMENT

Henryk M. Wisniewski and Jerzy Wegiel
New York State Institute for Basic Research in Developmental Disabilities,
Staten Island, New York

Neuropathological implications for Alzheimer disease (AD) treatment are based on several basic observations. There appears to be more than one cause of development of AD neuropathology and therefore, AD might be considered a syndrome. The duration of both the clinical and the preclinical course is very long. Discoveries of the proteins (ß-peptide, over-phosphorylated tau, apolipoprotein (Apo) E4 and other amyloid-associated proteins) and the cells (microglia, perivascular cells and myocytes) that participate in amyloid formation open a new avenue for development of therapeutic strategies in prevention and treatment of AD.

CLINICAL COURSE OF AD

The duration of AD may extend to 20 years. Empirical longitudinal observations permit differentiation between normal central nervous system (CNS) aging and AD on the basis of mental status, psychometric and other assessment measures as well as the description of the mean temporal course of each of the clinical stages of the disease (Reisberg et al., 1989). The incipient and mild AD stages comprise the first nine years. The moderate and moderately severe stages of AD encompass approximately the next 5 years. Severe changes may last for more than the next 6 years (GDS stage 7). This late stage of the disease is characterized by neuronal loss in many brain structures; loss is especially severe in the transentorhinal and entorhinal cortex, cornu Ammonis, subicular complex, amygdala and nucleus basalis Meynert (Braak et al., 1993; Scott et al., 1991; Vogels et al., 1990). Linear correlation between the stage of AD and the volume of brain structures (Bobinski et al., 1994) indicates gradual progress of neuropathological changes during the course of AD. It also suggests that successful therapeutic intervention might stop the further progress of pathological changes at any stage of disease. Intervention in the first half of the course of AD may leave the patient independent, in relatively good physical and mental status or needing only minimal assistance. Interruption in the progress of the disease in later stages reduces the misery of the patient and costs of the care. Theoretically, the progress of changes might be interrupted even in the late stage of the disease because neuropathological studies show that even at the end stage of AD, many neurons, terminals and neuronal processes show evidence of degeneration - not death. If progression of the disease could be stopped, the abnormal neuronal elements could in part recover and regain their function.

NEUROPATHOLOGICAL MARKERS OF AD

Alzheimer disease is characterized by (1) the presence of plaques, amyloid angiopathy and neurofibrillary tangles (NFTs) as well as neuronal loss and brain atrophy; (2) a specific time course of degenerative changes; and (3) the correlation of some measures of pathological changes with clinical course.

Correlations between plaque and NFT counts and psychometric tests (Blessed et al., 1968; Wilcock and Esiri, 1982), and between counts of the large neocortical pyramidal cells and clinical measures of AD pathology were found (Neary et al., 1986). However, the correlation between psychometric indices of AD and counts of neocortical synapses is much stronger than that between these indices and counts of plaques and NFTs (Terry et al., 1991). Neuropathological criteria of AD diagnosis are based on the number of plaques and tangles (Khachaturian, 1985; Mirra et al., 1993).

Neuropathological staging based on the onset of neurofibrillary pathology in brain structures and semiquantitative assessment of its severity shows expansion of neurofibrillary changes from the transentorhinal cortex to the entorhinal cortex and hippocampal formation. The first two transentorhinal stages of AD correspond to a clinically silent period (preclinical phase). Cases classified as belonging to the limbic stages (III and IV) show mild or moderately severe impairment of cognition as well as personality changes. In isocortical stages V and VI, the dementia is present, and devastating destruction of hippocampal formation and isocortex is observed (Braak et al., 1993). Our studies show that atrophy of the hippocampal formation subdivisions appears to be a function of the duration of pathological changes in individual structures. The changes in the volume of the hippocampal subdivisions correlate with stage and duration of AD (Bobinski et al., 1994).

Both clinical and neuropathological studies show a several-year-long period of incipient or mild changes in which successful treatment is possible.

MORPHOLOGICAL DIVERSITY OF AMYLOID DEPOSITS

The amyloid cascade hypothesis implies that deposition of the amyloid ß- protein is the causative agent of AD pathology and that neurofibrillary pathology, cell loss and dementia follow (Wisniewski et al., 1985; Hardy and Higgins, 1992). Deposits of thioflavin S-negative, non-fibrillar ß-protein are responsible for formation of cerebral diffuse plaques and diffuse deposits in the molecular layer of the cerebellum. The fibrillar thioflavin S-positive deposits of amyloid are responsible for development of neuritic classical and primitive plaques in the cerebral cortex and subcortical gray matter as well as globose deposits in the cerebellar Purkinje and granule cell layer. The morphological appearance of amyloid deposits and the response of the surrounding tissue depends on the site of amyloid deposits, the amount of amyloid, and pattern of distribution of amyloid-forming cells, the rate of formation and turn-over of amyloid deposits, the type and extent of the response of the surrounding tissue and the type of staining technique used (Wisniewski et al., 1989a). The broad spectrum of morphologically different types of amyloid deposits suggests (1) different mechanisms of their formation and (2) different impacts of amyloid on surrounding tissue.

Morphological studies show different tissue response in different types of ß-immunoreactive plaques. Diffuse plaques in the cerebellar cortex of AD subjects (Le et al., 1994), and diffuse plaques in 15- to 40-year old patients with Down syndrome are examples of ß-amyloid deposits with minimal or no impact on the neuropil (Wisniewski et al., 1994a). The second category of ß-immunoreactive plaques represents classical and primitive plaques with severe dystrophic pathology of neurites, many of which are filled with paired helical filaments (PHF). The characteristic feature of diffuse or benign plaques is accumulation of the nonfibrillar ß-protein in extracellular space. Neuritic or malignant plaques always contain fibrillar ß-protein. The differentiation of ß-protein deposits into fibrillar and nonfibrillar is essential for both the diagnosis and the therapy of AD.

Our studies show that amyloid deposition is a cell-associated event. Fibrillization is seen in the basal lamina of the smooth muscle cells in the wall of the arteries and veins in leptomeninges; in altered smooth endoplasmic reticulum; and in cytoplasmic infoldings of microglial cells and perivascular cells (Wisniewski et al., 1989b, 1992; Wisniewski and Wegiel, 1993, 1994). Diffuse deposit formation appears to be associated by and large with nerve cells and their terminals (Probst et al., 1991; Pappolla et al., 1991). However, the ß-protein of neuronal origin does not fibrillize, or fibrillization is very slow and the amount of fibrils is minimal (Joachim et al., 1989; Wisniewski et al., 1994a).

AMYLOID-ASSOCIATED PROTEINS

Amyloid deposits show the presence of other proteins that are called amyloid-associated proteins or pathological chaperons: glycosaminoglycans, component P, α1-antichymotrypsin, and the recently discovered apoE (Strittmatter et al., 1994; Kisielewski and Young, 1994; Wisniewski et al., 1994c). Chaperon proteins studies indicate that sequestration of the ß-protein by some chaperon proteins may prevent amyloid formation. The binding by others accelerates and/or stabilizes amyloid fibrils. Aggregation and polymerization of ß-protein appears to be the result of an imbalance of multiple extracellular factors. Local changes in the equilibrium of the ß-protein and the proteins participating in the sequestration of the ß-protein could facilitate amyloid formation. Apolipoprotein E4 appears to be the most important chaperon protein because it has been found that the allelic form of the apoE4/4 increases the risk of late-onset AD by eight times (Corder et al., 1994). ApoE4 not only accelerates fibrillization and stabilizes amyloid fibrils *in vitro*, but it also affects phosphorylation of tau, leading to PHF formation (Strittmatter et al., 1994). The risk of developing AD when the apoE3/4 allelic form is present is two times higher than in control group. Presence of the apoE2 allele appears to protect against AD (Corder et al., 1994).

THERAPEUTIC TARGETS

Morphological studies indicate that study of the cells that are engaged in amyloid fibril formation (microglia, perivascular cells and myocytes) should be of highest priority in the development of therapeutic strategies to prevent and treat AD. Understanding of how they process amyloid precursor protein and what chaperon proteins they produce is of critical importance. Our recent findings that in tissue culture, myocytes isolated from vessels affected by amyloid angiopathy can secrete ß-protein and make amyloid should accelerate studies on drugs affecting ß-protein amyloidogenesis (Wisniewski et al., 1994b). Because diffuse non-fibrillar plaques do not appear to damage brain tissue, understanding of and influencing by drugs of the process of ß-protein fibrillogenesis is another area that should be of high priority in research and development of treatment of AD.

ACKNOWLEDGEMENTS

This work was supported in part by funds from the New York State Office of Mental Retardation and Developmental Disabilities and grants PO1-AGO-4220 and P30-AGO-8051 from the National Institutes of Health, National Institute on Aging.

REFERENCES

Blessed G, Tomlinson BE and Roth M (1968): The association between quantitative measures of dementia and of senile change in the cerebral gray matter of elderly subjects. *Br J Psychiatry* 114:797-811.

Bobinski M, Wegiel J, Wisniewski HM, Tarnawski M, Reisberg B, Mlodzik B, de Leon MJ and Miller DC (1994): Atrophy of the hippocampal formation subdivisions correlates with duration and stage of Alzheimer disease. *Neurology* (In Press).

Braak H, Duyckaerts C, Braak E and Piette F (1993): Neuropathological staging of Alzheimer-related changes correlates with psychometrically assessed intellectual status.

In: *Alzheimer's Disease: Advances in Clinical and Basic Research*, Corain B, Iqbal K, Nicolini M, Winblad B, Wisniewski HM and Zatta P, eds. Chichester, England: John Wiley and Sons Ltd, pp. 131-137.

Corder EH, Saunders AM, Risch NJ, Strittmatter WJ, Schmechel DE, Gaskell PC Jr, Rimmler JB, Locke PA, Conneally PM, Schmader KE, Small GW, Roses AD, Haines JL and Pericak-Vance MA (1994): Apolipoprotein E4 type 2 allele decreases the risk of late-onset Alzheimer's disease. *Nature Genetics* 7:180-183.

Hardy JA and Higgins GA (1992): Alzheimer's disease: the amyloid cascade hypothesis. *Science* 256:184-185.

Joachim CL, Morris JH and Selkoe DJ (1989): Diffuse senile plaques occur commonly in the cerebellum in Alzheimer's disease. *Am J Pathol* 135:309-319.

Khachaturian ZS (1985): Diagnosis of Alzheimer's disease. *Arch Neurol* 42:1097-1105.

Kisielewsky R and Young ID (1994): Extracellular matrix constituents in Alzheimer's amyloid deposits. In: *Glycobiology and the Brain*. Nicolini M and Zatta PF, eds. Oxford, England: Pergamon Press, pp. 179-196.

Le Y-T, Woodruff-Pak DS and Trojanowski JQ (1994): Amyloid plaques in cerebellar cortex and the integrity of Purkinje cell dendrites. *Neurobiol Aging* 15:1-9.

Mirra SS, Hart MN and Terry RD (1993): Making the diagnosis of Alzheimer's disease. A primer for practicing pathologists. *Arch Pathol Lab Med* 117:132-144.

Neary D, Snowden JS, Mann DMA, Bowen DM, Sims NR, Northen B, Yates PO and Davison AN (1986): Alzheimer's disease: A correlative study. *J Neurol Neurosurg Psychiatry* 49:229-237.

Pappolla MA, Omar RA and Vinters HV (1991): Image analysis microspectroscopy shows that neurons participate in the genesis of subset of early primitive (diffuse) senile plaques. *Am J Pathol* 139:599-607.

Probst A, Langui D, Ipsen S, Robakis N and Ulrich J (1991): Deposition of ß/A4 protein along neuronal plasma membranes in diffuse senile plaques. *Acta Neuropathol* 83:21-29.

Reisberg B, Ferris SH, de Leon MJ, Kluger A, Franssen E, Borenstein J and Alba RC (1989): The stage specific temporal course of Alzheimer's disease: functional and behavioral concomitants based upon cross-sectional and longitudinal observation. In: *Alzheimer's Disease and Related Disorders*. Iqbal K, Wisniewski HM, Winblad B, eds. New York: Alan R. Liss Inc, pp. 23-41.

Scott SA, DeKosky ST and Scheff SW (1991): Volumetric atrophy of the amygdala in Alzheimer's disease: Quantitative serial reconstruction *Neurology* 41:351-356.

Strittmatter WJ, Weisgraber KH, Goedert M, Saunders AM, Huang D, Corder EH, Dong L-M, Jakes R, Alberts MJ, Gilbert JR, Han S-H, Hulette C, Einstein G, Schmechel DE, Pericak-Vance MA and Roses AD (1994): Hypothesis: Microtubule instability and paired helical filament formation in the Alzheimer disease brain are related to apolipoprotein E genotype. *Exp Neurol* 125:163-171.

Terry RD, Masliah E, Salmon DP, Butters N, De Teresa R, Hill R, Hansen LA and Katzman R (1991): Physical basis of cognitive alterations in Alzheimer disease. Synapse loss is the major correlate of cognitive impairment. *Ann Neurol* 30:572-580.

Vogels OJM, Broere CAJ, Ter Laak HJ, Ten Donkelaar HJ, Nieuwenhuys R and Schulte BPM (1990): Cell loss and shrinkage in the nucleus basalis Meynerti complex in Alzheimer's disease. *Neurobiol Aging* 11:3-13.

Wilcock GK and Esiri MM (1982): Plaques, tangles, and dementia. A quantitative study. *J Neurol Sci* 56:343-356.

Wisniewski HM, Currie JR, Barcikowska M, Robakis NK and Miller DL (1985): Alzheimer's disease, a cerebral form of amyloidosis. In: *Immunology and Alzheimer's disease*. Pouplard-Barthelaix A, Emile J, Christen Y, eds. Berlin: Springer-Verlag, pp. 1-6.

Wisniewski HM, Bancher C, Barcikowska M, Wen GY and Currie J (1989a): Spectrum of morphological appearance of amyloid deposits in Alzheimer's disease. *Acta Neuropathol* 78:337-347.

Wisniewski HM, Wegiel J, Wang KC, Kujawa M and Lach B (1989b): Ultrastructural studies of the cells forming amyloid fibers in classical plaques. *Can J Neurol Sci* 16:535-542.

Wisniewski HM, Wegiel J, Wang KC and Lach B (1992): Ultrastructural studies of the cells forming amyloid in the cortical vessel wall in Alzheimer's disease. *Acta Neuropathol* 84:117-127.

Wisniewski HM and Wegiel J (1993): Migration of perivascular cells into the neuropil and their involvement in ß-amyloid plaque formation. *Acta Neuropathol* 85:586-595.

Wisniewski HM and Wegiel J (1994): ß-amyloid formation by myocytes of leptomeningeal vessels. *Acta Neuropathol* 87:233-241.

Wisniewski HM, Wegiel J and Popovitch E (1994a): Age associated changes in ß-amyloid plaque fibrillization in Down syndrome. *Developmental Brain Dysfunction* (In Press).

Wisniewski HM, Frackowiak J and Mazur-Kolecka B (1994b): *In vitro* production of ß-amyloid in smooth muscle cells isolated from amyloid angiopathy-affected vessels. *Neurosci Lett* (In Press).

Wisniewski T, Ghiso J and Frangione B (1994c): Alzheimer's disease and soluble Aß. *Neurobiol Aging* 15:143-152.

Alzheimer Disease: Therapeutic Strategies
edited by E. Giacobini and R. Becker.
© 1994 Birkhäuser Boston

AMYLOID DEPOSITION AS THE CENTRAL EVENT IN THE ETIOLOGY AND PATHOGENESIS OF ALZHEIMER'S DISEASE

John Hardy and Karen Duff
Suncoast Alzheimer's Disease Laboratories, Department of Psychiatry
3515 East Fletcher Avenue, Tampa, FL 33613 USA

Over the last few years, and particularly since the identification of pathogenic mutations, the amyloid cascade hypothesis (Glenner and Murphy, 1989; Hardy and Higgins, 1992) has become the dominant hypothesis for the etiology and pathogenesis of Alzheimer's disease (AD). In the last two years, much work based on the cascade hypothesis has been published which offers more support for it as a framework for the development of an understanding of the disease. However, the amyloid cascade hypothesis has been extensively criticized on many grounds, some valid and some probably specious. More worrisome, it remains, at best, a mere framework of understanding. In this article, we review recent advances in our understanding of the disease (Progress), outline and discuss some of the criticisms of the cascade hypothesis (Problems) and point to some of the many gaping holes in our knowledge of the disease with respect to this hypothesis (Deficiencies).

PROGRESS

At the time that we sketched out the amyloid cascade hypothesis (Hardy and Allsop, 1991) there was a single known mutation which was thought to cause AD: APP717Val->Ile (Goate et al., 1991). Now there are three other mutations which are known to cause AD: APP717Val->Phe (Murrell et al., 1991), APP717Val->Gly (Chartier-Harlin et al., 1991) and APP670/1Lys/Met->Asn/Leu (Mullan et al., 1992). Together, the evidence that these mutations cause AD is now overwhelming. More recently the position of the second gene causing AD has been identified as the long arm of chromosome 14 (Schellenberg et al., 1992; St. George et al., 1992; Van Broeckhoven et al., 1992; Mullan et al., 1992). The nature of the gene product from this locus will be a sensitive, independent test of the cascade hypothesis.

Although we have interpreted the occurrence of mutations in amyloid precursor protein (APP) in AD as the basis for the amyloid cascade hypothesis, another interpretation of these data is that the mutations in APP alter its functional activity and this loss of function underlies the dementia. This hypothesis was implicit in the first report of the cloning of APP (Kang et al., 1987) and has recently been resurrected with the realization that APP is linked to the G-protein signalling system (Nishimoto et al., 1993). While it would seem likely that understanding the normal function of APP is going to be important in designing therapeutic strategies for AD and in understanding the control of APP expression, it would seem less likely that beta-amyloid deposition is merely an accidental marker of APP dysfunction.

The mechanism by which APP mismetabolism might lead to amyloid deposition has been experimentally addressed. Key to this understanding was the realization that beta-amyloid was a normal product of cellular metabolism (Hardy, 1992; Haass et al., 1992; Seubert et al., 1992; Shoji et al., 1992). The position of the AD-causing mutations framing the beta-amyloid sequence was also an important clue since it suggested that the mutations might alter processing of APP to beta-amyloid (Hardy, 1992). This proposal (Hardy and Mullan, 1992) has been shown to be true for the APP670/1 mutation. Transfection studies have shown that this mutation greatly increases the proportion of APP metabolized to beta-amyloid (Citron et al., 1992; Cai et al., 1993) presumably by facilitating the beta-secretase cleavage. While it does not seem that all the APP mutations cause disease by precisely the same mechanism (Cai et al., 1993; Wisniewski et al., 1991) it does seem likely that causing amyloid deposition is the key similarity between the pathogenic variants.

The data presented above mean that we now have some understanding of how APP mismetabolism may lead to beta-amyloid deposition. However, there has been much less progress in developing an understanding of how beta-amyloid deposits might lead to the rest of the pathology of AD. It is a clear prediction of the cascade hypothesis that beta-amyloid deposits must be either directly or indirectly neurotoxic. There has been a huge amount of work designed to test whether beta-amyloid is neurotoxic *in vivo* and *in vitro* but no consensus has been reached (see September 1992 issue of Neurobiology of Aging for review). Two factors have emerged as potentially important in the "neurotoxicity" of beta-amyloid: the first is its physical state as a paracrystalline aggregate and the second is the that presence of other factors bound to the aggregate might be of importance. *A priori*, it would seem unlikely that beta-amyloid would be massively neurotoxic because the very large quantities found in some AD brains would then be expected to kill all neurons.

PROBLEMS

The problem that is most frequently raised with respect to the amyloid cascade hypothesis of AD is that plaque numbers do not correlate as well with indices of premorbid dementia as do tangle numbers or cell and synapse counts (Terry et al., 1991). In fact, this is not a problem with the cascade hypothesis, indeed it is a prediction of the hypothesis. The proximal cause of the dementia in AD is circuitry damage; therefore, one would predict that this would correlate best with degree of dementia. By the cascade hypothesis, a marker of cell damage and one of the proximal causes of cell death is tangle formation, thus one would expect tangle counts to correlate less well with the degree of dementia than cell or synapse counts. Finally, by the cascade hypothesis, plaque deposits lead to tangle formation. Thus, one should expect plaque counts to correlate less well again with degree of dementia than either tangle number or cell and synapse counts. The problem with all these correlative studies is that they depend upon the (unlikely) assumption that plaques and tangles remain indefinitely in the tissue waiting to be counted. The occurrence of dementia with tangles, but not plaques (Ulrich et al., 1993) may relate, in part, to this, or may reflect the fact that tangles can be caused by other etiologies (Giaccone et al., 1989).

A second, and probably related problem, often quoted against the cascade hypothesis, is that there are many subjects who come to autopsy who have large numbers of neuritic plaques, but little or no evidence of dementia. The simplest, albeit weak, explanation for these cases are that they represent preclinical cases of AD: that is, they are persons in which the disease process is just beginning. However, there is real difficulty in understanding what is the relationship between the diffuse, apparently benign deposits of beta-amyloid (Masliah et al., 1990) which appear years before the disease process begins and the neuritic plaques which seem to mark the point of disease initiation (Giaccone et al., 1989; Verga et al., 1989; Mann et al., 1989).

DEFICIENCIES

The amyloid cascade hypothesis has many deficiencies as an explanation of the the etiology and pathogenesis of AD.

As an etiological hypothesis, we still have almost no information concerning the other causes of the disease besides the APP mutations and trisomy (Cai et al., 1993). Possibly, however, the epidemiological evidence linking head injury to AD (Mortimer et al., 1991) together with the work showing abnormal beta-amyloid staining in both chronic head injury (dementia pugilistica) and acute fatal head trauma (Roberts et al., 1990a,b, 1991) fit well with both the cascade hypothesis and with data showing upregulation of APP in response to neuronal injury (Kawarabayashi et al., 1991; Abe et al., 1991). These data, therefore, fit with the notion that AD might sometimes represent a chronic, injury-associated inflammatory reaction (Vandenabeele and Fiers, 1991).

As a pathogenetic explanation for the progress and clinical symptoms of AD, the cascade hypothesis has many deficiencies. The arrows in the cascade hypothesis (Hardy and Allsop, 1991) diagram are meant to represent defined biochemical or morphological processes. As indicated above, we have little or no information on what are the stages of beta-amyloid accumulation in neuritic plaques, little certain information on the relationship of the plaques to tangle formation, and little information beyond morphometric analysis on the effects of tangles on their host neuron (Sumpter et al., 1986). Crucially, AD has a defined clinical picture because "AD knows neuroanatomy" (Sumpter et al., 1986; Duyckaerts et al., 1986; Pearson et al., 1985; Saper et al., 1987; Arnold et al., 1991). We have, as yet, little idea why AD appears to start in the amygdala and progress along neuronal pathways; this is clearly a major deficiency in the cascade hypothesis (DeLacoste and White, 1993; Hardy, 1992).

In conclusion, the problem with the amyloid cascade hypothesis is not that evidence against the hypothesis outweighs the evidence for it; it does not. Rather, the problem remains that there is astonishingly little data to allow the biochemical and morphological processes in the disease process to be delineated. The major reason for these deficiencies is the lack of an animal model of the disease which go beyond diffuse beta-amyloid staining (Quon et al., 1991; Kammesheidt et al., 1993). It is to be hoped that the difficulties inherent in making an animal model of the pathology of AD can be overcome.

REFERENCES

Abe K, Tanzi RE and Kogure K (1991): *Neurosci Letts* 125:172-174.

Arnold SE, Hyman BT, Flory J, Damasio AR and Van Hoesen GW (1991): *Cereb Cortex* 1:103-106.

Cai XD, Golde TE and Younkin SG (1993): *Science* 259:514-516.

Chartier-Harlin MC, Crawford F, Houlden H et al. (1991): *Nature* 353:844-846.

Citron M, Oltersdorf T, Haass C et al. (1992): *Nature* 360:672-674.

DeLacoste MC and White CL (1993): *Neurobiol Aging* 14:1-16.

Duyckaerts C, Hauw JJ, Bastenaire F et al. (1986): *Acta Neuropathol Berl* 70:249-256.

Giaccone G, Tagliavini F, Linoli G et al. (1989): *Neurosci Lett* 97:232-238.

Giaccone G, Tagliavini F, Verga L et al. (1990): *Brain Res* 530;325-329.

Glenner GG and Murphy MA (1989): *J Neurol Sci* 94:1-28.

Goate A, Chartier-Harlin MC, Mullan M et al. (1991): *Nature* 349:704-706.

Haass C, Schlossmacher MG, Hung AY et al., (1992): *Nature* 359:322-325.

Hardy JA and Higgins GA (1992): *Science* 256:184-185.

Hardy J and Mullan M (1992): *Nature* 358:268-269.

Hardy J and Allsop D (1991): *Trends Pharmacol* 12:383-388.

Hardy J (1992): *Trends Neurosci* 15:200-201.

Hardy J (1992): *Nature Genet* 1:233-234.

Kammesheidt A, Boyce FM, Spanoyannis AF et al. (1993): *Proc Natl Acad Sci USA* 89:10857-10861.

Kang J, Lemaire HG, Unterbeck A et al. (1987): *Nature* 325:733-736.

Kawarabayashi T, Shoji M, Harigaya Y, Yamaguchi H and Hirai S (1991): *Brain Res* 563:334-338.

Mann DM, Brown A, Prinja D et al. (1989): *Neuropathol Appl Neurobiol* 15:317-329.

Masliah E, Terry RD, Mallory M, Alford M and Hansen LA (1990): *Am J Pathol* 137:1293-1297.

Mortimer JA, van Duijn CM, Chandra V et al. (1991): *Int J Epidemiol* 20(Suppl)2:S28-S35.

Mullan M, Crawford F, Axelman K et al. (1992): *Nature Genet* 1:345-347.

Mullan M, Houlden H, Windelspecht M et al. (1992): *Nature Genet* 2:340-343.

Murrell J, Farlow M, Ghetti B and Benson M (1991): *Science* 254:97-99.

Nishimoto I, Okamoto T, Matsuura Y, Takahashi S, Murayama Y and Ogata E (1993): *Nature* 362:75-79.

Pearson RC, Esiri MM, Hiorns RW, Wilcock GK and Powell TP (1985): *Proc Natl Acad Sci USA* 82:4531-4534.

Quon D, Wang Y, Catalano R, Marian Scardina J, Murakami K and Cordell B (1991): *Nature* 352:239-241.

Roberts GW, Allsop D and Bruton C (1990a): *J Neurol Neurosurg Psychiatry* 53:373-378.

Roberts GW, Whitwell HL, Acland PR and Bruton CJ (1990b): *Lancet* 335:918-919.

Roberts GW, Gentleman SM, Lynch A and Graham DI (1991): *Lancet* 338:1422-1423.

Saper CB, Wainer BH and German DC (1987): *Neuroscience* 23:389-398.

Schellenberg GD, Bird T, Wijsman E et al. (1992): *Science* 258:668-671.

Selkoe DJ (1991): *Neuron* 6:487-491.

Seubert P, Vigo-Pelfrey C, Esch F et al. (1992): *Nature* 359:325-329.

Shoji M, Golde TE, Cheung TT et al. (1992): *Science* 258:126-129.

St George Hyslop PH, Haines J, Rogaev E et al. (1992): *Nature Genet* 2:330 334.

Sumpter PQ, Mann DM, Davies CA, Yates PO, Snowden JS and Neary D (1986): *Neuropathol Appl Neurobiol* 12:305-319.

Terry RD, Masliah E, Salmon DP et al. (1991): *Ann Neurol* 30:572-580.

Ulrich J, Spillantini MG, Goedert M, Dukas L and Stahelin HB (1993): *Neurodegen* 1:281-288.

Van Broeckhoven C, Backhovens H, Cruts M, De Winter G, Bruyland M and Cras P (1992): *Nature Genet* 2:335-339.

Vandenabeele P and Fiers W (1991): *Immunol Today* 12:217-219.

Verga L, Frangione B, Tagliavini F, Giaccone G, Migheli A and Bugiani O (1989): *Neurosci Lett* 105:294-299.

Wisniewski T, Ghiso J and Frangione B (1991): *Biochem Biophys Res Commun* 179:1247-1254.

Alzheimer Disease: Therapeutic Strategies
edited by E. Giacobini and R. Becker.
© 1994 Birkhäuser Boston

ROLE OF ABNORMAL PHOSPHORYLATION OF TAU IN NEUROFIBRILLARY DEGENERATION: IMPLICATIONS FOR ALZHEIMER THERAPY

Khalid Iqbal and Inge Grundke-Iqbal
New York State Institute for Basic Research in Developmental Disabilities, Staten Island, NY

INTRODUCTION

Alzheimer disease probably has polyetiology, which include genetic, environmental, and metabolic factors. Independent of the etiologic agent, histopathologically, Alzheimer disease (AD) is characterized by the presence of two brain lesions, paired helical filaments (PHF) in the neurons and ß-amyloid in the extracellular space. At present, the exact relationship between PHF and ß-amyloid in the pathogenesis of AD is not understood. However, there is growing evidence from a number of laboratories that dementia in AD patients is associated with neurofibrillary degeneration (e.g. Dickson et al., 1988). Thus one of the most rational therapeutic approaches to AD is to inhibit the neurofibrillary degeneration. In this chapter the mechanism of Alzheimer neurofibrillary degeneration and a strategy to inhibit this type of degeneration is described. Detailed reviews on Alzheimer neurofibrillary pathology were published recently (e.g. Iqbal et al., 1993).

Description of Alzheimer Neurofibrillary Degeneration
For a neuron to function it must be able to transport materials between its cell body and synapses, and integrity of the microtubule system is essential for this axonal transport. In certain selected neurons in AD brain the microtubule system is disrupted and replaced by neurofibrillary tangles of PHF.

Based on solubility in detergents there are two general populations of Alzheimer neurofibrillary tangles (ANT), the readily soluble (ANT/PHF I) and the sparingly soluble (ANT/PHF II) types (Iqbal et al., 1984). Microtubule associated protein tau is the major protein subunit of PHF (Grundke-Iqbal et al., 1986a,b; Iqbal et al., 1989). Tau in PHF is present in abnormally hyperphosphorylated forms (Grundke-Iqbal et al., 1986b; Iqbal et al., 1989). In addition to the PHF, there is a significant pool of the abnormal tau present in soluble form in the AD brain (Iqbal et al., 1986; Köpke et al., 1993). Small amounts of ubiquitin ($< 5\%$) are associated with PHF II but neither with PHF I nor with the non-PHF soluble abnormally phosphorylated tau in AD brain (see Iqbal et al., 1993). Furthermore, the pretangle neurons can readily be immunolabeled for the abnormally phosphorylated tau but not for ubiquitin (Bancher et al., 1989).

Nature of Abnormal Hyperphosphorylation of Tau

Tau in AD brain is phosphorylated differently from normal brain tau (Grundke-Iqbal et al., 1986b; Iqbal et al., 1986, 1989). The abnormal tau isolated from AD brain contains 5 to 9 moles of phosphate/mole of protein, which is about three- to four-times the level in normal brain tau (Köpke et al., 1993). Tau in PHF is phosphorylated at multiple sites. The sites at which the abnormal tau is phosphorylated are Ser 46, Thr 123, Ser 199/Ser 202, Thr 231, Ser 235, Ser 396, and Ser 404 (see Iqbal et al., 1993).

Role of Abnormally Phosphorylated Tau in Neurofibrillary Degeneration

Tau stimulates microtubule assembly by polymerizing with tubulin and maintains the microtubule structure. The levels of tau in homogenates of frontal cortex from AD patients are several-fold higher than in age-matched controls, and that this increase is in the form of abnormally phosphorylated protein (Khatoon et al., 1992). Microtubule assembly is defective in AD brain. Microtubules can be assembled *in vitro* from the cytosol of normal fresh autopsy brain obtained within 5 h postmortem, but not from identically treated brains of AD cases. The microtubule assembly from the Alzheimer brains, however, is induced by the addition of DEAE dextran, a polycation that mimics the effect of tau for microtubule assembly (Iqbal et al., 1986). Because tau in AD brain cytosol is abnormally phosphorylated (Grundke-Iqbal et al., 1986b; Iqbal et al., 1986; Köpke et al., 1993) and phosphorylation of tau depresses tau's ability to promote microtubule assembly (Lindwall and Cole, 1984), it appears that this alteration of tau in the Alzheimer brain might have been the cause of the microtubule assembly defect. Both PHF-tau (Iqbal et al., 1991) and the non-PHF soluble abnormally phosphorylated tau (Alonso et al., 1994) when dephosphorylated with alkaline phosphatase stimulate *in vitro* microtubule assembly. Furthermore, the soluble abnormally phosphorylated tau isolated from AD brain binds to normal tau and not to tubulin, and inhibits the microtubule assembly (Alonso et al., 1994). These findings confirm the role of the abnormal phosphorylation in microtubule assembly defect in AD.

Role of Protein Phosphatases in the Abnormal Phosphorylation of Tau

Protein phosphorylation is one of the major mechanisms for regulation of cellular function. The state of phosphorylation of substrate proteins depends on the relative activities of protein kinases and phosphoprotein phosphatases. Seven of nine abnormal phosphorylation sites of the Alzheimer hyperphosphorylated tau are canonical sites for the proline-directed protein kinases, suggesting that more than one protein kinase are likely involved in the abnormal phosphorylation. At present, the nature of these protein kinases is not clearly understood. Both mitogen activated protein (MAP) kinase and glycogen synthase kinase-3 (GSK-3) have been shown to phosphorylate tau at several of the abnormal phosphorylation sites (e.g. Drewes et al., 1992; Ishiguro et al., 1993). However, the kinetics of phosphorylation at the abnormal site(s) are very slow, suggesting that tau (abnormal sites) is not a preferred substrate for these kinases.

Studies (Grundke-Iqbal et al., 1986b; Iqbal et al., 1986, 1989) showing the dephosphorylation of the abnormally phosphorylated sites of tau after treatment with alkaline phosphatase *in vitro* suggested that the protein phosphorylation/dephosphorylation defect might be the result, in part, of a deficiency in a protein phosphatase system or systems in the affected neurons in AD. The activities of the phosphoseryl/phosphothreonyl protein phosphatases (PP)-1 and -2A towards phosphorylase kinase, and phosphotyrosyl phosphatase towards poly (Glu, Tyr) 4:1 are decreased in brains of AD cases (Gong et al., 1993). Furthermore, by immunocytochemical studies it has been observed that PP-1, PP-2A, PP-2B and cytosolic phosphotyrosyl protein phosphatase PTP-1B are all present in pyramidal neurons in human brain (Pei et al., 1994). To date, all the tau abnormal phosphorylation sites identified are Ser or Thr, and no phosphorylation of Tyr have been observed. However, a decrease in phosphotyrosine phosphatase in AD brain might contribute to hyperphosphorylation of tau by keeping MAP kinase activated for extended periods; dephosphorylation of MAP kinase at either Ser/Thr or Tyr inactivates it (Pelech and Sanghera, 1992). Furthermore, treatment of cultured neuroblastoma cells with inhibitors of PP-2A and PP-2B leads to abnormal phosphorylation of tau (Tanaka et al., in preparation).

Studies on site-specific dephosphorylation by protein phosphatases have revealed that the soluble abnormally phosphorylated tau isolated from AD brain is rapidly dephosphorylated at the abnormal sites Ser 46, Ser 199/Ser 202, Ser 235, and Ser 396/Ser 404 by protein phosphatase PP-2B, at all the above sites except Ser 235 by PP-2A, and at only Ser 199/Ser 202 and Ser 396/Ser 404 by PP-1. The activities of all the three phosphatases, i.e. PP-2B, PP-2A and PP-1 towards the abnormally phosphorylated tau are markedly increased by the presence of Mn^{2+}. Dephosphorylation of the abnormal tau by PP-2C at none of the above sites has been detected (Gong et al., 1994a,b,c). Unlike the soluble abnormally phosphorylated tau, the PHF are less favorable substrate for dephosphorylation both by PP-2A and PP-2B. The two phosphatases, PP-2A and PP-2B, can dephosphorylate PHF at Ser 199/Ser 202 but not Ser 396 using the same conditions as used for the dephosphorylation of the soluble abnormally phosphorylated tau (Wang et al., in preparation).

CONCLUSIONS

Microtubule associated protein tau is abnormally phosphorylated in the brain of patients with AD and the abnormal tau is the major protein subunit of PHF (see Fig. 1). The abnormal phosphorylation of tau probably precedes its polymerization into PHF. The abnormal tau does not bind to tubulin but competes with tubulin in binding to normal tau and thereby inhibits the assembly of microtubules in the affected neurons. The abnormal tau can be dephosphorylated enzymatically and by this way its microtubule assembly promoting activity can be restored. The activities of protein phosphatases might be decreased in the affected neurons in AD brain, allowing the abnormal hyperphosphorylation of tau. Neurofibrillary degeneration can probably be inhibited by increasing the activities of protein phosphatases in the brain of patients with AD.

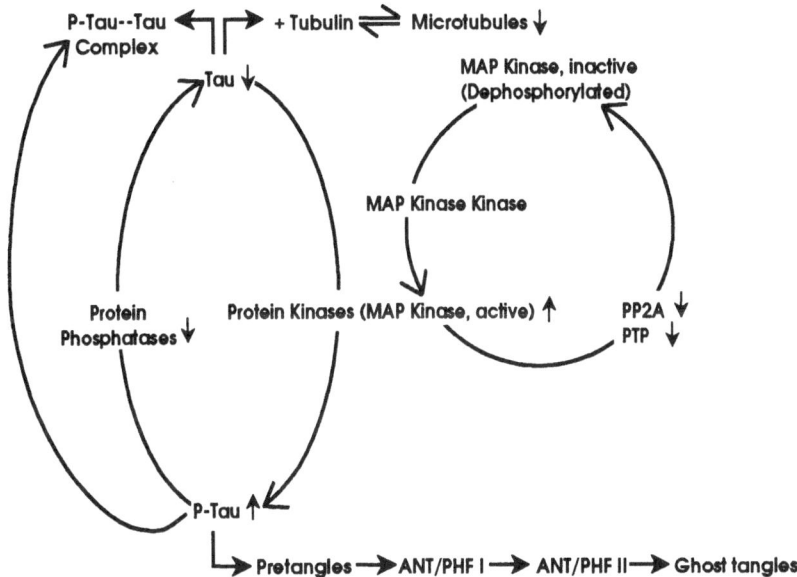

FIGURE 1. A hypothetical scheme showing the mechanism of neurofibrillary degeneration in AD.

Tau is phosphorylated by several protein kinases including MAP kinase. Because of a decrease in the activities of protein phosphatase 2A (2A) and phosphotyrosine protein phosphatases (PTP) in affected neurons, some of the protein kinases, including the MAP kinase, might remain active for extended periods of time, thereby producing hyperphosphorylated tau. The latter (1) does not bind to tubulin to promote assembly of microtubules, (2) binds to normal tau and makes it unavailable for the microtubule assembly, and (3) becomes stabilized and polymerizes into PHF. The affected neurons degenerate both as a result of the breakdown of the microtubule system, and because of the accumulation of PHF as Alzheimer neurofibrillary tangles (ANT) filling the entire cell cytoplasm, leaving behind ghost tangles in the extracellular space.

ACKNOWLEDGMENTS

Secretarial support was provided by Joanne Lopez and Padmini Reginald. This work was supported in part by funds from the New York State Office of Mental Retardation and Developmental Disabilities, National Institutes of Health Grants AG05892, AG08076, NS18105, and Zenith Award from the Alzheimer's Association, USA.

REFERENCES

Alonso A del C, Zaidi T, Grundke-Iqbal I and Iqbal K (1994): Role of abnormally phosphorylated tau in the breakdown of microtubules in Alzheimer disease. *Proc Natl Acad Sci USA* (In Press).

Bancher C, Brunner C, Lassmann H, Budka H, Jellinger K, Wiche G, Seitelberger F, Grundke-Iqbal I, Iqbal K and Wisniewski HM (1989): Accumulation of abnormally phosphorylated tau precedes the formation of neurofibrillary tangles in Alzheimer's disease. *Brain Res* 477:90-99.

Dickson DW, Farlo J, Davies P, Crystal H, Fuld P and Yen SH (1988): Alzheimer's disease. A double-labeling immunohistochemical study of senile plaques. *Am J Pathol* 132:86-101.

Drewes G, Lichtenberg-Kraag B, Döring F, Mandelkow E-M, Biernat J, Goris J, Doree M and Mandelkow E (1992): Mitogen activated protein (MAP) kinase transforms tau protein into an Alzheimer-like state. *EMBO J* 11:2131-2138.

Gong C-X, Singh TJ, Grundke-Iqbal I and Iqbal K (1993): Phosphoprotein phosphatase activities in Alzheimer disease. *J Neurochem* 61:921-927.

Gong C-X, Singh TJ, Grundke-Iqbal I and Iqbal K (1994a): Alzheimer disease abnormally phosphorylated τ is dephosphorylated by protein phosphatase-2B (calcineurin). *J Neurochem* 62:803-806.

Gong C-X, Grundke-Iqbal I and Iqbal K (1994b): Dephosphorylation of Alzheimer disease abnormally phosphorylated tau by protein phosphatase-2A. *Neurosci* (In Press).

Gong C-X, Grundke-Iqbal I, Damuni Z and Iqbal K (1994c): Dephosphorylation of microtubule-associated protein tau by protein phosphatase-1 and -2C and its implication in Alzheimer disease. *FEBS Lett* 341:94-98.

Grundke-Iqbal I, Iqbal K, Quinlan M, Tung Y-C, Zaidi MS and Wisniewski HM (1986a): Microtubule-associated protein tau: a component of Alzheimer paired helical filaments. *J Biol Chem* 261:6084-6089.

Grundke-Iqbal I, Iqbal K, Tung Y-C, Quinlan M, Wisniewski HM and Binder LI (1986b): Abnormal phosphorylation of the microtubule-associated protein tau in Alzheimer cytoskeletal pathology. *Proc Natl Acad Sci USA* 83:4913-1917.

Iqbal K, Zaidi T, Thompson CH, Merz PA and Wisniewski HM (1984): Alzheimer paired helical filaments: bulk isolation, solubility and protein composition. *Acta Neuropathol (Berl)* 62:167-177.

Iqbal K, Grundke-Iqbal I, Zaidi T, Merz PA, Wen GY, Shaikh SS, Wisniewski HM, Alafuzoff I and Winblad B (1986): Defective brain microtubule assembly in Alzheimer's disease. *Lancet* 2:421-426.

Iqbal K, Grundke-Iqbal I, Smith AJ, George L, Tung Y-C and Zaidi T (1989): Identification and localization of a tau peptide to paired helical filaments of Alzheimer disease. *Proc Natl Acad Sci USA* 86:5646-5650.

Iqbal K, Köpke-Secundo E and Grundke-Iqbal I (1991): Dephosphorylation of microtubule associated protein tau from Alzheimer disease brain increases its ability to promote *in vitro* assembly of microtubules. *J Neuropathol Exp Neurol Abstr* 50:316.

Iqbal K, Alonso A, Gong C-X, Khatoon S, Kudo T, Singh TJ and Grundke-Iqbal I (1993): Molecular pathology of Alzheimer neurofibrillary degeneration. *Acta Neurobiol Exp* 53:325-335.

Ishiguro K, Shiratsuchi A, Sato S, Omori A, Arioka M, Kobayashi S, Uchida T and Imahori K (1993): Glycogen synthase kinase 3ß is identical to tau protein kinase I generating several epitopes of paired helical filaments. *FEBS Lett* 325:167-172.

Khatoon S, Grundke-Iqbal I and Iqbal K (1992): Brain levels of microtubule-associated protein tau are elevated in Alzheimer's disease: a radioimmuno-slot blot assay for nanograms of the protein. *J Neurochem* 59:750-753.

Köpke E, Tung Y-C, Shaikh S, Alonso A del C, Iqbal K and Grundke-Iqbal I (1993): Microtubule associated protein tau: abnormal phosphorylation of a non-paired helical filament pool in Alzheimer disease. *J Biol Chem* 268:24374-24384.

Lindwall G and Cole RD (1984): Phosphorylation affects the ability of tau protein to promote microtubule assembly. *J Biol Chem* 259:5301-5305.

Pei J-J, Sersen E, Iqbal K and Grundke-Iqbal I (1994): Expression of protein phosphatases PP-1, PP-2A, PP-2B and PTP-1B and protein kinases MAP kinase and P34^{cdc2} in the hippocampus of patients with Alzheimer disease and normal aged individuals. *Brain Res* (In Press).

Pelech SL and Sanghera JS (1992): MAP kinases: charting the regulatory pathways. *Science* 257:1355-1356.

Alzheimer Disease: Therapeutic Strategies
edited by E. Giacobini and R. Becker.
© 1994 Birkhäuser Boston

OLFACTORY BULB INVOLVEMENT IN AD: AN EARLY CHANGE?

Robert G. Struble, Mona Ghobrial and Larry F. Hughes
Southern Illinois University School of Medicine, P.O. Box 19230,
Springfield, IL 62794

OVERVIEW

Olfactory function is severely compromised in the early stages of Alzheimer disease (AD). This compromise is particularly apparent in tasks requiring naming of the odorant (Serby et al., 1985; Peabody and Tinklenberg, 1985; Warner et al., 1986; Knupfer and Speigel, 1986; Doty et al., 1987). In contrast, detecting the presence of an odorant (i.e. detection) or discriminating that two odorants are different (discrimination) appear to be relatively spared early in the disease (Engen, 1977; St Clair et al., 1985; Rezek, 1987; Koss et al., 1988; Hughes et al., 1994). To date it has been unclear what lesion(s) might underlay the early deterioration of olfactory recognition function.

Olfactory system lesions in AD have not been well established. Cytoskeletal and amyloid preprotein abnormalities have been identified in the olfactory mucosa in patients with AD (Talamo et al., 1989; Tabaton et al., 1991; Wolozin et al., 1993) although many of the abnormalities may also be found in normal controls (Trojanowski et al., 1991). Olfactory mucosa biopsy samples, adequate to address a primary change in olfactory mucosa, are problematic in elderly individuals (Paik et al., 1992). Concluding that the olfactory receptor neurons are directly involved in the pathogenesis of AD may be premature.

The olfactory bulb (OB) proper is reported to display few senile plaques (SP) or neurofibrillary tangles (NFT), the classic markers of AD (Esiri and Wilcock, 1984). Senile plaques and NFT have been found in the anterior olfactory nucleus (AON), although this structure does not receive direct input from the olfactory receptors. Neuronal loss in the OB has been controversial (Davies et al., 1993; Hyman et al., 1991; Struble and Clark, 1992; ter Laak et al., 1994). Given early clinical deficits, we decided to evaluate both clinical function and olfactory bulb lesions in AD.

We have been interested in four questions: 1) Do recognition deficits represent discrimination *per se* or a higher order dysfunction in naming? 2) What anatomical substrates underlay these clinical deficits? 3) How early do the lesions appear in AD and could olfactory tests be used for early detection?

4) If OB lesions develop early in the course of AD, what predisposes the OB to develop these lesions? The following discussion relates to our recent work and speculations addressing these questions.

CLINICAL OLFACTORY TESTING

Two olfactory tests have been given in our clinics based on the University of Pennsylvania Smell Identification Test (UPSIT) (Doty et al., 1984). These odorants, equated for intensity and identifiability, were given to three groups: a) young subjects (age < 50); b) elderly controls (mean age = 74.6); and c) mild AD cases [Mini-Mental State Exam (MMSE) > 18] age-matched to the controls. In the first task, two odorants were presented sequentially and the patient responded whether they were the same or different. The second task was a recognition task. Each patient selected a verbal label from four choices for an odorant. Signal detection theory was then used to determine a d' for performance. Cognitively intact elderly compared favorably with young controls on recognition. Patients with mild AD performed at a chance level. In contrast, AD patients performed as well as either control group on discrimination. These data confirmed previous studies of deficits in the ability to name an odorant (smell recognition tasks) but found normal suprathreshold discrimination in the same subjects suggesting differential vulnerability of information processing in early AD.

ANATOMICAL SUBSTRATES

Our clinical data suggest that anatomical substrates subserving recognition and discrimination might be differentially disrupted in early AD. One possible explanation is that loss of mitral cells, which project to areas close to entorhinal cortex (ERC), functionally disconnects the OB from ERC and prevents integration between names and odors. Alternatively, early changes in ERC might disrupt the ability to name an odorant. Discrimination might be subserved by a more restricted system of primary olfactory cortex and orbital frontal cortex (Tanabe et al., 1975a,b) that could utilize the relatively preserved tufted cells (Struble and Clark, 1992). Threshold deficits might be related to degeneration of the olfactory nerve.

HOW EARLY DO OLFACTORY DEFICITS OCCUR?

Severe clinical olfactory deficits in mild AD patients suggest that olfactory deficits might be marked when other cognitive domains might be only mildly affected or unaffected. However, detection of early cognitive deficits in AD is problematic. Alzheimer disease is already advanced, at least to mild stages, when a patient is brought to the clinic for evaluation. These patients would not be suitable for detecting early olfactory changes. Testing "intact" elderly controls, some of whom are early in the course of dementia, could detect some with poor performance on recognition but sparing of discrimination. These cases might develop AD. However, the incidence of clinical AD is relatively low in cognitively intact individuals (e.g. 14-50/1000/year in the over 85 y/o group) (see Bachman et al., 1993) and large samples would be required to identify stable deficits. Nonetheless, this strategy is reasonable with a relatively stable elderly population amenable to retesting.

An alternative approach was to use neuropathologic criteria as an approximate guide to stage early AD. Our studies, started in 1989, used this strategy of neuropathologic findings to group patients into those with **few or no** AD lesions, those with a **mild** density of AD lesions (borderline AD) and those with clinical dementia and **definitive** densities of SP and NFT. We operationally defined a population of cases as "borderline" AD (Struble and Clark, 1992) displaying focal densities of NFT/SP of $15+/mm^2$, but densities in other neocortical areas insufficient for a neuropathologic diagnosis of AD (Khachaturian, 1985). We reported that mitral cells, the large projecting neurons of the OB, were substantially (ca. 70%) reduced from age-matched controls with no AD lesions. Mitral cells were also equivalently reduced in neuropathologically "borderline" AD cases (Struble and Clark, 1992). These cases also displayed olfactory nerve heteroplasia, diffuse β-APP-like immunoreactivity surrounding glomeruli, and over expression of growth cone associated protein (GAP43) (Struble and Ghobrial, 1993).

Defining early neuropathologic lesions in AD is difficult or impossible in the absence of clinical information (Katzman et al., 1988; Morris et al., 1991; Price et al., 1991). However, on the average, this grouping should give mean values of information applicable to understanding lesion progression in AD.

	N	AGED MEAN ± SEM	G-EPL MEAN ± SEM	I-EPL MEAN ± SEM	GCL MEAN ± SEM
CONT-Y	14	42.6 ± 5.6	2.22 ± 0.21	0.78 ± 0.34	0.22 ± 0.14
CONT-O	10	75.7 ± 1.8	2.08 ± 0.17	0.77 ± 0.25	0.23 ± 0.12
AD	13	76.1 ± 1.8	2.77 ± 0.12	2.46 ± 0.26	2.31 ± 0.23
PAD	10	77.0 ± 2.9	2.80 ± 0.13	2.40 ± 0.29	2.30 ± 0.28

TABLE I. GFAP Immunoreactivity in Olfactory Bulb. CONT-Y, controls, young; CONT-O, controls old; AD, Alzheimer disease and AD combined with Parkinson disease; PAD, possible AD.

To further evaluate these cases we examined glial reactivity. Reactive gliosis has been reported in the OB in AD (Hyman et al., 1991). Glial fibrillary acidic protein (GFAP) was assessed with a 0-3 rating scale in three zones: the interface of the external plexiform layer and the glomerular zone; the inner external plexiform layer; and the granule cell layer (Table I).

AD cases and AD/PD cases were equivalent, so they were pooled for analysis. Glial fibrillary acidic protein staining was approximately comparable among all four groups at the interface between the glomerular and outer external plexiform layers. In contrast, staining in the internal part of the external plexiform layer and in the granule cell layer of the AD and the PAD groups was substantially increased over either control group. In sum, our data suggested that individuals with mild cortical lesions, indicative of AD, might represent early AD and show substantial OB changes.

THE OLFACTORY BULB AS A MODEL IN AD

The important question for any model is what predisposing factors are present in the OB that make it susceptible to early AD changes? One possibility for vulnerability is plasticity. Plasticity is a striking feature of the OB. The olfactory system is unique in that the olfactory receptor is continuously regenerated throughout the life of the organism and must grow into the bulb and establish new synapses (Graziadei and Monti-Graziadei, 1980) requiring substantial plasticity in OB neurons. A juvenile form of microtubule associated protein (MAPII) is expressed by mitral cells in adult rats (Viereck et al., 1989). Developmental regulation of β-APP during development occurs in rats with high levels in neonatal rats decreasing during development. Levels of β-APP remain high in the OB in adult animals (Löffler et al., 1992). GAP43 is a peptide associated with axonal growth and is expressed, as would be expected, in the axons of olfactory nerve cells. It is also found in the internal plexiform layer in small axons suggesting plasticity (Verhaagen et al., 1989). High levels of β-APP are reported in ERC cells that are at risk to degenerate in AD (Roberts et al., 1993; Braak and Braak, 1991). Regions high in GAP43 message are at substantial risk in AD (Neve et al., 1988; Brun and Englund, 1981). Finally, numerous studies have suggested that SP represent abortive sprouting associated with β-APP and GAP43 (Masliah et al., 1991). If β-APP and GAP43 are associated with axonal growth and plasticity, then OB may express substantial of "plasticity".

We hypothesize that some proximal dysfunction in AD induces abortive attempts at neuronal repair and plasticity. The etiology of dysfunction or loss is probably manifold. Nonetheless, a cascade of lesions follows that manifest in the clinical and neuropathologic entity of AD (e.g. see Butcher and Woolf, 1989). Finding substantial damage in olfactory functioning and lesions in the OB might reflect the plasticity of this region. Using olfactory testing for diagnostic aid in AD may identify early changes. Testing efficacy in other dementing illnesses, e.g. Parkinson disease (PD), remains to be evaluated. Some patients with PD display olfactory recognition deficits (Doty et al., 1988). Some of these patients might develop AD or diffuse Lewy body disease.

However, too little literature exists on olfactory bulb changes in dementing illnesses to be able to anticipate possible neuropathological and clinical deficits.

REFERENCES

Bachman DL, Wolf PA, Linn RT, Knoefel JE, Cobb JL, Belanger AJ, White LR and D'Agostino RB (1993): Incidence of dementia and probable Alzheimer disease in a general population: The Framingham study. *Neurology* 43:515-519.

Braak H and Braak E (1991): Neuropathological staging of Alzheimer-related changes. *Acta Neuropathol* 82:239-259.

Brun A and Englund E (1981): Regional pattern of degeneration in Alzheimer disease: neuronal loss and histopathological grading. *Histopathology* 5:549-564.

Butcher LL and Woolf NJ (1989): Neurotrophic agents may exacerbate the pathologic cascade of Alzheimer disease. *Neurobiol Aging* 10:557-570.

Davies DC, Brooks JW and Lewis DA (1993): Axonal loss from the olfactory tracts in Alzheimer Disease. *Neurobiol Aging* 14:353-357.

Doty RL, Shaman P and Dann M (1984): Development of the University of Pennsylvania Smell Identification Test: A standardized microencapsulated test of olfactory function. Monograph: *Physiol Behav* 32:489-502.

Doty RJ, Reyes P and Gregor T (1987): Presence of both odor identification and detection deficits in Alzheimer disease. *Brain Res Bull* 18:597-600.

Doty RL, Deems DA and Stellar S (1988): Olfactory dysfunction in Parkinsonism: a general deficit unrelated to neurologic signs, disease stage or disease duration. *Neurology* 38:1237-1244.

Engen T (1977): Taste and Smell. In: *Handbook of the Psychology of Aging*, Birren JE, Schaie KW, eds. New York: Van Nostrand Reinhold, pp. 554-561.

Esiri M and Wilcock G (1984): The olfactory bulbs in Alzheimer disease. *J Neurol Neurosurg Psychiat* 47:56-60; 1984.

Graziadei PPC and Monti-Graziadei GA (1980): Neurogenesis and neuron recognition in the olfactory system of mammals. III. Deafferentation and reinnervation of the olfactory bulb following section of the *fila olfactoria* in rat. *J Neurocytol* 9:145-162.

Hughes LF, Shaffer CL and Struble RG (1994): Olfactory discrimination and identification functions in elderly normal and Alzheimer subjects. *Abst ARO* 34:9

Hyman BT, Arriagada PV, and Van Hoesen (1991): Pathologic changes in the olfactory system in aging and Alzheimer disease. *Ann NY Acad Sci* 640:14-19.

Katzman R, Terry R, DeTeresa R, Brown T, Davies P, Fuld P, Renbing X, and Peck A (1988): Clinical, pathological, and neurochemical changes in Dementia: a subgroup with preserved mental status and numerous neocortical plaques. *Ann Neurol* 23:138-144.

Khachaturian Z (1985): Diagnosis of Alzheimer disease. *Arch Neurol* 42:1097-1105.

Knupfer L and Speigel R (1986): Differences in olfactory test performance between normal aged, Alzheimer and vascular type dementia individuals. *Int J Geriat* 1:3-14

Koss E, Weiffenbach JM, Haxby JV and Friedland RP (1988): Olfactory detection and identification performance are dissociated in early Alzheimer disease. *Neurology* 38:1228-1232.

Löffler J and Huber G (1992): β-amyloid precursor protein isoforms in various rat brain regions and during brain development. *J Neurochem* 59:1316-1324.

Masliah E, Mallory M, Hansen L, Alford M, Albright T, DeTeresa R, Terry R, Baudier J and Saitoh T (1991): Patterns of aberrant sprouting in Alzheimer disease. *Neuron* 6:729-739.

Morris JC, McKeel DW Jr, Stroandt M, Rubin EH, Price JL, Grant EA, Ball MJ and Berg L (1991): Very mild Alzheimer disease: Informant-based clinical, psychometric and pathologic distinction from normal aging. *Neurology* 41:469-478.

Neve RL, Finch EA, Bird ED and Benowitz LI (1988): Growth-associated protein GAP-43 is expressed selectively in associative regions of the adult human brain. *Proc Natl Acad Sci USA* 85:3638-3642.

Paik SI, Lehman MN, Seiden AM, Duncan HJ and Smith DV (1992): Human olfactory biopsy: The influence of age and receptor distribution. *Arch Otolaryngol Head Neck Surg* 118:731-738.

Peabody CA and Tinklenberg JR (1985): Olfactory deficits and primary degenerative dementia. *Am J Psychiat* 142:524-525.

Price JL, Davis PB, Morris JC and White DL (1991): The distribution of tangles, plaques and related immunohistochemical markers in health aging and Alzheimer disease. *Neurobiol Aging* 12:295-312.

Rezek DJ (1987): Olfactory deficits as a neurologic sign in dementia of the Alzheimer type. *Arch Neurol* 44:1030-1032.

Roberts GW, Nash M, Ince PG, Roysotn MC and Gentleman SM (1993): On the origin of Alzheimer disease: a hypothesis. *Neuroreport* 4:7-9.

Serby M, Corwin J, Conrad P, and Rotrosen J (1985): Olfactory dysfunction in Alzheimer's disease and Parkinson's disease. *Am J Psychiatry* 142:781-782.

St. Clair DM, Simpson J, Yates CM and Gordon A (1985): Letter. *J Neurol Neurosurg Psychiat* 1985;48:849.

Struble RG and Clark HB (1992): Olfactory bulb lesions in Alzheimer disease. *Neurobiol Aging* 13:469-473.

Struble RG and Ghobrial M (1993): Growth cone associated protein (GAP43) and amyloid precursor protein (APP) in the olfactory bulbs (OB) in Alzheimer disease. *Soc Neurosci Abst* 19:430

Tabaton M, Cammarata S, Mancardi GL, Cordone G, Perry G and Loeb C (1991): Abnormal tau-reactive filaments in olfactory mucosa in biopsy specimens of patients with probable Alzheimer disease. *Neurology* 41:391-394.

Talamo B, Rudel R, Kosik K, Lee V, Neff S, Adelman L and Kauer J: Pathological changes in olfactory neurons in patients with Alzheimer disease. *Nature* 337:736-738

Tanabe T, Yarita H, Iino M, Ooshima Y and Takagi SF (1975a): An olfactory projection area in orbitofrontal cortex of the monkey. *J Neurophys* 38:1269-1283.

Tanabe T, Iino M and Takagi SF (1975b): Discrimination of odors in olfactory bulb, pyriform-amygdaloid areas, and orbitofrontal cortex of the monkey. *J Neurophys* 38:1284-1296.

ter Laak HJ, Renkawek K, and van Workum FPA (1994): The olfactory bulb in Alzheimer disease: A morphologic study of neuron loss, tangles and senile plaques in relation to olfaction. *Alz Dis Assoc Dis* 8:38-48.

Trojanowski JQ, Newman PD, Hill WD and Lee VM-Y (1991): Human olfactory epithelium in normal aging, Alzheimer disease and other neurodegenerative disorders. *J Comp Neurol* 310:365-376.

Verhaagen J, Oestreicher AB, Gispen WH and Margolis FL (1989): The expression of the growth associated protein B50/GAP43 in the olfactory system of neonatal and adult rats. *J Neurosci* 9:683-691.

Viereck C, Tucker RP and Matus A (1989): The adult rat olfactory system expresses microtubule-associated proteins found in the developing brain. *J Neurosci* 9:3547-3557

Warner MD, Peabody CA, Flattery JJ and Tinklenberg JR (1986): Olfactory deficits and Alzheimer Disease. *Biol Psychiat* 21:116-118.

Wolozin B, Lesch P, Lebovics R and Sunderland T (1993): Olfactory neuroblasts from Alzheimer donors: Studies on APP processing and cell regulation. *Biol Psychiat* 34:824-838.

Alzheimer Disease: Therapeutic Strategies
edited by E. Giacobini and R. Becker.
© 1994 Birkhäuser Boston

ALZHEIMER DISEASE -- A SPIROCHETOSIS?

Judit Miklossy
University Institute of Pathology, Division of Neuropathology,
1005 Lausanne, Switzerland

INTRODUCTION

Dementia associated with cortical atrophy and microgliosis has been observed in the late stages of two spirochetal diseases: Lyme disease, a late stage of neuroborreliosis caused by *Borrelia burgdorferi* (Burgdorfer et al., 1982; Pachner et al., 1989), and general paresis, tertiary stage of neurosyphilis caused by *Treponema pallidum*. Two cases of concurrent neocortical borreliosis and Alzheimer disease (AD) have been reported (MacDonald and Miranda, 1987; MacDonald, 1988): immunostaining showed *Borrelia burgdorferi* in brain tissue and the spirochetes were cultured from cerebral cortex. A careful study of 18 AD cases, using several methodological approaches, failed to support an association between *Borrelia burgdorferi* and AD, but the authors did not rule out the possibility that another spirochete, not detectable by their methods, may be responsible for AD (Pappolla et al., 1989).

From the beginning of this century, descriptions and illustrations of the distribution of *Treponema pallidum* in brains of patients with general paresis (Schlossberger and Brandis, 1958) show a striking similarity with the argyrophilic, senile plaques of AD. Neurofibrillary tangles have also been described in general paresis (Hirano and Zimmerman, 1962) and, finally, amyloid degeneration secondary to syphilitic infection is a well-known phenomenon (Mauric and Godel, 1949).

RESULTS

Twenty-seven autopsy cases were investigated. Blood, cerebrospinal fluid (CSF) and brain tissue samples from the frontal, parietal and temporal regions were taken under sterile conditions. A systematic evaluation of brain pathology based on a standardized protocol for tissue sampling and staining was performed to assure the neuropathological diagnosis of AD (Miklossy, 1993). Examination of the blood and CSF was carried out in all cases using dark field microscopy. In the blood and the CSF of 14 of the 27 cases, motile, coiled spirochetes were observed. Their diameter was approximately 0.2 to 0.3 μm and their length varied between 8 and 30 μm (Fig. 1A).

Histological changes typical of AD were observed in all 14 cases whose blood and CSF contained spirochetes. When silver methods described for the demonstration of spirochetes in tissue sections were used (Warthin and Starry, Bosma-Steiner), we found silver-stained filaments in senile plaques, neuropil threads and neurofibrillary tangles. In the remaining 13 cases, those without spirochetes in blood and CSF, the neuropathological examination revealed no signs of AD.

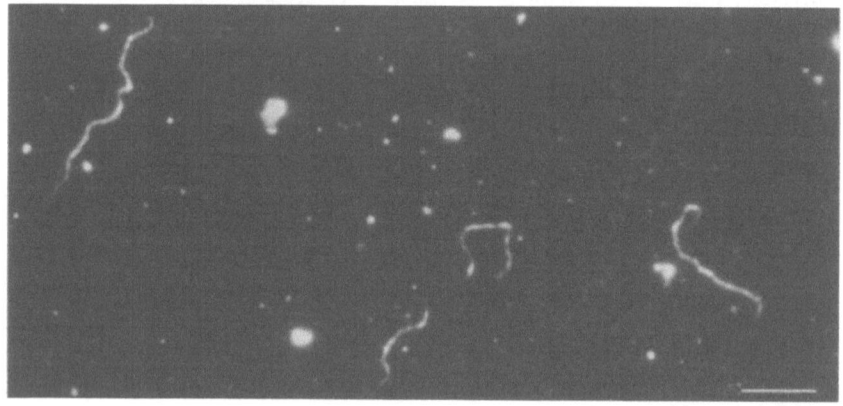

FIGURE 1. Spirochetes in the cerebrospinal fluid of an AD case as shown by dark field microscopy. Bar: 10 μm. Reproduced with the permission of *NeuroReport* [4(7):841-848, 1993].

Spirochetes were isolated from the unfixed brain tissue (Miklossy, 1993) of all 14 AD cases (Fig. 1B). In addition, we isolated spirochetes from the brains of two histologically confirmed familial AD cases. No spirochetes were found in four out of four arbitrarily chosen control cases tested. The spirochetes were cultured from the blood, in four out of five arbitrarily chosen AD cases, in a modified Noguchi medium and in three out of four AD cases from the brain in a BSK medium (Fig. 2A). No spirochetes could be cultured from the blood or from the brain in four cases tested without AD. The fact that the control cases were free of spirochetes and that we isolated the helically shaped microorganisms from 8 AD brains derived from another laboratory (unpublished data) seems to contradict the possibility of a contamination by spirochetes of the autopsy material in our laboratory. The presence of spirochetes in the blood of five living patients with Alzheimer's type dementia argues against a post mortem contamination (unpublished data).

A case of concurrent AD and serologically confirmed Lyme disease was used to investigate immunohistochemically whether *Borrelia burgdorferi* was present in brain tissue. Using a monoclonal antibody against *Borrelia burgdorferi* (Biodesign, C63780M), spirochetes were found in senile plaques, in leptomeningeal and cortical vessel walls, in neurons, and in microglial cells. They were also found as solitary elements in the neuropil.

An ultrastructural study of silver-stained and anti-APP-immunostained sections of the cerebral cortex in three AD cases tested also revealed coiled elements whose morphology was compatible with that of spirochetes (Miklossy, 1993). When using scanning electron microscopy and atomic force microscopy, both able to scan surfaces, we found that the helically shaped microorganisms isolated and cultured from the AD brains possess axial filaments (Fig. 2B). This indicates that these microorganisms taxonomically indeed belong to the order *Spirochaetales* (Miklossy et al., 1994).

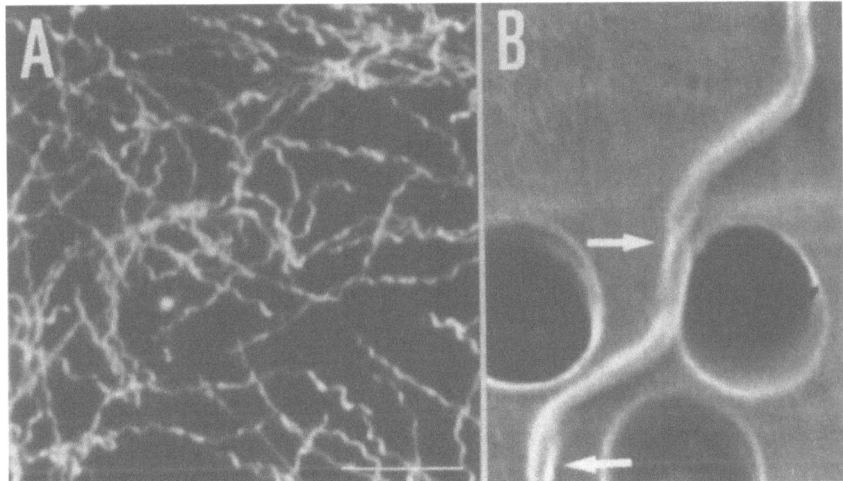

FIGURE 2. A: Cultured spirochetes from the cortex of one of the histologically confirmed AD cases. Bar: 10 μm. B: Scanning electron micrograph. Arrows point to the axial filament of this spirochete cultured from the brain, which taxonomically distinguishes spirochetes from other bacteria. The pore-size of the Millipore filter corresponds to 1.2 μm. B: Reproduced with the permission of *NeuroReport* (5:1201-1204, 1994).

The finding that spirochetes from reference strains of *Treponema pallidum* and *Borrelia burgdorferi* showed positive immunoreaction with a monoclonal antibody against the N-terminal part of the amyloid precursor protein (APP) suggests that the APP or at least an APP-like protein (APLP) may be an integral part of the infectious agent and thus may be the source of the excess of ßA4 deposited in the AD brain. This would be in agreement with the observations made by Jarrett and Lansbury (1992), who reported that a periplasmic outer membrane associated lipoprotein of the *Escherichia coli* resemble that of the C-terminal region of the β amyloid protein of AD. This peptide, called OsmB was shown to form amyloid fibrils and they bond Congo red. These data suggest that these gram negative bacteria contain in their outer sheaths an amyloidogenic protein which resembles the βA4.

DISCUSSION

The similar localization and distribution of the ßA4 deposited in the brain in both forms -familial and sporadic AD cases- and in late Down syndrome (DS) cases, as well as the isolation of spirochetes from the brain of two familial AD cases are difficult to explain on a genetic basis alone.   An alternative reconciliation of the genetic and infectious etiology of AD lie in the supposition that the genetic defects associated with AD and DS may lead to a predisposition for spirochetal infection, or may favor its progress.

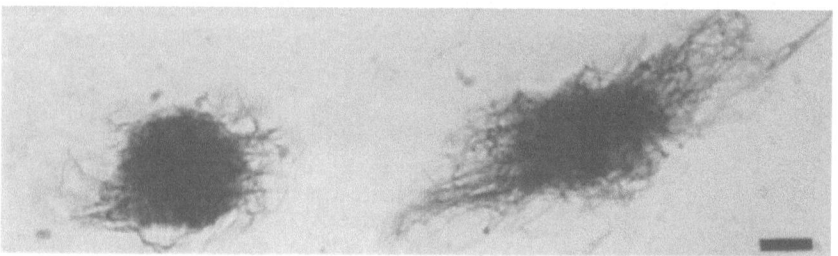

FIGURE 3. Cultured, reference spirochetes from the B 31 strain of *Borrelia burgdorferi* immunostained with an anti-APP monoclonal antibody. Bar: 10 μm.

Several authors have reported that spirochetes may invade the parenchyma without the challenge of an inflammatory reaction (Gastinel, 1949).   The presence of spirochetes in brain tissue sections in cases of Lyme disease with microgliosis and without inflammatory infiltrate was also reported (Pachner et al., 1989).   In addition, recent observations suggest that the amyloid-bearing plaques may be the sites of chronic inflammatory process (Selkoe, 1991).

All attempts to transmit the disease to animals have remained unsuccessful (Koch postulate 3).   Here, one may argue as do authors for the transgenic animal models inducing APP over-production, that an animal with a life-span as short as a mouse's can never develop a pathology that in man takes several decades.   In general paresis (tertiary stage of neurosyphilis) the latent stage between the primary infection and the development of dementia may take several decades (Storm-Mathisen, 1978).   The long latent stage would have to be taken into consideration in attempts to transmit the disease to chimpanzees.

Based on the observations reported here AD may correspond to the tertiary stage of neurospirochetosis. The characterization of the spirochetes found in AD is needed.   It would enable one to develop serological tests for early detection of the infection. The observations made for the treatment of Lyme disease show that the antibiotic therapy is particularly efficient in the earliest stages of the disease. In general paresis as in AD the pathological process is thought to begin long before the diagnosis "dementia" is made, and thus, appropriate antibiotic treatment should start early in order to prevent the development of dementia.

ACKNOWLEDGEMENTS

I am grateful to R. Berger, R. Kraftsik and J. Maillardet for their helpful assistance.

REFERENCES

Burgdorfer W, Barbour AG, Hayes SF, Benach JL, Grunwaldt E and Davis JP (1982): Lyme disease - a tick-borne spirochetosis? *Science* 216:1317-1319.

Gastinel P (1949): *Précis de bactériologie médicale.* Masson and Cie, eds. Paris, pp. 1040.

Hirano A and Zimmerman HM (1962): Alzheimer's neurofibrillary changes. A topographical study. *Arch Neurol* 7:227-242.

Jarrett JT and Lansbury T (1992): Amyloid fibril formation requires a chemically discriminating nucleation event: Studies of an amyloidogenic sequence from the bacterial protein OsmB. *Biochemistry* 31:12345-12352.

MacDonald AB (1988): Concurrent neocortical borreliosis and Alzheimer's disease. Demonstration of a spirochetal cyst form. *Ann NY Acad Sci* 539:468-470.

MacDonald AB and Miranda JM (1987): Concurrent neocortical borreliosis and Alzheimer's disease. *Human Pathol* 18:759-761.

Mauric G and Godel R (1949): La syphilis rénale. In: *Traité de Médecine*, Masson and Cie, eds. Paris, Vol XIV. pp. 685-713.

Miklossy J (1993): Alzheimer's disease - a spirochetosis? *NeuroReport* 4:841-848.

Miklossy J, Kasas S, Janzer RC, Ardizzoni F and Van der Loos H (1994): Further ultrastructural evidence that spirochetes may play a role in the etiology of Alzheimer's disease. *NeuroReport* 5:1201-1204.

Pachner AR, Duray PH and Steere AC (1989): Central nervous system manifestations of Lyme disease. *Arch Neurol* 46:790-795.

Pappolla MA, Omar R, Saran B, Andorn A, Suarez M, Pavia C, Weinstein A, Shank D, Davis K and Burgdorfer W (1989): Concurrent neuroborreliosis and Alzheimer's disease - analysis of evidence. *Human Pathol* 20:753-757.

Schlossberger H and Brandis H (1958): Ueber Spirochaetenbefunde im Zentralnerven system mit besonderer Beruecksichtigung der syphilogenen Erkrankungen. In: *Handbuch der speziellen pathologischen Anatomie und Histologie*, Lubarsch O, Henke F and Rössle R, eds. Berlin: Springer, Vol II. pp. 1048-1085.

Selkoe DJ (1991): The molecular pathology of Alzheimer's disease. *Neuron* 6:487-498.

Storm-Mathisen A (1978): Syphilis. In: *Handbook of Neurology*, Vinken PJ and Bruyn GW, eds. Amsterdam: Elsevier, Vol 33, Chapter 17, pp. 358-359.

PART II

THERAPEUTICAL STRATEGIES TO ARREST PRODUCTION AND PROCESSING OF AMYLOID

Alzheimer Disease: Therapeutic Strategies
edited by E. Giacobini and R. Becker.
© 1994 Birkhäuser Boston

BETA AMYLOID (Aβ) AS A THERAPEUTIC TARGET IN ALZHEIMER'S DISEASE

Ivan Lieberburg
Athena Neurosciences, Inc., South San Francisco, California, USA, 94080

Alzheimer's disease (AD) is a chronic, neurodegenerative disorder which is characterized by a loss of cognitive ability, severe behavioral abnormalities and ultimately death. It is the fourth leading cause of death in Western cultures, preceded only by heart disease, cancer and stroke. There are currently 2.5-4.0 million AD patients in the U.S. and 17-25 million worldwide. There is no definitive treatment or cure for this devastating disease (Selkoe, 1991).

At autopsy, the AD brain is characterized by a number of important pathological changes. There is a dramatic loss of neurons and synapses in many areas of the CNS, but particularly in regions involved in higher order cognitive functions, such as the hippocampus and association cortices. In addition, the levels of many neurotransmitters are greatly reduced, including but not limited to acetylcholine, serotonin, noradrenaline, dopamine, glutamate, and substance P. This dramatic and global reduction of a number of important CNS neurotransmitters is almost certainly responsible for the broad and profound clinical manifestations of AD, i.e., memory impairment, hallucinations, paranoia, restlessness and depression (Selkoe, 1991).

However, two microscopic deposits which were originally defined by Alois Alzheimer in 1907 - the neurofibrillary tangle (NFT) and the senile amyloid plaque - remain the pathological hallmarks that define the disease. Plaques and tangles are also highly concentrated in regions of substantial neuronal death in the AD brain, such as the hippocampus and association cortex. A debate still rages as to whether plaques and tangles are harmless by-products or tombstones of the neurodegeneration seen in AD, or if they are causal in the neuronal death (Selkoe, 1991). Our position at Athena is that these deposits, notably amyloid plaques, cause or greatly contribute to the neurodegeneration seen in AD.

The amyloid plaque as described by Alzheimer was isolated by Glenner and Wong in 1984. It is composed of an approximately 40 amino acid peptide (now known as Aβ) which becomes compacted into a fibrillar, β-pleated structure, and which appears green under polarized or fluorescent light after staining with Congo Red (Selkoe, 1991). It is this classic staining characteristic which defines the deposit as being amyloid.

Aβ has been hypothesized to be causally related to AD for a number of reasons: (1) In peripheral amyloidoses (such as primary light chain disease, or secondary AA amyloidosis), large amyloid burdens strongly correlate with tissue and organ dysfunction in those diseases; (2) In AD, amyloid plaque density is positively correlated with pre-mortem dementia scores (Selkoe, 1991); (3) Aβ deposition is the earliest neuropathological marker in AD and related disorders such as in Down's Syndrome, where it can precede NFT formation by two to three decades (Selkoe, 1991); (4) β-amyloidosis is relatively specific to AD and related disorders (Selkoe, 1991); (5) Aβ is toxic to neurons (Yankner et al., 1990; Mattson et al., 1992); (6) Rare missense mutations in the structural amyloid precursor protein (APP) gene cause early onset familial AD (Goate et al. 1991; Mullan et al., 1992). Notably one such mutation (Mullan, et al., 1992) causes dramatic Aβ overproduction (Citron et al., 1992).

In 1987 four groups independently cloned the gene from which Aβ is derived. The larger protein encoded by this gene, now known as the amyloid precursor protein (APP) is expressed in virtually all tissues. There are at least five splicing variants of APP, four of which contain the β-amyloid peptide sequence (Selkoe, 1991). Much of our work at Athena has been directed toward an understanding of how Aβ is released from this larger precursor molecule, and how the released peptide results in neuronal toxicity.

One of the initial approaches in studying Aβ formation was to observe the metabolism of APP in over-expressing transfected cells. APP exists in the cell as an integral membrane protein with a large amino terminal domain and a small carboxy-terminal cytoplasmic tail (Selkoe, 1991; Sinha and Lieberburg, 1992). The Aβ region is situated in the APP molecule partially embedded in the membrane and partially exposed in its N-terminus. Metabolic studies of endogenous and transfected APP in most transformed cell lines have revealed that the amino terminal domain of APP is rapidly secreted into the medium leaving behind a short, approximately 10 Kd membrane-bound fragment (Selkoe, 1991; Sinha and Lieberburg, 1992). This cleavage event, mediated by an enzyme dubbed "secretase" is dramatically increased by protein kinase C (PKC) activation (Sinha and Lieberburg, 1992). Sequencing analysis of this cleavage site reveals that this normal cleavage event occurs in the middle of the β-peptide sequence (at amino acid 17). Thus, normal processing of APP mitigates amyloid formation. Aβ deposition must therefore be the result of an alternative metabolic pathway.

Several laboratories subsequently demonstrated that a variable amount of APP is processed via the endosomal/lysosomal pathway resulting in the generation of potentially amyloidogenic fragments of APP (Sinha and Lieberburg, 1992). However appealing the lysosomal pathway may be for Aβ generation, no one has yet demonstrated the presence of Aβ in lysosomes or other vesicular compartments within the cell. More recently, three groups independently demonstrated that the Aβ is continuously generated both in vitro and in vivo (Shoji et al., 1992; Haass et al., 1992; Seubert et al., 1992).

Absolute proof of identity was obtained by direct sequencing, and in one report (Seubert et al., 1992) by mass spectrometry. Together these investigators showed that Aβ is produced by a variety of APP-transfected cells, human mixed brain cultures and is also present in CSF. In addition to the scientific novelty and therapeutic utility of this observation, there is also the possibility that Aβ levels in the CSF may have diagnostic utility. A rare disease-causing mutation of the APP gene found in a Swedish kindred (Mullan et al., 1992) causes 6-8 fold overproduction of Aβ when expressed in cells (Citron, et al., 1992). While this mutation is obviously very rare, the potential heuristic value of this observation cannot be overstated.

Finally, a recent paper by Seubert and colleagues (Seubert et al., 1993) has demonstrated that a major metabolic pathway of APP in human mixed brain cultures results in the production of a truncated secreted form of APP which ends precisely at the beginning of the Aβ sequence (aspartate 597). This alternatively cleaved form of APP may be the product of the crucial cleavage (by an enzyme called β-secretase) which then goes on to permit Aβ formation. In this scenario a further intra-membrane carboxy-terminal cleavage would then release intact Aβ. If this is true, a further implication of this is that the secretory pathway, which has so far been assumed to preclude the formation of Aβ, may actually play a role in the normal generation of amyloid (see Sinha and Lieberburg, 1992 for review of APP metabolism). We have been studying the interplay of these various APP-metabolizing pathways. In addition, we have been isolating APP cleaving enzymes from human tissues that are capable of producing Aβ. Inhibition of such an enzyme would be an obvious therapeutic target in treating AD.

Once formed, Aβ accumulates in certain regions of the brain, notably the association cortices. It is not known why this soluble peptide, which circulates in CSF at ~1nM, (Seubert et al., 1992) begins to form insoluble aggregates. Possibilities include regional overproduction, interaction with extracellular matrix molecules, inappropriate chaperoning, reduced clearance or some combination of these factors. The recent discovery of genetic disequilibrium between the APOE4 allele and the subsequent development of AD (Strittmatter, et al., 1993), has pointed to this important lipoprotein as a possible pathologic chaperone involved in the binding, folding, and/or clearance of Aβ. Drugs which alter the production of APOE in the CNS or which alter the clearance or toxicity of the APOE/Aβ complex may also represent fruitful therapeutic targets.

However, once higher concentrations of Aβ are achieved for whatever reason, neurotoxicity is likely to occur. Yankner was the first to describe the toxic effects of Aβ on neurons in culture (Yankner et al., 1990). This was later confirmed by a number of groups, including our own (Mattson, et al., 1992). In our hands (Mattson et al., 1992) we have found that Aβ will measurably increase intracellular free calcium levels in neurons, and will exacerbate the toxicity of a number of neurotoxic substances, such as excitatory amino acid neurotransmitters and the calcium ionophore, A23187, probably through a dysregulation of calcium homeostatic mechanisms. The precise mechanism of the Aβ-induced calcium dysregulation has not been clearly identified; however, a recent report by Arispe and colleagues (Arispe et al., 1993) suggests that Aβ is able to form calcium channels in lipid bilayer membranes. Whether this mechanism is responsible for Aβ-induced neurotoxicity remains to be determined. Recently, the Aβ-neurotoxicity debate has filled an entire issue of Neurobiology of Aging (1992, 13:535-630). Though there is reasonable consensus that Aβ neurotoxicity can be readily observed in vitro, there remains substantial debate concerning the extent of the in vivo toxicity which is induced by the peptide. Current thinking would argue that the peptide has limited in vivo toxicity in its own right, but that it clearly exacerbates the toxicity of a variety of CNS insults including exitotoxins (Mattson et al., 1992) glucose deprivation (Copani et al., 1991) and oxidative damage (Saunders et al., 1991). The role of Aβ as a synergistic co-toxin is clinically quite compatible with the prolonged and chronic deterioration seen in AD. Drugs capable of aborting or slowing this process would also represent therapeutic targets.

Finally, once deposited, the Aβ peptide likely induces a chronic inflammatory response in the AD brain. This process is still incompletely understood, but involves the activation of microglia, the overproduction of cytokines in involved brain regions, and the generation and activation of complement (Dickson and Rogers, 1992; Rogers et al., 1992), all of which can lead to neuronal dysfunction or death. This general area of chronic CNS inflammation also represents a major opportunity for drug discovery in AD.

REFERENCES

Arispe N, Roja E and Pollard HB (1993): Alzheimer's disease amyloid beta protein forms calcium channels in bilayer membranes: blockade by tromethamine and aluminum. *Proced. Natl. Acad. Sci.* 90:567-571.

Citron M, Oltersdorf T, Haass C, McConlogue L, Hung AY, Seubert P, Vigo-Pelfrey C, Lieberburg I and Selkoe DJ (1992): Mutation of the beta-amyloid precursor protein in familial Alzheimer's disease increases beta-protein production. *Nature* 360:672-674.

Copani A, Koh JY and Cotman CW (1991): Beta-amyloid increases neuronal susceptibility to injury by glucose deprivation. *Neurol. Rep.* 2:763-765.

Dickson DW and Rogers, J (1992): Neuroimmunology of Alzheimer's disease: a conference report. *Neurobiol. Aging* 13:793-798.

Glenner GG and Wong CW (1984): Alzheimer disease: initial report of the purification and characterization of a novel cerebrovascular amyloid protein. *Biochem. Biophys. Res. Commun.* 120:885-890.

Goate A, Chartier-Harlin MC, Mullan M, Brown J, Crawford F, Fidani L, Giuffra L, Haynes A, Irving N, James L et al. (1991): Segregation of a missense mutation in the amyloid precursor protein gene with familial Alzheimer's disease. *Nature* 349:704-706.

Haass C, Schlossmacher MG, Hung AY, Vigo-Pelfrey C, Mellon A, Ostaszewski BL, Lieberburg I, Koo EH, Schenk D, Teplow DB et al. (1992): Amyloid beta-peptide is produced by cultured cells during normal metabolism. *Nature* 359:322-325.

Mattson M, Cheng B, David D, Bryant K, Lieberburg I and Rydel RE (1992): Beta-amyloid peptides destabilize calcium homeostasis and render human cortical neurons vulnerable to excitotoxicity. *J. Neurosci.* 12:376-389.

Mullan M, Crawford F, Axelman K, Houlden H, Lilius L, Winblad B and Lannfelt L (1992): A pathogenic mutation for probable Alzheimer's disease in the APP gene at the N-terminus of beta-amyloid. *Nature Genetics* 1:345-347.

Rogers J, Cooper NR, Webster S, Schultz J, McGeer PL, Styren SD, Civin WH, Brachova L, Bradt B, Wart P et al. (1992): Complement activation by beta-amyloid in Alzheimer's disease. *Proced. Natl. Acad. Sci.* 89:10016-10020.

Saunders R, Luttman CA, Keith PT and Little SP (1991): Beta-amyloid protein potentiates H_2O_2-induced neuron degeneration in vitro. *Soc. Neurosci. Abst.* 17:1447.

Selkoe DJ (1991): The molecular pathology of Alzheimer's disease. *Neuron* 6:487-498.

Seubert P, Vigo-Pelfrey C, Esch F, Lee M, Dovery H, Davis D, Sinha S, Schlossmacher M, Whaley J, Swindlehurst C et al. (1992): Isolation and quantification of soluble Alzheimer's beta-peptide from biological fluids. *Nature* 359:325-327.

Seubert P, Oltersdorf T, Lee MG, Barbour R, Blomquist C, Davis DL, Bryant K, Fritz LC, Galasko D, Thal LJ et al. (1993): Secretion of beta-amyloid precursor protein cleaved at the amino terminus of the beta-amyloid peptide. *Nature* 361:260-263.

Shoji M, Golde TE, Ghiso J, Cheung TT, Estus S, Shaffer LM, Cai XD, McKay DM, Tintner R, Frangione B et al. (1992): Production of the Alzheimer amyloid beta protein by normal porteolytic processing. *Science* 258:126-129.

Sinha S and Lieberburg I (1992): Normal metabolism of the amyloid precursor protein (APP). *Neurodegeneration* 1:169-175.

Strittmatter WJ, Saunders AM, Schmechel D, Pericak-Vance M, Enghild J, Salvesen GS and Roses AD (1993): Apolipoprotein E: High avidity binding to β-amyloid and increased frequency of type 4 allele in late-onset familial Alzheimer disease. *Proced. Natl. Acad. Sci.* 90:1977-1981.

Yankner BA, Duffy LK and Kirschner DA (1990): Neurotrophic and neurotoxic effects of amyloid beta protein: reversal by tachykinin neuropeptides. *Science* 250:279-282.

Alzheimer Disease: Therapeutic Strategies
edited by E. Giacobini and R. Becker.
© 1994 Birkhäuser Boston

REGULATION OF APP PROCESSING BY FIRST MESSENGERS

Roger M. Nitsch and John H. Growdon
Department of Neurology, Massachusetts General Hospital and Harvard
Medical School, Boston, MA

Steven A. Farber, Meihua Deng and Richard J. Wurtman
Department of Brain and Cognitive Sciences, M.I.T., Cambridge, MA

INTRODUCTION

Brain amyloid deposits are invariant neuropathological hallmarks of Alzheimer's disease (AD) and Down's syndrome, and are sometimes also found in lesser amounts in brains of non-demented aged human subjects. Alzheimer disease-type brain amyloid consists of aggregated amyloid ß- (Aß) peptides which are self-aggregating molecules of 39-43 residues in length. Aß is derived, by proteolytic processing, from a larger amyloid ß-protein precursor (APP). The hydrophobic C-terminal region of the amyloidogenic Aß domain is located within the single transmembrane domain of APP, and its N-terminus extends 28 residues into the ectodomain (for review, see Selkoe, 1994). The APP gene is expressed at remarkably high levels in brain but is also expressed in many peripheral tissues. The biological function of APP is unclear and it is possible that individual proteolytic derivatives of APP have distinct biological consequences. For instance, accumulating evidence suggests that the full-length protein and its secreted N-terminal derivatives can promote cell adhesion (Schubert et al., 1989), stimulate neurite outgrowth (Milward et al., 1992), and protect cultured neurons from excitotoxic damage (Mattson et al., 1993). In contrast, Aß and its aggregates can be cytotoxic and induce cell death in cultured neurons (Yankner et al., 1990; Loo et al., 1993). Moreover, Aß inhibits the normal function of a potassium channel which appears to be impaired in fibroblasts obtained from AD patients (Etcheberrigaray et al., 1994). These initial data support the concept that large portions of the N-terminal ectodomain have trophic functions whereas the Aß domain can be cytotoxic. The biochemical mechanisms involved in the regulation of local brain tissue concentrations of particular proteolytic APP derivatives may thus play an important role in determining the actual functions of APP.

The APP holoprotein is normally processed rapidly by various alternative proteolytic pathways to yield both secreted and cell-associated products. These include the secreted 97-110kDa N-terminal ectodomain (APP^S) derived from α-secretase cleavage within the Aß region (Esch et al., 1990; Sisodia et al., 1990) and secreted p3, a 3kDa Aß fragment possibly generated by cleavage at both the α-secretase site and the γ-secretase site at the C-terminus of the Aß domain (Haass et al., 1993). Additionally ~4kDa Aß-peptides derived from two cleavage events both at the N-terminus (ß-secretase) and at the C-terminus of the Aß domain can be produced by normal cellular metabolism of APP (Haass et al., 1992a; Shoji et al., 1992.; Busciglio et al., 1993). Similar secretory APP processing pathways are likely to occur in human brain tissues because both APP^S and Aß are present in human cerebrospinal fluid at concentrations of 0.5-2.5 μg/ml and 5-25 ng/ml, respectively (Seubert et al., 1992; Nitsch et al., 1994). Amyloid precursor protein holoprotein can also be targeted to the endosomal-lysosomal system (Haass et al., 1992b) in which multiple fragments are generated some of which contain the intact Aß domain and thus are potentially amyloidogenic (Golde et al., 1992; Estus et al., 1992). In summary, α-secretase processing prevents the processing of APP into amyloid whereas APP holoprotein and its proteolytic derivatives generated by endosomal-lysosomal proteinases or the ß-secretase processing pathway are potentially amyloidogenic. It is thus important to understand the cellular mechanisms that regulate these proteolytic APP processing pathways.

MUSCARINIC RECEPTORS CAN INCREASE THE FORMATION OF APP^S AND DECREASE Aß PRODUCTION

Many cell-surface receptors can regulate the rates at which APP is hydrolyzed by individual proteolytic processing pathways (for review, see Nitsch and Growdon, 1994). For example, stimulation of muscarinic acetylcholine receptor (mAChR) subtypes m1 and m3 with carbachol increases the release of APP^S 6- to 8-fold within minutes in HEK 293 cell lines which were stably transfected with cDNA expression constructs encoding these receptors (Nitsch et al., 1992; Buxbaum et al., 1992). Increased APP^S secretion was paralleled by a decrease in levels both of cell-associated full-length APP and of C-terminal fragments. Carbachol also increased APP^S secretion in the presence of the translation inhibitor cycloheximide, indicating that muscarinic receptors can accelerate the cleavage of pre-existing, full-length APP independently of possible effects on the rate of APP synthesis. Moreover, carbachol caused a 60% decrease in the production and the secretion of Aß from the cell lines that over-express the m1 receptor subtype (Hung et al., 1993). Together these data suggest that muscarinic receptors can accelerate α-secretase processing of APP and concurrently inhibit the ß-secretase processing pathway. It is possible that stimulated α-secretase processing and the ß-secretase processing pathway simply *compete for* APP as a substrate to be metabolized. Alternatively, the (unknown) proteases involved in generating either APP[S] or Aß may be regulated differentially by signalling events initiated by muscarinic receptor activation. Secretion of Aß is increased 4- to 5-fold in cell lines expressing an APP gene that includes the double mutation found in the APP gene of a Swedish familial AD kindred (Citron et al., 1992; Cai et al., 1993). These results suggested a causal role of this mutation in contributing to amyloid formation in affected individuals. In cells transfected with cDNAs encoding both the muscarinic m1 receptors and this mutated APP695, receptor stimulation with carbachol blocked the increased Aß secretion (Hung et al., 1993). This result shows that the cleavage events regulated by m1 receptors are able to process both normal APP and the APP associated with the Swedish mutation. It also implies that even pathologically high Aß secretion associated with a disease-causing mutation can be suppressed by the activity of muscarinic m1 receptors. A clinical study in this Swedish family is needed to test whether specific m1-receptor agonists can decrease Aß levels and slow amyloid formation in brains of affected family members.

SEROTONIN 5-HT$_2$ AND 5-HT$_{1C}$, AND NEUROPEPTIDE RECEPTORS CAN INCREASE THE SECRETION OF APP[S]

Muscarinic m1 and m3 receptors are members of a large family of structurally and functionally related neurotransmitter and hormone receptors characterized by 7 transmembrane domains and 3 cytoplasmic loops (Bonner et al., 1987; Peralta et al., 1988). These receptors are coupled to G proteins and to signalling pathways that involve activation of phospholipases, and the consequent generation of diacylglycerol along with inositol trisphosphate. Additional members of this receptor family include the serotoninergic 5-HT$_2$ and 5-HT$_{1C}$ receptors (for review see Peroutka, 1993). To test whether such serotonin (5-HT) receptors can regulate proteolytic APP processing pathways, we used NIH 3T3 fibroblast lines that were stably transfected with cDNA expression constructs encoding 5-HT$_2$ and 5-HT$_{1C}$ receptors (Julius et al., 1988, 1990), stimulated them with 5-HT, and measured the release of APP[S] into the culture medium. 5-HT caused a dose-dependent 3- to 4-fold increase in APP[S] secretion from both cell lines. In control experiments with the untransfected parent NIH 3T3 cell line, 5-HT did not change the release of APP[S]. Increased APP[S] secretion in the transfected cell lines was blocked by the 5-HT receptor antagonists ritanserin, mianserin, and ketanserin. Hence stimulation of 5-HT$_2$ and 5-HT$_{1C}$ receptors can also regulate rates of APP[S] secretion. The data obtained so far imply that stimulation of these serotonin receptor subtypes accelerates α-secretase processing of APP. Vasopressin (V1a) (Morel et al., 1992) and bradykinin (B2) (McEachern et al., 1991) receptors also belong to the 7 transmembrane domain receptor family. To test whether these neuropeptide receptors could also regulate APP processing, we subcloned a rat kidney fibroblast (NRK 49F) line and a PC-12 cell line to express functionally intact receptors for vasopressin and bradykinin, respectively, as affirmed by agonist-induced acceleration (10-fold) of PI-turnover. Arginine-vasopressin caused a rapid 2- to 5-fold dose-dependent increase in APP^S secretion in NRK49F cells. This increase was blocked by the vasopressin receptor agonist [diamino-Pen^1, Val^4, Arg^8]-vasopressin, indicating that the vasopressin had increased APP^S release by stimulating endogenously expressed vasopressin receptors coupled to PI-turnover. Similarly, bradykinin caused a dose-dependent increase in APP^S release that was blocked by D-Arg-Arg-Pro-Hyp-Gly-Thi-Ser-D-Tic-Oic-Arg, a bradykinin receptor antagonist. These data show that bradykinin also can regulate APP processing via endogenously bradykinin receptors. Bradykinin stimulated APP^S secretion both in undifferentiated and in differentiated (50 g/ml 7S-NGF for 3 days prior to stimulation) PC-12 cells suggesting that both the undifferentiated and differentiated cell lines used in these experiments expressed sufficient levels of functionally intact bradykinin receptors to modulate APP processing pathways.

SIGNAL TRANSDUCTION: PKC-DEPENDENT AND PKC-INDEPENDENT SIGNALLING

Initial evidence showed that staurosporine, a protein kinase inhibitor, blocked the increase in the rates of APP^S secretion induced by m1- and m3-receptors (Nitsch et al., 1992). This finding suggested that receptor-coupled stimulation of protein kinases may be involved in the cellular signalling pathways that couple surface receptor activity to APP processing events. Moreover, phorbol myristate acetate (PMA), a potent activator of protein kinase C (PKC), also increases APP^S secretion from many cell lines (Caporaso et al., 1992; Slack et al., 1993) including these described in this report, underscoring the possibility that PKC might be involved in the signalling pathways that couple receptor activation to APP processing pathways. However, our data clearly indicate that down-regulation of PKC by chronic treatment with PMA, which blocked the PMA-mediated increase in APP^S secretion, did not inhibit the increase in APP^S secretion caused by 5-HT, for example, in 3T3 cells expressing 5-HT$_2$ or 5-HT$_{1C}$ receptors. Moreover, the protein kinase inhibitors chelerythrine and staurosporine did not block the increase in APP^S secretion caused by 5-HT in either cell line. These results demonstrate that stimulation of PKC can be sufficient but may not be necessary to increase APP^S release. Our data imply redundancy in cellular signalling pathways that couple 5-HT receptors to the regulation of APP metabolism.

ELECTRICAL DEPOLARIZATION INCREASES APP^S RELEASE IN MAMMALIAN BRAIN

Compared to the regulation of processing events in tissue culture experiments, regulation of APP processing in brain tissue is much more complex in that multiple surface receptors may interact simultaneously with various APP processing pathways. In an attempt to study receptor-coupled regulation of APP processing in brain tissue, we prepared fresh tissue slices from the hippocampus, the cortex, the striatum, and the cerebellum of young adult rats, and incubated them in superfusion chambers that were equipped with electrical field stimulation electrodes (Nitsch et al., 1993). Electrical stimulation with 10 to 30 Hz (individual pulse duration 1 ms) caused 3- to 10-fold increases in the release of such endogenous hippocampal neurotransmitters as glutamate and acetylcholine, for example. We controlled for the structural integrity of cells within the slices by monitoring the release of lactate dehydrogenase (an intracellular marker enzyme), which was unchanged before, during, and after the electrical stimulation periods. The increased release in endogenous neurotransmitters was paralleled by an averaged 2-fold increase in the rates of APP^S release during a 50 min stimulation period with 30 Hz. Individual brain regions varied slightly with respect to the magnitude of the increase in APP^S formation: in brain cortex, stimulation increased APP^S secretion 2.5-fold, in striatum 1.7-fold, in cerebellum 1.4-fold and in hippocampus 1.9-fold. The depolarization-induced increase in APP^S secretion was blocked by the sodium channel blocker tetrodotoxin, indicating that this release resulted from the formation of action potentials, and, probably, from depolarization-generated neurotransmitter release. The effect of electrical stimulation on APP^S secretion from hippocampal slices was frequency-dependent in a range from 0-30 Hz, and reached its maximum at 30 Hz. Together, these data suggest that APP processing pathways in brain may be regulated by neuronal activity. Pharmacological experiments showed that the muscarinic receptor agonist atropine partially blocked the depolarization induced increase in the rates of APP^S release. Moreover, receptor agonists which specifically stimulate m1 and m3 receptor subtypes (as opposed to m2 and m4) stimulated rates of APP^S release from cortical slices in a dose-dependent manner. The acetylcholinesterase (AChE)-inhibitor physostigmine (20 μM), however, did not change rates of APP^S release. These data show that muscarinic receptors in the mammalian brain cortex can regulate APP processing pathways and imply that muscarinic agonists, but not physostigmine, can stimulate non-amyloidogenic α-secretase processing of APP in brain.

HUMAN STUDIES

In an initial attempt to test whether pharmacological alterations of neurotransmission can influence APP metabolism in AD patients, we treated 10 patients with the AChE-inhibitor physostigmine (9-15 mg b.i.d.) for two weeks and measured CSF levels of APP derivatives before and after treatments. CSF levels of the major secreted APP derivatives, the 106kDa APP^S and a 25kDa N-terminal fragment, were not altered by this treatment. These results could imply that AChE-inhibitors may not be effective to modulate APP processing in human brain. The next phase of clinical trials should include the investigation of possible effects on specific muscarinic receptor agonists on APP processing.

IMPLICATIONS FOR ALZHEIMER'S DISEASE

The concept of receptor-coupled APP processing has two possible implications: First, the normal metabolism of APP and its processing into various non-amyloidogenic and amyloidogenic derivatives in AD brain may be compromised as a result of impaired neuronal signalling caused by a combination of diminished availability of chemical neurotransmitters, decreased number in synaptic receptors, and impaired post-synaptic signal transduction. Together, these abnormalities may result in changes of the relative rates of individual APP processing pathways in favor of amyloidogenic processing and the increased generation of possibly neurotoxic Aß peptides, which might eventually aggregate to form amyloid. Second, the neurotransmitter and neuromodulator systems that are capable of regulating brain metabolism of APP may provide potential targets for drugs designed to increase non-amyloidogenic APP processing pathways. Human studies will be necessary to test whether this treatment approach can decrease the amyloid burden in brain, slow the rate of progression of dementia, and ameliorate the clinical symptoms of AD.

ACKNOWLEDGMENTS

We thank Barbara E. Slack, Christine Bilmazes, U. Ingrid Richardson, Paul R. Borghesani and Jochen G. Schulz for their valuable contributions. This work was supported by the NIA, NIMH, the Center for Brain Sciences and Metabolism Charitable Trust and the Hoffman Fellowship in AD.

REFERENCE

Bonner I, Buckley NJ, Young AC and Brann MR (1987): Identification of a family of muscarinic acetylcholine receptor genes. *Science* 273:527-532.

Busciglio J, Gabuzda DH, Matsudeira P and Yankner BA (1993): Generation of ß-amyloid in the secretory pathway in neuronal and non-neuronal cells. *Proc Natl Acad Sci USA* 90:2092-2096.

Buxbaum JD, Oishi M, Chen HI, Pinkas-Kramarski R, Jaffe EA, Gandy SE and Greengard P (1992): Cholinergic agonists and interleukin 1 regulate processing and secretion of the Alzheimer ß/A4 amyloid protein precursor. *Proc Natl Acad Sci USA* 89:10075-10078.

Cai X-D, Golde TE and Younkin SG (1993): Release of excess amyloid ß-protein from a mutant amyloid ß-protein precursor. *Science* 259:514-516.

Caporaso GL, Gandy SE, Buxbaum JD, Ramabhadran TV and Greengard P (1992): Protein phosphorylation regulates secretion of Alzheimer ß/A4 amyloid precursor protein. *Proc Natl Acad Sci USA* 89:3055-3059.

Citron M, Oltersdorf T, Haass C, McConlogue L, Hung AY, Seubert P, Vigo-Pelfrey C, Lieberburg I and Selkoe DJ (1992): Mutation of the ß-amyloid precursor protein in familial Alzheimer's disease increases ß-protein production. *Nature* 360:672-674.

Esch FS, Keim PS, Beattie EC, Blacher RW, Culwell AR, Oltersdorf T, McClure, D and Ward P (1990): Cleavage of amyloid beta peptide during constitutive processing of its precursor. *Science* 248:1122-1124.

Estus S, Golde TE, Kunishita T, Blades D, Lowery D, Eisen M, Usiak M, Qu X, Tabira T, Greenberg BD and Younkin SG (1992): Potentially amyloidogenic, carboxy-terminal derivatives of the amyloid protein precursor. *Science* 255:726-728.

Etcheberrigaray R, Ito E, Kim CS and Alkon DL (1994): Soluble ß-amyloid induction of Alzheimer's phenotype for human fibroblast K$^+$ channels. *Science* 264:276-279.

Golde TE, Estus S, Younkin LH, Selkoe DJ and Younkin SG (1992): Processing of the amyloid protein precursor to potentially amyloidogenic derivatives. *Science* 255:728-730.

Haass C, Schlossmacher MG, Hung AY, Vigo-Pelfrey C, Mellon A, Ostaszewski BL, Lieberburg I, Koo EH, Schenk D, Teplow DB and Selkoe DJ (1992a): Amyloid ß-peptide is produced by cultured cells during normal metabolism. *Nature* 359:322-325.

Haass C, Koo EH, Mellon A, Hun, AY and Selkoe DJ (1992b): Targeting of cell-surface ß-amyloid precursor protein to lysosomes: alternative processing into amyloid-bearing fragments. *Nature* 357:500-503.

Haass C, Hung AY, Schlossmacher MG, Teplow DB and Selkoe DJ (1993): ß-amyloid peptide and a 3kDa fragment are derived by distinct cellular mechanisms. *J Biol Chem* 268:3021-3024.

Hung A, Haass C, Nitsch RM, Qiu W, Citron M, Wurtman RJ, Growdon JH and Selkoe DJ (1993): Activation of protein kinase C inhibits cellular production of the amyloid ß-protein. *J Biol Chem* 268:22959-22962.

Julius D, MacDermott AB, Axel R and Jessel T (1988): Molecular characterization of a functional cDNA encoding the serotonin 1C receptor. *Science* 241:558-564.

Julius D, Huang K, Livelli J, Axel R and Jessel TM (1990): The 5-HT$_2$ receptor defines a family of structurally distinct but functionally conserved serotonin receptors. *Proc Natl Acad Sci USA* 87:928-932.

Loo DT, Copani A, Pike CJ, Whittemore ER, Walencewicz AJ and Cotman CW (1993): Apoptosis is induced by ß-amyloid in cultured central nervous system neurons. *Proc Natl Acad Sci USA* 90:7951-7955.

Mattson MP, Cheng B, Culwell AR, Esch FS, Lieberburg I and Rydel RE (1993): Evidence for excitoprotective and intraneuronal calcium-regulating. *Neuron* 10:243-254.

McEachern AE, Shelton ER, Bhaka S, Obernolte R, Bach C, Zuppan P, Fujisaki J, Aldrich RW and Jarnagin K (1991): Expression cloning of a rat B$_2$ bradykinin receptor. *Proc Natl Acad Sci USA* 88:7724-7728.

Milward EA, Papadopoulos R, Fuller SJ, Moir RD, Small, D, Beyreuther K and Masters CL (1992): The amyloid protein precursor of Alzheimer's disease is a mediator of the effects of nerve growth factor on neurite outgrowth. *Neuron* 9:129-137.

Morel A, O'Carroll A-M, Brownstein MJ and Lolait SJ (1992): Molecular cloning and expression of a rat V1a arginine vasopressin receptor. *Nature* 356:523-526.

Nitsch RM, Slack BE, Wurtman RJ and Growdon JH (1992): Release of Alzheimer amyloid precursor derivatives stimulated by activation of muscarinic acetylcholine receptors. *Science* 258:304-307.

Nitsch RM, Farber SA, Growdon JH and Wurtman RJ (1993): Release of amyloid ß-protein precursor derivatives from hippocampal slices by electrical depolarization. *Proc Natl Acad Sci USA* 90:5191-5193.

Nitsch RM and Growdon JH (1994): Role of neurotransmission in the regulation of amyloid ß-protein precursor processing. *Biochem Pharmacol* 47:1275-1284.

Nitsch RM, Rebeck GW, Deng M, Richardson UI, Tennis M, Vigo-Pelfrey C, Lieberburg I, Schenk D, Wurtman RJ, Hyman BT and Growdon JH (1994): Cerebrospinal fluid levels of amyloid ß-protein are independent of apolipoprotein E genotype and are inversely correlated with severity of dementia in Alzheimer's disease (Submitted).

Peralta EG, Ashkenazi A, Winslow JW, Ramachandran J and Capon DJ (1988): Differential regulation of PI hydrolysis and adenylyl cyclase activity by muscarinic receptor subtypes. *Nature* 334:434-437.

Peroutka SJ (1993): 5-Hydroxytryptamine receptors. *J Neurochem* 60:408-416.

Schubert D, Jin L-W, Saitoh T and Cole G (1989): The regulation of amyloid beta precursor protein and its modulatory role in cell adhesion. *Neuron* 3:689-694.

Selkoe DJ (1994): Normal and abnormal biology of the ß-amyloid precursor protein. *Ann Rev Neurosci* 17:489-517.

Seubert P, Vigo-Pelfrey C, Esch F, Lee M, Dovey H, Davis D, Sinha S, Schlossmacher M, Whaley J, Swindlehurst C, McCormack R, Wolfert R, Selkoe D, Lieberburg I and Schenk D (1992): Isolation and quantification of soluble Alzheimer's ß-peptide from biological fluids. *Nature* 359:325-327.

Shoji M, Golde TE, Ghiso J, Cheung TT, Estus S, Shaffer LM, Cai X-D, McKay DM, Tintner R, Frangione B and Younkin SG (1992): Production of the Alzheimer amyloid ß-protein by normal proteolytic processing. *Science* 258:126-129.

Sisodia SS, Koo EH, Beyreuther K, Unterbeck A and Price DL (1990): Evidence that ß-amyloid protein in Alzheimer's disease is not derived by normal processing. *Science* 248:492-495.

Slack BE, Nitsch RM, Livneh E, Kunz Jr GM, Breu J, Eldar H and Wurtman RJ (1993): Regulation by phorbol esters of amyloid precursor protein release from Swiss 3T3 fibroblasts overexpressing protein kinase C. *J Biol Chem* 268:21097-21101.

Yankner BA, Duffy LK and Kirschner DA (1990): Neurotrophic and neurotoxic effects of amyloid beta protein: reversal by tachikinin neuropeptides. *Science* 250:279-282.

Alzheimer Disease: Therapeutic Strategies
edited by E. Giacobini and R. Becker.
© 1994 Birkhäuser Boston

IN VITRO PRODUCTION OF AMYLOID ß-PROTEIN: A ROUTE TO THE MECHANISM AND TREATMENT OF ALZHEIMER'S DISEASE

Dennis J. Selkoe
Harvard Medical School, Brigham and Women's Hospital, Boston, MA 02115

Progressive cerebral dysfunction in Alzheimer's disease and Down's syndrome is accompanied by the formation of innumerable extracellular amyloid deposits in the form of senile plaques and microvascular amyloid. The amyloid fibrils are composed of the 39-43 residue amyloid ß-protein (Aß), a fragment of the integral membrane polypeptide, ß-amyloid precursor protein (ßAPP). Evidence from several laboratories has shown that amorphous, largely nonfilamentous deposits of Aß ("diffuse or "pre-amyloid" plaques) precede the development of fibrillary amyloid, dystrophic neurites, neurofibrillary tangles, and other cytopathological changes in Down's syndrome and, by inference, in Alzheimer's disease. This finding suggests that ß-amyloidosis, like certain other amyloidoses, does not occur secondary to local cellular pathology (e.g., dystrophic neurites) but rather precedes it. The clearest evidence that the processing of ßAPP into Aß can actually cause Alzheimer's disease has come from the identification by several laboratories of missense mutations in the ßAPP gene within and flanking the Aß region in affected members of certain families having Alzheimer's disease or hereditary cerebral hemorrhage with amyloidosis of the Dutch type.

The mechanism of proteolytic release of the Aß fragment from ßAPP is incompletely understood. Because the normal secretion of the large extramembranous portion of ßAPP (APP$_s$) from cells involves a proteolytic cleavage within Aß, thus precluding amyloid formation, we searched for evidence of an alternate pathway of ßAPP processing that leaves Aß intact. In view of the presence of a consensus sequence (NPXY) in the cytoplasmic tail of ßAPP that could mediate internalization of the protein from the cell surface and its targeting to endosomes/lysosomes, we looked specifically for evidence of endocytotic trafficking of ßAPP. Incubation of an antibody to the extracellular region of ßAPP with living human cells led to binding of the antibody to cell-surface ßAPP and trafficking of the antigen antibody complex to endosomes/lysosomes (Haass et al., 1992a). The resultant ßAPP-immunoreactive pattern closely resembled that seen after incubating the same cells with rhodamine-tagged albumin, a marker for fluid-phase pinocytosis. Late endosomes/lysosomes purified from the cells contained abundant full-length ßAPP plus an array of low molecular weight fragments ranging from ~ 10 to ~ 22 kDa, most of which are of a size and immunoreactivity suggesting they contain the intact Aß peptide (Haass et al., 1992a). These results provided direct evidence that some ßAPP molecules are normally reinternalized from the cell surface and targeted to lysosomes. This second normal pathway for ßAPP processing is capable of producing potentially amyloidogenic fragments. However it is not yet clear whether this pathway, an alternative proteolytic cleavage occurring within the secretory pathway (Seubert et al., 1993), or another yet undescribed trafficking pathway is actually responsible for Aß formation.

During the aforementioned studies, we searched intensively for evidence of the production and release of the Aß peptide itself during normal cellular metabolism, based in part on the hypothesis that some Aß deposits (e.g., those in capillary walls and the subpial cortex) might arise from a circulating (plasma or CSF) form of the peptide. To this end, a series of antibodies to Aß were used to screen the conditioned media of several cell types for the presence of soluble Aß. These experiments demonstrated that Aß is continuously produced as a soluble 4 kDa peptide and is released into the media of normal cells (Haass et al., 1992b). Moreover, Aß-immunoreactivity has also been detected in human cerebrospinal fluid (Seubert et al., 1992; Shoji et al., 1992) and plasma (Seubert et al., 1992). The form in CSF has been purified and sequenced, confirming that it is authentic Aß (Seubert et al., 1992), whereas the plasma form is not yet characterized. Aß peptides of varying length are released by all ßAPP-expressing cells studied to date under normal culture conditions (Haass et al., 1992b; Seubert et al., 1992; Shoji et al., 1992; Haass et al., 1993; Busciglio et al., 1993). Aß in culture supernatants is entirely soluble and generally present in high picomolar to low nanomolar concentrations (Seubert et al., 1992). Pulse-chase and biological toxin experiments suggest that Aß is produced following full maturation of ßAPP and involves an acidic compartment other than lysosomes, e.g., early endosomes or the late Golgi (Haass et al., 1993). The two proteolytic cleavages generating Aß may therefore occur in an acidic vesicle near the cell surface, after which Aß is rapidly released into the medium, with very little or no Aß detected intracellularly (Haass et al., 1992b; Haass et al., 1993).

The relevance of such *in vitro* Aß production to the pathogenesis of Alzheimer's disease (AD) is demonstrated by the finding that a ßAPP missense mutation causing a Swedish form of familial AD, when expressed in cultured cells, leads to a marked increase in Aß production (Citron et al., 1992). The amyloidogenic mechanisms of other FAD-linked ßAPP mutations are now being elucidated in both transfected and primary (donor) cells. Effects of the recently identified FAD detected on chromosome 14 (Schellenberg et al., 1992) on ßAPP processing and Aß production can be searched for in cultured primary cells from these patients, even before the responsible gene is identified and characterized.

Importantly, transfected or primary cells expressing the Swedish mutant gene can readily be used to screen a variety of compounds and identify those capable of decreasing Aß secretion to normal levels in the absence of significant cytotoxicity. Such agents can then be tested in laboratory rodents or in aged animals (e.g., dogs, monkeys) which spontaneously develop Aß plaques to determine their effects on brain and CSF levels of Aß as well as their safety.

Thus, studies of *in vitro* Aß production should advance the fundamental understanding and ultimately the pharmacological treatment of ß-amyloidosis in Alzheimer's disease. Therapeutic approaches could include: (1) inhibiting amyloid-generating proteases; (2) diverting ßAPP from amyloidogenic to non-amyloidogenic processing pathways (3) preventing the aggregation of soluble extracellular Aß into fibrils; (4) interfering with the toxic response of neurons to aggregated Aß and its tightly associated proteins; and (5) inhibiting the chronic inflammatory process (including microgliosis and astrocytosis) that develops around amyloid plaques.

REFERENCES

Busciglio J, Gabuzda DH, Matsudaira P and Yankner BA (1993): Generation of ß-amyloid in the secretory pathway in neuronal and non-neuronal cells. *Proc Natl Acad Sci USA* 90:2092-2096.

Citron M, Oltersdorf T, Haass C, McConlogue L, Hung AY, Seubert P, Vigo-Pelfrey C, Lieberburg I and Selkoe DJ (1992): Mutation of the ß-amyloid precursor protein in familial Alzheimer's disease causes increased ß-protein production. *Nature* 360:672-674.

Haass C, Hung AY, Schlossmacher MG, Teplow DB and Selkoe DJ (1993): Amyloid peptide and a 3-kDa fragment are derived by distinct cellular mechanisms. *J Biol Chem* 268:3021-3024.

Haass C, Koo EH, Mellon A, Hung AY and Selkoe DJ (1992a): Targeting of cell surface ß-amyloid precursor protein to lysosomes: Alternative processing into amyloid-bearing fragments. *Nature* 357:500-503.

Haass C, Schlossmacher MG, Hung AY, Vigo-Pelfrey C, Mellon A, Ostaszewski BL, Lieberburg I, Koo EH, Schenk D, Teplow DB and Selkoe, DJ (1992b): Amyloid ß-peptide is produced by cultured cells during normal metabolism. *Nature* 359:322-325.

Schellenberg GD, Bird TD, Wijsman EM, Orr HT, Anderson L, Nemens E, White JA, Bonnycastle L, Weber JL, Alonso ME, Potter H, Heston LH and Martin GM (1992): Genetic linkage evidence for a familial Alzheimer's disease locus on chromosome 14. *Science* 258:668-671.

Seubert P, Oltersdorf T, Lee MG, Barbour R, Blomquist C, Davis DL, Bryant K, Fritz LC, Galasko D, Thal LJ, Lieberburg I and Schenk DB (1993): Secretion of ß-amyloid precursor protein cleaved at the amino-terminus of the ß-amyloid peptide. *Nature* 361:260-263.

Seubert P, Vigo-Pelfrey C, Esch F, Lee M, Dovey H, Davis D, Sinha S, Schlossmacher M, Whaley J, Swindlehurst C, McCormack R, Wolfert R, Selkoe D, Lieberburg I and Schenk D (1992): Isolation and quantification of soluble Alzheimer's ß-peptide from biological fluids. *Nature* 359:325-327.

Shoji M, Golde TE, Ghiso J, Cheung TT, Estus S, Shaffer LM, Cai X, McKay DM, Tintner R, Frangione B and Younkin SG (1992): Production of the Alzheimer amyloid ß protein by normal proteolytic processing. *Science* 258:126-129.

Alzheimer Disease: Therapeutic Strategies
edited by E. Giacobini and R. Becker.
© 1994 Birkhäuser Boston

APOLIPOPROTEIN E AND ALZHEIMER'S DISEASE: THERAPEUTIC IMPLICATIONS

Warren J. Strittmatter, David Y. Huang, Ann Saunders, Donald Schmechel, Margaret Pericak-Vance and Allen D. Roses
Department of Medicine (Neurology) Duke University Medical Center, Durham, NC

Karl H. Weisgraber
The J.D. Gladstone Institutes, University of California, San Francisco, CA

Michel Goedert
MRC Laboratory of Molecular Biology, Hills Road, Cambridge, UK

INTRODUCTION

Recent studies have implicated apolipoprotein E (apoE) in the pathogenesis of Alzheimer disease (AD). One of the apoE alleles, ε4, is highly associated with late-onset familial (Strittmatter et al., 1993a) and sporadic (Saunders et al., 1993) AD. Three major protein isoforms of apoE (apoE2, E3 and E4) are the products of three alleles ε2, ε3, ε4 at a single gene locus on the proximal long arm of chromosome 19q13.2 (Mahley, 1988), within the region previously associated with linkage of late-onset familial AD (Pericak-Vance et al., 1991). In patients with late-onset familial AD, the ε4 allele frequency was 0.50 ± 0.06, compared to age-matched controls, 0.16 ± 0.03. We found that ε4 was also highly associated with patients with sporadic AD, with an allele frequency of 0.40 ± 0.026. The apoE gene dose is a major risk factor for late onset AD, and in these families homozygosity for APOE4 is virtually sufficient to cause AD by age 80 (Corder et al.,1993). The apoE 2 allele decreases risk (Corder et al., 1994).

Apolipoprotein E accumulates extracellularly in the senile plaque and congophilic angiopathy of AD and intracellularly in neurofibrillary tangle-bearing neurons (Strittmatter et al., 1993a). In cerebrospinal fluid, apoE avidly binds to synthetic ßA peptide, the primary constituent of the senile plaque and congophilic angiopathy.

The increased frequency of the apoE4 allele in AD, and the localization of apoE to both characteristic extra- and intracellular lesions of AD implies that apoE may be central to a unifying hypothesis. Neurofibrillary tangles are a defining pathologic finding in AD brain, and the burden of tangles correlates with the severity of the dementia. Neurofibrillary tangles are formed from paired helical filaments of hyperphosphorylated tau (Goedert et al., 1991 for review). Because of the intracytoplasmic localization of apoE (Han et al., 1994) and tau in neurons, we are examining the ability of the apoE isoforms to interact with tau *in vitro*. Apolipoprotein E3, but not apoE4, irreversibly binds tau, forming a complex not dissociated by boiling with sodium dodecyl sulfate (Strittmatter et al., 1994). We are examining the hypothesis that such isoform-specific interactions of apoE and tau might alter tau metabolism, and its functions in microtubule assembly and stabilization, and may be central to disease mechanism.

The senile, or neuritic, plaque is another defining lesion in AD and contains βA peptide. The apoE isoforms E3 and E4 avidly and irreversibly bind βA peptide *in vitro*, resisting dissociation by sodium dodecyl sulfate (SDS) or guanidine hydrochloride (Strittmatter et al., 1993b). Apolipoprotein E4 binds βA peptide more rapidly, and with a different pH dependence than does apoE3. Apolipoprotein E associates with βA peptide to form novel monofibrils (Sanan et al., 1994). These *in vitro* differences in the binding of these apoE isoforms are paralleled by differences *in vivo* (Schmechel et al., 1993). In a study of the comparative neuropathology of brain tissue from AD patients homozygous for $\epsilon4$ or $\epsilon3$, congophilic staining of amyloid in senile plaques and blood vessels was greatly increased in $\epsilon4$ patients. In addition, βA immunoreactivity in plaques and blood vessels was also increased in $\epsilon4$ homozygotes.

The association of the apoE4 allele with both late-onset familial and sporadic AD suggests that isoform-specific interactions of apoE are important in the pathogenesis of the disease. The mechanism by which the presence of the apoE4 *protein isoform*, or the absence of the apoE3 (or E2) *isoform* contributes to increased risk of AD is central, and unresolved. The identification of isoform-specific interactions of apoE with other molecules, in cellular trafficking, and in microtubule function are critical to determine the mechanism by which apoE is involved in disease *pathogenesis*. In addition, the presence of apoE in the extracellular senile plaques and angiopathy and in neurons with intracellular neurofibrillary tangles, and the irreversible binding demonstrated *in vitro*, suggests that apoE is also involved in the formation of these defining pathologic lesions.

APOLIPOPROTEIN E ISOFORMS

The most common isoform of apoE in the general population, apoE3, is secreted as a 299 amino acid protein containing a single cysteine residue at position 112 (Weisgraber, 1994, for review). The other two common isoforms, apoE2 and apoE4, differ at one of two positions (residues 112 and 158) from apoE3 by cysteine-arginine interchanges: apoE2 contains a cysteine at position 158 and apoE4 contains an arginine at 112.   The single cysteine in apoE3 permits disulfide bond formation with other molecules, including itself. Heterodimer formation with apolipoprotein A-II and homodimers with another apoE3 molecule have been reported. The apoE4 isoform lacks a cysteine and cannot form these disulfide complexes. The isoforms of apoE also differ in their interactions with the low density lipoprotein (LDL) receptor with apoE3 and apoE4 binding normally and apoE2 binding approximately 1% of normal. Apolipoprotein E contains two independently folded domains that can be modeled by the thrombolytic fragments, residues 1-191 and 216-299.   The region of apoE that binds to the LDL receptor is contained in the amino-terminal domain (residues 1-191), while the carboxyl-terminal domain contains the major lipid binding region of the protein.   Recently it was demonstrated that residues that are carboxyl-terminal to 244 play a major role in lipoprotein binding.

Although the cysteine-arginine interchange at position 112 (which distinguishes apoE3 from apoE4) is not contained in the major lipid binding region of apoE, this position influences the distribution of these isoforms among the various classes, with apoE3 preferentially binding to the high density lipoproteins (HDL) while apoE4 strongly binds the triglyceride-rich lower density lipoprotein particles, both VLDL and IDL.   A domain:domain interaction has been suggested to account for the distribution effect. The recent elucidation of the three dimensional structure of the receptor-binding domain of apoE has helped model isoform-specific functional properties, including differences in LDL receptor binding.

IRREVERSIBLE, ISOFORM SPECIFIC BINDING OF APOE3 WITH THE MICROTUBULE BINDING PROTEINS TAU AND MAP-2

Dementia in AD is generally accepted to be better correlated with the neurofibrillary pathology than with the extent of βA deposition. Neurofibrillary lesions contain paired helical filaments whose principal constituent is hyperphosphorylated tau, a microtubule-associated protein (Goedert et al., 1991 for review).   Because of the genetic relevance of APOE4 and the presence of immunoreactive apoE in neurons containing neurofibrillary tangles, we examined isoform-specific interactions of apoE with recombinant tau before and after phosphorylation with a brain extract.

In vitro, purified human apoE3 binds to tau-40, forming a molecular complex which resists dissociation by boiling in 2% sodium dodecyl sulfate.   The apoE3/tau complex has an apparent molecular weight of approximately 105 kDa (tau-40, 68 kDa; apoE, 34 kDa) and is not observed in either protein preparation alone.   Tau also binds the disulfide-linked apoE3 homodimer.   Irreversible binding of tau and apoE3 is maximal within 30 min at 37°C and occurred between pH 4.6 - 7.6.   Binding of tau to apoE3 could be detected down to $3 \times 10^{-8}M$ apoE.   Apolipoprotien E4 does not irreversibly bind tau under identical conditions.   The SDS-stable apoE3/tau complex is dissociated by boiling in the reducing agent β-mercaptoethanol. However, the apoE3/tau was probably *not* complexed through disulfide bond formation since tau bound both the monomer and the homodimer of apoE3 . There is only insignificant SDS-stable binding of tau by apoE4 under a variety of conditions, including increased duration of incubation, increased concentration of apoE4, or pH values 7.6-4.6.

Apolipoprotein E contains two functionally important domains, one which binds the LDL receptor and the other which binds lipoprotein particles (VLDL or HDL). Thrombin cleaves apoE at residues 191 and 215, yielding a 22-kDa amino-terminal fragment and a 10-kDa carboxyl-terminal fragment. The receptor-binding domain is located within the 22-kDa amino-terminal fragment and both the lipid binding and the Aß peptide binding regions are within the 10-kDa fragment. Tau binds the 22-kDa amino-terminal fragment of apoE3. Recombinant apoE3 fragments, 1-244, 1-266, and 1-272, bind equivalent amounts of tau when compared with that bound by the 22-kDa fragment of native apoE (amino acids 1-191). Thus, tau binds irreversibly to the fragment of apoE3 which also binds the LDL receptor. This region is distinct from the region (between amino acids 245-272) that binds lipoprotein particles and the βA peptide. The 22-kDa amino-terminal fragment of apoE4 does not bind tau.

Paired helical filament tau is phosphorylated at a number of serine/threonine-proline sites. At least some of these sites are phosphorylated by incubating recombinant tau with a crude rat brain extract and ATP. Recombinant tau-40 phosphorylated in this manner did not bind either apoE3 or apoE4, even with a prolonged 12 hr incubation. Failure of apoE3 and apoE4 to bind tau phosphorylated by brain extract resulted from phosphorylation, since omission of ATP from the incubation mixture still permitted binding of apoE3 to the non-phosphorylated tau. In AD, hyperphosphorylated tau is believed to self-assemble into the paired helical filament by formation of anti-parallel dimers of the microtubule-binding repeat region. *In vitro*, the microtubule-bind repeats of tau self-assemble into paired helical-like filaments. Apolipoprotein E3 irreversibly binds the microtubule-binding repeat region of tau, whereas apoE4 did not bind with this avidity. Boiling apoE3 prior to incubation with the microtubule-binding repeats prevented binding, demonstrating conformational requirements for binding.

IRREVERSIBLE ISOFORM-SPECIFIC BINDING OF APOE WITH βA PEPTIDE

Incubation of purified, delipidated apoE4 or apoE3 with synthetic βA peptide (βA4$_{(1-28)}$) results in the formation of an apoE-βA peptide complex with an apparent molecular weight greater than apoE alone that is recognized by both an apoE antibody and by a βA peptide antibody (Strittmatter et al., 1993b). This complex is maintained even after boiling in 2% sodium dodecyl sulfate for five minutes. In contrast, boiling apoE prior to incubation with βA peptide prevents binding. The apoE3/βA peptide complex is first detectable after two hours incubation, and increases over the next twenty-four hours. In contrast the apoE4/βA complex is easily detected after five minutes incubation. The βA peptide binds to both the monomer of apoE3, and to the disulfide-linked homodimer of apoE3. After incubation for twelve hours, an additional, higher molecular weight apoE/βA complex is observed. Only a small percentage (less than 10%) of the total amount of apoE in the incubation binds βA peptide after twenty four hours, despite a large molar excess of βA peptide (βA peptide at 2.5×10^{-4} molar, apoE at 1.8×10^{-6} molar).

The incomplete formation of the apoE-βA peptide complex could be due either to the slow association of these molecules or to modification of protein prior to binding. Addition of the reducing agents dithiothreitol or β-mercaptoenthanol, either before or after incubation of apoE and βA peptide, prevents SDS-stable binding, suggesting that oxidation may be required. Oxygen-saturated buffer increases and nitrogen decreases the rate of SDS-stable binding. Prolonged incubation of apoE3 or apoE4 alone at 37°C results in the gradual loss of the ability of apoE to bind βA peptide. These results demonstrate that both apoE3 and apoE4 bind βA peptide, forming a complex which resists dissociation by boiling in SDS. Binding of βA by apoE appears to require the oxidation of apoE, and can be prevented or reversed by reduction with dithiothreitol or β-mercaptoethanol. The more rapid binding of βA by apoE4 than by E3 may be due to an increased rate of oxidation of E4 or other factors leading to differences in the oxidation of these isoforms.

The SDS-stable binding of βA peptides by apoE4 and by apoE3 is dose dependent. Apolipoprotein E3 and apoE4 bind $\beta A_{(1-40)}$, $\beta A_{(1-28)}$ and $\beta A_{(12-28)}$ and is maximal at 10^{-4} molar peptide. In all three cases half-maximal binding is approximately 10^{-5} molar. Binding of βA peptide by apoE is pH dependent. Binding of ßA peptide by apoE3 and apoE4 is observed at pH 7.5 and decreases at lower pH. Virtually no apoE4/βA peptide complex is observed at pH lower than 6.6. In contrast, apoE3/βA peptide complex is still detectable at pH 4.6, suggesting isoform-specific effects.

The domain of apoE which binds βA peptide was determined by examining various apoE fragments. The βA4 peptide does not bind to the 22-kDa thrombin-generated apoE3 fragment. Binding of βA to recombinant-expressed truncated apoE mutants was also investigated. Binding of βA peptide to $apoE3_{(1-244)}$ is very low or minimal. In contrast, $apoE3_{(1-266)}$ forms an SDS-stable βA peptide complex, which is further increased with $apoE_{(1-272)}$. Therefore, βA binding to apoE appears to require the domain of apoE between amino acids 244 to 272, within the region previously demonstrated to mediate binding to lipoprotein particles.

SUMMARY

Since the apoE4 allele is a risk factor or susceptibility gene in late-onset familial and sporadic AD, the mechanism of disease expression may involve metabolic effects that are isoform specific. Isoform-specific interactions of apoE therefore become critical in the mechanism of AD pathogenesis. Detailed characterization of the binding of the apoE isoforms with proteins and peptides relevant to the pathology of the disease may be critical in understanding disease pathogenesis. These critical isoform-specific interactions of apoE may involve interactions with proteins and peptides in the defining neuropathologic lesions of the disease, the neurofibrillary tangle and senile plaque. Other possible critical isoform-specific interactions include the mechanism of internalization, intracellular trafficking, and subsequent metabolism. In addition, differential post-translational modifications of apoE isoforms may determine differences in metabolism contributing to the pathogenesis of the disease. Oxidation of apoE may confer several isoform-specific, biochemically distinct properties. Since βA peptide binds apoE in the lipoprotein binding domain of the protein and not in the receptor-binding domain, apoE could target bound βA4 peptide to neurons via the LRP receptor. Internalization of the apoE/βA peptide complex into the cell, by the same route as the apoE-containing lipoproteins, would result in incorporation into primary lysosomes and pH dependent dissociation. The demonstration of apoE in the cytoplasm of neurons, with isoform-specific interactions of apoE with the microtubule-binding protein tau demonstrated *in vitro*, suggest additional, testable hypotheses of disease pathogenesis. Isoform-specific differences in binding of apoE illustrate only part of the differential repertoire that could lead to disease pathogenesis. The mechanisms that modulate apoE binding to tau, βA peptide and the LRP receptor may be important in determining the intracellular metabolism of these molecules, or their deposition in the extracellular space. Studying these processes *in vitro* may provide important insights into disease mechanisms.

REFERENCES

Corder EH, Saunders AM, Strittmatter WJ, Schmechel D, Gaskell P, Small GW, Roses AD, Haines JL and Pericak-Vance MA (1993): Apolipoprotein E gene dose affects the risk of Alzheimer disease. *Science* 261:921-923.

Corder EH, Haines JL, Saunders AM, Strittmatter WJ, Schmechel DM, Gaskill PC Jr, Rimmler JB, Conneally PM, Schmader KE, Small GW, Roses AD, Risch NJ and Pericak-Vance MA (1994): Apolipoprotein E type 2 allele decreases the risk of late onset Alzheimer disease. *Nature Genetics* (In Press).

Goedert M, Crowther RA and Garner CC (1991): Molecular characterization of microtubule-associated proteins tau and MAP-2. *Trends Neurosci* 14:193-199.

Han S-H, Hulette C, Saunders AM, Einstein G, Pericak-Vance M, Strittmatter WJ, Roses AD and Schmechel DE (1994): Apolipoprotein E is present in hippocampal neurons without neurofibrillary tangles in Alzheimer's disease and in age-matched controls. *Experimental Neurology* In Press.

Mahley RW (1988): Apolipoprotein E: Cholesterol transport protein with expanding role in cell biology. *Science* 240:622-628.

Pericak-Vance MA, Bebout JL, Gaskell PC Jr, Yamaoka LH, Hung WY, Alberts MJ, Walker AP, Bartlett RJ, Haynes CA, Welsh KA, Earl NL, Heyman A, Clark CM and Roses AD (1991): Linkage studies in familial Alzheimer disease: evidence for chromosome 19 linkage. *Am Hum Genet* 48:1034-1050.

Sanan D, Weisgraber KH, Mahley RW, Huang DY, Russell SJ, Saunders A, Schmechel D, Wisniewski T, Frangione B, Roses AD and Strittmatter WJ (1994): Apolipoprotein E associates with βA amyloid peptide to form novel monofibrils *in vitro*: Isoform apoE4 associates more efficiently than apoE3. *J Clin Invest* In Press.

Saunders AM, Strittmatter WJ, Schmechel D, St George-Hyslop PH, Pericak-Vance MA, Joo SH, Rosi BL, Gusella JF, Crapper-MacLachlan DR, Growden J, Alberts MJ, Hulette C, Crain B, Goldgaber D and Roses AD (1993): Association of apolipoprotein E allele c4 with late-onset familial and sporadic Alzheimer's disease. *Neurology* 43:1467-1472.

Schmechel DE, Saunders AM, Strittmatter WJ, Joo SH, Hulette C, Crain B, Goldgaber D and Roses AD (1993): Increased vascular and plaque βA4 amyloid deposits in sporadic Alzheimer disease patients with apolipoprotein E-e4 allele. *Proc Natl Acad Sci* 90:9649-9653.

Strittmatter WJ, Saunders AM, Pericak-Vance M, Salvesen GS, Enghild J and Roses AD (1993a): Apolipoprotein E: High affinity binding to βA amyloid and increased frequency of type 4 isoform in familial Alzheimer Disease. *Proc Natl Acad Sci* 90:1977-1981.

Strittmatter WJ, Weisgraber KH, Huang D, Dong L-M, Salvesen GS, Pericak-Vance M, Schmechel D, Saunders AM, Goldgaber DM and Roses AD (1993b): Binding of human apolipoprotein E to βA4 peptide: isoform-specific effects and implications for late-onset Alzheimer disease. *Proc Natl Acad Sci* 90:8098-8102.

Strittmatter WJ, Weisgraber KH, Goedert M, Saunders AM, Huang D, Corder EH, Dong L-M, Jakes R, Alberts MJ, Gilbert JR, Schmechel DE, Pericak-Vance MA and Roses AD (1994): Hypothesis: microtubule instability and paired helical filament formation in the Alzheimer disease brain as a function of apolipoprotein E genotype. *Exptl Neurol* 125:163-171.

Weisgraber KH (1994): Apolipoprotein E: structure-function relationships. *Advances in Protein Chemistry* 45:249-302.

Alzheimer Disease: Therapeutic Strategies
edited by E. Giacobini and R. Becker.
© 1994 Birkhäuser Boston

APOLIPOPROTEIN E4 AND CHOLINERGIC DYSFUNCTION IN ALZHEIMER'S DISEASE

Judes Poirier, Isabelle Aubert, Philippe Bertrand, Rémi Quirion, Serge Gauthier and Josephine Nalbantoglu
McGill Centre for Studies in Aging, Montreal Neurological Institute, and
Douglas Hospital Research Centre, McGill University,
Montréal, Québec, Canada

INTRODUCTION

Apolipoprotein E (apoE) is a well-characterized lipophilic protein associated with plasma and CSF lipoproteins. Apolipoprotein E is synthesized primarily by the liver, but also at other sites including brain, macrophages and adrenals (Elshourbagy et al., 1985). Furthermore, apoE is unique among apolipoproteins in that it has a special relevance to the central and peripheral nervous systems. It is a key determinant in the cellular recognition and internalization of cholesterol- and phospholipid-rich lipoproteins in the developing brain and in the response to neuronal injury (Boyles et al., 1989; Poirier et al., 1991a,b, 1993a). It was shown to play a fundamental role in the CNS during hippocampal synaptic plasticity induced by entorhinal cortex lesions in the rat (Poirier et al., 1991a,b, 1993).

Apolipoprotein E is synthesized and secreted by astrocytes in the deafferented zone of the hippocampus following lesions of the entorhinal cortex (Poirier et al., 1991a). Shortly after the peak in apoE synthesis, a time-dependent, cell specific induction of the [^{125}I]apoE/apoB (LDL) receptors in the granule cell layer of the dentate gyrus was shown to correlate closely with the cholinergic synaptogenesis resulting from the loss of entorhinal cortex projections (Poirier et al., 1993a). In contrast, hippocampal cholesterol synthesis fell by more than 60 % during the early phase of the cholinergic reinnervation process, during peak synthesis of apoE in the deafferented zone (Poirier et al., 1993a).

These changes were interpreted as evidences for a role of apoE and the LDL receptor in the process of cholinergic compensatory synaptogenesis caused by the loss of entorhinal cortex neurons, a pathophysiological process also observed in Alzheimer's disease (AD) (Hyman et al., 1984).

The human apoE gene on chromosome 19 has three common alleles (E2, E3, E4), which encode three major apoE isoforms. Recently, the frequency of the apoE4 allele was shown to be markedly increased in sporadic

(Poirier et al., 1993b; Saunders et al., 1993; Noguchi et al., 1993) and late onset familial AD (Corder et al., 1993; Payami et al., 1993). Most interestingly, a gene dosage effect was observed in both familial (Corder et al., 1993) and sporadic (Poirier et al., 1993b) cases (i.e. as age of onset increases, E4 allele copy number decreases). Women, who are generally at a greater risk of developing AD, showed increased apoE4 allele frequency when compared to age-matched men (Poirier et al., 1993b). A recent study reveals that apoE protein levels are significantly reduced in the hippocampus of AD subjects homozygous for apoE4 (Poirier et al., submitted).

It has been shown that apoE-like immunoreactivity was found to be associated with amyloid in senile plaques, cerebral vessels and neurofibrillary tangles (Namba et al., 1991). *In vitro*, amyloid ß binds more avidly to apoE4 than to apoE3 (Strittmatter et al., 1993). Increased amyloid ß peptide deposition was recently reported in the cerebral cortex (Schmechel et al., 1993) and hippocampus (Poirier et al., submitted) of late-onset AD subjects carrying one or two copies of the apoE4 allele.

Recently, we examined the impact of apoE4 on choline acetyltransferase (ChAT) activity, muscarinic "M1" and nicotinic binding site densities in the hippocampus of post-mortem subjects with different apoE genotypes.

RESULTS

On the basis of its well-recognized post-mortem stability, ChAT activity was examined in relation to apoE genotype in control and AD post-mortem subjects. Figure 1A illustrates that the loss in ChAT activity (as measured by the method of Tucek, 1978) in the hippocampus of control and AD cases is a function of apoE4 allele copy number [i.e. as apoE4 allele copy number increased, ChAT activity decreased (Poirier et al., submitted)]. These results indicate the existence of distinct genetic entities in sporadic AD which show differential degrees of alterations of cholinergic innervation, at least as revealed by ChAT activity. To further characterize the nature of cholinergic impairment in apoE4 AD carriers, the apoE genotype of 7 AD subjects for which we had previously documented (Etienne et al., 1985) the number of cholinergic neurons in the nucleus basalis of Meynert (NBM) and diagonal band of Broca (DBB) was determined by allele specific PCR. Figure 1B summarizes the results obtained so far in these post-mortem AD subjects. A marked reduction in the number of acetylcholinesterase-positive neurons was observed in apoE4 homozygote AD subjects group.

The duration of the disease was similar for both groups (AD-E3/3: 7 ± 3 years, AD-E4/4: 10 ± 4 years; mean $\pm$ S.D.). We also monitored the density of nicotinic (putative pre-synaptic) and muscarinic "M1" (putative post-synaptic) binding sites in the hippocampus of AD subjects as a function of apoE genotype.

Figure 2 illustrates the hippocampal binding site densities obtained using the methods described by Aubert et al. (1992) in genotyped AD subjects (n=17).

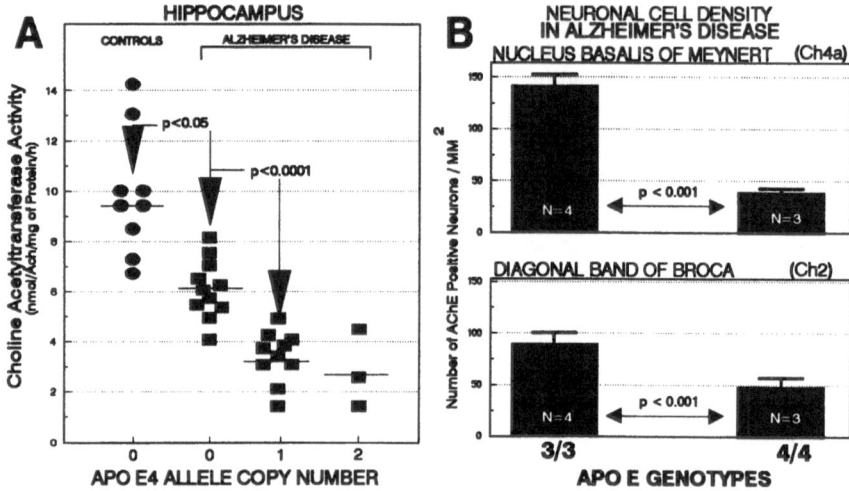

FIGURE 1. Choline acetyltranferase activity in the hippocampus and AChE-positive neuronal count in the nucleus basalis of control and Alzheimer's subjects. Genotype was determined as described in Poirier et al. (submitted).

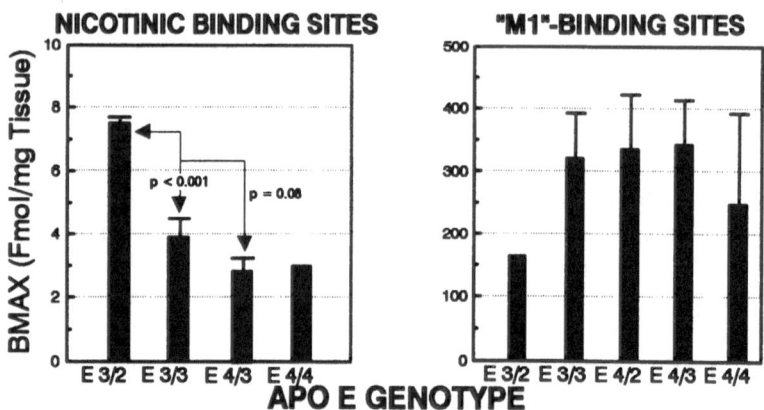

FIGURE 2. Hippocampal cholinergic binding sites density in apoE genotyped subjects with AD.

Nicotinic receptor binding site density decreases in AD according to genotype in the order of E3/2 >> E3/3 > E4/3 = E4/4, which is consistent with the known genotype-dependent metabolic rate of apoE in humans (for a review, see Davignon et al., 1988). These changes also support the concept that nicotinic receptors, like ChAT, have a pre-synaptic location in the hippocampal formation and that the loss of cholinergic neurons in the DBB and septal areas may account for the genotype-related loss of cholinergic function in this area in AD. In contrast, pirenzepine sensitive "M1" sites remain relatively unaltered in the hippocampus of AD subjects with different apoE genotypes.

Taken together, our data clearly suggest that cholinergic function in AD-E3/3 subjects may at least be partially spared when compared to AD-E4/3 and AD-4/4 carriers. Most importantly, this genetic susceptibility could result in sub-groups of AD patients which may respond differently to acetylcholine precursor-based therapies; E4 carriers having lost most of their ACh synthetic capacities. These results also suggest that "M1"-receptor-based therapies should not be affected by individual apoE genotypes.

ACKNOWLEDGEMENTS

The research from our laboratory reviewed here was supported by grants from the National Institute on Aging, AG-10003, American Alzheimer Association and from the Medical Research Council of Canada.

REFERENCES

Aubert I, Araujo DM, Cécyre D, Robitaille Y and Quirion R (1992): Comparative alterations of nicotinic and muscarinic binding sites in Alzheimer's and Parkinson's diseases. *J Neurochem* 58:529-541.

Boyles JK, Zoellner CD, Anderson LJ, Kosick LM, Pitas RE, Weisgraber KH, Hui DY, Mahley RW, Gebicke-Haeter PJ, Ignatius MJ and Shooter EM (1989): A role for apolipoprotein E, apolipoprotein A-1, and low density lipoprotein receptors in cholesterol transport during regeneration and remyelination of the rat sciatic nerve. *J Clin Invest* 83:1015-1031.

Corder EH, Saunders AM, Strittmatter WJ, Schmechel DE, Gaskell PC, Small GW, Roses AD and Pericak-Vance MA (1993): Gene dose of apolipoprotein E type 4 and risk of Alzheimer's disease in late onset families. *Science* 261:921-923.

Davignon J, Gregg RE and Sing CF (1988): Apolipoprotein E polymorphism and atherosclerosis. *Arteriosclerosis* 8:1-21.

Elshourbagy NA, Liao WS, Mahley RW and Taylor JM (1985): Apolipoprotein E mRNA is abundant in the brain and adrenals, as well as in the liver, and is present in other peripheral tissues of rats and marmosets. *Proc Natl Acad Sci* 82:203-207.

Etienne P, Robitaille Y, Wood P, Gauthier S, Nair NPV and Quirion R (1986): Nucleus basalis neuronal loss and choline acetyltransferase activity in advanced Alzheimer's disease. *Neuroscience* 4:1279-1291.

Hyman BT, Van Hoesen GW, Damasion AR and Barnes CL (1984): Alzheimer's disease: Cell-specific pathology isolates the hippocampal formation. *Science* 225:1168-1170.

Namba Y, Tomonaga M and Kawasaki H (1991): Apolipoprotein E immunoreactivity in cerebral amyloid deposits and neurofibrillary tangles in Alzheimer's disease and in Creutzfeld-Jacob disease. *Brain Res* 541:163-166.

Noguchi S, Murakami K and Yamada N (1993): Apolipoprotein E and Alzheimer's disease. *Lancet* (Letter) 342:737.

Payami H, Kaye J, Heston LL and Schellenberg GD (1993): Apolipoprotein E and Alzheimer's disease. *Lancet* (Letter) 342:738

Poirier J, Hess M, May PC and Finch CE (1991a): Cloning of hippocampal poly(A+) RNA sequences that increase after entorhinal cortex lesion in adult rat. *Mol Br Res* 9:191-195.

Poirier J, Hess M, May PC and Finch CE (1991b): Apolipoprotein E-and GFAP-RNA in hippocampus during reactive synaptogenesis and terminal proliferation. *Mol Brain Res* 11:97-106.

Poirier J, Baccichet A, Dea D and Gauthier S (1993a): Role of hippocampal cholesterol synthesis and uptake during reactive synaptogenesis in adult rats. *Neuroscience* 55: 81-90.

Poirier J, Davignon J, Bouthillier D, Bertrand P and Gauthier S (1993b): Apolipoprotein E and Alzheimer's disease. *Lancet* 342:697-699.

Saunders AM, Strittmatter WJ, Schmechel D, St George-Hyslop PH, Pericak-Vance MA, Joo SH, Rosi BA, Gusella JF, McClaclans DR, Alberts MJ and Roses AD (1993): Association of apolipoprotein E allele E4 with late onset familial and sporadic Alzheimer's disease. *Neurology* 43:1467-1472.

Schmechel D, Saunders AM, Strittmatter WJ, Crain BJ, Hulette CM, Joo SH and Roses AD (1993): Increased amyloid ß-peptide deposition in cerebral cortex as a consequence of apolipoprotein E genotype in late-onset Alzheimer's disease. *Proc Natl Acad Sci* 90:9649-9653.

Strittmatter WJ, Weisgraber KH, Huang DY, Dong LM, Salvesen GS, Pericak-Vance M, Schmechel D and Roses AD (1993): Binding of human apolipoprotein E to synthetic amyloid ß-peptide: isoform-specific effect and implication for late onset Alzheimer's disease. *Proc Natl Acad Sci* 90:8098-8102.

Tucek S (1978): Choline acetyltransferase. In: *Acetylcholine Synthesis in Neurons*, London: Chapman and Hall Ltd., pp. 29-42.

PART III
THE CHOLINERGIC SYSTEM OF HUMAN BRAIN

Alzheimer Disease: Therapeutic Strategies
edited by E. Giacobini and R. Becker.
© 1994 Birkhäuser Boston

BUTYRYLCHOLINESTERASE IN ALZHEIMER'S DISEASE

M.-Marsel Mesulam
Departments of Neurology and Psychiatry, Northwestern University Medical School, Chicago, Illinois

Butyrylcholinesterase (BChE, EC.3.1.1.8) is a hydrolytic enzyme of unknown function. Although it is usually considered in conjunction with acetylcholinesterase (AChE), BChE is the product of a different gene, has a much more restricted distribution in the mammalian brain and has no major role in conventional cholinergic neurotransmission. It is now definitively established that the two histopathological hallmarks of Alzheimer's disease (AD), neurofibrillary tangles and amyloid plaques, display intense BChE enzyme activity (Mesulam et al., 1987; Mesulam and Morán, 1987).

The origin of the plaque- and tangle-bound BChE is not yet fully identified. The neurons of the normal cerebral cortex contain very little BChE so that the enzyme activity in plaques and tangles could not be attributed to the passive entrapment of BChE within degenerated axons and perikarya. Furthermore, the amyloid precursor protein (APP) does not display significant BChE activity (Geula et al., 1994), so that the plaque-bound enzyme activity cannot be attributed to the presence of amyloid deposits. Recent observations indicate that the neuroglial cells of the brain may constitute a major source of the plaque and tangle-bound BChE in AD (Wright et al., 1993a).

We observed that BChE activity with pH preferences and inhibitor selectivities identical to those of the plaque and tangle-bound enzyme are found in the astrocytes and oligodendrocytes of control and AD brains. In non-AD control brains, the density of BChE-positive glia (especially in the deep layers of cortex and the subjacent white matter) was higher in entorhinal and inferotemporal cortex, two regions with a high susceptibility to the pathology of AD, than in primary somatosensory and visual cortex, two areas with a relatively lower susceptibility to the disease process. In comparison to age-matched control specimens, AD brains had a significantly higher density of BChE glia in entorhinal and inferotemporal regions but not in the primary somatosensory or visual areas. These results suggested that glia constitute a likely source for the BChE activity of plaques and tangles, and that a high density of BChE-positive glia may play a permissive or causative role in the neuropathology of AD. In control brains, the glial cholinesterases appear confined to the intracellular space whereas in AD they decorate plaques and tangles as well. It is interesting to note that AD is associated with a significant increase in the total BChE activity of the temporal lobes (Perry et al., 1978).

The brains of patients with AD display numerous pathological changes. Only the extracellular accumulation of Aß amyloid in the form of plaques is specific to AD and differentiates this condition from other dementing diseases. The Aß peptide is a 4 kd fragment of a membrane spanning, naturally occurring amyloid precursor protein (APP). Increased production, point mutations, deviant sequestration and abnormal processing of APP have been invoked as causative mechanisms for plaque formation and AD (Yankner and Mesulam, 1991; Citron et al., 1992; Mullan et al., 1993; Saunders et al., 1993).

Although amyloid deposits constitute necessary elements in the pathogenesis of AD, numerous observations indicate that they are not by themselves sufficient for triggering the neural degeneration and dementia characteristic of this disease. The deposition of amyloid does not initially cause tissue pathology (Yamaguchi et al., 1989) and may need to go on for years before the emergence of clinically recognizable dementia (Rumble et al., 1989). There is also very little correlation between dementia severity and plaque formation (Arriagada et al., 1992; Berg et al., 1993), and many non-demented elderly individuals have plaque densities in the range seen in AD (Dayan, 1970; Katzman et al., 1988; Dickson et al., 1991; Mizutani and Shimada, 1992; Delaère et al., 1993).

One possibility is that amyloid plaques undergo a lengthy process of transformation at the site of deposition before they become pathogenic. Our recent observations suggest that BChE reactivity may be a factor that participates in the "ripening" and eventual pathogenicity of Aß deposits in AD. In an unselected sample of 4 demented and 4 age-matched non-demented brains, the total cortical area covered by plaque-like Aß amyloid and (BChE) deposits was measured at two regions of the temporal cortex with the help of computerized densitometry. Demented as well as age-matched non-demented brains contained Aß and BChE positive plaques. The total cortical area covered by the Aß precipitates was higher in demented individuals but there was overlap with the values seen in the specimens from non-demented individuals. The proportional plaque area displaying BChE reactivity was very significantly and 5-6 fold higher in the demented than in the non-demented group and there was no overlap between the two populations (Mesulam and Geula, 1994).

These results suggest that the progressively more extensive BChE reactivity of plaques may participate in their transformation from a relatively benign form to pathogenic structures associated with neuritic degeneration and dementia.

The physiological role served by BChE remains mysterious. Detoxifying, growth promoting and morphogenetic functions have been described (Massoulié et al., 1993). The BChE in plaques and neuroglia is selectively inhibited by indoleamines, carboxypeptidase inhibitor and other protease inhibitors such as bacitracin (Wright et al., 1993b). In keeping with these inhibitor responses, BChE has been shown to display a serotonin-sensitive aryl-acylamidase and perhaps also metalloprotease activity (Rao and Balasubramanian, 1993). Butyrylcholinesterase thus joins a number of other substances such as a_1-antichymotrypsin (Abraham et al., 1990), protease nexin 1 (Rosenblatt et al., 1989), and a_1-antitrypsin (Gollin et al., 1992) which are found in association with the amyloid plaque deposits and which may disrupt the delicate local balance between proteases and their inhibitors.

The excessive deposition of insoluble Aß amyloid in the cerebral cortex is a necessary and specific factor in the pathogenesis of AD. This conclusion needs to be reconciled with the inconsistent temporal and quantitative relationship between Aß deposits and either tissue injury or dementia. One explanation is that the deposition of Aß is a necessary but not sufficient factor and that additional downstream events are required for the development of AD.

Our findings identify the increase of BChE reactivity as a potentially significant downstream event in the complex life cycle of Aß plaques. The initially diffuse Aß deposits induce little or no tissue pathology in the brain (Yamaguchi et al., 1989) and may, in fact promote neurite outgrowth (Koo et al., 1993). At these early or benign stages of plaque formation, no more than 17% of the surface area covered by the amyloid deposit is BChE-reactive. At later or more pathogenetic stages of plaque formation, the proportional plaque area displaying BChE reactivity increases by a factor of 5-6 and may reach values that are as high as 87% (Mesulam and Geula, 1994). The BChE may become inserted into the area of Aß deposits through the mediation of neuroglia and may alter the pathogenicity of amyloid plaques. This potential sequence of events suggests that BChE-inhibitors may play an important and hitherto unexpected role in the prevention of AD. Human BChE displays numerous allelic polymorphic variants (Soreq et al., 1992) and it would be of considerable interest to determine if some of these are more closely associated with AD.

REFERENCES

Abraham C, Shirahama T and Potter H (1990): a1-Antichymotrypsin is associated solely with amyloid deposits containing the ß-protein: Amyloid and cell localization of a1-antichymotrypsin. *Neurobiol Aging* 11:123-129.

Arriagada PV, Growdon JH, Hedley-Whyte ET and Hyman BT (1992): Neurofibrillary tangles but not senile plaques parallel duration and severity of Alzheimer's disease. *Neurol* 42:631-639.

Berg L, McKeel DW, Miller JP, Baty J and Morris J (1993): Neuropathological indexes of Alzheimer's disease in demented and nondemented persons aged 80 years and older. *Arch Neurol* 50:349-358.

Citron M, Oltersdorf T, Haass C, McConlogue L, Hung AY, Seubert P, Vigo-Pelfrey C, Lieberburg I and Selkoe DJ (1992): Mutation of the ß-amyloid precursor protein in familial Alzheimer's disease increases ß-protein production. *Nature* 360:672-674.

Dayan AD (1970): Quantitative histological studies on the aged human brain. II. Senile plaques and neurofibrillary tangles in senile dementia (with an appendix on their occurrence in cases of carcinoma). *Acta Neuropathol* 16:95-102.

Delaère P, He Y, Fayet G, Duyckaerts C and Hauw J-J (1993): ßA4 deposits are constant in the brain of the oldest old: An immunohistochemical study of 20 French centenarians. *Neurobiol Aging* 14:191-194.

Dickson DW, Crystal HA, Mattiace LA, Masur DM, Blau AD, Davies P, Yen SH and Aronson MK (1991): Identification of normal and pathological aging in prospectively studied nondemented elderly humans. *Neurobiol Aging* 13:179-189.

Geula C, Greenberg BD and Mesulam M-M (1994): Cholinesterase activity in the plaques, tangles and angiopathy of Alzheimer's disease does not emanate from amyloid. *Brain Res* (In Press).

Gollin PA, Kalaria RN, Eikelenboom P, Rozemuller A and Perry G (1992): Alpha-1-antitrypsin and alpha-1-antichymotrypsin are in lesions of Alzheimer's disease. *Neuroreport* 3:201-203.

Katzman R, Terry R, DeTeresa R, Brown T, Davies P, Fuld P, Renbing X and Peck A (1988): Clinical, pathological and neurochemical changes in dementia: A subgroup with preserved mental status and numerous neocortical plaques. *Ann Neurol* 23:138-144.

Koo EH, Park L and Selkoe DJ (1993): Amyloid ß-protein as a substrate interacts with extracellular matrix to promote neurite outgrowth. *Proc Natl Acad Sci (USA)* 90:4748-4752.

Massoulié J, Pezzementi L, Bon S, Krejci E and Vallette F-M (1993): Molecular and cellular biology of cholinesterases. *Prog Neurobiol* 41:31-91.

Mesulam M-M and Geula C (1994): Butyrylcholinesterase reactivity differentiates the amyloid plaques of aging from those of dementia. *Ann Neurol* (In Press).

Mesulam M-M, Geula C and Morán A (1987): Anatomy of cholinesterase inhibition in Alzheimer's disease: Effect of physostigmine and tetrahydroaminoacridine on plaques and tangles. *Ann Neurol* 22:683-691.

Mesulam MM and Morán A (1987): Cholinesterases within neurofibrillary tangles related to age and Alzheimer's disease. *Ann Neurol* 22:223-228.

Mizutani T and Shimada H (1992): Neuropathological background of twenty-seven centenarian brains. *J Neurol Sci* 108:168-177.

Mullan M, Tsuji S, Miki T, Katsuya T, Naruse S, Kaneko K, Shimizu T, Kojima T, Nakano I, Ogihara T, Miyatake T, Ovenstone I, Crawford F, Goate A, Hardy J, Roques P, Roberts G, Luthert P, Lantos P, Clark C, Gaskell P, Crain B and Roses A (1993): Clinical comparison of Alzheimer's disease in pedigrees with the codon 717 Val-Ile mutation in the amyloid precursor protein gene. *Neurobiol Aging* 14:407-419.

Perry EK, Perry RH, Blessed G and Tomlinson BE (1978): Changes in brain cholinesterases in senile dementia of Alzheimer type. *Neuropath Appl Neurobiol* 4:273-277.

Rao RV and Balasubramanian AS (1993): The peptidase activity of human serum butyrylcholinesterase: Studies using monoclonal antibodies and characterization of the peptidase. *J Prot Chem* 12:103-110.

Rosenblatt DE, Geula C and Mesulam M-M (1989): Protease nexin I immunostaining in Alzheimer's disease. *Ann Neurol* 26:628-634.

Rumble B, Retallack R, Hilbich C, Simms G, Multhaup G, Martins R, Hockey A, Montgomery P, Beyreuther K and Masters CL (1989): Amyloid A4 protein and its precursor in Down's syndrome and Alzheimer's disease. *New Eng J Med* 320:1446-1452.

Saunders AM, Strittmatter WJ, Schmechel D, St. George-Hyslop PH, Pericak-Vance MA, Joo SH, Rosi BLG JF, Crapper-McLachlan DR, Alberts MJ, Hulette C, Crain B, Goldgaber D and Roses AD (1993): Association of apolipoprotein E allele E4 with late-onset familial and sporadic Alzheimer's disease. *Neurol* 43:1467-1472.

Soreq H, Gnatt A, Loewenstein Y and Neville LF (1992): Excavations into the active-site gorge of cholinesterases. *Trends Biochem Sci* 17:353-358.

Wright CI, Geula C and Mesulam MM (1993a): Neuroglial cholinesterases in the normal brain and in Alzheimer's disease: relationship to plaques, tangles, and patterns of selective vulnerability. *Ann Neurol* 34:373-84.

Wright CI, Geula C and Mesulam MM (1993b): Protease inhibitors and indoleamines selectively inhibit cholinesterases in the histopathologic structures of Alzheimer disease. *Proc Natl Acad Sci USA* 90:683-686.

Yamaguchi H, Nakazato Y, Hirai S, Shoji M and Harigaya Y (1989): Electron micrograph of diffuse plaques. Initial stages of senile plaque formation in the Alzheimer brain. *Amer J Path* 135:593-597.

Yankner BA and Mesulam M-M (1991): ß-amyloid and the pathogenesis of Alzheimer's disease. *New Eng J Med* 325:1849-1856.

Alzheimer Therapy: Therapeutic Strategies
edited by E. Giacobini and R. Becker.
© 1994 Birkhäuser Boston

MODULATING CHOLINERGIC NEUROTRANSMISSION THROUGH TRANSGENIC OVEREXPRESSION OF HUMAN CHOLINESTERASES

Hermona Soreq, Rachel Beeri, Shlomo Seidman, Rina Timberg, Yael Loewenstein, Meira Sternfeld and Christian Andres
Department of Biological Chemistry, The Life Sciences Inst.,
The Hebrew University, Jerusalem 91904, Israel

Moshe Shani
Department of Genetic Engineering, The Inst. of Animal Science,
Agricultural Research, 906, Beit Dagan 50250, Israel

INTRODUCTION

Impaired cholinergic metabolism has been associated with several neurodegenerative disorders of the central (Wurtman, 1992) and peripheral nervous system (Harding, 1992), suggesting that experimental modulation of cholinergic neurotransmission can serve to study the relationship between cholinergic deficits and neuropathology. To this end, we established transgenic models for overexpressing human cholinesterases (ChEs) (Soreq and Zakut, 1993) in cholinergic synapses of *Xenopus laevis* tadpoles and mice. Cholinesterase over-expression should create a local deficit of acetylcholine at the "engineered" synapses and initiate feedback responses from which one may learn about the role of cholinergic neurotransmission in regulating synaptic structure and function.

There are two genes in humans encoding ChEs. These are designated ACHE and BCHE and encode acetylcholinesterase (AChE) and butyrylcholinesterase (BuChE), respectively. Molecular cloning of these two genes revealed the primary sequence of their closely related protein products and *in situ* hybridization mapped these two genes to the distinct chromosomal positions of 7q22 (ACHE) and 3q26 (BCHE). Several point mutations abundant in the Israeli population were discovered in the BCHE gene (Ehrlich et al., 1994) and a complex pattern of alternative splicing was found to be unique to the human ACHE gene. Alternative splicing modifies the C-terminus of the AChE protein and its anchoring potential in 3 different ways (Karpel et al., 1994). It was therefore of interest to determine which of all of these AChE and BuChE variants would be correctly targeted to synapses and what should be the outcome of such synaptic targeting.

RESULTS

To elucidate the biochemical properties and biological functions of the large array of human ChE variants, schematically presented in Fig. 1, we first employed microinjected oocytes of *Xenopus laevis*. The natural variants of the BCHE gene were all efficiently expressed. The common allelic substitution of aspartate at position 70 in BuChE by glycine created an enzyme incapable of hydrolyzing succinylcholine. This structure-function analysis revealed the molecular basis for "succinylcholine apnea", the well known clinical syndrome where patients subjected to muscle relaxation by succinylcholine experience delayed post surgical recovery of diaphragm function and independent breathing (Neville et al., 1992). To examine the peptide domain harboring Asp70 for its role in determining substrate and inhibitor interactions in ChEs, we replaced a 78 amino acid peptide including Asp70 in BuChE with the corresponding peptide from AChE. Although the resultant catalytically active chimera carried only 12 non-conserved amino acid substitutions, this analysis was able to attribute many of the differences between AChE and BuChE with respect to inhibitor sensitivities to this peptide domain (Loewenstein et al., 1993). A population diversity study then revealed 11% heterozygotes for Asp/Gly 70 among Israelies and shed new light on variabilities in individual responses toward anti-AChE drugs examined for their potential in Alzheimer therapy (Ehrlich et al., 1994).

Once the biochemical characteristics of the human ChE variants were determined, we moved on to initiate transgenic ChE overexpression in *in vivo* milieus. When microinjected into fertilized *Xenopus* eggs, DNA and/or mRNA sequences encoding for human BuChE or the brain and muscle form of human AChE that includes the alternative 3' exon E6 (E_6AChE) induced a several-days-long accumulation of the heterologous human enzymes in neuromuscular junctions of these transiently transgenic tadpoles (Seidman et al., 1994). No major differences were observed in gross development or movement. However E_6AChE caused, within 2 days, an increase of up to 4-fold in the post-synaptic length of neuromuscular junctions in which it accumulated as compared with control junctions, and doubled the content of nicotinic acetylcholine receptors in these tadpoles (Shapira et al., 1994).

Placed under control of the human ACHE promoter (Ben Aziz et al., 1993) and stably introduced into the mouse genome by techniques detailed elsewhere (Beeri et al., 1994), E_6AChE was faithfully overexpressed and assembled in cholinergic brain neurons of adult mice, which displayed 2-fold increased AChE activities in central brain nuclei as compared with controls (Andres et al., 1994). Using a species-specific mAb, multimeric assembly of this human AChE was observed to be identical to that of the mouse brain enzyme. *In situ* hybridization revealed transcription patterns resembling those of the host mouse gene.

However, no gross changes were apparent in normal development and behavior of these mice.

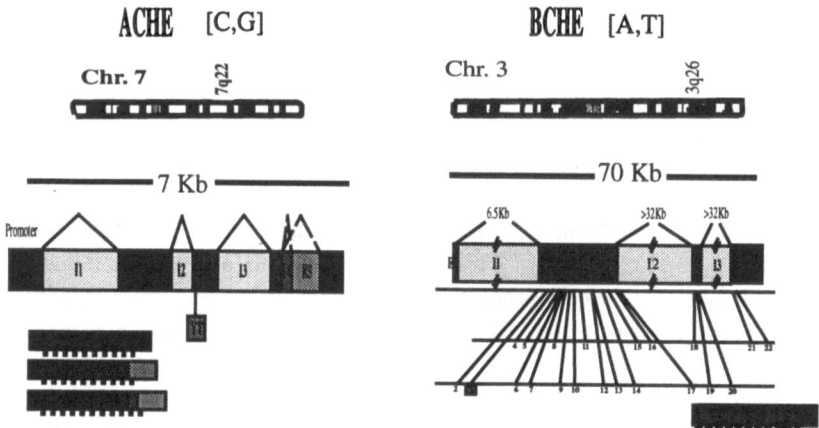

FIGURE 1. Human cholinesterase genes and their variants. The two human genes, ACHE and BCHE, differ in their nucleotide composition (ACHE being G,C-rich and BCHE-A,T-rich), chromosomal position (Chr. 7q22 for ACHE and 3q26 for BCHE), total length [7 and 70 kilobase (kb) for ACHE and BCHE, respectively], tendency for phenotypically effective point mutations (one known for ACHE, over 20 for BCHE) and the no. of alternatively spliced mRNA transcripts they express into (3 for ACHE, 1 for BCHE). Yet, the length of the open reading frames (dotted underlines) is rather similar for all of these variants.

Cross-species tolerance of excessive ChE activities suggests the existence of adjustment mechanism(s) which may restore balanced cholinergic functioning under conditions of imbalance. While *Xenopus* tadpoles should be most useful to search for such mechanisms as they operate in early vertebrate embryogenesis, the transgenic mouse model can shed new light on the adjustment mechanisms operating in the mammalian brain.

ACKNOWLEDGEMENTS

The research from our laboratory reviewed here was supported by grants from the U.S. Army Medical Research and Development Command and the Israel Basic Research Fund (to H.S). C.A. received an INSERM fellowship.

REFERENCES

Andres C, Beeri R, Lev-Lehman E, Timberg R, Shani M and Soreq H (1994): Transgenic overexpression of human acetylcholinesterase in mouse brain. *J Neurochem (Abst. Suppl.)* (In Press).

Beeri R, Gnatt A, Lapidot-Lifson Y, Ginzberg D, Shani M, Zakut H and Soreq H (1994): Testicular amplification and impaired transmission of human butyrylcholinesterase cDNA in transgenic mice. *Human Reprod* (In Press).

Ben Aziz-Aloya R, Seidman S, Timberg R, Sternfeld M, Zakut H and Soreq H (1993): Expression of a human acetylcholinesterase promoter-reporter construct in developing neuromuscular junctions of *Xenopus* embryos. *Proc Natl Acad Sci (USA)* 90:2471-2475.

Ehrlich G, Ginzberg D, Loewenstein Y, Glick D, Kerem B, Ben-Ari S, Zakut H, Soreq H (1994): Population diversity and distinct haplotype frequencies associated with ACHE and BCHE genes of Israeli Jews from Trans-Caucasian Georgia and from Europe. *Genomics* (In Press).

Harding AE (1992): Molecular genetics and clinical aspects of inherited disorders of nerve and muscle. *Curr Opin Neurol Neurosurg* 5:600-604.

Karpel R, Ben Aziz-Aloya R, Sternfeld M, Ehrlich G, Ginzberg D, Tarroni P, Clementi F, Zakut H and Soreq H (1994): Expression of 3 alternative acetylcholinesterase messenger RNAs in human tumor cell lines of different tissue origins. *Exptl Cell Res* 210:268-277.

Loewenstein Y, Gnatt A, Neville LF and Soreq H (1993): A chimeric human cholinesterase: identification of interaction sites responsible for sensitivity to acetyl or butyrylcholinesterase-specific ligands. *J Mol Biol* 238:289-296.

Neville LF, Gnatt A, Loewenstein Y, Seidman S, Ehrlich G and Soreq H (1992): Intramolecular relationships in cholinesterases revealed by oocyte expression of site-directed and natural variants of human BCHE. *EMBO J* 11:1641-1649.

Seidman S, Ben-Aziz Aloya R, Timberg R, Loewenstein Y, Velan B, Shafferman A, Liao J, Norgaard-Pedersen B, Brodbeck U and Soreq H (1994): Overexpression of human acetylcholinesterase monomers induces subtle ultrastructural modifications in *Xenopus laevis* neuromuscular junctions. *J Neurochem* (In Press).

Shapira M, Seidman S, Sternfeld M, Timberg R, Kaufer D, Patrick JW and Soreq H (1994): Transgenic engineering of neuromuscular junctions in *Xenopus laevis* embryos transiently overexpressing key cholinergic proteins. (Submitted).

Soreq H and Zakut H (1993): Human cholinesterases and anti-cholinesterases. San Diego: Academic Press, pp. 1-314.

Wurtman RJ (1992): Choline metabolism as a basis for the selective vulnerability of cholinergic neurons. *Trends in Neurosci* 5:117-122.

Alzheimer Disease: Therapeutic Strategies
edited by E. Giacobini and R. Becker.
© 1994 Birkhäuser Boston

STRUCTURE-FUNCTION RELATIONSHIPS IN THE BINDING OF REVERSIBLE INHIBITORS IN THE ACTIVE-SITE GORGE OF ACETYLCHOLINESTERASE

I. Silman[†], M. Harel[*], J. Eichler[†] and J.L. Sussman[*]
Departments of [†]Neurobiology and [*]Structural Biology,
The Weizmann Institute of Science, Rehovot 76100, Israel

A. Anselmet and J. Massoulié
Laboratoire de Neurobiologie, Ecole Normale Supérieure, Paris 75230, France

INTRODUCTION

Acetylcholinesterase (AChE) terminates transmission at cholinergic synapses by rapid hydrolysis of acetylcholine (ACh) (Quinn, 1987). Anti-cholinesterase agents are used in treatment of various disorders (Taylor, 1990), and have been proposed as therapeutic agents for managing Alzheimer's disease (AD) (Becker and Giacobini, 1991). The AChE active site contains a catalytic subsite and a so-called 'anionic' subsite, which binds the quaternary group of ACh (Quinn, 1987). A second, 'peripheral' anionic site is so named since it is distant from the active site (Taylor and Lappi, 1975). Bisquaternary AChE inhibitors derive their enhanced potency, relative to homologous monoquaternary ligands (Main, 1976), from their ability to span these two 'anionic' sites, which are *ca.* 14 Å apart.

The 3D structure of *Torpedo* AChE reveals that, like other serine hydrolases, it contains a catalytic triad at the bottom of a deep and narrow cavity (Sussman et al., 1991) named the 'aromatic gorge', since >50% of its lining is composed of the rings of 14 conserved aromatic amino acids (Sussman et al., 1991; Axelsen et al., 1994). Docking studies indicate that the quaternary group of ACh at the active site interacts with the indole of conserved Trp84 (Sussman et al., 1991), in agreement with affinity labeling (Weise et al., 1990).

X-ray crystallography of drug-AChE complexes can show which residues are important for ligand binding, this being crucial for structure-based drug design. Valuable information is also obtained by site-directed mutagenesis (Harel et al., 1992), or by utilizing natural mutations in which certain amino acid residues display species variation. We here present X-ray data showing the structures of complexes of AChE with three drugs, and a comparative study of inhibition of *Torpedo* and chicken AChE by various ligands (Eichler et al., 1994), which exploits the fact that chicken AChE lacks two aromatic residues within the 'peripheral' anionic site involved in binding of quaternary ligands by *Torpedo* AChE (Anselmet et al., in preparation).

RESULTS AND DISCUSSION

Crystalline complexes were obtained by soaking three ligands into native AChE crystals. These ligands were: decamethonium (DECA), a bisquaternary ligand which is both a neuromuscular blocker and an anti-cholinesterase; edrophonium (EDR), a powerful competitive AChE inhibitor (Wilson and Quan, 1958), which acts peripherally (Taylor, 1990); and tacrine (THA), also a potent inhibitor (Heilbronn, 1961), a promising candidate for treating AD (Gauthier and Gauthier, 1991).

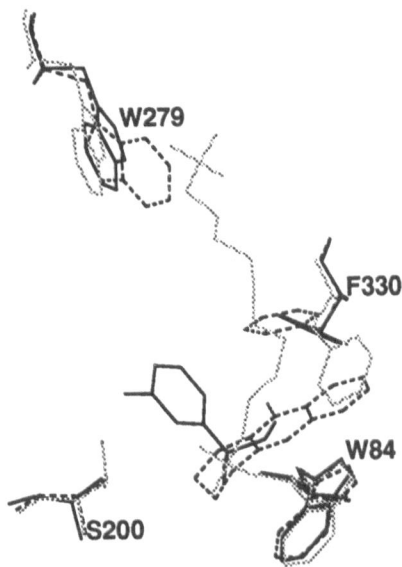

FIGURE 1. Superimposed representations of the conserved aromatics and the inhibitor molecules in the refined structures of DECA-AChE (gray), EDR-AChE (bold) and THA-AChE (dash).

Figure 1 shows the orientation of all three ligands, within the 'aromatic gorge', with respect to some important aromatic residues. The active-site-serine, Ser200, is also shown. Crystals of the AChE-DECA complex display an elongated electron density in the gorge consistent with that expected for DECA. Apart from space adequate to accommodate five or six waters, DECA defines and fills the gorge. Both its quaternary groups are in van der Waals contact with tryptophan indoles; one with that of Trp84, at the base of the gorge, and the other with that of Trp279, *ca.* 12 Å distant, near the top. The crystallographic data thus identify the 'peripheral' anionic site as being at the top of the gorge, and indicate that here, too, an aromatic group, in this case the indole of Trp279, is an important component of the binding site.

In the EDR complex, the quaternary group assumes a position adjacent to the Trp84 indole virtually equivalent to that of the proximal quaternary group of DECA. Trp84 is covalently labeled by aziridinium, which is similar in structure to EDR (Weise et al., 1990). Thus, there is good correspondence between the crystal structure and that in solution. The m-hydroxyl group of EDR makes hydrogen bonds with His440N$^{\varepsilon2}$ and Ser200O$^{\gamma}$. This provides a structural basis for the observation that $meta$-substituted anilinium ions are much more potent AChE inhibitors than the homologous ligand lacking the hydroxyl (Wilson and Quan, 1958).

In the THA-AChE complex, THA is stacked against the indole of Trp84. This agrees with the observation that N-methylacridinium forms a charge-transfer complex with a tryptophan in the active site (Shinitzky et al., 1973).

The overall conformations of AChE in the three complexes are similar to that of native AChE. In all three, only Phe330 undergoes conspicuous conformational change (Fig. 1). In DECA-AChE it lies parallel to the methylene chain of DECA, and thus to the gorge axis. In EDR-AChE, it is slightly rotated, and contacts the ethyl substituent of EDR. In THA-AChE, the Phe330 ring is rotated to lie parallel to and in contact with THA, which is thus sandwiched between the rings of Phe330 and Trp84. The direct involvement of Phe330 in binding these ligands is in excellent agreement with photoaffinity labeling experiments in solution (Schalk et al., 1992; Harel et al., 1993). The differences in orientation of Phe330 in the different complexes must be taken into account in designing novel anti-cholinesterase drugs. Trp279 also undergoes affinity labeling (Harel et al., 1993; Schalk et al., 1994). Here, too, the solution studies agree with the crystallographic data showing the distal quaternary group of DECA contacts the Trp279 indole.

Sequencing of the cDNA for chicken AChE (Anselmet et al., in preparation), shows that it lacks two aromatic residues of the gorge, which are conserved in $Torpedo$ and mammalian AChEs, but absent in butyrylcholinesterase (BChE) (Harel et al., 1992). These two residues are Trp279 and Tyr70, both near the top of the gorge. Propidium, and d-tubocurarine, typical 'peripheral' site inhibitors, inhibit chicken AChE much more weakly than $Torpedo$ AChE (Eichler et al., 1994). In contrast, EDR inhibits $Torpedo$ and chicken AChE very similarly. DECA has a K_i for chicken AChE $ca.$ 70-fold higher than for $Torpedo$ AChE; and BW284c51, another bisquaternary compound, used to inhibit AChE selectively in the presence of BChE (Austin and Berry, 1953), inhibits chicken AChE $> 10^2$ more poorly than $Torpedo$ AChE. However, hexamethonium (HEXA), a DECA analog in which only 6 methylenes separate the quaternary groups, as compared to 10 in DECA, inhibits AChE from the two species very similarly. Crystallographic data for both DECA [see Figs. 1 and 2 (left)] and BW284c51 (Harel et al., in preparation) show that both bisquaternary ligands span the gorge; their affinity is apparently reduced by the absence of Trp279 and Tyr70 from chicken AChE. Docking of HEXA shows that if one of its quaternary groups is bound to the 'anionic' subsite of the active site, the other will not be in contact with either of these two aromatics in *Torpedo* AChE [Fig. 2 (right)]; their absence in chicken AChE should not affect its capacity to bind HEXA, as the kinetic data confirm. The comparative studies on chicken and *Torpedo* AChE are in good agreement with site-directed mutagenesis data (Harel et al., 1992; Vellom et al., 1993).

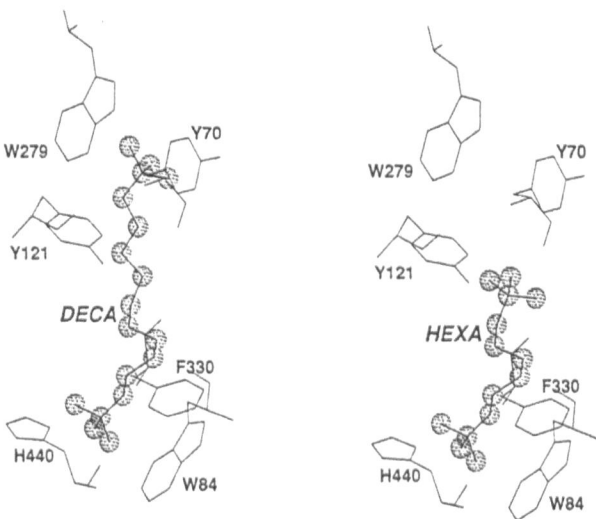

FIGURE 2. Representations of decamethonium (DECA, left) and of hexamethonium (HEXA, right) in the active site gorge of AChE. The DECA-AChE structure represents a portion of the crystal structure, whereas the HEXA-AChE model was constructed on the basis of the DECA-AChE structure (cf. Eichler et al., 1994).

Growing evidence implicates π electrons of aromatic residues in polar interactions within proteins (Sussman and Silman, 1992). Moreover theoretical considerations (Dougherty and Stauffer, 1990) invoke aromatic groups as a general feature of quaternary-ligand-binding sites. Our data clearly implicate aromatic residues in binding quaternary ligands both at the 'anionic' subsite of the active site and at the 'peripheral' site. These assignments should be invaluable in designing drugs targeted to the active site of AChE. Electrostatic calculations indicate that AChE has a strong electrostatic dipole aligned with the aromatic gorge (Ripoll et al., 1993). A positively charged substrate will be drawn towards the active site by the electrostatic field. Within the gorge, the aromatic groups appear to shield substrate from direct interaction with the negatively charged residues giving rise to the dipole. The affinity of quaternary ammonium compounds for aromatic rings, coupled with field, may work in concert to create a selective and efficient substrate-binding site in AChE, thus explaining why the active site is near the bottom of a deep gorge lined with aromatic rings.

ACKNOWLEDGEMENTS

This work was supported by the U.S. Army Medical Research and Development Command Contract DAMD17-89-C-9063, the Kimmelman Center and the Minerva Foundation.

REFERENCES

Austin L and Berry WK (1953): *Biochem J* 54:695-700.

Axelsen PH, Harel M, Silman I and Sussman JL (1994): *Protein Sci* 3:188-197.

Becker R and Giacobini E (1991): *Cholinergic Basis for Alzheimer Therapy*, Boston: Birkhäuser.

Dougherty DA and Stauffer DA (1990): *Science* 250:1558-1560.

Eichler J, Anselmet A, Sussman JL, Massoulié J and Silman I (1994): *Mol Pharmacol* 45:335-340.

Gauthier S and Gauthier L (1991): In: *Cholinergic Basis for Alzheimer Therapy*, Becker R and Giacobini E, eds. Boston: Birkhäuser, pp. 224-230.

Harel M, Sussman JL, Krejci E, Bon S, Chanal P, Massoulié J and Silman I (1992): *Proc Natl Acad Sci USA* 89:10827-10831.

Harel M, Schalk I, Ehret-Sabatier L, Bouet F, Goeldner M, Hirth C, Axelsen PH, Silman I and Sussman JL (1993): *Proc Natl Acad Sci USA* 90:9031-9035.

Heilbronn E (1961): *Acta Chem Scand* 15:1386-1390.

Main AR (1976): In: *Biology of Cholinergic Function*, Goldberg AM and Hanin I, eds. New York: Raven, pp. 269-353.

Quinn DM (1987): *Chem Rev* 87:955-979.

Ripoll DR, Faerman CH, Axelsen PH, Silman I and Sussman JL (1993): *Proc Natl Acad Sci USA* 90:5128-5132.

Schalk I, Ehret-Sabatier L, Bouet F, Goeldner M and Hirth C (1992): In: *Multidisciplinary Approaches to Cholinesterase Functions*, Shafferman A and Velan B, eds. New York: Plenum Press, pp. 121-130.

Schalk I, Ehret-Sabatier L, Bouet F, Goeldner M and Hirth C (1994): *Eur J Biochem* 219:155-159.

Shinitzky M, Dudai Y and Silman I (1973): *FEBS Lett* 30:125-128.

Sussman JL and Silman I (1992): *Current Opinion Structural Biol* 2:721-729.

Sussman JL, Harel M, Frolow F, Oefner C, Goldman A, Toker L and Silman I (1991): *Science* 253:872-879.

Taylor P (1990): In: *The Pharmacological Basis of Therapeutics*, 8th Ed., Gilman A, Rall TW, Nies A and Taylor P, eds. New York: Pergamon, pp. 131-149.

Taylor P and Lappi S (1975): *Biochemistry* 14:1989-1997.

Vellom DC, Radic Z, Li N, Pickering NA, Camp S and Taylor P (1993): *Biochemistry* 32:12-17.

Weise C, Kreienkamp HJ, Raba R, Pedak A, Aaviksaar A and Hucho F (1990): *EMBO J* 9:3885-3888.

Wilson IB and Quan C (1958): *Arch Biochem Biophys* 73:131-143.

Zaimis E and Head S (1976): In: *Handbuch der Experimentellen Pharmakologie*, *Vol. 42*, Zaimis E, ed. Berlin: Springer, pp. 365-419.

Alzheimer Disease: Therapeutic Strategies
edited by E. Giacobini and R. Becker.
© 1994 Birkhäuser Boston

CHOLINERGIC CHANGES AND SYNAPTIC ALTERATIONS IN ALZHEIMER'S DISEASE

Steven T. DeKosky, Scot D. Styren and Mark E. O'Malley
University of Pittsburgh ADRC and Western Psychiatric Institute and Clinic, 3811 O'Hara Street, Pittsburgh PA 15213

INTRODUCTION

The cholinergic deficit in Alzheimer's disease (AD) brain has given rise to numerous pharmacological strategies designed to enhance cholinergic metabolism and efficacy and improve cognition. Although the cholinergic system is important to cognition we know that correlations between cortical cholinergic function and level of cognition are relatively weak (DeKosky and Scheff, 1990). Synapse loss is more robustly linked to decline in cognition (DeKosky and Scheff, 1990; Terry et al., 1991; DeKosky et al., 1992). Ultrastructural assessment of cortical biopsy samples from AD patients showed a strong correlation with cognition (DeKosky and Scheff, 1990). Confocal immunohistochemical examination of postmortem brain confirmed this correlation between synapse loss and (antemortem) measurements of cognition (Terry et al., 1991). Thus, therapeutic strategies must consider both cholinergic status and the degree of synaptic loss in AD brain.

Both presynaptic and postsynaptic measures indicate enlargement of residual synapses in AD (Scheff et al., 1990; DeKosky and Scheff, 1990; Masliah et al., 1991). Antibodies to synaptophysin, a 38 kDa synaptic vesicle membrane protein, have enabled immunohistochemical quantification of synapses (for review see Thiel, 1993). Synaptophysin antibodies have been used to examine synaptic changes in experimental paradigms and neurodegenerative diseases (for review see Masliah and Terry, 1993). We wished to see if homogenate assays would reflect the synapse changes demonstrated by ultrastructural and confocal microscopic studies. Would the compensatory enlargement of synapses observed in AD cortex (Fig. 1) (Scheff et al., 1990) mask synapse loss if analyzed by ELISA? If so, homogenates might underestimate the synapse loss observed by ultrastructural and confocal analyses. Our ELISA methodology reliably assesses synaptophysin in normal and AD brain, and we have assessed synapse loss in AD cortex by this method.

Normal   Alzheimer's Disease

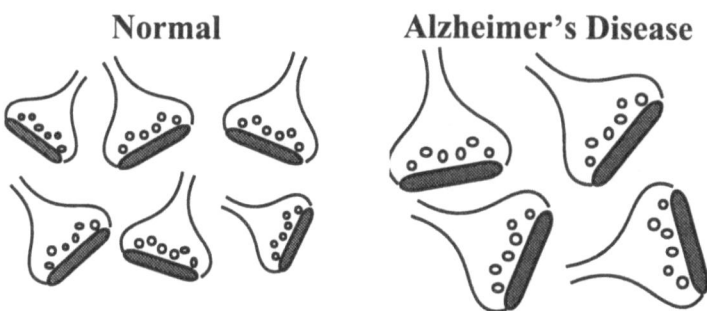

FIGURE 1. Graphical representation of cortical synapse loss and compensatory enlargement in Alzheimer's disease.

MATERIALS AND METHODS

Patients
Tissue from 30 AD (75.7 $\pm$ 1.43 yr) and 8 neurologically normal (70.25 $\pm$ 2.21 yr) patients was obtained at autopsy through the Alzheimer's Disease Research Center at the University of Pittsburgh. Tissue samples from middle frontal and temporal cortex were stored at -70°C prior to examination.

ELISA Analysis
Brain homogenates were prepared by sonication; samples were diluted to 50 μg/ml and stored at -70°C. Triplicate 50 μl samples were aliquoted into 96-well plates. To monitor intra- and interassay variability, a dilution curve (0-10 μg/well) consisting of a pooled tissue homogenate of cerebellum (AD/control, n=3/group) was co-incubated with frontal and temporal cortices. Samples were dried and blocked with 5% non-fat dry milk. SY38 (Boehringer Mannheim, Indianapolis, IN) was added to each well, and plates incubated at 4°C overnight. The next day, wells were rinsed and alkaline-phosphatase conjugated sheep anti-mouse IgG (Organon Teknika, Durham, NC) was added to each well (two hours at 22°C). Plates were rinsed and incubated for one hour with substrate [2.23 mg p-nitrophenyl phosphate/ml glycine buffer (pH 10.4)]. Sample (100 μl) was removed and read at 410 nm on a plate reader.

Statistical Analysis
Mean optical density (OD) values were assessed by analysis of variance (ANOVA) in each brain region.

RESULTS

All assays were performed with samples from each brain region run at the same time and on the same plate. Cerebellar tissue was run as a standard. Interassay correlation was 0.799.

BRAIN REGION	n (AD, CTL)	% loss of SY38
middle frontal	(25,5)	30.55 *
middle temporal	(29,8)	18.72 *

TABLE I. Percent loss of synaptophysin relative to controls in affected cortical regions in Alzheimer's disease (* p < 0.002).

Middle Frontal Cortex

Analysis revealed significant differences between AD and control samples (p = 0.0013; Table I). Optical density values for control samples (n=5) were 0.599 ± 0.054 (mean ± SEM). Alzheimer disease samples (n=25) had values of 0.416 ± 0.021. There were no significant correlations between OD and patient age, brain weight, or post mortem interval.

Middle Temporal Cortex

Comparison of OD values from AD and control revealed highly significant differences (p = 0.0001; Table I). There were no significant correlations between OD and age or brain weight. Postmortem interval and O.D. revealed a significant correlation (p=0.0335).

DISCUSSION

There is significant decline in synaptophysin protein in AD cortex. This overall reduction in synaptic integrity as assessed by ELISA, is in agreement with our ultrastructural observations (DeKosky and Scheff, 1990; Scheff et al., 1990; Scheff and Price, 1993), and previous confocal (Masliah et al., 1991) and homogenate assessments of synaptic loss in AD (Honer et al., 1992; Alford et al., 1994). While this new ELISA analysis of synaptophysin is a readily applied, reliable technique, some caveats must be considered. Affected and less affected cortical lamina are mixed together. White matter must be excluded during dissection to prevent dilution of synaptophysin protein. There is no "standard" for synaptophysin, therefore pooled brain homogenates must be employed as described above.

The significance of dynamic changes in synaptic structure and efficacy remain unclear. Why do the remaining synapses in cortex, but not hippocampus, increase in volume? Is synaptic efficacy enhanced by increasing synaptic contact area? Can synaptic connections, including cholinergic synapses, be stabilized and if so, would that slow the onset or severity of symptoms in AD? The neuropharmacologic efforts to enhance and preserve neurotransmitter function must be supported by efforts to slow synapse loss and neuronal death, maintaining the substrate on which neurotransmitter function takes place.

REFERENCES

Alford MF, Masliah E, Hansen LA and Terry RD (1994): A simple dot-immunobinding assay for quantification of synaptophysin-like immunoreactivity in human brain. *J Histochem Cytochem* 42:283-287.

DeKosky ST and Scheff SW (1990): Synapse loss in frontal cortex biopsies in Alzheimer's disease: correlation with cognitive severity. *Ann Neurol* 27:457-464.

DeKosky ST, Harbaugh RE, Schmitt FA, Bakay RE, Chui HC, Knopman DS et al. (1992): Cortical biopsy in Alzheimer's disease: diagnostic accuracy and neurochemical, neuropathological and cognitive correlations. *Ann Neurol* 32:625-632.

Honer WG, Dickson DW, Gleeson J and Davies P (1992): Regional synaptic pathology in Alzheimer's disease. *Neurobiol Aging* 13:375-382.

Masliah E and Terry R (1993): The role of synaptic proteins in the pathogenesis of disorders of the CNS. *Brain Path* 3:77-85.

Masliah E, Terry RD, Alford M, DeTeresa R and Hansen LA (1991): Cortical and subcortical patterns of synaptophysin-like immunoreactivity in Alzheimer's disease. *Amer J Pathology* 138:235-246.

Scheff SW and Price DA (1993): Synapse Loss in the temporal lobe in Alzheimer's disease. *Ann Neurol* 33:190-199.

Scheff SW, DeKosky ST and Price DA (1990): Quantitative assessment of cortical synaptic density in Alzheimer's disease. *Neurobiol Aging* 11:29-37.

Terry RD, Masliah E, Salmon DP, Butters N, De Teresa R, Hill R, Hansen LA and Katzman R (1991): Physical basis of cognitive alterations in Alzheimer's disease: synapse loss is the major correlate of cognitive impairment. *Ann Neurol* 30:572-580.

Thiel G (1993): Synapsin I, synapsin II, and synaptophysin: Marker proteins of synaptic vesicles. *Brain Path* 3:87-95.

PART IV

CHOLINESTERASE INHIBITORS IN AD TREATMENT

Alzheimer Disease: Therapeutic Strategies
edited by E. Giacobini and R. Becker.
© 1994 Birkhäuser Boston

INTRODUCTION TO CHOLINESTERASE INHIBITORS USED IN ALZHEIMER'S DISEASE THERAPY

Vinod Kumar
Department of Psychiatry, University of Miami,
300 Alton Road, Miami, FL 33140

Alzheimer's disease patients show deficits in cholinergic as well as in several other neurotransmitter and neuropeptide systems (Kumar and Calache, 1991; Kumar and Becker, 1989). Cholinergic system deficits cause decreases in: a) choline acetyltransferase; b) acetylcholinesterase (AChE) activity; c) release of and synthesis of acetylcholine (ACh); and d) presynaptic nicotine receptor binding. It is known that ACh is needed in sufficient amount for neuronal transmission. It is not possible to administer ACh directly to patients. The best approach to increase ACh has been by reducing the hydrolysis of ACh by means of cholinesterase inhibitors (ChEI).

The most studied ChEI have been physostigmine and tacrine. Physostigmine is very short acting with a half life of 30 minutes to 1 1/2 hours, while tacrine has a comparatively longer half life of about 3 hours. Both of these drugs have shown limited efficacy and serious cardiovascular and gastrointestinal side effects. Tacrine has been approved by the U.S. Food and Drug Administration in October of 1993. The approval of tacrine by the Food and Drug Administration has intensified the race among the pharmaceutical companies to introduce other ChEI into the market. There are nine to twelve ChEI being developed by various pharmaceutical companies; some of these compounds are listed in Table I.

Several chapters in this book describe basic and clinical data on some of these compounds. Available data on physostigmine, tacrine, velnacrine, E-2020 and heptylphysostigmine are not able to answer several important questions related to the development of ChEI as an anti-dementia medication. It is important to discuss these questions in depth so that we can plan further basic as well as clinical studies appropriately. These questions are:

1) <u>Do we know enough about efficacy of the ChEI?</u> Available data on physostigmine, tacrine, and velnacrine suggest that about 15-40% of AD patients show a variable degree of improvement while taking these medications (Becker and Giacobini, 1988; Kumar and Becker, 1989;

Kumar and Calache, 1991; Schneider et al., 1991; Schneider and Tariot, 1994). These improvements are mostly in the cognitive function area. Some patients show improvement also in the clinical global impression of clinicians. The results of the individual studies are discussed in the chapters on tacrine, velnacrine, E-2020, etc.

Ideally, we would need a drug which can improve both cognitive and behavioral symptoms in at least 70-80% of patients as we have seen antidepressant medication in depressive disorders. The reasons for this limited response are still unknown.

COMPOUND	COMPANY
Suronacrine HOE 427	Hoechst-Roussel
Mentane, velnacrine, HP 029	Hoechst-Roussel
Synapton sustained-release physostigmine salicylate	Forest Laboratories
Heptylphysostigmine	Mediolanum
Metrifonate	Miles Inc.
ENA 713	Sandoz
E-2020	Eisai
MDL-73,745	Marion Merrell Dow
Galanthamine	CIBA-Geigy

TABLE I. Cholinesterase Inhibitors for AD Treatment. (Modified from Schneider and Tariot, 1994)

2)   Who are the non-responders to ChEI? The exact answer to this question is not known but there are several factors which may be responsible for this very high rate (60-80%) of non-responders:

A. Alzheimer's disease (AD) is a very heterogeneous disorder. Patients are clinically, neuropathologically, and neurochemically different, and it is not surprising that all of those patients do not respond to ChEI. We need to divide AD patients according to neurochemical and possibly neuropathological characteristics while enrolling in various research protocols. The most difficult task has been to establish the markers that divide the patients into various groups that may respond to different treatments. There is a need to develop cost-effective imaging techniques to study cholinergic and adrenergic structural and functional changes in pre- and post-treatment periods.

B. Genetic heterogeneity in AD patients has drawn a great deal of attention in the past few months. We know now that at least three chromosomes (21, 19, and 14) and several genes including gene expressing ApoE (2,3,4) are involved. We do not know the effect of this genetic heterogeneity on the response to the ChEI therapy. A need exists to study enough AD patients in each genetically distinct group to reach a meaningful conclusions.

C. We may be under-treating these patients to avoid serious side effects. We should try to study the metabolites of the ChEI, their plasma levels, and activity of the AChE while developing these drugs. This approach may help us to understand the reasons why patient might not improve with ChEI. We also need to study the relationship between inhibition, clinical improvement and possibly the degree of increase in ACh in the brain. The different ChEI have a tendency to vary in their potency to increase AChE in the brain while achieving the similar AChE inhibition. Somehow we should investigate the optimum magnitude of the ACh increase or AChE inhibition to achieve the maximum improvement in cognition and behavior of AD patients.

3) What is the role of combination therapies? Cholinesterase inhibitors have been used in combination with choline, deprenyl, and yohimbine (Bierer et al., 1993; Gauthier et al., 1990; Schneider et al., 1991; Schneider and Tariot, 1994). The results seem to indicate that it is a safe strategy and there are some patients who may show an added improvement while taking deprenyl and tacrine.

However, the combination of choline and ChEI has not shown a distinctly better response compared to the response when used alone. The theoretical evidence to combine ChEI with choline is strong (Wurtman et al., 1988), but the actual results of the drug trials have been negative. As AD patients have the deficits of adrenergic, dopaminergic, and serotonergic systems, it is rational to consider various combinations. There may be a group of patients with combined deficits of these systems, requiring combination therapies.

4) What is the effect of ChEI on the decline of AD patients? This is one of the most asked questions by clinicians, researchers, and even by the patient's families. Unfortunately, we do not know the answer. There are some indications (Becker, 1994) suggesting that we should study the effect

of ChEI on the decline of AD before reaching a firm conclusion. It is important to remember that to study the decline of AD patients, one has to study these patients for a longer period of time -maybe up to one year- before being able to answer this question. The protocols have to be designed with appropriate outcome measures and sufficient number of patients to be included to achieve enough power to reach a meaningful conclusion. Some of the problems and solutions to the outcome measures and decline issues are discussed by Dr. Thal and Dr. Mohs.

CONCLUSION

Cholinesterase inhibitors are the first group of compounds showing some promise in the treatment of AD. One of the drugs, tacrine, was approved by the FDA in 1993. Several new compounds of this group are being studied at present. It would help if new and the current protocols would include some of the suggestions made in this paper. It is not difficult to do ApoE typing even in the ongoing protocols. We hope there will be more responders than non-responders to various treatments and ChEI will continue to play a role in the treatment of AD in the appreciable future.

REFERENCES

Becker RE and Giacobini E (1988): Mechanisms of cholinesterase inhibition in senile dementia of the Alzheimer type: clinical, pharmacological, and therapeutic aspects. *Drug Dev Res* 12:163-195.

Bierer LM, Aisen PS, Davidson M, Ryan TM, Stern RG, Schmeidler J and Davis KL (1993): A pilot study of oral physostigmine plus yohimbine in patients with Alzheimer disease. *Alzheimer Disease Associated Disorders* 7(2):98-104.

Gauthier S, Bouchard R, Lamontagne A et al. (1990): Tetrahydroaminoacridine-lecithin combination treatment in patients with intermediate-stage Alzheimer's disease. *New Engl J Med* 322(18):1272-1276.

Kumar V and Becker RE (1989): clinical pharmacology of tetrahydroaminoacridine: A possible therapeutic agent for Alzheimer's disease. *Intl J Pharmacol and Toxicol* 27:478-485.

Kumar V and Calache M (1991): Treatment of Alzheimer disease with cholinergic drugs. *Intl J Clin Pharmacol Ther and Toxicol* 29(1):25-37.

Schneider LS, Pollock VE, Zemansky MF et al. (1991): A pilot study of low dose L deprenyl in AD. *J Geriat Psych and Neurol* 4:143-148.

Schneider LS and Tariot PN (1994): Emerging drugs for Alzheimer's disease. Mechanisms of action and prospects for cognitive enhancing medication. In: *Medical Clinics of North America*, Eisdorfer and Olsen, eds. Philadelphia: Saunders (In Press).

Wurtman RJ, Blusztajn JK, Growdon JH and Ulus IH (1988): Cholinesterase inhibitors increase the brain's need for free choline. In: *Current Research in Alzheimer's Therapy*, Giacobini E and Becker R, eds. New York: Taylor and Francis, pp. 95-100.

Alzheimer Disease: Therapeutic Strategies
edited by E. Giacobini and R. Becker.
© 1994 Birkhäuser Boston

A PHARMACODYNAMIC STRATEGY TO OPTIMIZE THE CLINICAL RESPONSE TO EPTASTIGMINE (MF-201)

Bruno P. Imbimbo and Paolo E. Lucchelli
Medical Department, Mediolanum Farmaceutici, Milan, Italy

INTRODUCTION

Clinical results obtained over the past 20 years with acetylcholinesterase (AChE) inhibitors in Alzheimer's disease (AD) have been contradictory. This is mainly due to the short duration of action and poor systemic tolerability of current drugs. A further open issue is that the ideal AChE inhibition level (peripheral or central) to be reached in AD patients is unknown.

Eptastigmine is a highly lipophilic AChE inhibitor. The drug is less toxic in rodents than physostigmine at corresponding levels of AChE inhibition (Brufani et al., 1986). Studies in rodents have shown that eptastigmine enters the brain readily and produces long-lasting inhibition of AChE (DeSarno et al., 1989). Studies in monkeys have shown a good correlation between peripheral (red blood cells) and central (cerebrospinal fluid) AChE inhibition induced by the drug (Rupniak et al., 1992). Studies in animals have identified AChE inhibition thresholds for both toxicity and activity on cognitive and behavioral performance (Dawson et al., 1991). Although animal toxicity thresholds correspond to those found in human studies, animal efficacy thresholds cannot be easily extended to AD patients. Thus, in order to optimize the clinical response to eptastigmine, the relationship between AChE inhibition and the corresponding cognitive and behavioral effects in the individual patient must be identified.

MATERIALS AND METHODS

Since multiple blood samplings in AD patients are problematic, both from a practical and ethical point of view, we developed an automated device that measures AChE from 10 μL capillary blood (Cazzola et al., 1993). The activity of the enzyme is measured indirectly from the changes in pH generated by the hydrolysis of acetylcholine. This non-invasive technique allows for multiple measurements of AChE activity in the individual patient and leads to a precise estimate of individual pharmacodynamic parameters (maximum, minimum and daily average AChE inhibition, recovery half-life of the enzyme, time to reach steady-state inhibition, etc.).

Studies in Young Healthy Volunteers
We investigated the relationship between the given dose and AChE inhibition, the duration of AChE inhibition and the presence or absence of acute tolerance on AChE activity. Eight young, healthy volunteers received rising single oral doses of eptastigmine (0, 10, 20 and 30 mg). Multiple blood samples were collected up to 24 h post-dose to measure AChE activity and eptastigmine plasma levels.

Studies in Alzheimer Patients
We correlated the extent of AChE inhibition with tolerability and efficacy during prolonged treatment with eptastigmine. Eighty patients were treated with eptastigmine (30-60 mg/day) and 20 with placebo for 4 weeks. Patients had the option to enter an 8-week open extension treatment with eptastigmine at the end of the 4-week double-blind phase. At least 16 AChE measurements were performed in each patient. Individual pharmacodynamic parameters were estimated by modeling the AChE values with a bi-exponential equation.

RESULTS

Studies in Healthy Volunteers
Eptastigmine plasma concentrations increased proportionally with the dose. The inhibition of AChE was dose-dependent and long-lasting (Fig. 1).

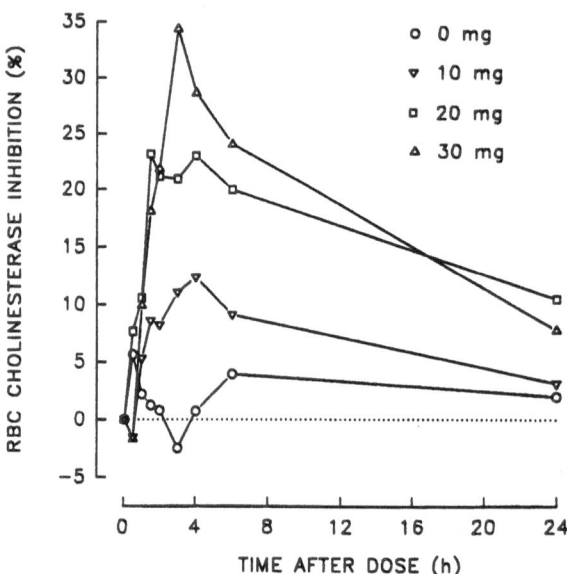

FIGURE 1. Dose-response effect of eptastigmine on AChE in healthy volunteers.

AChE inhibition and drug plasma levels were related over time with a counter-clockwise hysteresis curve indicating a formation of active metabolites and/or a slow association to and dissociation from the compound to the enzyme in red blood cells.

Studies in Alzheimer Patients

Peak AChE inhibition generally occurred after 2-4 h from drug ingestion. After the first dose, the maximum mean ($\pm$ SEM) inhibition of the enzyme was 33 $\pm$ 2%. At steady-state, the mean of individual maximum values of AChE inhibition was 55 $\pm$ 1% and was reached after 3.7 $\pm$ 0.7 days (Fig. 2).

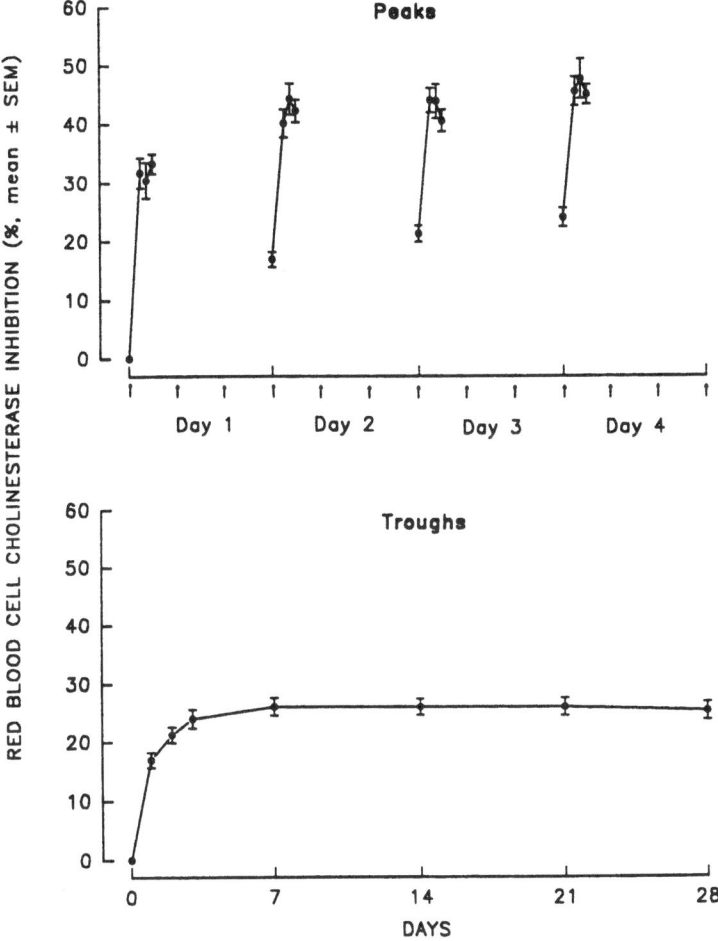

FIGURE 2. Peak and trough AChE inhibitions measured in 80 Alzheimer patients receiving eptastigmine (30-60 mg/day) for 4 weeks.

Trough inhibition of AChE activity increased during the first four days of treatment, reaching a mean value of 24 $\pm$ 2% at Day 4. This value remained constant throughout the study period (25 ± 2% at Day 29). The average daily AChE inhibition (area under the AChE inhibition divided by dose interval) at steady-state was 38 ± 1%. Mean recovery half-life of enzyme activity was 7.4 ± 0.8 h. Trough levels of AChE inhibition measured in the 36 patients who entered the open extension phase with eptastigmine remained around 25% for the entire 12-week study period. There was a significant linear relationship between the dose per body weight and AChE inhibition at 4 h (r=0.810) or at steady-state (r=0.881). Cholinergic adverse events occurred in 19 patients treated with eptastigmine and were generally associated to peak AChE inhibition exceeding 50% after the first dose or 70% at steady-state. At Day 29, 34% of patients on eptastigmine versus 0% on placebo improved according to Physician Clinical Global Impression of Change, a seven-point scale from "very much improved" to "very much worse" (p=0.006). This percentage increased to 46% in a subgroup of patients with average daily AChE inhibition ranging from 25-35% (Fig. 3). Performances on Logical Memory, Semantic Word Fluency and Trail Making tests improved with an inverted U-shaped relation to average steady-state AChE inhibition.

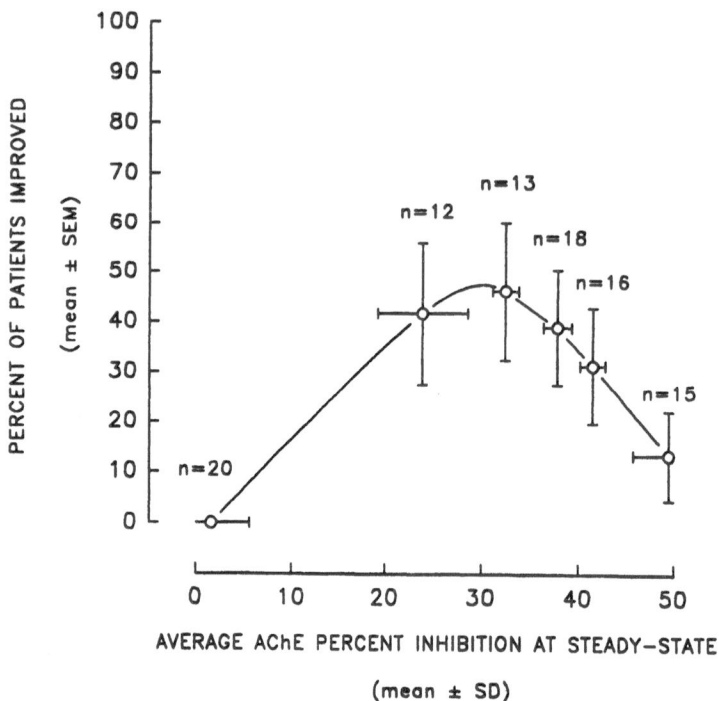

FIGURE 3. Relationship between average AChE inhibition at steady-state and Physician Clinical Global Impression of Change in 94 Alzheimer patients treated with eptastigmine (30-60 mg/day, n=74) or placebo (n=20) for 4 weeks.

CONCLUSIONS

Studies in healthy volunteers indicate that, after oral administration, eptastigmine is absorbed linearly, produces a dose-dependent, long-lasting inhibition of AChE without developing acute tolerance. The drug undergoes a significant first-pass effect with the formation of active metabolites which are responsible for the prolonged duration of action of the drug.

Studies in AD patients indicate that moderate steady-state AChE inhibition is associated to maximal cognitive and clinical improvement with eptastigmine. These studies support previously reported hypotheses (Peters et al., 1977; Mohs et al., 1985; Becker et al., 1991) that an inverted U-shaped dose-response curve is likely for AChE inhibitors in AD patients, with no effect at low doses, improvement at moderate doses and impairment at higher doses.

The long duration of action of eptastigmine, its predictable pharmacodynamic activity and the simple method for individual pharmacodynamic monitoring may maximize the clinical response to this drug in the treatment of AD patients.

REFERENCES

Becker RE, Moriearty P and Unni L (1991): The second generation of cholinesterase inhibitors: clinical and pharmacological effects. In: *Cholinergic Basis for Alzheimer Therapy*, Becker R and Giacobini E, eds. Boston: Birkhauser, pp. 211-215.

Brufani M, Marta M and Pomponi M (1986): Anticholinesterase activity of a new carbamate, heptylphysostigmine, in view of its use in patients with Alzheimer-type dementia. *Eur J Biochem* 157:115-120.

Cazzola E, Lattuada N, Zecca L, Radice D, Luzzana M, Imbimbo BP, Auteri A and Mosca A (1993): Rapid potentiometric determination of cholinesterases in plasma and red cells: application to eptastigmine monitoring. *Chem Biol Interact* 87:265-268.

Dawson GR, Bentley G, Draper F, Rycroft W, Iversen SD and Pagella PG (1991): The behavioral effects of heptyl-physostigmine, a new cholinesterase inhibitor, in tests of long-term and working memory in rodents. *Pharmacol Biochem Behav* 39:865-871.

De Sarno P, Pomponi M, Giacobini E, Tang XC and Williams E (1989): The effect of heptyl-physostigmine, a new cholinesterase inhibitor, on the central cholinergic system of the rat. *Neurochem Res* 14:971-977.

Peters BH and Levin HS (1977): Memory enhancement after physostigmine treatment in the amnesic syndrome. *Arch Neurol* 34:215-219.

Rupniak NMJ, Tye SJ, Brazell C, Heald A, Iversen SD and Pagella PG (1992): Reversal of cognitive impairment by heptylphysostigmine, a long lasting cholinesterase inhibitor, in primates. *J Neurol Sci* 107:246-249.

Mohs RC, Davis BM, Johns CA, Mathe AA, Greenwald BS, Horvath TB and Davis K (1985): Oral physostigmine treatment of patients with Alzheimer's disease. *Am J Psychiatry* 142:28-33.

Alzheimer Disease: Therapeutic Strategies
edited by E. Giacobini and R. Becker.
© 1994 Birkhäuser Boston

EPTASTIGMINE (MF-201).
A DOUBLE-BLIND, PLACEBO-CONTROLLED,
CLINICAL TRIAL IN ALZHEIMER DISEASE PATIENTS

Nicola Canal, Massimo Franceschi and the Italian Eptastigmine Investigators*
Neurology Department, Milan University School of Medicine, Scientific Institute, H. S. Raffaele, Milan, Italy

INTRODUCTION

Cholinergic drugs have a well established role in the symptomatic treatment of patients with Alzheimer's disease (AD) (Becker et al., 1991). The most extensively studied cholinergic compounds are anticholinesterase agents such as physostigmine and tacrine.

Eptastigmine (heptyl-physostigmine tartrate, MF-201) is a new anticholinesterase drug derived from physostigmine with a carbamoyl-heptyl group in position 5 of the indole ring (Brufani et al., 1986). Compared to previous anticholinesterase drugs, eptastigmine has a longer duration of action both in brain and red blood cells (RBC) and lower cholinomimetic or hepatic toxicity. Phase I studies have demonstrated that eptastigmine has good cholinergic tolerability in healthy volunteers. However, Phase II studies employing high doses of the drug (up to 120 mg/day) have revealed reversible neutropenia in two patients with AD.

In order to better define the tolerability and safety profile of eptastigmine in AD patients, a double-blind, placebo-controlled, parallel group, multicenter study was carried out. The pharmacokinetics, pharmacodynamics and preliminary efficacy of the drug were also evaluated.

---

* Sirio Bassi, Cinisello Balsamo; Carlo A. De Fanti, Bergamo; Francesco Erminio, Milan; Cesare Fieschi, Rome; Ludovico Frattola, Monza; Angelo Mamoli, Bergamo; Stelio Marforio, Como; Remigio Montanini, Gallarate; David Zerbi, Milan.

METHODS

Study Design

One-hundred patients were randomized to receive eptastigmine or placebo according to a double-blind, parallel group design. Patients with body weight ≤ 65 kg were given eptastigmine 20 mg b.i.d. or placebo b.i.d. and patients with body weight > 65 kg were randomized to eptastigmine 20 mg t.i.d. or placebo t.i.d. Treatment assignment was unbalanced, eptastigmine and placebo being given at a ratio of 4:1. Thus, 80 patients received eptastigmine and 20 received placebo.

Patients were hospitalized from Study Day -1 through Study Day 4 and were monitored daily for vital signs and white blood cell (WBC) count. At Day 5 patients continued treatment at home where the test drug was administered by a responsible caregiver. Patients returned to the clinic at Days 8, 15, 22 and 29 during treatment and at follow-up (Day 36) for WBC count and laboratory safety tests.

Red blood cell cholinesterase was measured from 10 μL capillary blood with an automated device at each center at baseline (Day -1), at Days 1, 4, 8, 15, 22 and 29 during treatment and at follow-up (Day 36). Blood specimens for drug level assays were collected at baseline (Day -1), at Days 1, 4, 8, 15, 22 and 29 during treatment and at follow-up (Day 36).

Patients had the option to enter an 8-week open extension treatment with eptastigmine at the end of the 4-week double-blind phase.

Patients

Patients with a diagnosis of probable AD according to the definition of the National Institute of Neurological and Communicative Disorders and Stroke and the Alzheimer's Disease and Related Disorders Association (NINCDS-ADRDA) (McKhann et al., 1984) were eligible for enrollment. Exclusion criteria included severe dementia (Mini-Mental State Examination, MMSE score < 10), the absence of a responsible caregiver, neutrophil count < 2,000/μL at baseline and/or other severe medical or surgical conditions.

All centers obtained approval for the study from their local Ethics Committee. Patients and responsible caregivers gave informed consent prior to the start of the study.

Outcome Measures For Preliminary Efficacy

Although this study was primarily aimed at evaluating the safety, tolerability and pharmacokinetics of eptastigmine, simple efficacy outcome measures were employed in order to obtain preliminary data on the possible therapeutic value of the test drug in AD patients. A 7-point scale (Clinical Global Impression) was performed at Day -1 and at Day 29 to rate the severity of the disease. In addition, the Physician and Caregiver Clinical Global Impression of Change (CGIC) were recorded at Day 29 to evaluate change from baseline. The WAIS

Logical Memory Test (LMT), the Semantic Word Fluency Test (SWFT) and the Trail Making Test A (TMT-A) were administered to the patient at Day -1 and Day 29. The Index of Independence in Daily Living (ADL) and the Instrumental Activities of Daily Living Scale (IADL) were administered to the caregiver at Day -1 and at Day 29.

Changes in efficacy outcome measures from baseline were statistically analyzed with the Mann-Whitney test.

RESULTS

Ten Italian centers enrolled a total of 100 patients over a 10 month period.

The eptastigmine group included 80 patients (43 males and 37 females), with a mean age of 68 years (range 48-85), mean body weight of 64 kg (range 39-100), and a mean MMSE score of 17.5 (range 10-25). The placebo group included 20 patients (10 males and 10 females), with a mean age of 67 years (range 52-82), mean body weight of 67 kg (range 45-104) and a mean MMSE score of 16.7 (range 10-24).

Six patients from the eptastigmine group dropped out, three due to cholinergic side effects and three due to reasons unrelated to drug treatment. Twenty-two (27.5%) patients reported adverse events; of which 18 were of the cholinergic type (nausea, vomiting, faintness, bradycardia, etc.) and were associated to peak cholinesterase inhibition exceeding 50% after the first dose, or 70% at steady-state. A reversible increase in liver transaminases was observed in 9 (11%) patients on eptastigmine (only in three more than two-fold the normal value) and in 2 (10%) placebo-treated patients.

One patient (1.3%) in the eptastigmine 20 mg b.i.d. group showed asymptomatic and transient neutropenia with a neutrophil count of $1,370/\mu L$ at Day 29. This patient had a neutrophil count of 2,000 and $2,500/\mu L$ at the two baseline measurements. Since the caregiver reported a slight cognitive improvement, the patient entered the open extension phase with a weekly monitoring of WBC count. During this phase, the patient had a neutrophil count which fluctuated between 1,500 and $7,000/\mu L$.

Thirty-six patients (25 in the eptastigmine group and 11 in the placebo group) entered the 8-week open extension phase. No adverse events were observed.

Overall, according to the Physician CGIC, 25 patients (34%) improved on eptastigmine compared to no patient on placebo (p=0.006). According to the Caregiver CGIC, 33 patients (45%) improved on eptastigmine as compared to 5 patients (25%) on placebo (p=0.118). Of the 33 patients who improved on eptastigmine, 4 were judged to be "much improved".

All tests and scales showed an improvement at Day 29 in the eptastigmine group as compared to baseline. Conversely, there was a mild deterioration or no change in patients' performance on tests and scales in the placebo group (Table I). Compared to placebo, the improvement in the eptastigmine group reached statistical significance on the Physician CGIC (p=0.006, see above) and

IADL (p=0.019) scales (Table I). Patients' performance on all tests and scales improved with an inverted U-shaped relation to average steady-state RBC cholinesterase inhibition (Fig. 1). In a subgroup of 43 patients with an average daily RBC cholinesterase inhibition ranging from 25-40%, improvement on all tests and scales reached statistical significance, with the exception of the LMT. In the same subgroup, the percentage of patients improved according to the Physician CGIC increased from 34% to 46%.

	Placebo	Eptastigmine	P
Physician CGIC	4.10 (0.07)	3.68 (0.06)	0.006
Caregiver CGIC	3.75 (0.10)	3.54 (0.08)	0.180
LMT	0.15 (0.72)	1.48 (0.42)	0.157
SWFT	-0.75 (0.54)	0.65 (0.43)	0.087
TMT-A	-4.60 (5.13)	-17.00 (4.70)	0.252
ADL	0.35 (0.32)	-0.08 (0.10)	0.427
IADL	0.65 (0.40)	0.41 (0.19)	0.019

TABLE I. Changes in outcome measures (mean and S.E.M.) for preliminary efficacy at Day 29 in placebo and eptastigmine groups.

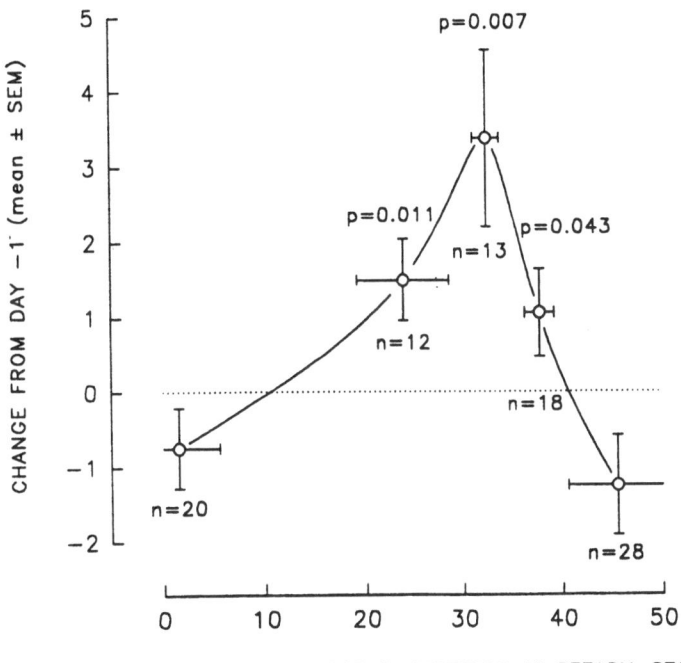

FIGURE 1. Relationship between average AChE inhibition at steady-state and Semantic Word Fluency test in 91 Alzheimer patients treated with eptastigmine (30-60 mg/day, n=71) or placebo (n=20) for 4 weeks.

CONCLUSIONS

This study shows that oral daily doses up to 60 mg eptastigmine are safe and well tolerated for up to 13 weeks.

Preliminary clinical data suggest that behavioral measures, such as Physician CGIC and IADL, are more sensitive to improvement than psychometric measures of memory (LMT), semantic fluency (SWFT) or frontal lobe functioning (TMT-A).

Moderate (25-40%) RBC cholinesterase inhibition at steady-state is associated with maximal cognitive and behavioral improvements. Higher levels of RBC cholinesterase inhibition are associated with subjective discomfort and cholinergic adverse events. Eptastigmine doses higher than 60 mg/day may also lead to excessive accumulation of unchanged drug in plasma and/or bone marrow of AD patients. This may have an inhibitory effect on granulocyte cells and consequently lead to neutropenia. The use of lower daily eptastigmine doses and frequent monitoring of WBC counts during the early stages of treatment may prevent the occurrence of neutropenia and assure a good safety profile of the drug.

Further trials are warranted to evaluate long-term clinical efficacy of eptastigmine in AD patients.

REFERENCES

Becker RE, Moriearty P and Unni L (1991): The second generation of cholinesterase in inhibitors: clinical and pharmacological effects. In: *Cholinergic Basis for Alzheimer Therapy*, Becker RE and Giacobini E, eds. Boston: Birkauser, pp. 211-215.

Brufani M, Mara M and Pomponi M (1986): Anticholinesterase activity of a new carbamate, heptylphysostigmine, in view of its use in patients with Alzheimer-type dementia. *Eur J Biochem* 157:115-120.

McKhann G, Drachman D, Folstein M, Katzman R, Price D and Stadlan E (1984): Clinical diagnosis of Alzheimer's disease: report of the NINCDS-ADRDA work group under the auspices of the Department of Health and Human Services Task Force on Alzheimer's disease. *Neurology* 34:939-944.

Alzheimer Therapy: Therapeutic Strategies
edited by E. Giacobini and R. Becker.
© *1994 Birkhäuser Boston*

COGNITION IMPROVEMENT BY ORAL HUPERZINE A: A NOVEL ACETYLCHOLINESTERASE INHIBITOR

Xi Can Tang and Zhi Qi Xiong
Department of Pharmacology, Shanghai Institute of Materia Medica,
Chinese Academy of Sciences, Shanghai 200031, China

Bo Chu Qian and Zhi Fang Zhou
Zhejiang Academy of Medical Sciences, Hangzhou 310013, China

Ci Lu Zhang
Zhejiang Jiaojiang People's Hospital, Jiaojiang 317700, China

INTRODUCTION

Alzheimer's disease (AD) is one of the most severe mental health problems commonly found in the aged population. The dementia disorders will continue to constitute a major burden upon social and medical care systems due to the mean age of the population as it continues to rise. Hence, a cure or prevention for the disease would be most desirable. Current efforts to develop an effective drug treatment for AD are in large part based upon the consistent finding that patients with this disease suffer from marked reduction of cholinergic neuronal function resulting in a deficiency in acetylcholine (ACh) concentration in the central nervous system (Whitehouse et al., 1982; Davies and Maloney, 1976; Coyle et al., 1983), and that these reductions have been associated with changes in memory (Giacobini, 1991). Of all the attempts at symptomatic therapy for AD based on the cholinergic hypotheses, studies using cholinesterase inhibitor (ChEI) has been the most encouraging up to now (Pomponi et al., 1990). Several ChEIs such as physostigmine (Phys) (Thal, 1991) and tacrine (THA) (Summers et al., 1986) have recently been the focus of extensive clinical investigation in patients who had AD (Becker and Giacobini, 1988). However, the liver toxicity with a higher dose of THA and short duration of action as well as a narrow dosing range with Phys were viewed as serious limitations to the development of these compounds as therapeutics. At present there is no therapeutic ChEI that has been shown to be both effective and safe in the treatment of AD. Thus the search for a potent, long-acting ChEI which exerts minimal side effects in the clinic for the treatment of AD is still most active.

Huperzine-A (Hup-A) was first isolated from clubmoss *Huperzia serrata* which is known as the Chinese folk medicine *Qian Chen Ta* (Liu et al., 1986). Huperzine-A, an alkaloid chemically unique from other agents under study for AD, is a reversible and mixed competitive ChEI, its potency rivals that of Phys, galanthamine (Gal) (Wang et al., 1986) and THA (DeSarno et al., 1989).

The duration of acetylcholinesterase (AChE) inhibition by a single dose of Hup-A in rats was over 6 hrs (Tang et al., 1989). Huperzine-A has been found to be an effective cognition enhancer in a number of different animal species (Tang et al., 1988; Vincent et al., 1987). Preliminary clinical trials conducted in China have indicated that intramuscular injection of Hup-A induced significant efficacy in the improvement of memory disruption in the aged and AD patients (Zhang, 1986; Zhang et al., 1991) being devoid of any remarkable side effects. In this paper, we report improving effects on cognition by oral Hup-A in rodents and in dementia patients.

RESULTS AND DISCUSSION

Effects in Rodent Behavioral Model

By using step-down passive avoidance task, effects of Hup-A, Phys, Gal and THA on learning and memory retention in mice were compared. Step-down latency was used as parameter of learning and memory retention performance (Kameyama et al., 1986). In learning trials, each dose of Hup-A (0.05-0.4 mg/kg), Phys (0.025-0.3 mg/kg), Gal (0.05-3 mg/kg) or THA (2-20 mg/kg) were orally administered 30 min before training task, respectively. The active dose on learning was 0.2-0.3 mg/kg (Hup-A), 0.05 mg/kg (Phys), 1 mg/kg (Gal) and 10-14 mg/kg (THA), respectively. Facilitation of learning performance exhibited the inverted U-shaped dose-response curve that is characteristic of known cognitive performance enhancing agents. Figure 1 shows the time course of each ChEI on learning tested with effective dosage. It is clear that Hup-A produced enhancing effect on learning lasts for up to 3 hrs. The longest enhancing effect of Hup-A was also observed in memory retention performance. Huperzine-A exhibited facilitating effect on memory retention up to 96 hrs (Table I). These results show that the effect of oral Hup-A on learning and memory retention processes are longer than those of Phys, Gal and THA.

Figure 2 shows that the amnesic action of $NaNO_2$, indicated by the reduced step-down latency, was reversed significantly by Hup-A. The improving effect of Hup-A on $NaNO_2$-induced amnesia was about 3-30 times stronger than those of Phys and Gal, respectively. The magnitude of improving effect produced by oral and intraperitoneal administration were nearly equivalent. Huperzine-A had a higher efficacy with oral route than that of Phys (Beller et al., 1985). The result coincides with previous data reported by Wang et al. (1988).

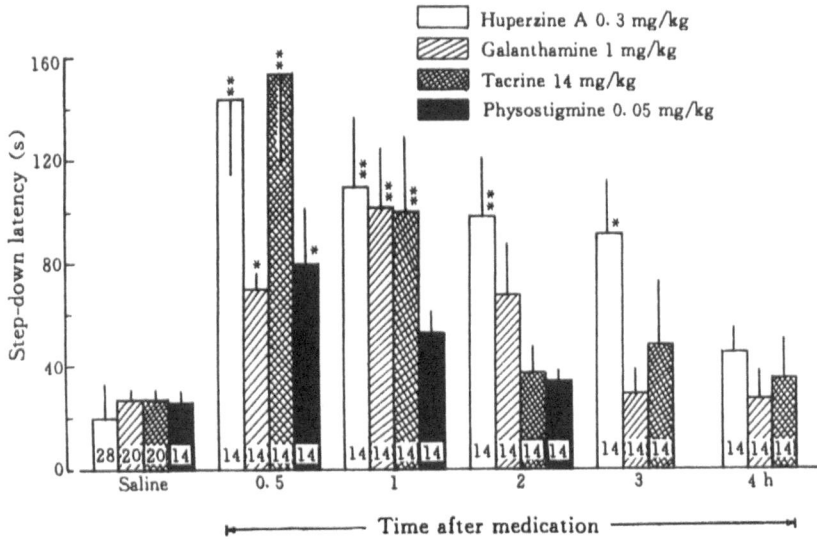

FIGURE 1. Facilitation of learning of a passive avoidance task in mice. A dose of ChEI or saline (10 ml/kg) was administered orally before training performance. Number of mice in bars. * p < 0.05; ** p < 0.01 vs saline.

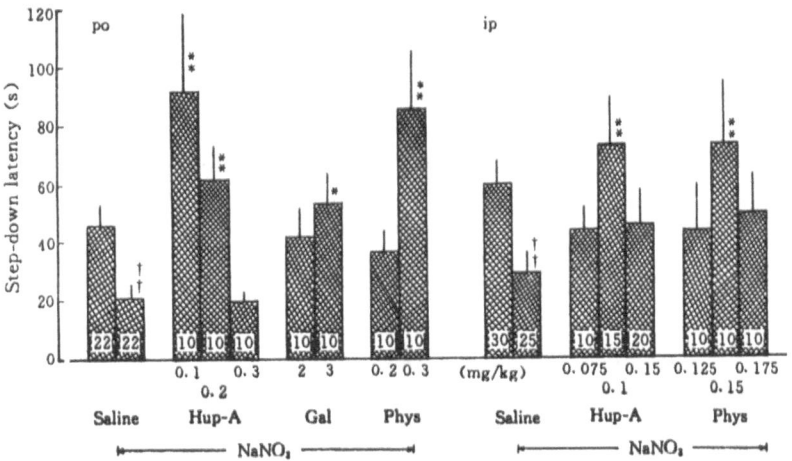

FIGURE 2. Reversal of NaNO₂-induced disruption of the retention of a passive avoidance task in mice treated with Hup-A (X ± SEM). The retention test was performed 24 hr after training. NaNO₂ (120 mg/kg, s.c.) immediately after training. Huperzine-A or saline (10 ml/kg) was administered immediately after NaNO₂. Number of mice in bars. ++ p < 0.01 vs saline. * p < 0.05; ** p < 0.01 vs saline + NaNO₂.

ChEI	Dose (mg/kg)	Step-down latency (s ± SEM)			
		24	48	72	96 (hr)
Saline	-	16.8 ± 2.5	19.2 ± 2.2	24.6 ± 3.2	22.5 ± 5.6
Hup-A	0.2	78.8 ± 16.0**	34.5 ± 5.9	67.1 ± 19.9*	50.8 ± 8.9*
Phys	0.3	66.0 ± 13.1**	22.2 ± 3.7	29.0 ± 5.2	37.5 ± 7.7
Saline	-	19.4 ± 1.6	34.3 ± 4.7	21.4 ± 19.5	37.3 ± 5.3
Gal	2.0	48.5 ± 9.9**	67.8 ± 11.8**	44.4 ± 40.1	60.6 ± 10.5
THA	16.0	44.6 ± 6.1**	70.9 ± 15.0*	31.5 ± 33.7	59.1 ± 14.0

TABLE I. Facilitation effect of ChEI on memory retention of a passive avoidance task in mice (n = 10-14). * $p < 0.05$, ** $p < 0.01$ *vs* saline. An oral dose of ChEI or saline (10 ml/kg) was administered immediately after training. The retention test was performed 24, 48, 72, or 96 hr after training.

The effect of oral Hup-A on radial maze performance was evaluated using a 4-out-of-8 baiting procedure. Rats were trained to find and eat the dustless pellet (45 mg). At the start of each session, the four predetermined arms were baited at their distal end. Each rat was placed on the platform and left until all the four baited arms were collected or 10 min had elapsed, whichever came first. Rats choice accuracy stabilized over four days. An arranged criterion of 87% or better was used in the test. Scopolamine (Scop) pretreatment produced significant increase in error numbers of reference memory (RM), working memory (WM) as well as reference and working memory (RWM). However, when Scop-treated rats were pretreated orally with Hup-A, maze performance was improved (Fig. 3). The results also showed single dose and seven multiple doses of oral Hup-A did not exhibit difference on improving the amnesia induced by Scop ($p > 0.05$). These results indicated that Hup-A can significantly reverse effects of central cholinergic impairment of spatial memory. Huperzine-A induced improving effect was as potent after chronic, as it was after acute treatment indicating that no tolerance to the drug occurred.

Effects in Human and Patients with Dementia
Phase I clinical studies of safety, tolerance and pharmacokinetics of oral Hup-A have been conducted in 22 young healthy volunteers. No significant side effects were observed at doses of 0.18-0.54 mg. Plasma levels of Hup-A determined by an HPLC method with electrochemical detector indicated that Hup-A is fairly rapidly absorbed following oral administration, with an average T_{max} of 1.27 hr. The terminal half-life is 349 min. Peak plasma levels after oral 0.99 mg dose was 8.1 ng/ml. Huperzine-A has a low plasma clearance of 14.4 L/hr and volume of distribution of 104.5 L in volunteers. Compared with THA and Phys (Hartvig et al., 1991), the terminal half-life of Hup-A was at least 4-17 times longer.

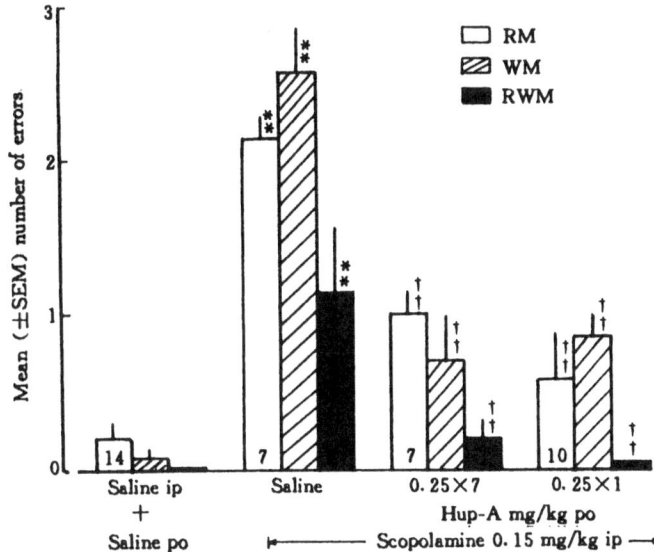

FIGURE 3. Improving effect of acute and 7 chronic administrations of Hup-A on Scop-induced amnesia on radial maze performance in rats (X ± SEM). Scopolamine and Hup-A were administered 30 min before test. Number of rats in bars. ** p < 0.01 *vs* saline + saline; ++ p < 0.01 *vs* saline + Scop.

To examine the efficacy of oral Hup-A, cognitive function was studied in a sample of 20 patients with senile dementia impairment over 2-6 years. The subjects were ten males and 10 females in the range of 50-68 years. A double-blind design was used to compare efficacy of different dose levels. Tables of 50 μg of Hup-A were given t.i.d. in three consecutive days, then three days abrupt washouts were made between next dosage. The treatment response was evaluated by Buschke Selective Reminding (BSR) task. Comparison of all rating scores from oral Hup-A and placebo show significant difference (Table II). It can also be seen from Table II that an inverted U-shaped dose-response curve in memory as measured by objective verbal memory tests was observed. The results coincide with animal results (Tang et al., 1986) and oral Phys in human (Beller et al., 1985). The improving effect of oral Hup-A on memory has about 10 times more potency compared with physostigmine. Side effects that were recorded at doses of 0.2 mg were unremarkable. The most frequently occurring side effects with Hup-A were related to the cholinergic property of the compound. Some mild side effects, i.e. dizziness, nausea and sweating occurred in a few patients at doses over 0.2 mg. During the increase in Hup-A dose up to 0.4 mg fasciculation was recorded in two of 10 patients. There was no toxicity on liver and kidney at 0.5 mg dose tested.

Phase II clinical trials are in progress.

Dosage (mg, t.i.d.)	Group n=10	Rating Scores (X ± SD)			
		ΣR	LTR	LTS	CLTR
0	C	49 ± 9	27 ± 8	37 ± 8	19 ± 5
	M	50 ± 9	28 ± 8	37 ± 8	19 ± 5
0.1	C	50 ± 9	28 ± 8	37 ± 8	18 ± 5
	M	54 ± 9	34 ± 8	40 ± 8	24 ± 5
0.15	C	49 ± 9	27 ± 8	36 ± 8	18 ± 5
	M	63 ± 9**	44 ± 8**	46 ± 9**	39 ± 6**
0.25	C	50 ± 9	27 ± 8	37 ± 8	18 ± 5
	M	74 ± 9**	68 ± 9**	69 ± 9**	60 ± 7**
0.4	C	50 ± 9	28 ± 8	37 ± 8	18 ± 5
	M	55 ± 9	37 ± 8*	47 ± 9*	41 ± 6**

TABLE II. Memory improvement by oral Hup-A in patients with senile dementia. * $p < 0.05$; ** $p < 0.01$ *vs* premedication. ΣR = ΣRecall; LTR = Long-term retrieval; LTS = Long-term storage; CLTR = consistent LTR; C = control; M = medication, double-blind measurement.

On the basis of these findings, it is reasonable to expect that oral Hup-A is a promising candidate for clinical development as second generation of anticholinesterase in the treatment of cholinergic related neurodegenerative disorders such as AD.

REFERENCES

Becker R and Giacobini E (1988): Mechanisms of cholinesterase inhibition in senile dementia of the Alzheimer type: Clinical, pharmacological, and therapeutic aspects. *Drug Dev Res* 12:163-195.

Beller SA, Overall JE and Swann AC (1985): Efficacy of oral physostigmine in primary degenerative dementia. A double-blind study of response to different dose level. *Psychopharmacology* 87:147-151.

Coyle JT, Price DL and DeLong MR (1983): Alzheimer's disease: a disorder of cortical cholinergic innervation. *Science* 219:1184-1190.

Davies P and Malone AJF (1976): Selection loss of central cholinergic neurons in Alzheimer's disease. *Lancet* 11:1403

DeSarno P, Pomponi M, Giacobini E, Tang XC and Williams E (1989): The effect of heptyl-physostigmine, a new cholinesterase inhibitor, on central cholinergic system of the rat. *Neurochem Res* 14:971-977.

Giacobini E (1991): The second generation of cholinesterase inhibitors: pharmacological aspects. In: *Cholinergic Basis for Alzheiomer Therapy*, Becker R and Giacobini E, eds. Boston: Birkhauser, pp. 247-262.

Hartvig P, Wiklund L, Aquilonius SM and Lindstrom B (1991): Clinical pharmacology of centrally acting cholinesterase inhibitors. *Second Intl Springfield Symp Advances in Alzheimer Therapy Abst*, pp. 16.

Kameyama T, Nabeshima T and Kozawa T (1986): Step-down-type passive avoidance- and escape-learning method. *J Pharmacol Method* 16:39-52.

Liu JS, Zhu YL, Yu CM, Han YY, Wu FW and Qi BF (1986): The structure of huperzine A and B, two new alkaloids exhibiting marked anticholinesterase activity. *Can J chem* 64:837-839.

Pomponi M, Giacobini E and Brufani M (1990): Present state and future development of the therapy of Alzheimer disease. *Aging* 2:125-153.

Summers W, Majovski LV, Marsh GM, Tachiki K and Kling A (1986): Oral tetrahydroaminoacridine in long-term treatment of senile dementia, Alzheimer type. *New Engl J Med* 315:1241-1245.

Tang XC, Zhu XD and Lu WH (1988): Studies on the nootropic effects of huperzine A and B: two selective AChE inhibitors. In: *Current Research in Alzheimer Therapy: Cholinesterase Inhibitors*, Giacobini E and Becker R, eds. New York: Taylor and Francis, pp. 289-293.

Tang XZ, DeSarno P, Sugaya K and Giacobini E (1989): Effect of hyperzine A, a new cholinesterase inhibitor, on the central cholinergic system of the rat. *J Neurosci Res* 24:276-285.

Thal LJ (1991): Physostigmine in Alzheimer's disease. In: *Cholinergic Basis for Alzheimer Therapy*, Becker R and Giacobini E, eds. Boston: Birkhauser, pp. 209-215.

Vincent GP, Rumennik L, Cumin R, Martin J and Sepinwall J (1987): The effects of huperzine A, an acetylcholinesterase inhibitor, on the enhancement of memory in mice, rats and monkeys. *Neurosci Abst* 13:844.

Wang YE, Yue DX and Tang XC (1986): Anti-cholinesterase activity of huperzine A. *Acta Pharmacol Sin* 7:110-113.

Wang YE, Feng J, Lu WH and Tang XC (1988): Pharmacokinetics of huperzine A in rats and mice. *Acta Pharmacol Sin* 9:193-196.

Whitehouse PJ, Price DL, Struble RG, Clark AW, Coyle JT and DeLong MR (1982): Alzheimer's disease and senile dementia: loss of neurons in the basal forebrain. *Science* 215:1237-1239.

Zhang CL (1986): Therapeutic effects of huperzine A on the aged with memory impairment. *New Drugs and Clinical Remedies* 5:260-262.

Zhang RW, Tang XC, Han YY, Sang GW, Zhang YD, Ma YX, Zhang CL and Yaug RM (1991): Drug Evaluation of huperzine A in the treatment of senile memory disorder. *Acta Pharmacol Sin* 12:250-252.

Alzheimer Disease: Therapeutic Strategies
edited by E. Giacobini and R. Becker.
© 1994 Birkhäuser Boston

IN VITRO AND IN VIVO EFFECTS OF A DUAL INHIBITOR OF ACETYLCHOLINESTERASE AND MUSCARINIC RECEPTORS, CI-1002

Mark R. Emmerling, Vlad E. Gregor, Roy D. Schwarz, Jeff D. Scholten, Michael J. Callahan, Chitase Lee, Catherine J. Moore, Charlotte Raby, William J. Lipinski, Juan Jaen and Robert E. Davis
Parke-Davis Pharmaceutical Research, Division of Warner-Lambert Co., Ann Arbor, MI 48105

INTRODUCTION

The observed loss of cholinergic innervation in the frontal cortex and hippocampus of Alzheimer's Disease (AD) brains prompted the testing of centrally acting anticholinesterases to restore cholinergic tone and to produce cognitive improvement. The success of the anticholinesterase tacrine (THA, Cognex®) in benefitting the cognitive function of many individuals with AD (Knapp et al., 1994) validates this approach and encourages us to find even better compounds with which to treat the disease. Currently, a number of anticholinesterases, both reversible and irreversible inhibitors of acetylcholinesterase (AChE), are being studied for the treatment of AD (Jaen and Davis, 1993). However, many appear to be limited in their therapeutic usefulness by the production of peripheral cholinergic side-effects at the same drug concentrations that also improve cognitive performance (Kumar and Calache, 1991)). In an effort to overcome this limitation, we synthesized and characterized a series of substituted dihydroquinazolines that show anticholinesterase activity. The most potent of this series, CI-1002 (1,3-dichloro-6,7,8,9,10,12-hexahydroazepino[2,1-b]quinazoline),has a potency similar to tacrine in inhibiting AChE, but unlike tacrine acts like an antagonist at muscarinic receptors at higher concentrations. The novelty of this dual action prompted us to characterize the *in vitro* and *in vivo* effects of CI-1002 to determine if it could be useful in the treatment of AD. Our data suggest that CI-1002 enhances performance of animals on cognitive tasks while producing few, if any, overt peripheral cholinergic side-effects. Thus, the combined effects of CI-1002, as an anticholinesterase and as a muscarinic antagonist, may improve the therapeutic potential of the compound.

RESULTS

Anticholinesterase Activity of CI-1002

CI-1002 is a potent inhibitor of AChE, but not butyrylcholinesterase (BuChE). The inhibition of human erythrocyte AChE by CI-1002 has an IC_{50} value the same as tacrine and greater than that of the specific AChE inhibitor, BW284C51 (Table I). However, CI-1002 inhibits BuChE from horse and monkey at much higher concentrations than needed for its inhibition of AChE, and than is required by tacrine and by the specific BuChE inhibitor, ethopropazine (Table I). The inhibition of AChE by CI-1002 is fully reversible with all the activity of the enzyme being restored upon removing CI-1002 from the AChE. Changes in the enzyme kinetics of AChE treated with CI-1002 reveals a reduction in both the affinity of the enzyme for its substrate (competitive inhibition) and the rate at which product is formed (noncompetitive inhibition). This type of inhibition indicates that CI-1002 is a mixed competitive inhibitor of AChE, the same as tacrine.

	Human AChE	Horse BuChE	Monkey BuChE
CI-1002	0.019	20.0	3.14
Tacrine	0.020	0.0052	0.0075
BW284C51	0.0034	nd*	16.85
Ethopropazine	>100.00	nd	0.048

TABLE I. Concentration producing 50% inhibition of enzyme activity, (IC_{50}) μM, measured by a modified Ellman assay (Ashour et al., 1987). * nd = not determined.

CI-1002 Acts Like a Muscarinic Antagonist

CI-1002 displaces the binding of the muscarinic antagonist, [^{3}H]-quinuclidinyl-benzylate (QNB), and the muscarinic agonist, [^{3}H]-cis-methyldioxolane (CMD), from rat neocortex membranes with IC_{50} values, respectively, of 398 nM and 209 nM. The ratio of the QNB/CMD values is 1.9, similar to that of the muscarinic antagonist scopolamine (QNB/CMD = 1). In comparison, tacrine displaces QNB and CMD with IC_{50} values of 759 nM and 36 nM, respectively, giving it a QNB/CMD ratio of 21. CI-1002 interacts with all known human muscarinic receptor subtypes transfected into Chinese Hamster Ovary (CHO) cells as indicated by the displacement of [^{3}H]-N-methylscopolamine (Table II). CI-1002 shows a slightly greater affinity for m2, m3 and m5 than for m1 and m4 muscarinic receptors. CI-1002 displaces ligand binding to these receptors with IC_{50} values that are about ten-fold greater than the IC_{50} value for its inhibition of human AChE.

Our studies show that CI-1002 antagonizes muscarinic receptor function *in vivo* and *in vitro*. CI-1002 reduces carbachol-stimulated phosphatidyl-inositol (PI) turnover in m1 transfected CHO cells with an IC_{50} value of 1.6 μM.

(PI) turnover in m1 transfected CHO cells with an IC_{50} value of 1.6 μM. Reversal of an arecoline-induced decrease in acetylcholine release from brain slices occurs at 1.0 μM CI-1002, further indicating CI-1002's antagonism toward the function of muscarinic receptors. *In vivo*, CI-1002 inhibits the normal passage of material through the gastrointestinal (GI) tract at oral doses of 10 mg/kg or greater. This decrease is typical of muscarinic antagonists (Schworer and Kilbinger, 1988) and is opposite to the actions of tacrine. The increased GI-motility induced by treatment with the balanced muscarinic agonist CI-979 is reversed by CI-1002, consistent with CI-1002 being a muscarinic antagonist (data not shown). Other signs of peripheral muscarinic antagonism are not evident in our animal studies outside the GI system. Possibly, insufficient levels of CI-1002 are achieved in organs and tissues other than the GI-tract to produce the antagonism.

	m1	m2	m3	m4	m5
CI-1002	410	330	340	530	300

TABLE II. Subtype selectivity of muscarinic receptor binding by CI-1002 (IC_{50} values in nM).

CI-1002 Is a Centrally Active Cholinomimetic That Improves Cognitive Performance

Despite its antagonism of muscarinic receptor function peripherally, CI-1002 acts as an indirect cholinomimetic centrally. Changes in body temperature and cortical EEG provide an indirect indication of central cholinergic function. CI-1002 when administered orally to rats lowers core body temperature with maximal effects seen at 17.8 mg/kg and decreases significantly the total power of cortical EEG at doses of between 10 mg/kg and 32 mg/kg. The effect on rat cortical EEG lasts for more than two hours and correlates temporally with the inhibition of cortical AChE activity measured *ex vivo* (data not shown).

Microdialysis studies provide further evidence that CI-1002 reaches the brain after oral administration. Injection of 10 mg/kg or 17.8 mg/kg of CI-1002 subcutaneously in anesthetized rats results in about a 2- to 3-fold increase in acetylcholine levels in the frontal cortex after 2 to 3 hours postdose (Fig. 1). This increase is similar to that of tacrine. The levels of CI-1002 (or its metabolites), detected in the microdialysate by an AChE inhibition assay, peak at the same time as acetylcholine (Fig. 1).

The effects of CI-1002 on cognitive performance was assessed in mice and monkeys. C57Bl/10SnJ (B10) mice have an inherited loss of neurons in the hippocampus (Symons et al., 1988). This cell loss is associated with poor spatial learning abilities. CI-1002 dose-dependently improves the ability of B10 mice to find a hidden platform in a spatial water maze task. Significant improvements in performance are seen after oral doses of CI-1002 of 10.0 and 17.8 mg/kg. Lower and higher doses of CI-1002 are less effective.

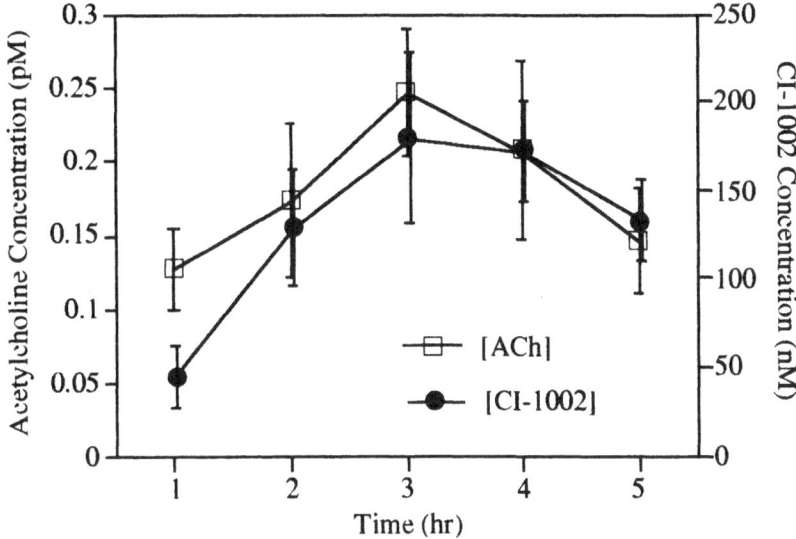

FIGURE 1. Concentration of acetylcholine (ACh) and CI-1002 in microdialysate from rat frontal cortex after oral dosing with 17.8 mg/kg of CI-1002. Values are the mean $\pm$ S.E. for acetylcholine levels (n=8) or for CI-1002 levels (n=3). ACh levels were determined by electrochemical detection after microdialysis. CI-1002 levels were determined indirectly by measuring the amount of AChE inhibition caused by the microdialysate.

CI-1002 also improves short-term memory abilities of aged rhesus monkeys. Performance on a delayed match-to-sample task was improved maximally on trials with long delays ($\geq$ 5 sec) following an intramuscular dose of 0.1 mg/kg. At this dose performance was improved to the level attained by these monkeys on trials with short delays (1 sec) and is most likely equivalent to the theoretical maximum performance on this test when delays are interposed between stimulus presentation and the opportunity to respond. The level of improvement produced by CI-1002 in this test is even greater than that caused by tacrine (data not shown).

DISCUSSION

To our knowledge the dihydroquinazoline CI-1002 is the first anticholinesterase of its type. Our *in vitro* characterization shows that in addition to inhibiting AChE, the compound at higher concentrations is a functional antagonist of muscarinic receptors. There is about a ten-fold separation in the IC_{50} values between the two activities. This difference may help to explain the pharmacology of the compound. It is expected that higher levels of CI-1002

M. R. Emmerling et al.

will be reached in the GI-tract than the brain after oral administration. Presumably, the level in the stomach and intestines is sufficient to antagonize the resident muscarinic receptors, thereby reducing gastric transit.

The effects of CI-1002 on GI-physiology, however, do not prevent the passage of compound into the blood or subsequently into the brain. The central effects of CI-1002 are clearly that of a cholinomimetic. Reduced body temperature and decreased cortical EEG activity imply that CI-1002 acts as a (indirect) cholinomimetic in the brain. These cholinergically-mediated responses are consistent with the ability of CI-1002 to raise the extracellular levels of brain acetylcholine, measured by microdialysis. The level of CI-1002 achieved extracellularly in brain appears to be around 200 nM after a subcutaneous injection of 17.8 mg/kg. This concentration would favor the compound functioning primarily as an anticholinesterase. A point underscored by the positive effects that CI-1002 has in our animals models of cognition.

Experience from clinical trials with anticholinesterases show that one of the major reasons for noncompliance with the treatment is peripheral cholinergic side effects (Knapp et al., 1994). If our animal studies are predictive, it appears that CI-1002 will produce fewer peripheral side effects than other anticholinesterases. In theory, this reduction should improve patient compliance with treatment as well as quality of life.

REFERENCES

Ashour A, Gee SJ and Hammock BD (1987): Use of a 96-well microplate reader for measuring enzyme activities. *Anal Biochem* 166:353-360.

Jaen J and Davis RE (1993): Cholinergic therapies for Alzheimer's disease: Acetylcholinesterase inhibitors of current clinical interest. *Curr Opin Invest Drugs* 2:363-377.

Knapp MJ, Knopman DS, Solomon PR, Pendlebury WW, Davis CS, Gracon SI (1994): A 30-week randomized controlled trial of high-dose tacrine in patients with Alzheimer's Disease. *JAMA* 271: 985-991.

Kumar V and Calache M (1991): Treatment of Alzheimer's Disease with cholinergic drugs. *Int J Clin Pharm Ther Tox* 29:323-337.

Schworer H and Kilbinger H (1988): Enhancement of guinea-pig intestinal peristalsis by blockade of muscarinic M1-receptors. *Br J Pharmacol* 93:715-720.

Symons JP, Davis RE and Marriot JG (1988): Water-maze learning and effects of cholinergic drugs in mouse strains with high and low hippocampal pyramidal cell counts. *Life. Sci.* 42:373-383.

Alzheimer Disease: Therapeutic Strategies
edited by E. Giacobini and R. Becker.
© 1994 Birkhäuser Boston

EFFECTS OF NOVEL CHOLINESTERASE INHIBITORS BASED ON THE MECHANISM OF ENZYME INHIBITION

Albert Enz[1], Dieter Meier[2] and René Spiegel[2]
Preclinical[1] and Clinical[2] CNS Research, SANDOZ PHARMA LTD.,
Basel, Switzerland

INTRODUCTION

The most extensively investigated acetylcholinesterase inhibitors (AChEI) in Alzheimer's disease (AD) are physostigmine and tacrine (THA). Studies by several investigators (see Thal et al., 1991) in the eighties showed that physostigmine applied intravenously can transiently improve memory and psychological functions to a small extent in AD patients. The response to oral physostigmine was less conclusive. Thal attempted to monitor the distribution of physostigmine to the central nervous system (CNS) by measuring acetylcholinesterase (AChE) activity in the CSF of AD patients and found a correlation between the fall in AChE level and the decrease in intrusions (a measure of incorrect responses) (Thal et al., 1986). This finding suggests that the failure of physostigmine to induce improvements in many of the patients reported in the literature may be due to failure to achieve adequate CNS AChE inhibition. The partial efficacy of THA in AD led the Food and Drug Administration (FDA) to approve of this drug. However, while its beneficial effects are encouraging, THA exhibits intrinsic liver toxicity, although the elevation of liver enzyme activity is reversible following withdrawal of the drug. Metrifonate, a drug initially used in the treatment of schistosomiasis in the tropics, was examined in clinical studies in AD by the group of Becker and Giacobini. This organophosphorus compound is not itself a cholinesterase inhibitor (ChEI) but is broken down non-enzymatically *in vitro* and *in vivo* to the active inhibitor dichlorvos. Becker et al. (1990) treated AD patients with metrifonate (2.5-15 mg/kg/week orally). A significant improvement in performance in psychological tests was observed with the intermediate dose of 5 mg/kg/week, while both lower and higher doses were less effective.

PROPERTIES OF INDIVIDUAL ACHE INHIBITORS

Several difficulties exist with the AChEI examined to date in AD treatment. These may be related to the intrinsic individual properties of these drugs: i) Non-selective inhibitors have a low therapeutic index, and the inhibition of peripheral cholinesterases in heart, muscle and plasma contribute to adverse peripheral effects; ii) rapid and multiple-path drug metabolism has the potential to cause organ toxicity and can impair sustained effective AChE inhibition; iii) the desired enzyme inhibition is dependent on the mechanism of inhibition both in terms of duration and selectivity. Based on the different mechanisms of inhibition, the compounds can be divided into three main classes: reversible inhibitors (aminoacridines), pseudo-irreversible inhibitors (carbamates) and irreversible inhibitors (organophosphorus compounds).

MECHANISM OF ACHE INHIBITION

The pioneering work performed by the group of Sussman et al. (1991) in elucidating the three-dimensional structure of AChE confirmed that this enzyme has multiple binding sites in a "gorge" which can interact with inhibitors in many different ways.

Tacrine

In kinetic studies the mechanism of AChE inhibition by THA was found to be linear mixed inhibition with respect to both the AChE and butyrylcholinesterase (BChE), reflecting both competitive and non-competitive components. The apparent inhibition constants (K_i values) for AChE and BChE are in the nM range, indicating high affinity for both enzymes (Berman and Leonard, 1992). However, the doses used *in vivo* are much higher (up to 160 mg in humans) than that needed to provide such an inhibitor concentration. The need for such high doses might be explained either by competitive interaction with the cholinesterases and/or by rapid metabolism. Tacrine causes truly reversible cholinesterase inhibition, the duration of which is, however, short and directly dependent on drug concentration.

Metrifonate

Following conversion to the organophosphorus compound dichlorvos, metrifonate seems to have some advantages regarding duration of action. As a prodrug of dichlorvos, metrifonate acts like a slow release ChEI. Although the half-life of metrifonate is very short, the inhibition of AChE in mouse brain was more than 3 hours (Nordgren and Holmstedt, 1988).

Carbamates

The mechanism of the carbamates as inhibitors of cholinesterase was established a long time ago using the representative compound physostigmine. This class of inhibitors interacts with the enzyme active site, with transfer of the carbamoyl group to the hydroxyl function of the active serine residue. Until the enzyme is regenerated by hydrolysis of the carbamoylated complex the enzyme is unable to degrade acetylcholine (ACh).

SDZ ENA 713

The compound known as SDZ ENA 713 [(-)(S)-N-ethyl-3-[(1-dimethyl-amino)ethyl]-N-methylphenylcarbamate] is a carbamate and belongs to a series of miotine derivatives all having AChE inhibitory activity *in vitro* and *in vivo*. *In vitro*, SDZ ENA 713 is 100-1000 times less potent than physostigmine and THA. It has no affinity for muscarinic, α- or ß-adrenergic, dopaminergic or opioid receptors.

Cardiovascular Effects
Effects of SDZ ENA 713 on the cardiovascular system of the rat, cat and squirrel monkey were minimal and only seen at doses which caused marked central nervous system effects. In the rat a slight decrease in heart rate and rise in blood pressure occurred after a high dose of SDZ ENA 713 (5.7 mg/kg p.o.).

In the anesthetized cat doses up to 1.5 mg/kg i.v. had minimal effects on blood pressure and heart rate, although central cholinergic effects (tremors) were evident at 0.7 mg/kg i.v.

In the squirrel monkey only a slight increase in blood pressure was observed, even at doses inducing marked tremor and emesis (1 mg/kg p.o.).

In conclusion: in the rat, cat and squirrel monkey SDZ ENA 713 exhibits no significant effects on cardiovascular parameters at doses at which clear central effects can be demonstrated.

AChE Inhibition Ex Vivo
The effect of SDZ ENA 713 and physostigmine on AChE activity in different rat brain regions was measured *ex vivo* following administration at several dose levels and after various time intervals. The effect of SDZ ENA 713 differed from that of physostigmine. The difference in inhibitory potency between the two drugs *in vitro* was less marked measured *ex vivo* following systemic administration. Furthermore, SDZ ENA 713 inhibited AChE in cortex and hippocampus more strongly than in other brain regions (e.g. striatum and pons/medulla). This brain region selectivity of SDZ ENA 713 is maintained over the entire time course of inhibition following oral administration (> 6 hrs). Moreover, whereas in the brain inhibition of the enzyme was *ca.* 80%, AChE activity in peripheral organs such as liver, lung and heart was only slightly affected. A physiological consequence of central AChE inhibition is the accumulation of ACh in the brain, and such accumulation was observed with physostigmine, THA and SDZ ENA 713 (Enz et al., 1993). Again, regarding

this parameter, SDZ ENA 713 exerted a more potent effect in cortical tissue compared with other brain regions.

Effect of Various AChE Inhibitors on Different Forms of the Enzyme Found in the Human Brain

The existence of different molecular forms of AChE is well established (Massoulie and Bon, 1982). In the human brain, the most abundant form is the tetrameric G4. This form is functionally important for the degradation of ACh at cholinergic synapses. The monomeric G1 form is also present in smaller amounts in the human brain.

During aging and, more dramatically, in AD, levels of the G4 form are decreased in neocortex and hippocampus, whereas there is no change or a smaller decrease in levels of the G1 form (Siek et al., 1990). We studied the effect of SDZ ENA 713, physostigmine, heptylphysostigmine and THA on the G1 and G4 forms of AChE *post mortem* in brain tissue samples from AD patients.

Effect of Different Inhibitors

With pooled fractions of either G1 or G4 enzyme from control and AD brains, *in vitro* inhibition experiments were performed with the different inhibitors. The inhibitory effect of physostigmine and THA on the G1 and the G4 forms of AChE was equipotent and the degree of inhibition was similar in both cortex and hippocampus.

In contrast, SDZ ENA 713 — and to a lesser extent heptylphysostigmine — preferentially inhibited the G1 form in both brain regions (Enz et al., 1993).

In summary, while physostigmine and THA inhibited the G1 and G4 forms equally, a clear difference was found for SDZ ENA 713 and heptylphysostigmine, with SDZ ENA 713 four and six times, respectively, and heptylphysostigmine two and four times, respectively, more potent in inhibiting the G1 as compared to the G4 form of AChE in cortex and striatum.

There are several implications of preferential inhibition of the G1 form. The membrane-bound G4 form located presynaptically at cholinergic nerve endings may be directly involved in the regulation of ACh transmission. It seems therefore that the loss of G4 represents a selective depletion of the membrane pool, reflecting the state of degeneration of cholinergic terminals in AD. On the other hand, the activity of the G1 form, reflecting ACh degradation unrelated to ACh release, remains unchanged. Preferential inhibition of this enzyme could be beneficial in situations of cholinergic hypofunction.

Study in Humans to Assess the Relationship Between Central and Peripheral Effects of SDZ ENA 713

Eight patients with a mean age of 72 years from two centers were included in this study. They were suffering from mild to moderate suspected normal pressure hydrocephalus and undergoing temporary external CSF drainage for diagnostic or therapeutic reasons.

Single doses of 3 mg SDZ ENA 713 induced sustained inhibition of AChE in the CSF lasting for at least 10 hrs. Mean maximal inhibition was 35% and occurred 2-3 hours after dosing. The inhibition of BChE in plasma followed a similar time course of AChE inhibition in the CSF, but at a lower level (mean maximal inhibition 20%).

SUMMARY AND CONCLUSIONS

It could be argued that clinical experience with cholinergic drugs in the treatment of AD has not yet shown relevant symptomatic improvements. The main reasons for this might be the peripheral cholinergic effects and liver toxicity of some of these drugs, which limit their use and prevent confirmation of the cholinergic hypothesis. The main disadvantages of the ChEIs investigated in clinical trials are short duration of action in the case of physostigmine and potential liver toxicity in the case of the aminoacridine derivatives. The results obtained with SDZ ENA 713 suggest that the disadvantages of AChE inhibitors might be overcome by improving CNS selectivity and thereby decreasing the peripheral cholinergic effects and toxicity. The brain selectivity observed in animals is confirmed in ongoing human studies by sustained inhibition of CSF enzyme levels with no effect on plasma BChE. To date 400 patients have been exposed for up to two years. Side effects observed include nausea and vomiting. No relevant liver toxicity or effects on cardiac parameters have been seen.

REFERENCES

Becker RE, Colliver J, Elble R, Feldman E, Giacobini E, Kumar V, Markwell S, Moriearty P, Parks R, Shillcutt SD, Unni L, Vicari S, Womack C and Zec RF (1990): Effect of metrifonate, a long-acting cholinesterase inhibitor in Alzheimer's disease. *Drug Dev Res* 19:425-434.

Berman HA and Leonard K (1992): Interaction of tetrahydroaminoacridine with acetylcholinesterase and butyrylcholinesterase. *Mol Pharmacol* 41:412-418.

Enz A, Amstutz R, Boddeke H, Gmelin G and Malanowsky J (1993): Brain selective inhibition of acetylcholinesterase: a novel approach to therapy for Alzheimer's disease. In: *Cholinergic Function and Dysfunction, Progress in Brain Research* Vol. 98, Cuello AC, ed. Amsterdam: Elsevier Science Publisher, pp. 431-438.

Massoulie J and Bon S (1982): The molecular forms of cholinesterase and acetylcholinesterase in vertebrates. *Ann Rev Neurosci* 5:57-106.

Nordgren I and Holmstedt B (1988): Metrifonate: a review. In: *Current research in Alzheimer Therapy*. Giacobini E and Becker RE, eds. New York: Taylor and Francis, pp. 281-288.

Siek GC, Katz LS, Fishman EB, Korosi TS and Marquis JK (1990): Molecular forms of acetylcholinesterase in subcortical areas of normal and demented (Alzheimer-type) patients. *Biol Psychiatry* 27:573-580.

Sussman JL, Harel M, Frolow F, Oefner C, Toker L and Silman I (1991): Atomic structure of acetylcholinesterase from Torpedo californica: a prototypic acetylcholine-binding protein. *Science* 253:872-879.

Thal LJ, Masur DM, Sharpless NS, Fuld PA and Davies P (1986): Acute and chronic effects of oral physostigmine and lecithin in Alzheimer's disease. *Prog Neuropsychopharmacol Biol Psychiatry* 10:627-636.

Thal LJ (1991): Physostigmine in Alzheimer's disease. In: *Cholinergic Basis of Alzheimer Therapy*. Becker RE and Giacobini E, eds. Boston: Birkhäuser, pp. 209-215.

Alzheimer Disease: Therapeutic Strategies
edited by E. Giacobini and R. Becker.
© 1994 Birkhäuser Boston

BIOCHEMISTRY, PHARMACOKINETICS AND PHARMACODYNAMICS OF MDL 73,745: A POTENT AND SELECTIVE INHIBITOR OF ACETYLCHOLINESTERASE

Jean-Marie Hornsperger, Jean-Noël Collard, Daniel Schirlin, James Dow, Jean-Georges Heydt and Bertrand Duléry
Marion Merrell Dow Research Institute, 16, rue d'Ankara, 67080 Strasbourg Cédex, France

INTRODUCTION

Acetylcholinesterase inhibitors (AChEI) as palliative agents in the treatment of Alzheimer's disease (AD) have been most widely studied so far. Novel compounds with higher lipophilicity, better selectivity and longer duration of inhibition are more promising candidates for a cholinomimetic therapy of AD.

Here, we report the *in vitro* and *in vivo* properties of MDL 73,745, a silylated aromatic trifluoromethylketone inhibitor of acetylcholinesterase (AChE) based on the concept of transition state analog inhibitors (Fig. 1). The distinct feature of this compound is the replacement of the trimethyl-ammonium group by a trimethylsilyl moiety in a trifluoromethylketone analogue of acetylcholine (ACh). This compound combines reactivity with the active-site serine of AChE (Brodbeck et al., 1979) and high lipophilicity. The study indicates that MDL 73,745 has interesting central cholinomimetic properties, and its pharmacological profile fits more closely with the established criteria for an ideal cholinesterase inhibitor to be used in clinical studies.

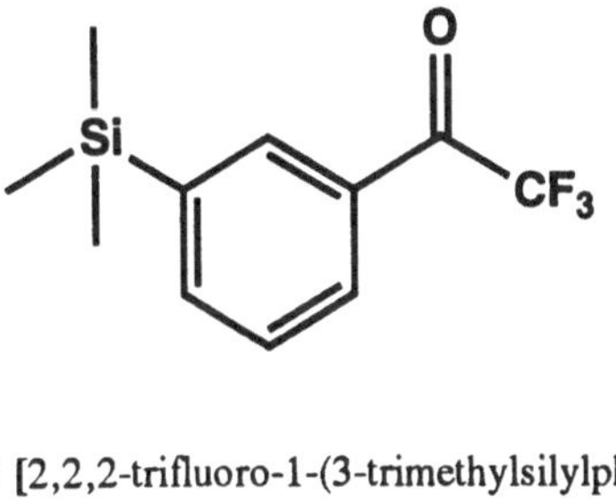

FIGURE 1. MDL 73,745 [2,2,2-trifluoro-1-(3-trimethylsilylphenyl)ethanone]

RESULTS

Effects of MDL 73,745 on In Vitro AChE Activity

Acetylcholinesterase and butyrylcholinesterase (BuChE) activities were determined according the method of Ellman et al. (1961).

Incubation of electric eel AChE (Type III) with MDL 73,745 resulted in a time- and concentration-dependent loss of enzyme activity which followed pseudo-first-order kinetics. By plotting the time of half inactivation ($t_{1/2}$) as a function of the reciprocal of the inhibitor concentration (1/I) according to the method of Kitz and Wilson (1962), a straight line was obtained. This line passes through the origin, suggesting a tight-binding inhibition (Cha, 1975). An association rate constant k_{on} of 1 x 10^5 $M^{-1}s^{-1}$ was calculated. The value of k_{off} was also determined by dilution of the enzyme-inhibitor complex after complete inactivation of the enzyme. A time of half-reactivation of 41 hrs was calculated leading to a rate constant k_{off} of 3.6 x $10^{-6}s^{-1}$. Qualitatively similar results were obtained from the rat and mouse brain enzymes as well as from the G1 and G4 molecular forms of the enzyme isolated from rat hippocampus (Table I). MDL 73,745 was found to be a slow-binding inhibitor of horse serum BuChE (Table I). On the basis of K_i values, the ratio (horse serum BuChE/rat brain AChE) obtained *in vitro*, showed a 63-fold selectivity for AChE versus BuChE.

Enzyme	k_{on} $(M^{-1}s^{-1})$	k_{off} (s^{-1})	K_i (pM)	$t_{1/2}$ reactivation (hrs)
Electric eel AChE (Type III)*	1.0 x 10^5	4.7 x 10^{-6}	47	41
Mouse brain AChE*	3.0 x 10^4	4.0 x 10^{-6}	130	48
Rat brain AChE*	1.5 x 10^4	3.9 x 10^{-6}	260	50
Horse serum BuChE**	2.8 x 10^4	4.6 x 10^{-4}	16400	0.25

TABLE I. Kinetic parameters determined for the *in vitro* inhibition of AChE and BuChE from different species by MDL 73,745. * time-dependent (or tight-binding) inhibition. ** slow-binding inhibition.

The compound shows low toxicity compared to other AChEI. Acute LD_{50} in mice and rats is 250 mg/kg [oral (p.o.), subcutaneous (s.c.)] and 180 mg/kg by intra-peritoneal injection.

Effects of MDL 73,745 on Ex Vivo AChE and BuChE Activities in Rats

The duration of action of a single dose of MDL 73,745 was studied in rat brain as well as in some other tissues. The maximal inhibition (65%) of AChE in brain produced by a dose of 10 mg/kg of MDL 73,745 (s.c.) occurred 3 hrs after drug administration (Fig. 2). Inhibition was maintained over a time-period of 24 hrs (40% inhibition is still observed after 24 hrs). Thereafter, the enzyme activity returned to control values which were reached within 48 hrs. Butyrylcholinesterase activity was measured in parallel in brain but was less affected. A maximum inhibition of 21% was reached 4 hrs after drug administration. In contrast, rat heart AChE and BuChE activities were inhibited to a lesser extent. Maximum inhibition (25%) occurred after two hours. Twenty-four hrs later, control levels of AChE and BuChE activities were reached (Fig. 2).

The effect of MDL 73,745 in rat brain is long-lasting after s.c. administration (about 60% inhibition of AChE activity was maintained for at least 8 hrs) but shorter acting after p.o. administration (about 30% inhibition of AChE activity was observed 4 hrs post-dose).

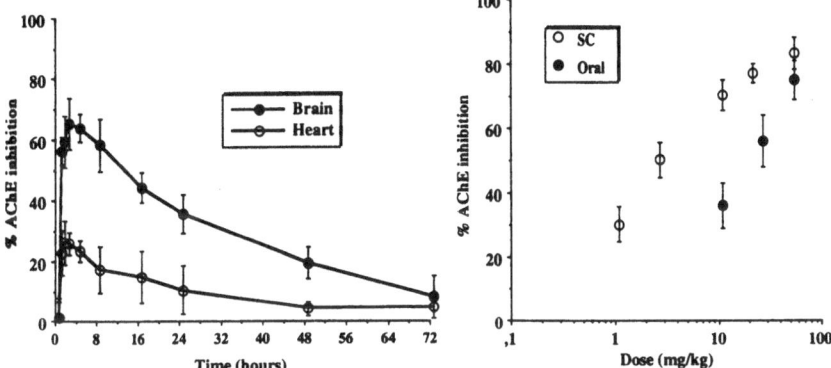

FIGURE 2. Time-course of effect of a single dose of MDL 73,745 (10 mg/kg, s.c.) on brain and heart AChE activities in the rat (mean $\pm$ SD, n = 5).

FIGURE 3. Dose-effect on rat brain AChE, 3 hrs after s.c. and p.o. administration of MDL 73,745 (mean $\pm$ SD, n = 5).

Dose-Effect of MDL 73,745 on Brain AChE and BuChE Activities

The dose dependent effects of MDL 73,745 on AChE and BuChE activities was investigated, 3 hrs after administration of the drug, in brain and peripheral tissues. In brain, s.c. administration of MDL 73,745 produced a dose-dependent inhibition of AChE activity with an ED_{50} of 2.5 mg/kg (Fig. 3). Similarly a dose-dependent inhibition of BuChE activity was observed with an ED_{50} value of 100 mg/kg. The ED_{50} for AChE, after p.o. administration of MDL 73,745 is about 20 mg/kg. This value is eight times greater than the value determined at the same time after s.c. administration.

Effect of MDL 73,745 Administration on the Concentration of ACh in Rat Brain and on the Extracellular Release of ACh

MDL 73,745 was given s.c. to rats at a dose of 10 mg/kg, and the animals were sacrificed by microwave irradiation of the head 0.5, 1, and 4 hrs later. A 30% increase in ACh level was observed in total rat brain 0.5 hrs post-dose. The increase after 1 hr is about 40%, and 4 hrs later, ACh level was 20% above control values.

The microdialysis technique was used to evaluate the effect of MDL 73,745 on the extracellular release of ACh in the rat cerebral cortex. A single dose of 10 mg/kg (s.c.) of the drug produced an 8-fold increase in the release of ACh. Maximal increase occurred 1-2 hrs after injection followed by a progressive return to basal level within 8 hrs (Zhu and Giacobini, 1994).

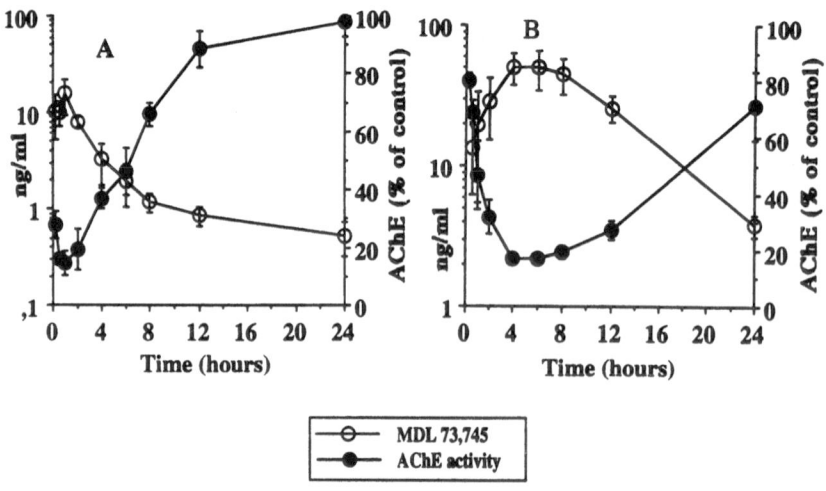

FIGURE 4. Plasma concentrations of MDL 73,745 (ng/ml) and AChE activity in dog (n = 3) after p.o. (A) and s.c. (B) administration of the drug (10 mg/kg).

Pharmacokinetics in Dogs

After p.o. administration of MDL 73,745 (10 mg/kg), a rapid and potent inhibition of plasma AChE was observed (> 80% at 1 hr), AChE activity recovered by 12 hr post-dose (Fig. 4A). A longer-lasting effect on AChE was seen after a single s.c. dose of MDL 73,745 (10 mg/kg). Four hrs post-dose, plasma AChE was inhibited by 80% and did not return to baseline levels until 36 hrs after drug administration (Fig. 4B). Plasma AChE inhibition could be significantly correlated with the concentration of parent drug for both routes of administration, suggesting that the parent drug is responsible for activity.

The s.c. administration improved bioavailability compared to the p.o. administration (34% versus 4%) by reducing the important first-pass effect seen with the compound. *In vitro* studies have shown that MDL 73,745 can be rapidly reduced to its alcohol metabolite when incubated in rat liver 10,000 g supernatant.

Pharmacokinetic parameters of MDL 73,745, calculated after intravenous administration, showed a terminal elimination half-life of 24 hrs, total body plasma clearance of around 70 ml/min/kg and an apparent volume of distribution of 150 l/kg. These results indicate that the compound has a rapid clearance and a large volume of distribution.

After transdermal administration of MDL 73,745 there was a rapid percutaneous absorption of the parent drug ($t_{1/2}$ abs: 0.58 hr) and t_{max} was reached 3.7 hrs after application of a patch equivalent to 50 mg/kg. A plateau for plasma concentrations of MDL 73,745 was observed from around 4-12 hrs together with a sustained inhibition of plasma AChE (55%) (Fig. 5). The patch can thus act as a rate control reservoir for drug delivery. Plasma concentrations of MDL 73,745 were correlated with plasma AChE inhibition. Transdermal application of MDL 73,745 also increased its bioavailability (13.7%) compared to p.o. administration (4%). A comparison of mean plasma concentrations of MDL 73,745 in dog (n = 3) after p.o., transdermal, and s.c. administration of 10 mg/kg is shown in Fig. 6. Again, transdermal delivery leads to more constant plasma concentrations of drug and avoids the peaks and troughs associated with other routes of administration.

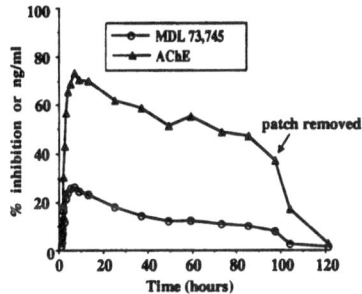
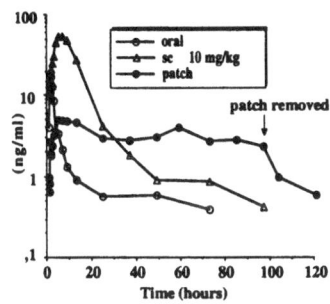

FIGURE 5. Plasma concentrations of MDL 73,745 and inhibition of AChE in dogs after application of a 150 cm² patch (50 mg/kg).

FIGURE 6. Comparison of plasma concentrations of MDL 73,745 after p.o., s.c. and patch administration in dogs.

CONCLUSION

MDL 73,745 is a highly selective and tight-binding inhibitor of AChE. In animals, MDL 73,745 produces a long-lasting inhibition of brain AChE and increases the extracellular ACh concentrations. The compound possesses a number of advantages over other AChE inhibitors: longer duration of action, lower toxicity, and the potential to be used in a transdermal delivery system, which would lead probably to fewer side-effects and a better therapeutic ratio. MDL 73,745 has entered clinical phase II evaluation.

REFERENCES

Brodbeck U, Schweikert K, Gentinetta R and Rottenberg M (1979):   Fluorinated
    aldehydes and ketones acting as quasi-substrate inhibitors of acetylcholinesterase.
    Biochem Biophys Acta 567:357.
Cha S (1975): Tight-binding inhibitors I. *Biochem Pharmacol* 24:2177.
Ellman GL, Courtney DK, Andres V and Featherstone RM (1961): A new and rapid
    colorimetric determination of acetylcholinesterase activity. *Biochem Pharmacol* 7:88.
Kitz R and Wilson IB (1962): Esters of methanesulfonic acid as irreversible inhibitors
    of acetylcholinesterase. *J Biol Chem* 237:3245.
Zhu X-D and Giacobini E (1994): Second generation cholinesterase inhibitors: the
    effect of MDL-73,745 on cortical acetylcholine. *Third Intl Springfield Alzheimer
    Symp Abst* p. 118(#P19).

Alzheimer Disease: Therapeutic Strategies
edited by E. Giacobini and R. Becker.
© 1994 Birkhäuser Boston

CLINICAL EXPERIENCE WITH MDL 73,745; PHARMACOKINETICS, PHARMACODYNAMICS, AND CLINICAL TOLERANCE IN NORMAL VOLUNTEERS

Margo M. Schleman, Stephen S. Songer and Olo J. Szylleyko
Marion Merrell Dow Inc., Kansas City, MO

Randall D. Seifert and Neal R. Cutler
California Clinical Trials, Beverly Hills, CA

INTRODUCTION

Alzheimer's disease (AD) represents one of the major debilitating illnesses facing our elderly population today (Jellinger et al., 1990). The magnitude of the financial and social costs associated with this progressive disorder is expected to increase dramatically as the numbers of people reaching their seventies, eighties and nineties continue to grow (Evans et al., 1989). There is clearly a pressing need for new therapies; those which can bring about symptomatic relief, those which can slow down the disease process, and those that can prevent onset of the disease itself. One clinical strategy being explored to relieve symptoms of dementia is to increase levels of the neurotransmitter, acetylcholine (ACh). The scientific rationale is based on the known cholinergic deficit found on post mortem examination (Perry et al., 1978) and clinical observations of improvement using acetylcholinesterase (AChE) inhibitors in the setting of cholinergic deficit (Thal et al., 1989; Davis et al., 1992).

MDL 73,745 is a selective and potent AChE inhibitor which has been shown to increase cortical ACh levels after subcutaneous administration in rats (Hornsperger et al., 1992). It is lipid soluble and has long-lasting but reversible binding properties for the AChE enzyme. MDL 73,745 was recently evaluated in normal male volunteers for safety, tolerance and pharmacological activity.

PHASE 1 TRIAL DESIGN

Fifty six normal male volunteers (mean age 27 ± 5.9 years) were recruited for this single, ascending oral dose, safety and tolerance trial. Nine dose levels were examined with each dose administered to 6 subjects (4 active and 2 placebo). The initial series of doses included 10, 30, 60, 90, 120 and 150 mg. Three additional doses were added by protocol amendment and included 200,

250 and 300 mg. Subjects were observed for 24 hrs post-dose and serial measurements of vital signs, ECGs, and chemistries were done. Plasma levels of parent compound were obtained prior to dosing and at 1/2, 1, 2, 3, 4, 6, 12, 16 and 24 hrs post-dosing. Red blood cell (RBC) AChE and plasma butyrylcholinesterase (BuChE) activity was measured by a standard calorimetric assay (Whitiker, 1983) and modified for use in a micro plate format. Measurements were made at the same time points as the plasma levels of MDL 73,745.

RESULTS

MDL 73,745 produced a dose dependent inhibition of RBC AChE activity ranging from 20% at the lowest doses to 61% at the highest dose. A strong correlation between RBC AChE inhibition and plasma levels of MD 73,745 was found. The effect on BuChE was small and not dose related. Single oral doses of MDL 73,745 were well tolerated up to doses of 250 mg. The proportion of subjects reporting adverse events was similar between the active treatment group (41.7%) and the placebo treatment group (38.9%). Adverse events were, in general, mild and transient. Headache was the most common complaint and was observed in both groups (MDL 73,745, 11.1%, Placebo, 16.7%). Dizziness was also noted in both treatment groups (MDL 73,745, 5.6%, Placebo 16.7%). Taste perversion was noted in 3 subjects (8.3%) all on active compound. Other events reported once by subjects on MDL 73,745 included abdominal distention, nausea, asthenia, increase in SGPT (less than twice normal), aggressive reaction, agitation, and drowsiness. Events reported once by subjects on placebo included abdominal pain, euphoria, fever, bradycardia, and increased sweating. One subject experienced an episode of syncope 4 hrs after receiving a 300 mg dose. This was associated with orthostatic blood pressure changes. The subject improved within a few hrs after fluid administration and bed rest. Because of the severity of this event after 300 mg, the maximally tolerated dose was felt to be 250 mg in this normal population. Clinical laboratory studies remained within normal limits except for one subject who developed a rise in SGPT to 89 U/L one day after dosing. This value returned to normal on follow-up. No changes were noted in the ECG, seated blood pressure or heart rate.

CONCLUSIONS

MDL 73,745 was well tolerated up to single oral doses of 250 mg. Adverse events related to excessive stimulation of the cholinergic system were not prominent. Pharmacodynamic measurements found good activity as measured in the RBC. Central activity was not measured in this study. Additional trials to further evaluate safety and the pharmacokinetic properties of this new compound appear warranted.

REFERENCES

Davis KL, Thal LJ, Gamzu ER, Davis CS et al. (1992): A double-blind, placebo-controlled multicenter study of Tacrine for Alzheimer's disease. *New Engl J Med* 327:1253-1259.

Evans DA, Funkenstein HH, Albert MS et al. (1989): Prevalence of Alzheimer's disease in a community population of older persons is higher than previously reported. *J Amer Med Assoc* 262:2551-2556.

Hornsperger JM, Collard JN, Moran PM, Dow J et al. (1992): Biochemical and pharmacological profile of MDL 73,745, a novel inhibitor of acetylcholinesterase for potential use in the treatment of cholinergic deficit in AD patients. *Neurobiology of Aging Abstr* 13:130.

Jellinger K, Danielczyk W, Fisher P and Gabriel E (1990): Clinical pathological analysis of dementia disorders in the elderly. *J Neuroscience* 95:239-258.

Perry EK, Tomlinson BE, Blessed G, Bergmann K et al. (1978): Correlation of cholinergic abnormalities with senile plaques and mental scores in senile dementia. *Br J Med* 2:1457-1459.

Thal LJ, Masur DM, Blau AD et al. (1989): Chronic oral physostigmine without lecithin improves memory in Alzheimer's disease. *J Am Geriatr Soc* 37:42-48.

Whitiker M (1983): Cholinesterases, calorimetric Method. In: *Methods of Enzymatic Analysis,* Third ed. Bergmeyer, Bergmeyer and Crassel, eds. Deerfield Beach, Florida: Verlag Chemie, Weinheim, pp. 57-73.

Alzheimer Disease: Therapeutic Strategies
edited by E. Giacobini and R. Becker.
© 1994 Birkhäuser Boston

GALANTHAMINE IN ALZHEIMER'S DISEASE

Helmut Kewitz
Institute of Clinical Pharmacology, Charite of Humboldt-University,
10098 Berlin, Schumannstr. 20/21, Germany

Gordon Wilcock
Department of Care of the Elderly, Frenchay Hospital,
Bristol BS2 8HW, U.K.

Bonnie Davis
Synaptic Inc., P.O. Box 157, Cold Spring Harbor, New York 11724 USA

Substantial efforts have been made in neurobiology and molecular biology but we are still far from a causal therapy of Alzheimer's disease (AD). In the interim, and perhaps ultimately as an adjunct to a progression inhibitor which may not be absolute, symptomatic treatment has to be optimized. Tacrine's approval by the FDA has stimulated a search for a less toxic and more efficacious agent. In this context, we report on the safety and efficacy of galanthamine in clinical trials.

PRECLINICAL CHARACTERISTICS OF GALANTHAMINE

Chemically, galanthamine is a naturally-occurring alkaloid, unrelated to the acridines. It is 50 times more potent at inhibiting acetylcholinesterase (AChE) in neurons and erythrocytes than butyrylcholinesterase (BuChE) in plasma, there being no BuChE inhibition at plasma levels sufficient to inhibit erythrocyte AChE by 50-70%. Tacrine is 10 times more potent at BuChE than AChE inhibition (Thomsen and Kewitz, 1990; Thomsen et al., 1991).

Unlike tacrine, galanthamine is a competitive inhibitor (Köster et al., in preparation). This has therapeutic implications. In the synapse, ACh concentrations are high at the presynaptic and low at the postsynaptic membranes. Galanthamine will therefore bind to AChE less presynaptically than postsynaptically. Acetylcholine will be increased less presynaptically, where the receptors inhibit ACh release, than postsynaptically, where the therapeutic effect is mediated. On an anatomic scale, the greater the cholinergic deficit in a particular area, the more cholinesterase inhibition will occur; conversely, the more normal areas will have less increase of ACh. Theoretically, an improved ratio of therapeutic to side effects could occur.

Oral bioavailability of galanthamine has been estimated to be about 90% (Bickel et al., 1991; Köster et al., in preparation). In contrast, tacrine's bioavailability is less than 5% (Forsyth et al., 1989). Thus, variations of a few percent in drug absorption or presystemic metabolism could produce much greater fluctuations in plasma tacrine levels and clinical effects than they could produce for galanthamine.

One of the metabolites of galanthamine is O-demethylgalanthamine which, like galanthamine, is eliminated 25% via the kidney. The formation of O-demethylgalanthamine (also called sanguinine) is due to the activity of cytochrome P4502D6 which can be inhibited by a number of different drugs but specifically by quinidine in therapeutic doses. It has been shown, however, that a block of O-demethylation leads to an increase of galanthamine in the blood which is little enough not to be of any clinical effect. While O-demethylgalanthamine is a three-fold stronger inhibitor of acetylcholinesterase than galanthamine itself, it is obviously glucuronidated as soon as it is formed (Bachus and Kewitz, in preparation).

With a terminal half-life of 6 hours, galanthamine permits dosing intervals of 8-12 hours, whereas tacrine, with a half life of 3-4 hours, requires at least 4 daily doses which interferes significantly with patients' compliance (Bickel et al., 1991; Westra et al., 1986; Knapp et al., 1994).

CLINICAL

An open pilot study was conducted in which 19 patients received predetermined doses of 30-60 mg galanthamine per day for two six-week periods separated by a three-week drug withdrawal. Patients were taken to the target dose in three-day increments of 10-15 mg per day. Six early patients experienced cholinergic side effects on this regimen and were discontinued. A seventh patient's caretaker became noncompliant during the second drug period. Thus, 11 patients completed the trial.

There were no laboratory abnormalities; one patient had a rash.

In the ADAS-cognitive (ADAS-cog), galanthamine produced a 5.4 point improvement in the first 6 weeks, a 1.8 point deterioration during three weeks of washout and a 2.5 point improvement from the elevated baseline of the second period to its completion. The total ADAS-cog improvement from baseline to the end of the study was 6.0 points ($p < .03$, Fig. 1)

In the Mini-Mental Sate Exam (MMSE), a 1.4 point increase occurred in the first period, a 0.5 point deterioration in the three-week withdrawal, and a 0.9 point improvement in the second period, for a total improvement of $1.7 \pm .7$ points ($p < .04$).

A four-point clinician's global rating (CGI) of each study period was performed at its end. In this scale, "2" represented no change, and higher numbers signified improvement. During the first period, a .36 ± .20 point improvement was nonsignificant. At withdrawal, there was a 0.73 ± .32 point exacerbation (t = 2.43, p < .04) and retreatment produced an improvement of 0.70 ± .26 (t = 2.69, p < .05).

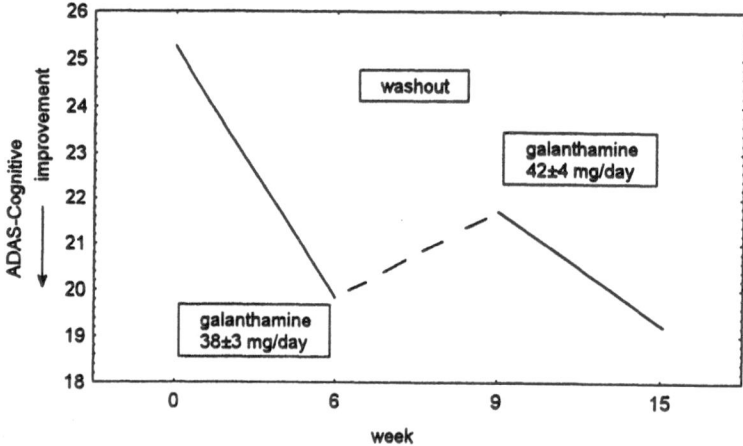

FIGURE 1. ADAS-Cognitive Response to Galanthamine. Baseline to week 15 effect 6.04 ± 2.16, t = 2.60, p = .0267, n = 11

Substantial carryover effects were present at three weeks, amounting to the persistence of about 2/3 of the therapeutic effect as measured on the ADAS-cog and the MMSE.

In a separate study, 143 patients received 20-50 mg galanthamine per day for three weeks, single-blind. Seventy-eight percent showed evidence of response and were randomized to receive galanthamine or placebo double-blind for 10 further weeks. ADAS-cog scores improved 5.1 points during the first three weeks, comparable to the 5.4 points in the first six weeks of the pilot study. Responders receiving galanthamine had a total 8.3 point improvement on the ADAS-cog at the end of the double-blind. MMSE scores improved 1.72 points for the unenriched population during the first three weeks, similar to the 1.73 point improvement in the unenriched pilot study. The responder subgroup had a total 2.5 point increase at the end of the double-blind. CGI scores were highly significant, with 72% of all patients felt to be improved, 30% of the total "much or very much improved." Thus, cognitive and global scales yielded clinically and statistically significant results, and the two separate studies were in remarkable accord.

Cholinergic symptoms not present at baseline were predominantly mild to moderate, transient, and a function of the rate of dose escalation. For the 81 patients receiving an average maximal dose of 29.4 mg/day during the first three weeks, nausea or vomiting occurred in 21%. For those receiving 34.7 mg, it was 29% (n = 58), and 15 of the 24 (63%) who reached an average of 37.9 mg/day had nausea or vomiting. By the last visit, there was no correlation between cognitive improvement and dose ($r = .04$). Thus, it does not seem justified to institute galanthamine therapy rapidly.

Overall new onset of other cholinergic symptoms were: diarrhea (4%), anorexia (3%), dyspepsia (0.6%), abdominal pain (4%), and weight loss (1.2%). There was neither liver nor other laboratory test toxicity.

The therapeutic effects reported here are consistent with other early studies of galanthamine in AD (Ranier et al., 1989; Dal Bianco et al., 1991), including a separate report on these patients, analyzed from a different statistical perspective (Wilcock et al., 1993).

Comparisons to tacrine are approximate because of differences in study design. It is difficult to know how the minority (27%) of patients completing the best dose (160 mg) represent those initially randomized. However, on the primary outcome measures of the ADAS-cog and CGI scales, the data suggest that galanthamine is more beneficial. Reported cholinergic side effects are fewer. Galanthamine did not demonstrate any of tacrine's liver toxicity or laboratory test abnormalities.

Differences in chemistry surely account for galanthamine's lack of toxicity. Its specificity of action for AChE as opposed to BuChE and for the substrate site suggested a cleaner therapeutic effect relative to side effects, and the comparison to tacrine supports this hypothesis. Galanthamine's half-life and almost complete absorption probably contribute to predictable and uniform effects. Thus, preclinical chemical, enzymatic and pharmacokinetic differences are consistent with the apparently greater safety, efficacy and tolerability of galanthamine than other cholinesterase inhibitors.

ACKNOWLEDGEMENTS

Clinical Investigators: P. Dal Bianco, Universitaelsklinik Neurologie, Wien, Austria; H. Berzewski, Klinikum Steglitz, Berlin; E. Deisenhammer, Wagner Jauregg Krankenhaus, Linz, Austria; R. Engel, Nervenklinik der Universität München, München, Germany; E.J. Friedel, Psychiatrisches Krankenhaus der Stadt Wein, Wien, Austria; J.P. Kummer, Landesklinik Nordschwarzwald, Calw, Germany; M. Rainer, Psychiatrisches Krankenhaus der Stadt Wein, Wien, Austria; D. Uebelhack, Charite - Nervenklinik, Berlin, Germany.

REFERENCES

Bickel U, Thomsen T, Weber W, Fischer PF, Bachus R, Nitz M and Kewitz H (1991): Pharmacokinetics of galanthamine and corresponding cholinesterase inhibition. *Clin Pharmacol Ther* 50:420-428.

Dal Bianco P, Maly J, Woeber C, Lind C, Koch G, Hufgard J, Marschall I, Mraz M and Deecke L (1991): Galanthamine treatment in Alzheimer's disease. *J Neurol Transm Suppl* 33:59-63.

Forsyth DR, Wilcock GK, Morgan RA, Truman CA, Ford JM and Roberts CJC (1989): Pharmacokinetics of tacrine hydrochloride in Alzheimer's disease. *Clin Pharmacol Ther* 46:634-641.

Knapp MJ, Knopman DS, Solomon PR, Pendlebury WW, Davis CS and Gracon SI (1994): A 30-week randomized controlled trial of high-dose tacrine in patients with Alzheimer's disease. *JAMA* 271:985-991.

Rainer M, Mark Th and Haushofer A (1989): Galanthamine hydrobromide in the treatment of senile demential of Alzheimer's type. In: *Pharmacological Interventions on Central Cholinergic Mechanisms in Senile Dementia (Alzheimer's Disease)*. Kewitz H, Thomsen T and Bickel U, eds. San Francisco: W. Zuchschwerdt Verlag München, pp. 233-237.

Thomsen T and Kewitz H (1990): Selective inhibition of human acetylcholinesterase by galanthamine *in vitro* and *in vivo*. *Life Sci* 46:1553-1558.

Thomsen T, Kaden B, Fischer JP, Bickel U, Barz H, Gusztony A, Cervos-Navarro J and Kewitz H (1991): Inhibition of acetylcholinesterase activity in human brain tissue and erythrocytes by galanthamine, physostigmine and tacrine. *Eur J Clin Chem Clin Biochem* 29:487-492.

Westra P, Van Thiel MJS, Vermeer GA, Soeterbroek AM, Scaf AHJ and Claessens HA (1986): Pharmacokinetics of galanthamine (a long acting anticholinesterase drug) in anaesthetized patients. *Br J Anaesth* 58:1303-1307.

Wilcock GK, Scott M, Pearsall T, Neubauer K, Boyle M and Razay G (1993): Letter to the Editor. Galanthamine and the treatment of Alzheimer's disease. *Int J Geriat Psychiat* 8:781-782.

Alzheimer Disease: Therapeutic Strategies
edited by E. Giacobini and R. Becker.
© 1994 Birkhäuser Boston

TACRINE: AN OVERVIEW OF EFFICACY IN TWO PARALLEL GROUP STUDIES

Stephen I. Gracon and Margaret J. Knapp
Clinical Research Department, Parke-Davis Pharmaceutical Research
Ann Arbor, MI

INTRODUCTION

Tacrine (Cognex®) is the first drug approved in the United States for the treatment of Alzheimer's disease (AD). The public response to the results of a small study of tacrine doses up to 160 mg/day (Summers et al., 1986) resulted in the initiation of a collaborative study of tacrine using an enrichment design (Davis et al., 1992). The total daily tacrine dose was limited to 80 mg as a result of the occurrence of asymptomatic alanine aminotransferase (ALT) elevations which, at the time, were thought to be dose-related.

The results of the collaborative study, and several other studies of enrichment and crossover design (Eagger et al., 1991; Wilcock et al., 1993) demonstrated a measurable, positive effect on several outcome assessments; however, the complicated nature of the study designs made it impossible to estimate, with any certainty, the exact magnitude of the treatment effect and its "clinical meaningfulness" given the restrictions on total daily dose and the relatively short duration of treatment. Two parallel group studies of 12 and 30 weeks' duration (Farlow et al., 1992; Knapp et al., 1994) were thus initiated to address concerns inherent to enrichment and crossover design trials. These two studies provide unequivocal proof of the efficacy of tacrine in treating patients with AD.

METHODS

In both the 12- and 30-week studies, men or women at least 50 years of age with a diagnosis of probable AD of mild-to-moderate severity (Mini-Mental State Examination [MMSE] scores of 10 to 26 [Folstein et al., 1975]) were randomly assigned to receive placebo or tacrine.

The 12-week study comprised 6 treatment groups; 3 of the groups maintained the same dosage throughout the 12 week study (placebo, tacrine 20 mg/day, or tacrine 40 mg/day). The other 3 groups escalated in tacrine dosage at week 6 (placebo to 20 mg/day, 20 mg/day to 40 mg/day, and 40 mg/day to 80 mg/day). Efficacy was assessed at weeks 4, 6, 10, and 12. The 30 week study comprised

4 treatment groups; group 1 received placebo for 30 weeks, groups 2, 3, and 4 received tacrine 40 mg/day for 6 weeks, followed by 80 mg/day for 6 weeks. Group 2 continued to receive 80 mg/day for the remaining 18 weeks, while Group 3 escalated to 120 mg/day for the remaining 18 weeks. Group 4 escalated to 120 mg/day for 6 weeks, followed by 160 mg/day for the remaining 12 weeks of study. An unbalanced scheme (3:1:3:4 for Groups 1, 2, 3, and 4, respectively) was used in randomizing patients to treatment due to expectations of a larger number of dropouts due to side effects in the highest dosage group. Efficacy was assessed at weeks 6, 12, 16, 18, 22, 24, and 30.

The primary outcome measures included the Alzheimer's Disease Assessment Scale, cognitive subscale [ADAS-Cog] (Rosen et al., 1984) and a clinician-rated global evaluation: the Clinical Global Impression of Change (CGIC) and Clinician Interview-Based Impression [CIBI] (Knopman et al., 1994) for the 12- and 30-week studies, respectively. A second global evaluation which allowed caregiver input, the Final Comprehensive Consensus Assessment (FCCA), was included as a primary outcome measure in the 30 week study.

A large number of patients failed to complete both studies, primarily as a result of side effects. In addition to the evaluatable patient analyses described in previous reports (Farlow et al., 1992; Knapp et al., 1994), a last observation carried forward (LOCF) analysis was conducted to address the issue of the high dropout rate and to provide confirmation of the conclusions drawn from planned analyses. The LOCF analysis utilized data from all patients randomized to treatment who had received at least 1 dose of study medication and had at least 1 post-treatment efficacy assessment. For the 12-week study, the LOCF analysis was limited to patients originally assigned to placebo for 12 weeks (N = 77) or a final tacrine dose of 80 mg/day (N = 77).

The estimated mean treatment differences, 90% and 95% confidence intervals for the treatment difference, and parametric p-values for each of the primary efficacy variables were computed from an analysis of variance model. Each model included effects for treatment group and center. The dose-trend and categorical variables (e.g. CGIC and CIBI scores), were analyzed using the Cochran-Mantel-Haenszel procedure. For all analyses, results were considered statistically significant if $p \leq 0.05$.

RESULTS

In the 12- and 30-week studies, 468 and 663 patients were randomized to treatment, respectively. There were no significant differences between treatment groups at baseline; 326 and 279 patients completed the entire 12- and 30-week study periods, respectively. In tacrine-treated patients, the primary reasons for early withdrawal were asymptomatic elevations in ALT (of which 90% occurred by week 12) and dose-related gastrointestinal side effects, primarily occurring in the higher dose groups (120 and 160 mg/day) in the 30-week study. Included

	ADAS-Cog		Global Measures		
	Week 12[a]	Week 30[b]	CGIC[a]	CIBI[b]	FCCA[b]
Dose-Trend[c] p-value	0.03*	< 0.001*	0.08	< 0.001*	< 0.001*
80 mg/d vs. Pbo					
N Pbo/N Tacrine	71/72	167/48	72/74	170/50	152/33
Tx Difference	-2.4	-1.9	-0.3	-0.3	-0.3
95% CI[d]	(-4.1, -0.8)	(-4.0, 0.2)	(-0.5, 0.1)	(-0.6, -0.01)	(-0.7, 0.08)
p-value	0.01*	0.07	0.06	0.04*	0.12
120 mg/d vs. Pbo					
N Pbo/N Tacrine	N/A	167/143	N/A	170/144	152/81
Tx Difference		-3.3		-0.4	-0.4
95% CI		(-5.0, -2.0)		(-0.6, -0.2)	(-0.7, -0.1)
p-value		< 0.001*		< 0.001*	0.004*
160 mg/d vs. Pbo					
N Pbo/N Tacrine	N/A	167/184	N/A	170/187	152/97
Tx Difference		-3.7		-0.4	-0.5
95% CI		(-5.0, -2.3)		(-0.6, -0.2)	(-0.8, -0.3)
p-value		< 0.001*		< 0.001*	< 0.001*

TABLE I. LOCF Analysis of Primary Outcome Measures. [a]Farlow et al., 1992; [b]Knapp et al., 1994; [c]Dose-trend p-values computed using CMH methods; [d]For the 12-week study, the 90% CI is presented; * p ≤ 0.05

in the LOCF analyses are 146 and 562 patients in the 12- and 30-week studies, respectively.

The results of the LOCF analyses for the primary outcome measures in each study are presented in Table I. Significant dose-response trends ($p \leq 0.05$) were observed for the ADAS-Cog in both studies. In the 12-week study, the 80 mg/day vs placebo comparison was significant with a mean treatment difference of -2.4 points based on a sample size of 72 patients receiving tacrine, while this comparison approached significance in the 30-week study ($p = 0.07$) with a mean treatment difference of -1.9 points and a sample size of 48 patients. Results for tacrine 120 and 160 mg/day vs placebo on the ADAS-Cog were highly significant ($p < 0.001$) with mean treatment differences of -3.3 and -3.7 points, respectively.

On the global measures, the dose-trend analysis approached significance in the the 12-week study ($p = 0.08$), and reached significance for both the CIBI and FCCA in the 30-week study ($p < 0.001$). In both studies, the mean treatment differences between tacrine 80 mg/day and placebo were identical (-0.3 points), and the primary determining factor on the significance level relates to the sample size within the placebo and tacrine-treated groups. For the tacrine 120 and 160 mg/day comparisons in the 30-week study, significance was achieved on both the CIBI and FCCA ($p \leq 0.004$) with mean treatment differences of -0.4 to -0.5 points.

DISCUSSION

In these two parallel group studies, statistically significant differences in favor of tacrine were demonstrated on an objective measure of cognitive function (ADAS-Cog) and clinician-rated global evaluations (CGIC, CIBI, and FCCA). A significant dose-response trend was evident. Although there were a large number of patients who could not complete the studies, the fact that the LOCF analysis supported the evaluable patient analysis suggests that the differential dropout rate between placebo- and tacrine-treated groups did not contribute significant bias to the overall conclusions of study results.

The double-blind phases in the studies reported herein are longer than the six week treatment periods in previously reported enrichment design studies (Davis et al., 1992), and at least as long as the 3-month treatment period in the crossover study described by Eagger et al. (1991). The parallel design avoids the methodological limitations of enrichment and crossover design studies by controlling for confounding factors such as in-study effects, learning effects, and practice effects. In addition, the 30-week study included evaluation of higher tacrine doses of 120 and 160 mg/day which were initially reported as effective by Summers et al. (1986).

The majority of patient withdrawals were due to asymptomatic ALT elevations and dose-related cholinergic events (e.g. nausea, vomiting, dyspepsia). The dose-related events generally occurred after patients reached a new dosage level;

therefore, the last observation on treatment was determined on a dose which the patient was clearly tolerating. Thus, the LOCF analysis provides a reasonable, but conservative estimate of the treatment effects of tacrine. The majority of patients who withdrew due to ALT elevations and dose-related side effects were able to resume treatment and titrate to higher daily doses using a more flexible dosing regimen.

REFERENCES

Davis KL, Thal LJ, Gamzu ER et al. (1992): A double-blind, placebo-controlled multicenter study of tacrine for Alzheimer's disease. *N Engl J Med* 327:1253-1259.

Eagger SA, Levy R, and Sahakian BJ (1991): Tacrine in Alzheimer's disease. *Lancet* 337:989-992.

Farlow M, Gracon SI, Hershey LA et al. (1992): A controlled trial of tacrine in Alzheimer's disease. *JAMA* 268:2523-2529.

Folstein MF, Folstein SE and McHugh PR (1975): Mini-Mental State: a practical method for grading the cognitive state of patients for the clinician. *J Psychiatr Res* 12:189-198.

Knapp MJ, Knopman DS, Solomon PR et al. (1994): A 30-week randomized controlled trial of high-dose tacrine in patients with Alzheimer's disease. *JAMA* 271:985-991.

Knopman DS, Knapp MJ, Gracon SI and Davis CS (1994): The Clinician Interview-Based Impression (CIBI): a clinician's global change rating scale in Alzheimer's disease. *Neurology* (Submitted).

Rosen WG, Mohs RC and Davis KL (1994): A new rating scale for Alzheimer's disease. *Am J Psychiat* 141:1356-1364.

Summers WK, Majovski LV, Marsh GM et al. (1986): Oral tetrahydroaminoacridine in long-term treatment of senile dementia, Alzheimer type. *N Engl J Med* 315:1241-1245.

Wilcock GK, Surmon DJ, Scott M et al. (1993): An evaluation of the efficacy and safety of tetrahydroaminoacridine (THA) without lecithin in the treatment of Alzheimer's disease. *Age and Aging* 22:316-324.

Alzheimer Disease: Therapeutic Strategies
edited by E. Giacobini and R. Becker.
© 1994 Birkhäuser Boston

CLINICAL UPDATE OF VELNACRINE RESEARCH

Klaudius Siegfried
Clinical Neuroscience/Europe, Corporate Clinical Research, Hoechst AG,
Frankfurt (M), Germany

Rich Civil
Clinical Neuroscience, SBU Neuroscience, Hoechst-Roussel
Pharmaceuticals Inc., Somerville, NJ USA

INTRODUCTION

Velnacrine is a 1,2,3,4-tetrahydro-9-aminoacridine-1-ol maleate which acts
biochemically as a potent cholinesterase inhibitor (ChEI). Due to its ability to
enhance cholinergic functions, it has been developed as an Alzheimer's disease
(AD) agent. Pharmacological studies in rodents demonstrated that the compound
can improve learning and memory functions and reverse learning deficits caused
either by scopolamine or lesions of the nucleus basalis magnocellularis (NBM)
(which in rats is the equivalent of the nucleus basalis of Meynert complex in
man) (Fielding et al., 1989). In pharmacokinetic studies in humans, plasma
peak levels were reached within one hr after oral administration, and the drug
was rapidly eliminated with a half-life of about two to three hrs. Steady-state
plasma levels were reached after approximately three days of repeated dose
(t.i.d.) treatment. There were dose-related increases in peak plasma
concentrations (Cmax), areas under the plasma concentration - time curves
(AUC) and the amount of drug excreted in the urine (Puri et al., 1988). Results
from a food interaction study suggest that food may delay time to peak
concentration and reduce Cmax, but not significantly alter the amount of
absorbed substance.

EFFECTS OBSERVED IN PHARMACODYNAMIC AND PHASE II EFFICACY STUDIES

Pharmacodynamic trials with single doses of velnacrine in both healthy, young
subjects and patients with AD were able to demonstrate statistically significant
effects, relative to placebo, on attentional, short-term memory, and recent
memory functions. The effects were apparent from approximately two hrs after
oral administration onwards (Siegfried, 1993, 1994). Single doses of 75 mg

velnacrine also significantly increased regional cerebral blood flow in the superior frontal and right parietal cortical areas in patients with AD (Reference area for SPECT evaluation: Calcarine cortex) (Ebmeier et al., 1992).

Patients selected for velnacrine studies, had to fulfill the criteria of 'probable AD' (McKhann et al., 1984) and to show a mild to moderate degree of dementia. The first repeated-dose study in patients was a European double-blind, placebo-controlled cross-over trial with fairly short treatment periods (2 times 10 days) and a wash-out time of four days in between the periods (Siegfried and Murphy, 1993). Of the 45 patients enrolled, 34 were available for efficacy analysis. In spite of the short treatment duration, this pilot project showed statistically significant treatment effects on various outcome measures: on the cognitive behavior subscale of the Alzheimer Disease Assessment Scale (ADAS) (Rosen et al., 1984) ($p = 0.013$); on an immediate word recognition task ($p = 0.048$), and a choice reaction time task ($p = 0.0024$). An aggregate measure (assessment on days 1, 4 and 10 of each treatment period) of the Clinical Global Impression of Change (CGI-Change) rating just failed to become significant ($p = 0.054$).

A pivotal source of evidence for short-term (or subchronic) efficacy of velnacrine in patients with AD was the US enrichment study No. 201 (Murphy et al., 1991; Siegfried and Murphy, 1993). Following a five-week dose-ranging and a two-week wash-out phase, patients who responded (i.e. had an improvement of $\geq$ 4 points on the ADAS-Cog) and tolerated the drug, were allowed to enter a six-week double-blind, placebo-controlled parallel-group treatment segment ('replication phase') receiving either their 'best' dose of velnacrine (in the majority of cases 50 or 75 mg t.i.d.) or placebo. Out of the 735 patients treated in the dose-ranging segment, 309 (i.e. approximately 42%) qualified for the replication phase. The efficacy analyses ('intention-to-treat analyses') brought about highly significant effects on both (pre-defined) primary outcome variables, the ADAS-Cog (in both completer and last observation carried forward analyses) and the CGI-Change (at week six of treatment).

PHASE III EFFICACY STUDIES

Two Phase III studies have been completed. One of them was a European enrichment study with a four-month double-blind, placebo-controlled replication phase, the other a six-month US double-blind, placebo-controlled parallel-group study. The efficacy results of both studies favored velnacrine.

In the European study, a total of 236 patients were enrolled at 12 study sites (in Austria, Belgium, France, Germany, the Netherlands, UK). Two hundred eight patients entered the three-week open-labelled 'test treatment' with velnacrine (150 mg/day) which was followed by a four-week placebo wash-out phase. Responders to test treatment (defined in the study protocol as an improvement of $\geq$ 4 points on ADAS-Cog) which also tolerated the drug, were randomized in a 2:1 ratio to a four-month double-blind, parallel-group treatment ('replication phase') of either velnacrine (50 mg t.i.d.) or placebo. One hundred eleven out of 203 analyzable patients (or 54.7%) qualified for the replication phase treatment. All efficacy evaluations were intention-to-treat analyses. None of the patients dropped out for efficacy problems during the replication phase. Therefore, completer analyses appeared to be the most adequate type of efficacy evaluations. An analyses of covariance, using the Folstein MMS screen score as a covariate, revealed a significant difference between the treatment groups (p = 0.038; n = 81) in favor of velnacrine. No significant differences in CGI-Change were found. Since, however, the CGI-Change significantly correlated with the ADAS Cog scores (r = 0.60; p=0.0001; n = 81) and measures considered indicators of clinical relevance (IADL, see below) which showed clear treatment effects, it was concluded that the CGI was not sensitive enough, possibly due to shifting reference points inherent to enrichment design studies (see similar problems in one of the tacrine studies: Davis et al., 1992). The following secondary outcome measures rendered significant treatment effects: the NOSGER (Nurses Observation Geriatric Scale: Spiegel, 1984) subscales 'Memory' (p=0.03) and 'Instrumental Activities of Daily Living' (p = 0.03), (IADL), both completed by patients' caregivers. In addition, significant effects (p < 0.05) or trends (0.05 < p ≤ 0.1) were observed with specific cognitive performance tests, such as the Digit Symbol Substitution Test (Wechsler, 1955), the Paired Associate Learning Test (Inglis, 1959) and the Block Design Test (Wechsler, 1955).

In the six-month US parallel-group study which compared velnacrine (150 and 225 mg/day) to placebo, 449 patients were enrolled, 297 received velnacrine and 152 placebo. One hundred sixty-seven out of the 297 velnacrine patients (56.2%) completed the study; the proportion of completers in the placebo group was 74.3%. The most common reason for discontinuation in the velnacrine group was abnormal clinical laboratory values. There was a baseline heterogeneity which was adjusted for by covariance analyses. Both completor and last observation carried forward analyses showed statistically significant (p < 0.05) results in favor of velnacrine on the two primary outcome variables (ADAS-Cog and CGI-Change) and in two caregiver-based assessments, the Patient Global Improvement Ratio (PGIR) and the 'Physical Self-Maintenance Scale' (PSMS). In a 'Caregiver Activities Time Survey' (CATS), an instrument developed by Duke University which requests caregivers to provide information on time usually allocated to patient cases such as feeding, toileting, bathing and general supervision, a comparison of week 24 of treatment with baseline, revealed marked differences between the treatment groups. In the velnacrine group, time spent on care was reduced by 45% (or 3.2 hrs per day) in comparison to baseline; whereas in the placebo group a statistically insignificant reduction of 25 mins only was observed (Moore and Clipp, 1994).

The most common safety-relevant observation in phase III studies were abnormal liver function tests - essentially significant transaminase increases. SGPT/SGOT increases of at least twice the upper limit of normal occurred in the two studies in an average of approximately 31% of patients treated with velnacrine. The most common symptoms reported as adverse events belonged to the central nervous system (CNS). There was, however, no important difference in the frequency of CNS symptoms between the treatment groups. The most common three events considered as possibly related to the study drug were diarrhea, dizziness and headache. Each of them occurred on average in 5-10% of the patients. In rare cases, neutropenia occurred.

CONCLUSION

The four velnacrine efficacy studies described consistently rendered favorable results. Significant treatment effects were observed on a performance-based scale of cognitive symptoms (ADAS-Cog), on the CGI-Change, on caregivers' ratings of patients' everyday behavior (e.g. IADL, ADL), in specific cognitive performance tests of attentional, recent memory and constructional praxis, and in a measure of caregivers time allocated to patient care. The consistency across the studies and the various types of measures, in particular the changes observed in patients everyday behavior and on caregivers' time, suggest clinical relevance of the effects. The average serum-placebo differences were generally of a modest size but there is a subgroup of patients which appear to have a clear benefit from treatment. These findings indicate a pharmacological heterogeneity of the population of patients having AD. Future research efforts must be directed at finding clinical and biological markers to subtype patients and predict response.

The safety problems appear to be acceptable for a first-generation of effective drugs provided patients are required to undergo regular frequent safety controls.

REFERENCES

Davis KL, Thal LJ, Gamzu ER, Davis CS, Woolson RF, Gracon SI, Drachman DA et al. (1992): A double-blind, placebo-controlled multicenter study of tacrine for Alzheimer's disease. *New Engl J Med* 327(18):1253-1259.

Ebmeier KP, Hunter R, Curran SM, Dougal N, Murray CL, Wyper D, Siegfried K, Goodwin G (1992): Effects of a single dose of the acetylcholinesterase inhibitor velnacrine on recognition memory and regional cerebral blood flow in Alzheimer's disease. *Psychopharmacol* 108:103-109.

Fielding S, Cornfeldt ML, Szewczak MR et al. (1989): HP 029, a new drug for the treatment of Alzheimer's disease; its pharmacological profile. In: *Pharmacological Intervention in a Central Cholinergic Meachanism in Senile Dementia (Alzheimer's Disease)*, Kewitz H, Thomson T and Bickel K, eds. Zuckschwerdt Verlag: Munchen-Bern-Wien-San Francisco, pp. 107-117.

Inglis J (1959): A paired-associate learning test for use with elderly psychiatric patients. *J Mental Sci* 105:440-443.

McKhann G, Drachman D, Folstein M, Katzman R, Price D and Stadlan E (1984): Clinical diagnosis of Alzheimer's disease: Report of the NINCDS-ADRDA work group under the auspices of the development of health and human services task force on Alzheimer's Disease. *Neurology* 34:939-944.

Moore MJ and Clipp EC (1994): Alzheimer's disease and caregiver time. *Lancet* 343(8891):239-240.

Murphy MF, Hardiman ST, Nash RJ et al. (1991): Evaluation of HP 029 (velnacrine maleate) in Alzheimer's disease. *Ann NY Acad Sci* 640:253-262.

Puri SK, Hsu R, Ho I and Lassman HB (1988): Single-dose, tolerance, and pharmacokinetics of HP 029 in elderly men: a potential Alzheimer's agent. *Curr Ther Res* 44:766-780.

Rosen WR, Mohs RC and Davis KL (1984): A new rating scale of Alzheimer's disease. *Am J Psychiatry* 141:1356-1354.

Siegfried K (1993): The Pharmacodynamics of velnacrine: results and conclusions from clincal studies in healthy subjects and patients with Alzheimer's disease. In: *The Management of Alzheimer's Disease*, Wilcock GK, ed. *Wrightson Biomedical Publishing Ltd.*, pp. 189-201.

Siegfried K (1994): The cholinergic hypothesis in Alzheimer's disease - Clinical evidence gained with velnacrine. In: *Alzheimer's disease: Clinical and treatment aspects*. Cutler N, Gottfries C-G and Siegfried K, eds. Chichester: John Wiley & Sons Ltd. (In Press).

Siegfried K and Murphy MF (1993): The cholinergic approach to the treatment of Alzheimer's disease. In: *Alzheimer's disease*. Wolters B and Scheltens K, eds. Amsterdam: Vrije Universiteit, pp. 97-106.

Spiegel R (1989): The NOSGER (Nurses' Observation Scale for Geriatric Patients). Distributed by the author.

Wechsler, D.; (1955): The measurement and appraisal of adult intelligence. Baltimore: Williams and Williams

Alzheimer Disease: Therapeutic Strategies
edited by E. Giacobini and R. Becker.
© 1994 Birkhäuser Boston

SECOND AND THIRD GENERATION CHOLINESTERASE INHIBITORS: FROM PRECLINICAL STUDIES TO CLINICAL EFFICACY

Ezio Giacobini and Gabriel Cuadra
Department of Pharmacology, Southern Illinois University School of
Medicine, Springfield, IL 62794-9230

Pharmacological Effects of Cholinesterase Inhibitors and Alzheimer Disease Therapy
Four main pharmacological effects of cholinesterase inhibitors (ChEI) constitute the theoretical basis for therapy of Alzheimer disease (AD): 1) functional improvement of central cholinergic synapses mediated through muscarinic and nicotinic mechanisms (Summers et al., 1994; Cuadra et al., 1994); 2) protection against neuronal degeneration mediated through nicotinic receptor activation (Janson and Moller, 1993; Sjak-shie et al., 1990); 3) modification of amyloid precursor protein (APP) processing mediated through muscarinic M_1 receptor activation (Nitsch et al., 1993; Buxbaum et al., 1992); and 4) regional enhanced synthesis of neurotrophic molecules [nerve growth factor (NGF) and brain derived nerve factor (BDNF)] via muscarinic receptor stimulation (Lindfors et al., 1992; Berzaghi et al., 1993).

The Second Generation Cholinesterase Inhibitors: The Last Three Years
Preclinical and clinical research on development of new ChEI has strongly advanced during the last five years and since our last meeting (Giacobini, 1991). A total of 13 ChEI (Table I) is presently being tested clinically throughout the world. Tacrine is the compound at the most advanced stage of clinical research. At least 2,000 AD patients treated with this drug have already been studied (Table II). Other amino acridine derivatives and active metabolites of tacrine such as velnacrine (1-0H metabolite) (HP029) and suronacrine (HP128) are also being tested in AD therapy. Multi-center trials are in progress for other ChEI to define their efficacy, safety and dose response relationships (Table I). The diversity of chemical structures and pharmacological characteristics among these compounds is striking. Both reversible (carbamates or non-carbamate compounds) and irreversible (e.g. organophosphate) inhibitors (metrifonate) are being tested. A new derivative of physostigmine (PHY), heptyl-physostigmine (HEP) (eptastigmine, MF-201) is also in clinical trial. Together with PHY, two other ChEI natural products, the Huperzines and galanthamine are being tested.

Second generation ChEI are characterized by their high penetration through the
blood brain barrier, potent, long-lasting and selective inhibition of
acetylcholinesterase (AChE) with low peripheral cholinergic side effects. The
appearance of hematologic complications (neutropenia or agranulocytosis) is a
new finding that together with hepatotoxicity needs to be considered carefully
in future drug development (Table I).

Compound	Country	Company	Clinical Phase	Side Effects Comments
Physostigmine retard	USA	Forest	II	N.A.
ENA 713	Europe	Sandoz	II	N.A.
Heptyl-physostigmine	Italy/USA	Mediolanum	II	Hematology**
E-2020	USA/Japan	Eisai	II	Mild side effects
MDL 73,745	USA/ Europe	Marion-Merrell Dow	II	Mild side effects
Metrifonate	USA/ Germany	Bayer/ Miles	II	Mild side effects
Tacrine (THA) *	USA/ Europe	Warner-Lambert	III	Hepatotoxicity
Velnacrine (HP029) Suronacrine (HP128)	USA/ Europe	Hoechst-Roussel	II	Hematology*** Hepatotoxicity
Galanthamine	Germany USA	Waldheim Ciba-Geigy	II	Mild side effects
Huperzine A	China	Chinese Acad. Sci.	III	N.A.
HP290	England	Astra Arcus	I	N.A.
ChEI	USA	Pfizer	II	NA

TABLE I. Cholinesterase inhibitors: AD clinical trials (1994). * other indications:
HIV, tardive dyskinesia; ** neutropenia or *** agranulocytosis; N.A. = data not
available.

New molecules are being designed to avoid both hematologic and hepatic
toxicity as well as to produce higher CNS AChE inhibition at a low level of side

effects and toxicity. Several new drugs are being studied preclinically. Whether or not they will reach the clinical phase will depend largely on the success of their parent compounds in the patient.

Efficacy of Cholinesterase Inhibitors in AD Therapy. Cholinesterase Inhibition or Acetylcholine Levels?

On the basis of preclinical and clinical studies we proposed that both cholinesterase (ChE) inhibition and increase in brain acetylcholine (ACh) would be directly related to the clinical efficacy of the inhibitor (Becker and Giacobini, 1988a,b). These suggestions were in agreement with the initial hypothesis (Becker and Giacobini, 1988a,b) postulating that steady-state high ChE inhibition measurable in plasma or RBC (but not drug concentration) would relate directly to a favorable clinical response. Yet, we found in animal experiments an inconsistent relationship among the degree of ChE inhibition, changes in brain ACh concentrations, behavioral changes and therapeutic and adverse effects following administration of ChEI in humans (Becker and Giacobini, 1988a,b) (Table III). Based on recent clinical data, Becker et al. (1991) proposed a hypothetical therapeutic window for RBC AChE inhibition in the range of 30-60% with a mid-point of 40% producing at least 50% clinical improvement.

This hypothesis is supported by three sets of clinical results related to three different ChEI. Thal et al. (1983) demonstrated an inverted "U" dose response curve for PHY (i.v.) effect on retrieval from long-term storage versus percent CSF ChE inhibition. Peak performance was at 40-50% ChE inhibition. A similar but less pronounced phenomenon was seen for orally administered PHY. Becker et al. (1990) reported a similar relation with metrifonate (5 mg/kg/week oral dose) associated to a 58% RBC AChE inhibition. Imbimbo and Lucchelli (this publication) (HEP, 30-60 mg/day oral dose) described an inverted U-shaped relation of performance to steady-state RBC AChE inhibition with an optimal effect at around 40% AChE inhibition. The three studies confirm a range of therapeutic efficacy with a window of 40-60% of AChE or ChE inhibition as postulated by the hypothesis of Becker et al. (1991).

Our animal experiments have shown that changes in brain ACh concentration that follow ChE inhibition are not solely the direct result of the percentage of ChE inhibition but are affected by the specific pharmacological properties of individual drugs (DeSarno et al., 1989; Giacobini, 1993) (Table III). These properties include effects on the inhibition of ChE as well as on neurotransmitter release (DeSarno et al., 1989; Messamore et al., 1993c). Table III presents a comparison of effects of six ChEI on cortical ChE activity and ACh release measured with microdialysis in non-anesthetized awake rats with no ChEI in the probe. It can be seen that following PHY administration, a maximal ChE inhibition in cortex of 60% will produce a maximal increase in ACh release of 4000% while a 50% ChE inhibition produced by HUP-A (L-Huperzine-A) or THA (tacrine) will cause only a 230-500% increase in ACh. At the 50% level of ChE inhibition, cholinergic side effects will also be more pronounced with

AUTHORS (year)	TYPE OF STUDY*	NR. OF PAT.	MAX DOSE (mg); DURATION (wk)	Points Difference from placebo MMSE	ADAS	DETERIORATION GAIN (mo)	% PAT. IMPROVED
Gauthier et al. (1990)	DB-CO-M	52	100 / 8	1		2	(75)
Eagger et al. (1991-1992)	DB-CO-PC	65	150 / 13	3-4		6-12	45
Davis et al. (1992)	DB-PC-M	632	80 / 8		2.4	5	34
Farlow et al. (1992)	DB-PC-M	468	80 / 12		4	6	51
Alhainen (1992)	DB-PC	25	100 / 7	≥3		≥6	44
Knapp et al. (1994)	DB-PC-M	663	160 / 30	4	3	>6	40
	Total	1905					

TABLE II. Clinical efficacy of Tacrine for Alzheimer disease. * DB = double-blind; CO = crossover; PC = placebo controlled; M = multicenter; MMSE = Mini-Mental State Examination (0-30); ADAS = Alzheimer Disease Assessment Scale (0-70) (ADAS-Cognitive)

Drug	Dose mg/kg	% Max. AChE Inhibition	Peak time AChE Inhibition (min)	Duration AChE Inhibition (hrs)	% ACh Maximum Increase	Peak time ACh Effect (min)	Duration ACh Effect (hrs)	Cholinergic Side Effects *
Physostigmine	.3	60	30	2	4000	60	1.5	+++
Heptyl-physostigmine	5	90	60	27	3000	90	10	++
Metrifonate **	80	70	60	24	1800	60	6	+
MDL-73,745	10	80	60	>9	1100	60	7	++
THA	5	50	60	10	500	90	3	+
Huperzine A	.5	50	30	>6	220	60	6	+

TABLE III. Comparison of effects of cholinesterase inhibitors on AChE activity and ACh release in rat cortex (Messamore et al., 1993a,b,c; Cuadra et al., 1994; Zhu and Giacobini (submitted). * fasciculations, tremor, splay; ** active metabolite = DDVP

PHY than with the other two drugs. Duration of ACh increase will also vary with different drugs from a minimum of 1.5 hrs for PHY to a maximum of 10 hrs for HEP (Table III). Based on these experimental data, it seems too restrictive to use ChE inhibition in plasma or RBC as the target of therapeutic effects. A restatement of the therapeutic strategy in terms of CNS ACh concentration and steady-state duration of ACh levels rather than ChE inhibition seems to be justified (Becker and Giacobini, 1988a,b).

Many ChEI already tested clinically, such as PHY and THA, do not fully express the potential of ChEI to induce long-lasting ACh concentrations with low side effect frequency. With these drugs, inhibition of ChE exceeding 50% is associated to strong side effects. We suggest to step up ACh CNS concentrations more effectively using drugs such as second generation ChEI which produce long-lasting changes in ACh CNS concentrations. It becomes an important priority to identify or design inhibitors free of adverse effects and with predictable effects on ACh brain concentrations. The recent study of Knapp et al. (1994) with THA demonstrating a dose-response effect of the drug (80-160 mg dose) illustrates the importance of reaching high-enough ChE CNS inhibition in order to produce therapeutic levels. However, for some new second generation ChEI it is still doubtful whether even 80% RBC AChE inhibition may effectively boost ACh concentrations to produce clinical efficacy.

Clinical Efficacy of Cholinesterase Inhibitors
Most data on ChEI efficacy studies are not yet available (Table I). The best documented studies of ChEI clinical efficacy in AD are related to the effect of THA administration for periods of time up to 30 weeks (Table II). Table II summarizes the results of six major double-blind, placebo-controlled trials using similar methods of assessment of cognitive function in a total of 1,905 patients during the period 1990-1994.

Based on point differences from placebo in cognitive scoring, a gain ranging from 2-12 months [Mini-Mental State Examination (MMSE)] to 5-6 months [Alzheimer Disease Assessment Scale (ADAS)] in deterioration can be seen for THA treatments lasting 2-6 month. A dose response (20-80 mg/kg) effect is described with a 4-point improvement on the ADAS cognitive scale after 3 month treatment (Farlow et al., 1992). Similarly, a more recent study of THA (Knapp et al., 1994) demonstrates a mean improvement of four points at 160 mg/kg dose on ADAS-Cog and at least 3.0 points on the MMSE after 6 months. These results suggest a positive effect of the drug on patient deterioration with a significant gain of several months per year of treatment. These results need to be confirmed with longer trials up to 24-36 months in order to demonstrate a real slow down of the disease course.

An attenuation of disease progression corresponding to a 12-month gain with a 24 month long ChEI therapy would represent a significant therapeutic effect. There are limitations with the present THA therapy. About one third of the patients entering the THA trial can not continue the treatment because of toxicity. Within this selected population of patients, only 30-50% is improved (Table II). The development of new ChEI with lower rate of side effects and toxicity will allow a higher level of prolonged steady-state inhibition promoting a functional level of cholinergic transmission.

Which Type of Cholinesterase Should be Inhibited in Order to Improve Cholinergic Function in AD Patients?

The concentration of ACh present in the cholinergic synapse is a main factor for the function of the synapse. It remains remarkably constant in spite of ample variations in functional activity and rate of release of ACh from the terminal. A rapid hydrolysis of the released ACh is catalyzed by AChE. The stability of ACh concentrations is maintained by short-term adjustments of the rate of synthesis in relation to the rate of release (Tucek, 1993). Because it is difficult to modify pharmacologically, functional activity, rate of synthesis or rate of release of ACh, the most efficient approach is to inhibit AChE activity (Messamore et al., 1993a,b). This will rapidly adjust ACh concentrations to near-physiological levels (Messamore et al., 1993a,b).

In animal experiments *in vivo* or *in vitro*, AChE inhibition enhances the action of ACh directly administered to the preparation and potentiates the effect of ACh released by electrical stimulation. This enhancement of synaptic transmission is a consequence of the stimulation of cholinergic muscarinic and nicotinic receptors extending over an area larger than the point of release. By delaying the termination of ACh action, AChE inhibition promotes a longer-lasting depolarization. Under pathological conditions such as AD, a pharmacologically enhanced concentration of ACh would allow for stimulation of a larger number of cholinergic receptors and facilitate transmission. Both AChE and butyrylcholinesterase (BuChE) are present in the CNS, however, the first type is mainly represented in axons and perikarya, the second in glia (Giacobini, 1959). The function of BuChE which is also present in the CNS is unknown. In AD, both enzyme activities can be histochemically demonstrated not only in cortical axons or perikarya but also in neuritic plaques (Mesulam and Geula, 1991) colocalized with amyloid deposits, abnormal neurites and paired helical filaments (Carson et al., 1991; Arendt et al., 1992). New inhibitors are available with selectivity for various isoform of ChEs as well as specificity for AChE or BuChE (Ogane et al., 1992a,b). It is unlikely that accumulation of either BuChE or AChE in or around neuritic plaques could play a physiological role. It is also unlikely that appreciable amounts of ACh may diffuse out from the synapse to reach these abnormal localization sites of the enzymes. Therefore, a rational approach to AD therapy should target the AChE forms which are associated with the basal lamina of the external surface of the synapse and which react with the released ACh. Based on this assumption, the basic requirements for a ChEI to be useful therapeutically in AD are: 1) penetrability of the compound to reach the synaptic area; and 2) good selectivity for AChE *and its membrane*-located isoform. The present knowledge of the molecular structures of the enzyme and of inhibitor-enzyme interaction allows us to design and develop such a class of selective AChE inhibitors (see Silman et al., this publication).

Effects of Cholinesterase Inhibitors on Cortical Neurotransmitters

The basic principle utilized in cholinomimetic therapy of AD with ChEI is an increase in extracellular synaptic ACh concentration in order to restore cholinergic hypofunction (Becker and Giacobini, 1988a,b).   Clinical and experimental evidence indicates involvement and   interactions between the cholinergic system and biogenic amine systems in the cognitive impairments observed in AD (Hardy et al., 1985; Decker and McGaugh, 1991). A brain region of particular interest is the frontal cortex since both in humans and rodents it represents the major cholinergic projection of the nucleus basalis magnocellularis (NBM) of the basal forebrain (Mesulam and Geula, 1988). Similarly, the major, if not sole, noradrenergic projection to the cortex is the locus coeruleus (LC) (Parnavelas, 1990).   Pharmacological alleviation of combined cholinergic (NBM)/noradrenergic (LC) lesion-induced memory deficits in rats has been reported (Santucci et al., 1991).   Interactions between norepinephrine (NE) and ACh in cortex are well known (Decker and McGaugh, 1991; McGaugh et al., 1992) (Fig. 1).

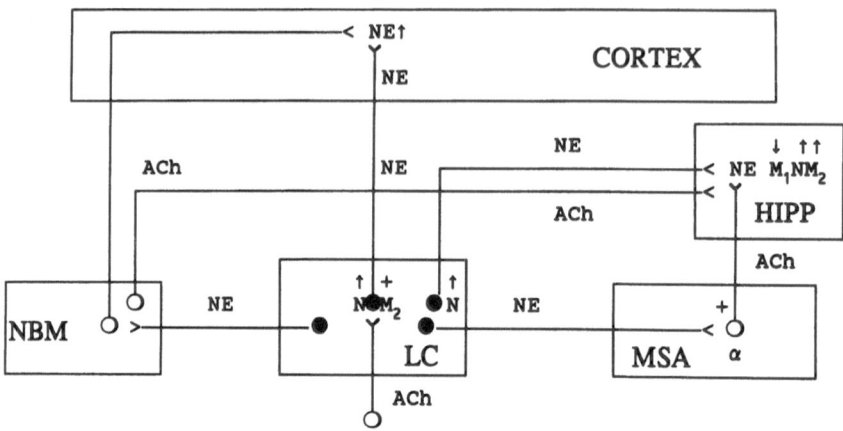

FIGURE 1. Effects of ACh on norepinephrine. M = muscarinic stimulation; N = nicotinic stimulation; ↓↑ = decreased/increased NE release; + = increased firing; NBM = nucleus basalis magnocellularis; LC = locus coeruleus; MSA = medial septal area; HIPP = hippocampus; ACh = acetylcholine; NE = norepinephrine; α = alpha-adrenoceptors; ● = adrenergic neurons; ○ = cholinergic neurons

We have compared the effect of PHY, a short-acting reversible carbamate inhibitor with its analogue HEP, a long-acting ChEI, administered systemically (s.c.) or by local perfusion into the cortex via a microdialysis probe, on extracellular levels of several biogenic amines including ACh, NE, dopamine

(DA) and 5-hydroxytryptamine (5-HT) in the same sample of perfusate (Cuadra et al., 1994) (Table IV) (Figs. 2 and 3).

Drug	Dose mg/kg	% Max. AChE Inhib.	Percent Increase and Peak Time (hrs)			
			ACh	NE	DA	5-HT
Physostigmine	.3	50	4000 (1)	75 (1.0)	120 (2)	0
Heptyl-physostigmine	2	70	2500 (1.5)	25 (1.5)	75 (2)	0

TABLE IV. Effect of two carbamate cholinesterase inhibitors on cortical neurotransmitters in rat cortex after systemic (s.c.) administration.

Our results show a dose-dependent increase in endogenous ACh levels in frontal cortex for both ChEIs (Table IV) (Figs. 2 and 3). This is in agreement with the results of previous studies demonstrating an increase of extracellular ACh after ChEI systemic administration of these compounds (Kosasa et al., 1990; Xu et al., 1991; Messamore et al., 1993b).

We observed differences between the two drugs in peak values of ACh and in time to peak and return to baseline. Physostigmine (300 μg/kg) produced its maximal ACh elevation between 30 and 60 min while HEP (5 mg/kg) effect peaked between 60 and 90 min (Table III) (Figs. 2 and 3). The most long-lasting effect on ACh levels (10 hrs) was seen after HEP treatment. At 360 min after the injection, ACh concentration was still significantly increased above baseline.

After systemic administration of PHY and HEP, we observed that the increase in ACh levels was followed in time by a significant elevation of extracellular NE levels (Table IV) (Figs. 2 and 3). However, only PHY at both doses elicited a significant NE increase. This effect was weaker after HEP (2 mg/kg) and not measurable at the high dose. If PHY and HEP were administered locally in the cortex they did not significantly modify NE levels. Norepinephrine decreases the release of ACh from cholinergic terminals in cortex (Vizi, 1980; Moroni et al., 1983). This effect is mediated both directly via alpha-adrenergic receptors on cholinergic terminals and indirectly via NE modulation of GABA release (Beani et al., 1986). There is also evidence that NE and ACh interact with each other influencing learning and memory (Santucci et al., 1991). The interaction between ACh and NE seems to be reciprocal, as also ACh is able to regulate NE function (Fig. 1). It is possible that the NE elevation seen in our experiments could down-regulate ACh levels and decrease the therapeutical effect of these drugs.

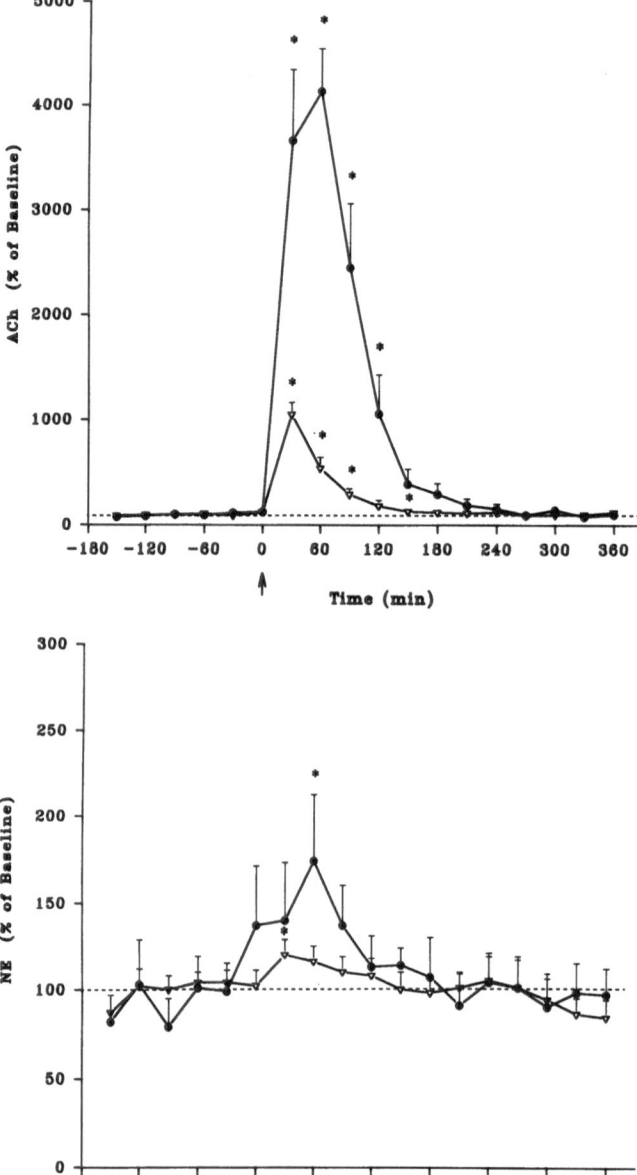

FIGURE 2A and 2B. Effect of systemic administration of PHY [30 μg/kg (∇) and 300 μg/kg (●)] on extracellular levels of (A) ACh and (B) NE in microdialysis samples from cerebral cortex of conscious, freely moving rats. Physostigmine was injected subcutaneously at time zero (↑). Data are expressed as percent of control levels (average of six samples prior to injection = 100%); mean ± S.E.M.; n=7. * p < 0.05 compared to baseline by paired t-test. No ChEI in the probe.

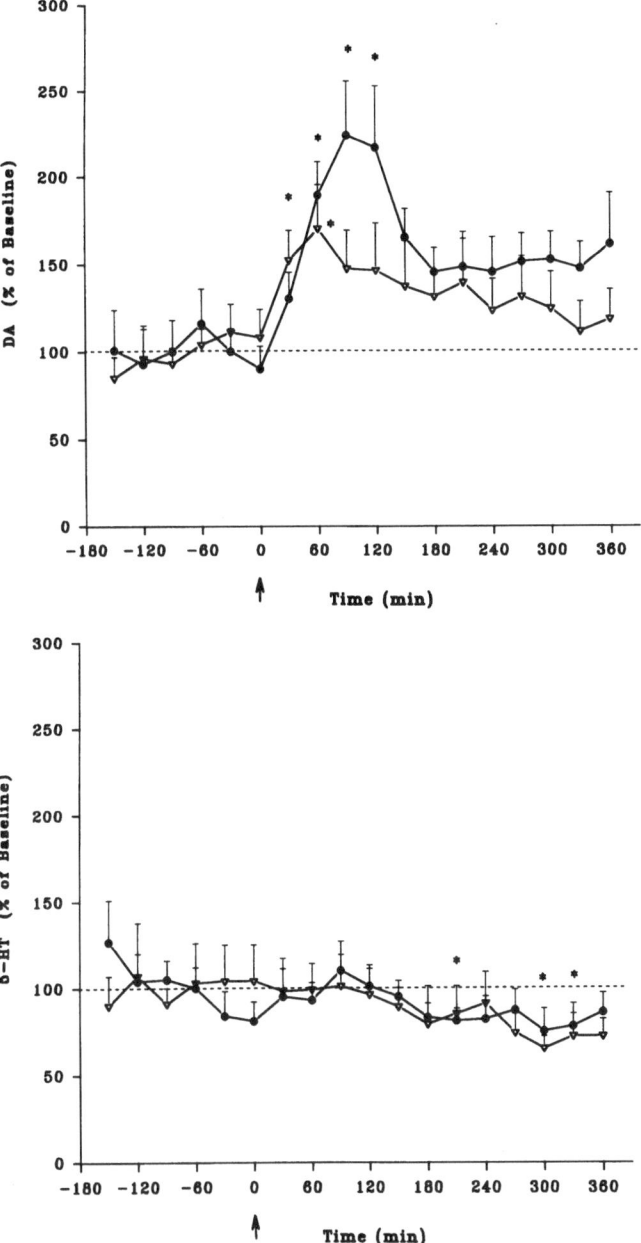

FIGURE 2C and 2D. Effect of systemic administration of PHY [30 μg/kg (∇) and 300 μg/kg (●)] on extracellular levels of (C) DA and (D) 5-HT in microdialysis samples from cerebral cortex of conscious, freely moving rats. Physostigmine was injected subcutaneously at time zero (↑). Data are expressed as percent of control levels (average of six samples prior to injection = 100%); mean ± S.E.M.; n=7.   *p < 0.05 compared to baseline by paired t-test. No ChEI in the probe.

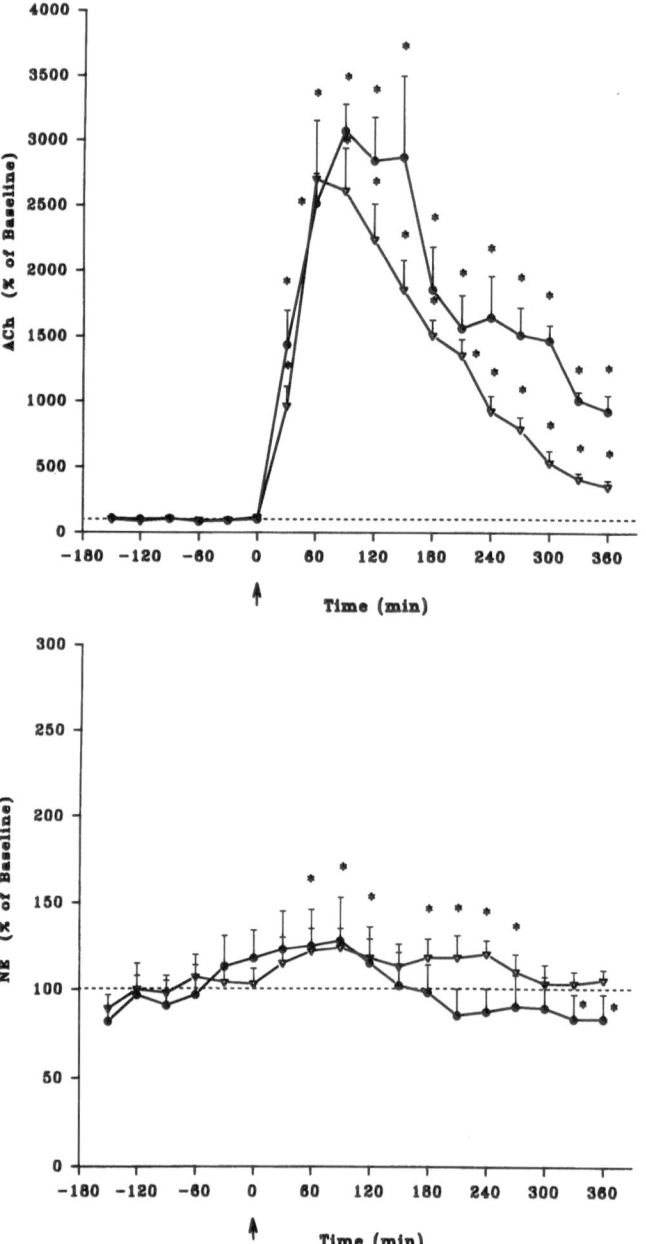

FIGURE 3A and 3B. Effect of systemic administration of HEP [2 mg/kg (∇) and 5 mg/kg (●)] on extracellular levels of (A) ACh and (B) NE in microdialysis samples from cerebral cortex of conscious, freely moving rats. Heptylphysostigmine was injected subcutaneously at time zero (↑). Data are expressed as percent of control levels (average of six samples prior to injection = 100%); mean ± S.E.M.; n=7. * p < 0.05 compared to baseline by paired t-test. No ChEI in the probe.

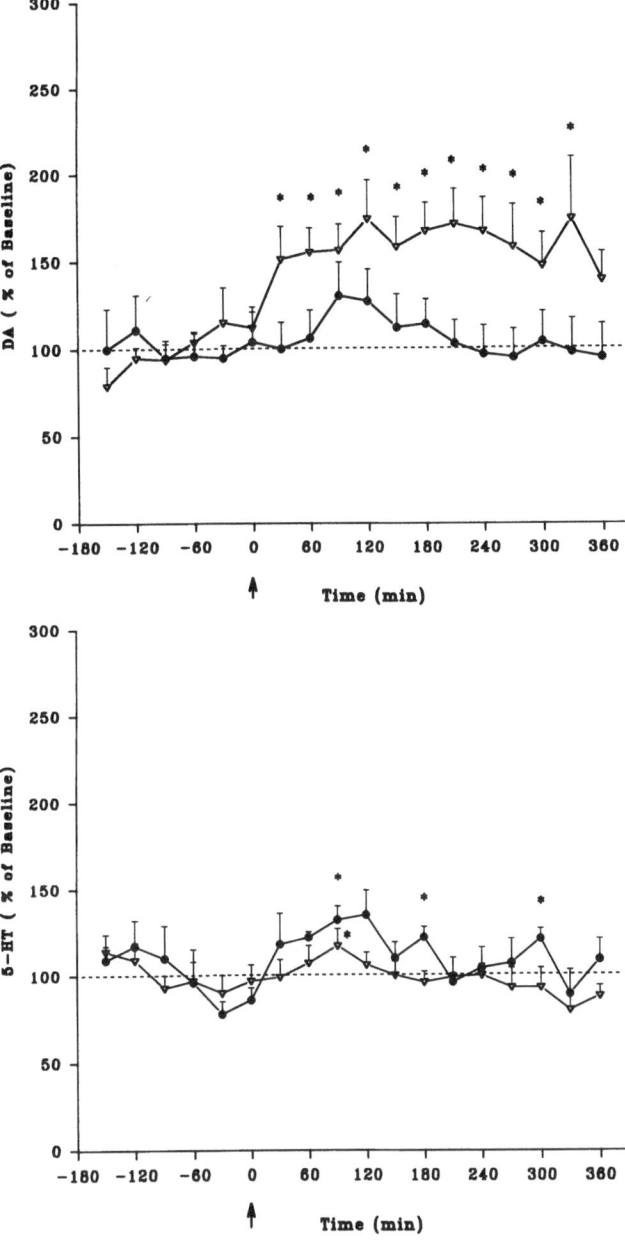

FIGURE 3C and 3D. Effect of systemic administration of HEP [2 mg/kg (∇) and 5 mg/kg (●)] on extracellular levels of (C) NE and (D) 5-HT in microdialysis samples from cerebral cortex of conscious, freely moving rats. Heptylphysostigmine was injected subcutaneously at time zero (↑). Data are expressed as percent of control levels (average of six samples prior to injection = 100%); mean ± S.E.M.; n=7. *p < 0.05 compared to baseline by paired t-test. No ChEI in the probe.

After systemic administration of both doses of the two ChEIs, DA levels are also increased over control values (Table IV) (Figs. 2 and 3). Dopamine elevation, unlike NE elevation, does not overlap in time with ACh increment and the effect on DA is longer than that observed for NE. Local administration of HEP in cortex produced a significant increase in extracellular DA.

Interactions between cholinergic and dopaminergic systems appear to play a role in modulation of memory processes. The participation of DA in learning and memory is suggested by the role of DA in attention and reward mechanisms (Wise, 1978; Beninger, 1983). There is also evidence that DA affects cholinergic neurons. Activity of cortically projecting neurons in the nucleus basalis is regulated in an excitatory manner by central dopaminergic neurons (Day and Fibiger, 1992). The elevation of DA levels observed in our study, and the reciprocal interaction of DA and ACh, suggests an additive therapeutical effect.

In agreement with previous observations, which demonstrated no effects of ChEI (tacrine) on 5-HT concentrations in frontal cortex (Baldwin et al., 1991), we detected no consistent changes of cortical 5-HT release after systemic or local administration (Figs. 2 and 3) of PHY and HEP (Table IV).

ACKNOWLEDGEMENTS

The author wishes to thank Diana Smith for typing and editing the manuscript. Supported by National Institute on Aging #P30 AG08014; Mediolanum Farmaceutici (Milan, Italy).

REFERENCES

Alhainen K (1992):   Anticholinesterase drug, tacrine, in Alzheimer's disease. Discrimination of responders and nonresponders. *Neurologia klinikian julkaisusarja; Series of Reports*, No. 27. Department of Neurology, University of Kuopio, Finland, p. 78.

Arendt T, Bruckner MK, Lange M and Bigl V (1992): Changes in acetylcholinesterase and butyrylcholinesterase in Alzheimer's disease resemble embryonic development - a study of molecular forms. *Neurochem Int* 21(3):381-396.

Baldwin HA, De Souza RJ, Sarna GS, Murray TK, Green AR and Cross AJ (1991): Measurements of tacrine and monoamines in brain by in vivo microdialysis argue against release of monoamines by tacrine at therapeutic doses. *Brit J Pharmacol* 103:1946-1950.

Beani L, Tanganelli S, Antonelli T and Bianchi C (1986): Noradrenergic modulation of cortical acetylcholine release is both direct and γ-aminobutyric acid-mediated. *J Pharmacol Exp Ther* 236:230-236.

Becker R and Giacobini E (1988a): Mechanisms of cholinesterase inhibition in senile dementia of the Alzheimer type: clinical, pharmacological and therapeutic aspects. *Drug Dev Res* 12:163-195.

Becker R and Giacobini E (1988b): Pharmacokinetics and pharmacodynamics of acetylcholinesterase inhibition: can acetylcholine levels in teh brain be improved in Alzheimer's disease? *Drug Dev Res* 14:235-246.

Becker R, Colliver J, Elble R, Feldman E, Giacobini E *et al.* (1990): Effects of metrifonate, a long-acting cholinesterase inhibitor, in Alzheimer disease: report of an open trial. *Drug Dev Res* 19:425-434.

Becker R, Moriearty P and Unni L (1991): The second generation of cholinesterase inhibitors: clinical and pharmacological effects. In: *Cholinergic Basis for Alzheimer Therapy*, Becker RE and Giacobini E, eds. Boston: Birkhauser, pp. 263-296.

Beninger RJ (1983): The role of dopamine in locomotor activity and learning. *Brain Res Rev* 6:173-196.

Berzaghi M, Cooper J, Castren E, Zafra F, Sofroniew M, Thoenen H and Lindholm D (1993): Cholinergic regulation of brain-derived neurotrophic factor and nerve growth factor but not neurotrophin-3 mRNA levels in the developing rat hippocampus. *J Neurosci* 13:3818-3826.

Buxbaum JD, Oishi M, Chen HI, Pinkas-Kramarski R, Jaffe EA, Gandy SE and Greengard P (1992): Cholinergic agonists and interleukin 1 regulate processing and secretion of the Alzheimer β/A4 amyloid protein precursor. *Proc Natl Acad Sci USA* 89:10075-10078.

Carson KA, Geula C and Mesulam M-M (1991): Electron microscopic localization of cholinesterase activity in Alzheimer's brain tissue. *Brain Res* 540:204-208.

Cuadra G, Summers K and Giacobini E (1994): Cholinesterase inhibitors effects on neurotransmitters in rat cortex in vivo. *J Pharmacol Exptl Therapeutics* 270:(In Press).

Davis KL, Thal LJ, Gamzu ER, Davis CS, Woolson RF, Gracon SI, Drachman DA, Schneider LS, Whitehouse PJ, Hoover TM, Morris JC, Kawas CH, Knopman DS, Earl NL, Kumar V and Doody RS (1992): A double-blind, placebo-controlled multicenter study of tacrine for Alzheimer's disease. *New Engl J Med* 327:1253-1259.

Day J and Fibiger HC. (1992): Dopaminergic regulation of cortical acetylcholine release. *Synapse* 12:281-286.

Decker MW and McGaugh JL (1991): The role of interactions between cholinergic system and other neuromodulatory systems in learning and memory. *Synapse* 7:151-168.

DeSarno P, Pomponi M, Giacobini E, Tang XC and Williams E (1989): The effect of heptyl-physostimgine, a new cholinesterase inhibitor, on the central cholinergic system of the rat. *Neurochemical Res* 14(10:971-977.

Eagger S, Morant N, Levy R and Sahakian B (1992): Tacrine in Alzheimer's disease - time course of changes in cognitive function and practice effects. *Brit J Psychiatry* 160:36-40.

Farlow M, Gracon S, Hershey LA, Lewis KW, Sadowsky CH and Dolan-Ureno J (1992): A controlled trial of tacrine in Alzheimer's disease. *J Amer Med Assoc* 268:2523-2529.

Gauthier S, Bouchard R, Lamontagne A, *et al.* (1990): Tetrahydroaminoacridine-lecithin combination treatment in patients with intermediate-stage Alzheimer's disease. *New Engl J Med* 322:1272-1276.

Giacobini E (1959): The distribution and localization of cholinesterases in nerve cells. Academic dissertation. *Acta Physiol Scand* 45(Suppl 156):1-45.

Giacobini E (1991): The second generation of cholinesterase inhibitors: pharmacological aspects. In: *Cholinergic Basis for Alzheimer Therapy*, Becker RE and Giacobini E, eds. Boston: Birkhauser, pp. 247-262.

Giacobini E (1993): Pharmacotherapy of Alzheimer's disease: new drugs and novel strategies. In: *Alzheimer's Disease: Advances in Clinical and Basic Research*, Corain B, Iqbal K, Nicolini M, Winblad B, Wisniewski H and Zatta P, eds. John Wiley & Sons Ltd., New York, pp. 529-538.

Hardy J, Adolfsson R, Alafuzoff I, Bucht G, Marcusson J, Nyberg P, Perdahl E, Wester P and Winblad B (1985): Transmitter deficits in Alzheimer's disease. *Neurochem Int* 7:545-563.

Janson AM and Moller A (1993): Chronic nicotine treatment counteracts nigral cell loss induced by a partial mesiodiencephalic hemitransection: an analysis of the total number and mean volume of neurons and glia in substantia nigra of the male rat. *Neuroscience* 57(4):931-941.

Knapp MJ, Knopman DS, Solomon PR, Pendlebury WW, Davis CS and Gracon SI (1994): A 30-week randomized controlled trial of high-dose tacrine in patients with Alzheimer's disease. *Journal Amer Med Assoc* 271(13):985-991.

Kosasa T, Yamanishi Y, Ogura H and Yamatsu K (1990): Effect of E2020 on the extracellular level of acetylcholine in the rat cerebral cortex measured by microdialysis without addition of cholinesterase inhibitor. *Eur J Pharmacol* 183:19-36.

Lindfors N, Ernfors P, Falkenberg T and Persson H (1992): Septal cholinergic afferents regulate expression of brain-derived neurotrophic factor and beta-nerve growth factor mRNA in rat hippocampus. *Exp Brain Res* 88:78-90.

McGaugh JL, Introini-Collison I and Decker MW (1992). Interaction of hormones and neurotransmitters in the modulation of memory storage. In: *Memory Function and Aging-Related Disorders*, Morley JE, Coe RM, Strong R and Grossberg GT, eds. New York: Springer Publishing Company, pp. 37-64.

Messamore E, Ogane N and Giacobini E (1993a): Cholinesterase inhibitor effects on extracellular acetylcholine in rat striatum. *Neuropharmacology* 32(3):291-296.

Messamore E, Warpman U, Ogane N and Giacobini E (1993b): Cholinesterase inhibitor effects on extracellular acetylcholine in rat cortex. *Neuropharmacology* 32(8):745-750.

Messamore E, Warpman U, Williams E and Giacobini E (1993c): Muscarinic receptors mediate attenuation of extracellular acetylcholine levels in rat cerebral cortex after cholinesterase inhibition. *Neuroscience Letters* 158:205-208.

Mesulam M-M and Geula C (1988): Nucleus basalis (Ch4) and cortical cholinergic innervation in the human brain: observations based on the distribution of acetylcholinesterase and choline acetyltransferase. *J Comp Neurol* 275:216-240.

Mesulam M-M and Geula C (1991): Cortical cholinesterases in Alzheimer's disease: anatomical and ezymatic shifts from the normal pattern. In: *Cholinergic Basis for Alzheimer Therapy*, Becker RE and Giacobini E, eds. Birkhauser Boston, pp. 25-30.

Moroni F, Tanganelli S, Antonelli T, Carlá V, Bianchi C and Beani L (1983): Modulation of cortical acetylcholine and gamma-aminobutyric acid release in freely moving guinea pigs: effects of clonidine and other adrenergic drugs. *J Pharmacol Exp Ther* 236:230-236.

Nitsch RM, Farber SA, Growdon JH and Wurtman RJ (1993): Release of amyloid β-protein precursor derivatives by electrical depolarization of rat hippocampal slices. *Proc Natl Acad Sci USA* 90:5191-5193.

Ogane N, Giacobini E and Messamore E (1992a): Preferential inhibition of acetylcholinesterase molecular forms in rat brain. *Neurochemical Res.* 17(5):489-495.

Ogane N, Giacobini E and Struble R (1992b): Differential inhibition of acetylcholinesterase molecular forms in normal and Alzheimer disease brain. *Brain Research* 589:307-312.

Parnavelas JG (1990): Neurotransmitters in the cerebral cortex. In: *Progress in Brain Research*, Vol. 85, Uylings HBM, Van Eden CG, De Bruin JPC, Corner MA and Feenstra MGP, eds., Netherlands: Elsevier, pp. 13-29.

Santucci AC, Haroutunian V and Davis KL (1991): Pharmacological alleviation of combined cholinergic/noradrenergic lesion-induced memory deficits in rats. *Clin Neuropharmacol* 14:1-8.

Sjak-shie NN, Burks JN and Meyer EM (1990): Long-term actions on nicotinic receptor stimulation in nucleus basalis lesioned rats: blockade of trans-synaptic cell loss. In: *Advances in Behavioral Biology, Vol. 2*, Nagatsu T, Fisher A and Yoshida M, eds. New York: Plenum Press, pp. 471-475.

Summers KL, Cuadra G, Naritoku D and Giacobini E (1994): Effects of nicotine levels on acetylcholine and biogenic amines in rat cortex. *Drug Dev Res* 31:108-119.

Thal LJ, Maasur DM, Fuld PA, Sharpless NS and Davies P (1983): Memory improvement with oral physostigmine and lecithin in Alzheimer's disease. In: *Banbury Report: Biological Aspects of Alzheimer's Disease*, Vol. 15, Katzman R, ed. Cold Spring Harbor, pp. 461-469.

Tucek S (1993): Short-term control of the synthesis of acetylcholine. *Prog Biophys Molec Biol* 60:59-69.

Vizi ES (1980): Modulation of cortical release of acetylcholine by noradrenaline released from nerves arising from the rat locus coeruleus. *Neuroscience* 5:2139-2144.

Wise RA (1978): Catecholamine theories of reward: a critical review. *Brain Res* 152:215-247.

Xu M, Nakamura Y, Yamamoto T, Natori K, Irie T, Utsumi H and Kato T (1991): Determination of basal acetylcholine release in vivo by rat brain dialysis with a U-shaped cannula: Effect of SM-10888, a putative therapeutic drug for Alzheimer's disease. *Neurosci Lett* 123:179-182.

Alzheimer Disease: Therapeutic Strategies
edited by E. Giacobini and R. Becker.
© 1994 Birkhäuser Boston

SECOND AND THIRD GENERATION CHOLINESTERASE INHIBITORS: CLINICAL ASPECTS

Robert E. Becker, Pamela Moriearty, Rita Surbeck, Latha Unni, Andrew Varney and Sandra K. Vicari
Departments of Psychiatry and Medicine (AV), Southern Illinois University School of Medicine, Springfield, Illinois 62794-9230

Loss of cholinergic neurons in the basal forebrain occurs early in Alzheimer's disease (AD). This loss and the memory deficit generated by administration of cholinergic antagonists, e.g. scopolamine, suggest a potential for the development of cholinergic therapy for AD. Unfortunately, studies of physostigmine and tacrine (THA) have shown encouraging, but only transient improvement in memory and other cognitive measures in AD patients (Becker and Giacobini, 1991). One of the major limitations to use of these cholinesterase inhibitors (ChEI) is the appearance of adverse effects, including nausea, vomiting, diarrhea, and abdominal cramps. We reviewed the status of early cholinergic studies and determined that the appearance of adverse effects and toxicity were not related to the level of cholinesterase (ChE) inhibition or the concentration of acetylcholine (ACh) in brain tissue (Becker and Giacobini, 1988). Rather, the appearance of toxicity seemed to be related to the individual compounds, which suggested to us the possibility that ChEIs could be identified which would be free of interfering adverse events. Other characteristics that we selected as important for the successful use of ChEIs were the ability to achieve a full range of ChE inhibition and a long duration of action. After animal studies, we selected metrifonate (MTF), an organophosphate ChEI, that spontaneously hydrolyses to the active ChEI dichlorvos (DDVP). In initial open studies in 20 AD patients, we found we could achieve up to 88% inhibition of red blood cell (RBC) acetylcholinesterase (AChE) and plasma butyrylcholinesterase (BuChE) without interfering side effects. Using the Alzheimer's Disease Assessment Scale (ADAS), we found an inverted "U" shaped dose-response curve comparing dose of MTF to percent of individuals responding (Becker et al., 1990). By plotting the dose-response relationship level of RBC AChE inhibition and ADAS response for 14 responders, we calculated an estimated optimal level of inhibition of 45%. This relationship was consistent with the report of Thal et al. (1986) who found ChE inhibition in the CSF of five patients had a "U" shaped relationship to improvement in memory. Based on these initial findings, we hypothesized that using MTF, a

40-60% level of RBC AChE inhibition was required to achieve an optimal cognitive response. This range of inhibition places each patient about three standard deviations from the mean level of AChE activity prior to the administration of MTF. To prepare for a double-blind, placebo-controlled evaluation of MTF, with ChE inhibition within the 40-60% range, we developed a dosing model to administer MTF.

A Mathematical Model for Cholinesterase Inhibitor Drugs

We constructed a mathematical model to predict the daily and weekly dosages necessary to achieve different levels of response after drug administration. Experimental data needed to construct the model were the equation for the dose-effect relationship and enzyme recovery half-time. The model can be applied to study the response of any enzyme inhibitor drug if one of the dose-related effects is enzyme inhibition. The user inputs desired steady state, the maximum allowable dose, maximum number of weeks before steady state is to be achieved, and dose intervals (daily or weekly) during loading and steady state phases.

Based on pharmacokinetics and pharmacodynamics of MTF and DDVP in 19 AD patients after oral MTF, a plot of log MTF dose versus effect at seven days after dosing gave the equation: RBC AChE inhibition = 32.68 log (MTF dose) - 1.25. We also measured the enzyme levels of subjects exposed to multiple MTF doses for 10 weeks followed by a recovery period of seven weeks, obtaining a half time of RBC AChE enzyme recovery of 40.3 days. Validity of the model, using a weekly loading dose and weekly steady state dose, was tested by comparing experimental and predicted values for RBC AChE inhibition in AD patients treated with placebo or MTF. A close correspondence between predicted and observed inhibition was obtained (Fig. 1).

Peripheral and Central Inhibitor Effects

Our measurements of RBC AChE activity are used to estimate drug effects in the central nervous system, a technique with obvious limitations. We have complemented our *in vivo* data with development of an *in vitro* assay system to compare inhibition and recovery of membrane-bound AChE from human brain and RBC sources. In a comparison of effects of three inhibitors we found that human brain enzyme recovers from inhibition by physostigmine, and recovery from DDVP can be promoted by the presence of 2-PAM, while this oxime (not surprisingly) has no effect on recovery from the carbamate heptylphysostigmine. In the case of heptylphysostigmine, human RBC enzyme recovers almost completely from inhibition within 24 hours; in contrast the brain enzyme remains inhibited (Moriearty and Becker, 1992).

We also compared oral and transdermal administration of inhibitors. In the case of DDVP, patch application produced predictable dose-dependent central nervous system inhibition within 24 hours. Advantages of transdermal *administration are reduction of* first pass effects and attenuation of rapid inhibition peaks which are associated with side effects. A single intramuscular (i.m.) dose of DDVP to rats resulted in an early inhibition peak in brain, followed by recovery. Patch administration resulted in sustained inhibition for one week, even when the patch was left in place for only 24 hours. For heptylphysostigmine a patch reduced the early peak seen after i.m. dosing, and inhibition in brain was sustained at the same levels for both routes of administration up to 5 days after a 24 hour patch (Moriearty et al., 1993).

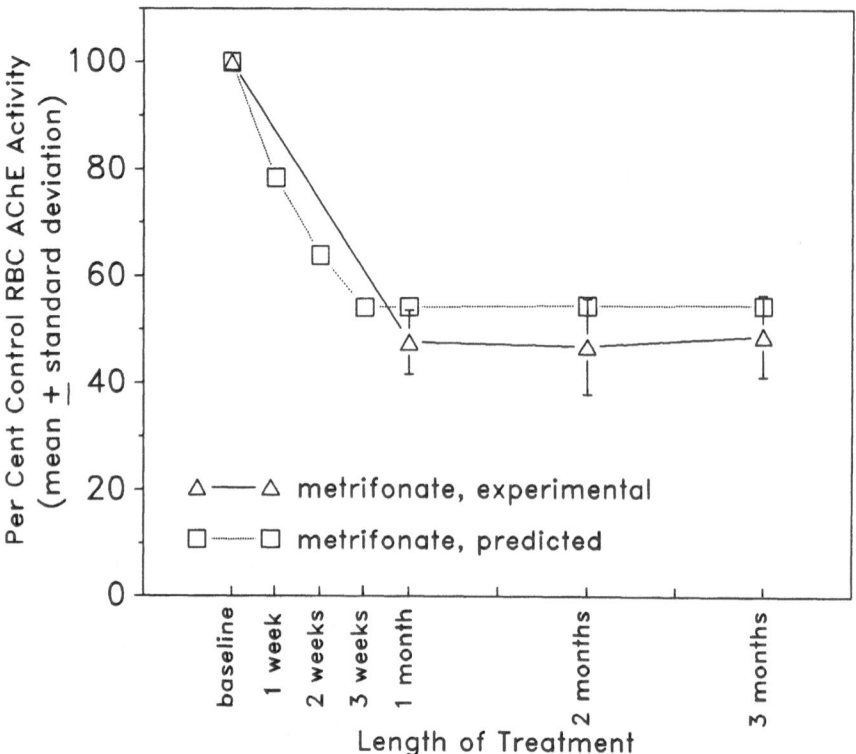

FIGURE 1. RBC AChE activity during weekly oral MTF treatment; observed results (20 patients) agreed with predicted values.

One limiting factor in clinical application of transdermal administration of inhibitors is drug potency; this must be considered in extrapolating feasible patch sizes from smaller experimental animals to man. We calculated that for MTF, a patch producing 50% inhibition in a 50 kg human would need to contain 28 grams; i.e., a full ounce of the drug. Actually patch administration would not offer significant advantages for MTF, whose slow transformation to DDVP mimics a sustained release administration mode. Characteristics of drugs favorable for patch administration are low molecular weight, favorable solubility partition coefficients and low melting point (Izumoto et al., 1992). Interestingly, of the drugs we tested DDVP has theoretically favorable physicochemical properties; in fact its profile (MW = 221; mp < 4°C) is in some ways similar to that of nitroglycerin (MW = 227; mp = 13.5°C) for which successful patch administration technology has been developed.

Current Status of MTF Clinical Trials

We have recently completed a preliminary interim analysis of data from a double-blind, placebo-controlled comparison of MTF and placebo. The success of our dosing model is reflected in 40-60% inhibition of RBC AChE inhibition over three months in 19 out of the 20 subjects analyzed to date. After three months' treatment with MTF, we found statistically significant differences in the ADAS, Mini-Mental State Examination (MMSE), and caregiver ratings of patient overall behavior scores. These differences were primarily due to a statistically significant deterioration in performance in the placebo-treated group. What is interesting in this study is the suggestion that effective levels of ChE inhibition using MTF may affect deterioration rate in AD. If ChEIs can be shown to have an effect on the rate of decline in AD, as our data suggest may be possible, this would open the possibility that cholinomimetic therapy may be more than a brief chapter in treatment of AD.

Direct evidence of a dose-response relationship between ChE inhibition and cognitive performance is reported in the paper by Imbimbo et al. (this publication). They found an optimal level of ChE activity at 35% inhibition in RBC's. We find that heptylphysostigmine has more prolonged inhibitory effect on AChE in brain than in RBC's. The relation of RBC AChE activity to central AChE activity, and thus the clinically optimal inhibition level, must be determined experimentally for each drug. Central AChE activity may be within a similar range in our studies using MTF and in the Imbimbo studies using heptylphysostigmine. The report of Knapp et al. (this publication) also suggests increased benefit from higher doses of THA. This is consistent with our concerns that use of many ChEIs involves too low levels of inhibition because of the appearance of side effects.

Metrifonate may affect AD by inhibiting AChE and/or BuChE inhibition. Most studies to date have focused on the effects of AChE inhibition; however, BuChE is also present in brain. Giacobini (1959) identified the presence of BuChE in CNS neuroglia, and Mesulam (this publication) has described a potential pathological role of BuChE in plaques. MTF is also an effective inhibitor of BuChE (Unni et al., 1994), a mechanism which Mesulam has proposed could affect the pathogenesis of AD.

CONCLUSION

There is no question that progress has been made in the field of cholinergic therapy since our last review of this field three years ago (Becker and Giacobini, 1991) - witnessed by the fact that the only approved treatment for AD is a ChEI. However, the contributions to this publication illustrate that as many questions remain as have been answered, and that a rational, concerted effort is needed to bring a more rapid pace of progress.

All drug development must be based on clearly defined treatment goals, which in turn determine definition of patient profiles, efficacy profiles and safety profiles to be incorporated in clinical trials. Now both preclinical and clinical evidence is accumulating that not only symptomatic improvement, but also alteration of decline rates, should be investigated as possible consequences of cholinergic therapy.

Chapters by Gauthier, Thal and Mohs (this publication) set forth observations of several groups concerning effects of disease stage on decline rate and on functioning in different testing paradigms. Careful selection and reporting of disease stage inclusion criteria and baseline functioning will help comparative analysis and interpretation of findings with different inhibitors. Newer information on genetic factors in AD risk and clinical patterns will make genetic characterization a necessary feature in defining patient profiles for clinical trials. Specifically, it will be very interesting to see if apolipoprotein E genotype is related to variability in responses to ChEIs and other treatment modes in AD (Strittmatter et al., this publication).

Several features of efficacy studies will depend on which treatment goals are sought. Trial duration will depend both on treatment goal and on the targeted physiological outcomes of treatment. But first, the desired pharmacological outcome of treatment must be delineated. We still do not know if steady state inhibition, as produced by MTF, or cyclic inhibition, as produced by physostigmine or THA, is preferable; possibly, one type of pharmacokinetics would favor symptomatic improvement while another would affect decline rates. Certainly controlled release or patch versus oral administration is relevant in this context and may provide a means to distinguish effects of pharmacokinetics and pharmacodynamics.

If the only goal of treatment were symptomatic relief and if improvement depended only on short term increases in amount of intrasynaptic ACh, then very short treatment schemes would test most relevant hypotheses. We know that is not the case - most clinical improvements are seen over weeks or months, suggesting that more complex homeostatic adjustments are occurring. This is not surprising, since many neuropharmacological treatments affecting cognitive functioning show similar lags. This means we must define critical physiological outcome measures, a task which will require close interactive work between preclinical and clinical studies. We have noted the limitations of peripheral ChE determinations for describing what is occurring in the central compartment. The observed clinically optimal peripheral ChE inhibition range for heptylphysostigmine is somewhat lower than we found for MTF. This difference may be due to differences in central versus peripheral enzyme recovery rates of the two drugs.

Giacobini et al. (this publication) have confirmed that central ChE inhibition and ACh levels are not necessarily correlated and now report that individual inhibitors are affecting aminergic systems in different ways. Quite probably, up-regulation or down-regulation of cholinergic and other receptors is one effect of prolonged treatment, so complete receptor binding profiles of candidate drugs and characterization of receptors after long term treatment with each drug are essential in order to interpret clinical results.

Clinical outcome measures themselves warrant further scrutiny, as we attempt to balance logistics, statistics and economics, while trying not to try the patience of our patients. The report by Knapp (this publication) on the multicenter THA trials brings home the limitations of our study designs and rationales. Certainly the interval between drug administration and evaluations should be rigorously controlled, especially for reversible or short-acting inhibitors; and patients should be re-examined at intervals which might identify changes in response due to receptor regulation or second messenger-driven alterations in synaptic connections over time. Optimization of the test instruments is covered in detail in chapters by Thal and Zec (this publication).

Our ideas about safety profiles have also evolved in the last three years. Mediolanum's automated measurements have permitted confirmation that cholinergic adverse events with heptylphysostigmine are associated with peak inhibition exceeding 50% on an initial dose or 70% at steady state (Imbimbo et al., this publication). These findings are in agreement with our own and are comforting, because adequate dosing schemes can easily be calculated to avoid these values while achieving therapeutically-targeted inhibition levels. The results also confirm our earlier assertions that adverse events appearing at lower levels of enzyme inhibition are probably due to non-cholinergic effects of the drugs.

As our clinical trials become longer, we are monitoring our patients for side effects which might only become apparent after months of treatment. Specifically with MTF, we know that hematological parameters remain normal (Moriearty et al., 1991) and that we have found no evidence of ChE gene amplification after up to two years of treatment in an ongoing study. Again, the enzyme inhibition itself appears to be quite benign, though each drug must be monitored for unique adverse effects.

Finally, we would like to make a plea to all who are investigating these drugs to undertake a thorough characterization of any patient who shows idiosyncratic responses to the drugs. Clear demonstration that such events are indeed idiosyncratic is in the interest of all, and the natural experiments provided by these individuals potentially can provide a great deal of information not only about the drugs we are studying, but perhaps about AD itself.

REFERENCES

Becker RE and Giacobini E (1988): Mechanisms of cholinesterase inhibition in senile dementia of Alzheimer's type - clinical, pharmacological, and therapeutical aspects. *Drug Dev Res* 12:163-195.

Becker R, Colliver J, Elble R, Feldman E, Giacobini E, Kumar V, Markwell S, Moriearty P, Parks R, Shillcutt S, Unni L, Vicari S, Womack C and Zec R (1990): Effects of metrifonate, a long acting cholinesterase inhibitor in Alzheimer disease: Report of an open trial. *Drug Dev Res* 9:425-434.

Becker R and Giacobini E (editors) (1991): *Cholinergic Basis of Alzheimer Therapy.* Cambridge: Birkhäuser.

Giacobini E (1959): The distribution and localization of cholinesterases in nerve cells. *Acta Physiol Scand* 45(Suppl 156):1-45.

Izumoto T, Aioi A, Uenoyama S, Kuriyama K and Axuma M (1992): Relationship between the transference of a drug from a transdermal patch and the physicochemical properties. *Chem Pharm Bull* 40(2):456-458.

Moriearty P, Womack C, Dick B, Colliver J, Robbs R and Becker R (1991): Stability of peripheral hematological parameters after chronic acetylcholinesterase inhibition in man. *Amer J Hematology* 37:280-282.

Moriearty PL and Becker RE (1992): Inhibition of human brain and RBC acetylcholinesterase (AChE) by heptylphysostigmine (HPTL). *Meth Find Exp Clin Pharmacol* 14(8):615-621.

Moriearty PL, Thornston SL and Becker RE (1993): Transdermal patch delivery of acetylcholinesterase inhibitors. *Meth Find Exp Clin Pharmacol* 15(6):407-412.

Thal LJ, Masur DM, Sharpless NS, Fuld PA and Davies P (1986): Acute and chronic effects of oral physostigmine and lecithin in Alzheimer's disease. *Prog Neuropsychopharmacol Biol Psychiatry* 10:627-636.

Unni LK, Womack C, Hannant ME and Becker RE (1994): Pharmacokinetics and pharmacodynamics of metrifonate in humans. *Meth Find Exp Clin Pharmacol* 16(4):285-289.

PART V

NICOTINIC AGONISTS AS DRUGS FOR AD TREATMENT

Alzheimer Disease: Therapeutic Strategies
edited by E. Giacobini and R. Becker.
© 1994 Birkhäuser Boston

NICOTINIC RECEPTORS IN HUMAN BRAIN

Hannsjörg Schröder, Andrea Wevers, Christina Birtsch
Institut II für Anatomie, Universität zu Köln, Köln, F.R.G.

Mona Ghobrial and Ezio Giacobini
Departments of Pathology and Pharmacology, Southern Illinois University
School of Medicine, Springfield, IL 62794-9230 USA

Alfred Maelicke
Institut für Physiologische Chemie und Pathobiochemie,
Universität Mainz, F.R.G.

INTRODUCTION

A vast knowledge is currently available on the molecular biology and the
pharmacology of nicotinic acetylcholine receptors (nAChR) in the mammalian
central nervous system (CNS) (Sargent, 1993). Only few attempts have been
made to approach the expression of nAChRs at the level of functional systems,
considering the different cell types involved and their connectivity. This aspect
is of particular importance in order to evaluate nAChR expression under
pathological conditions. Histochemical techniques have proven to be useful
since immunohistochemistry and *in situ* hybridization can be performed on
human autopsy tissue and allow for a cell type-specific localization of nAChR
proteins and nAChR mRNAs. Furthermore, morphometry enables the
quantitative assessment of receptor expression at the cellular level.

In this chapter we will discuss, (i) how nAChRs can be visualized at the
cellular and subcellular level, (ii) how molecular histochemistry can be applied
in order to study pathological entities and (iii) which new perspectives are
opened by the use of these techniques for studies on the human CNS.

Immunohistochemical Localization of nAChRs
Light microscopic detection of nAChR-expressing CNS structures became
possible with the arrival of monoclonal antibodies (mAb) to the nAChR
(cf. Schröder, 1992). The existence in the rat cerebral cortex of nAChR-bearing
pyramidal neurons was first shown by Deutch et al. (1987) using mAb 35
directed to the nAChR α-subunit, and an immunoperoxidase (PO) system. A
similar distribution of the nAChR ß-subunit was shown by Swanson et al. (1987)

using radiolabeled mAb 270. Definite evidence for rodent pyramidal neurons to bear mAb 270-immunoreactivity was provided by Marks et al. (1991) by use of mAb 270 and a PO system. Using mAb WF6 that detects the nAChR α-subunit, comparable light microscopic distribution patterns were seen in both, rat and human cerebral cortex (Schröder, 1992). Ultrastructurally, WF6 mainly decorated post-synaptic thickenings of synaptic complexes, microtubuli of neuronal dendrites and different perikaryal organelles (outer nuclear membrane, rough endoplasmic reticulum, Golgi apparatus). Thus, immunohistochemistry revealed the cell type-specific localization of the receptor and sites of receptor protein synthesis (perikaryon), transport (dendrites) and membrane location (post-synaptic thickenings).

Cellular Expression of nAChRs in Alzheimer's and Parkinson's Dementia
The quantitation in a standard volume of immunoreactive neurons together with the assessment of total neuron numbers serves as a measure of receptor expression (cf. Schröder, 1992). This technique has been applied to the cell type-specific assessment of nAChR expression in cortices of Parkinson dementia and Alzheimer patients as compared to age-matched controls. In both types of dementia a marked decrease of nAChR-expressing neurons was observed (Table I) being of statistical significance, however, only for the Alzheimer cortices. No significant differences were seen for total neuron numbers (Schröder, 1992).

		nAChR-bearing neurons / mm^3	mAChR-bearing neurons / mm^3
Controls	n=3	3960 ± 220^a	2393 ± 499^e
Alzheimer patients	n=6	900 ± 160^b	5070 ± 1008^f
Controls	n=3	5605 ± 1357^c	no data available
Parkinson dementia patients	n=5	2700 ± 853^d	no data available

a vs. b $p < 0.0001$ c vs. d $p < 0.05$ e vs. f $p < 0.05$

TABLE I. Quantitative assessment of AChR-immunopositive neurons in the frontal cortex of Alzheimer (b,f) and Parkinson dementia (d) in comparison to controls (a,c,e) (cf. Schröder, 1992).

Taking into account the expression pattern of muscarinic acetylcholine receptor (mAChRs) in Alzheimer cortices (Table I) (Schröder, 1992) these findings point to a selective impairment of nAChR protein expression and are in agreement with the findings of nicotinic binding studies in Alzheimer's and Parkinson's disease (Whitehouse et al., 1988).

A hypothetical cause of nAChR deficiency may be present at the transcriptional as well as at the translational / post-translational level. This cannot be clarified by techniques monitoring the protein level. The assessment of receptor subunit mRNAs may help to further elucidate this therapeutically important issue.

FIGURE 1. α4-1 nAChR-subunit mRNA expression in human cerebro-cortical neurons (A 4, L.V). Magnifi-cation bar 100 μM.

Molecular Histochemistry of nAChR Subunit-Specific mRNA Expression
In situ hybridization has enabled the assessment of mRNAs in tissue sections. While isotopic labels yield a resolution similar to that of receptor autoradiography, non-isotopic markers, e.g. digoxigenin (dig), allow to identify individual cells that express distinct mRNAs. As for immunopositive neurons (vide supra) the density of labeled cells can be assessed quantitatively. Furthermore, the combined demonstration of mRNA and of relevant markers by immunohistochemistry becomes possible in the same neuron. In our laboratory, dig-labeled cRNA probes complementary for the α3 and α4-1 subunit of the nAChR were used to study the mRNA expression (Wevers et al., 1994). The

mRNA is mainly found in neurons - in particular pyramidal cells - of layer III-IV of the human frontal cortex for the $\alpha3$-subunit-specific probe; $\alpha4$-1 mRNA is present in neurons of all cortical layers (Fig. 1).

Studies of the human frontal cortex are under way to examine two working hypotheses: (i) the nAChR deficiency in neurodegenerative diseases may be related to a decrease in one or more nAChR-subunit mRNAs. Preliminary studies using an $\alpha4$-1 subunit-specific probe do not support this assumption; (ii) intracellular tangles impair nAChR mRNA expression. Preliminary data suggest that tangles and $\alpha4$-1 transcripts do not coexist in cortical neurons. The absence of nAChR mRNA in tangle-bearing neurons supports the idea that Alzheimer-related pathology selectively impairs receptor expression in individual neurons. It is also possible, though, that tangle-bearing neurons belong a priori to a population that does not express nAChRs. The third possibility to be tested is an overall arrest of gene expression in diseased neurons.

CONCLUSIONS

The immunohistochemical and *in situ* hybridization studies reported above show that these approaches must be an integral part of the effort to elucidate the complex inter-relationship between Alzheimer pathology and nAChR expression. The subunit-specificity of *in situ*-hybridization will provide important clues as to the topographic localization of receptor subtypes available for pharmacological manipulation.

ACKNOWLEDGEMENTS

This work was supported by the Deutsche Forschungsgemeinschaft (Schr 283/6-1, 8-1, 8-2; H.S.; Ma 599/12; A.M.).

REFERENCES

Deutch AY, Holliday J, Roth RH, Chun LLY and Hawrot E (1987):   Immuno-histochemical localization of a neuronal nicotinic acetylcholine receptor in mammalian brain. *Proc Natl Acad Sci USA* 84:8697-8701.

Marks R, Schröder H and Lindstrom J (1991):   Die Verteilung nicotinischer. Acetylcholinrezeptoren im Cortex cerebri der Maus: Eine. *Immunhistochemische Darstellung Anat Anz Suppl* 168:603-604.

Sargent PB (1993): The diversity of neuronal acetylcholine receptors. *Ann Rev Neurosci* 16:403-443.

Schröder H (1992): Immunohistochemistry of cholinergic receptors. *Anat Embryol* 186:407-429.

Swanson LW, Simmons DM, Whiting PJ and Lindstrom J (1987): Immunohistochemical localization of neuronal nicotinic receptors in the rodent central nervous system. *J Neuroscience* 7:3334-3342.

Wevers A, Jeske A, Lobron Ch, Birtsch Ch, Heinemann S, Maelicke A, Schröder R and Schröder H (1994): Cellular distribution of nicotinic acetylcholine receptor subunit mRNAs in the human cerebral cortex as revealed by non-isotopic *in situ* hybridization. *Mol Brain Res* (In Press).

Whitehouse PJ, Martins AM, Wagster MV, Price DL, Mayeux R, Atack JR and Kellar KJ (1988): Reductions in [^{3}H]-nicotinic acetylcholine binding in Alzheiner's disease and Parkinson's disease: An autoradiographic study. *Neurology* 38:720-723.

Alzheimer Disease: Therapeutic Strategies
edited by E. Giacobini and R. Becker.
© 1994 Birkhäuser Boston

DEVELOPMENT OF NICOTINIC AGONISTS FOR THE TREATMENT OF ALZHEIMER'S DISEASE

Patrick M. Lippiello and William S. Caldwell
Research and Development Department, R.J. Reynolds Tobacco Company, Winston-Salem, NC

Michael J. Marks and Allan C. Collins
Institute for Behavioral Genetics, University of Colorado, Boulder, CO

Anatomical, physiological, and pharmacological evidence has implicated the cholinergic systems of the brain in memory function (Becker, 1991). Not surprisingly, these systems are severely compromised in Alzheimer's disease (AD), including deficiencies in the acetylcholine (ACh) synthesizing enzyme choline acetyltransferase, in the high affinity choline uptake system, and in the synthesis and release of ACh (Becker, 1991). These deficiencies correlate with the loss of memory function associated with the disease. As a result, many therapeutic strategies have focused on boosting ACh levels. Much attention has also been given to *muscarinic* cholinergic receptors as potential targets for AD therapeutics. More recent findings have established that *nicotinic* cholinergic receptors are severely altered in AD brains, being decreased by 50% or more (Nordberg et al., 1989). Animal studies have shown that activation of nicotinic receptors by nicotine can evoke ACh release (Rowell and Winkler, 1984), improve learning and memory (Hodges et al., 1992), prevent degeneration of cortical neurons (Sjak-Shie et al., 1990) and increase the number of CNS receptors (Marks et al., 1987). Two groups have experimented with nicotine as a treatment for AD. Newhouse et al. (1988) administered nicotine to AD patients and observed a decrease in intrusion errors during cognitive testing. Likewise, Jones et al. (1992) administered nicotine to AD patients and reported improvements in attention and information processing. These findings suggest that nicotinic agonists may have therapeutic potential for the treatment of AD.

METHODS

Development of nicotinic compounds was based on a number of structural themes, including the following: S-(-)-nicotines, R-(+)-nicotines, alpha- and gamma-nicotines, pseudooxynicotines, metanicotines, phenylpyrrolidines, myosmines, anabas(e)ines, tropanes, cytisines, cotinines and pyridyl-methylpyrrolidines (PMP). Nicotinic activity was assessed using the following assays/tests: L-[^{3}H]-nicotine binding (Lippiello and Fernandes, 1986); [^{125}I]-α-bungarotoxin binding (Marks et al., 1986); Dopamine release from rat brain striatal synaptosomes (Grady et al., 1992); ^{86}Rb$^+$ efflux from mouse brain thalamic synaptosomes (Marks et al., 1993); behavioral effects using a physiological and behavioral test battery in mice, including body temperature, Y-maze locomotor activity, acoustic startle response and changes in respiration (Marks et al., 1987).

RESULTS

The results of *in vitro* and *in vivo* testing for six representative nicotinic agonists, including S(-)-nicotine, R(+)-nicotine, anatabine, anabaseine, PMP and noranhydroecgonine, are summarized in Table I.

Receptor Binding

The binding affinities of these compounds for high affinity nicotinic receptors (α4β2 subtype) ranged from 2 nM for S(-)-nicotine to 870 nM for the tropane compound. The ratio of affinities for low affinity ([^{125}I]-α-bungarotoxin binding) receptors to high affinity ([^{3}H]-nicotine binding) receptors varied widely, ranging from 1.7 for anatabine to 300 for S(-)-nicotine. Pyridyl-methyl-pyrrolidine was the most potent inhibitor of [^{3}H]-nicotine binding, while the two compounds with anabas(e)ine-like structures (i.e., having a six-membered ring in place of the pyrrolidine ring of nicotine) competed more effectively for α-bungarotoxin binding.

In Vitro Function

Despite the wide range of binding affinities demonstrated by these compounds (around 200-fold for α-bungarotoxin binding and 400-fold for nicotine binding), their potencies for dopamine release and Rb$^+$ ion efflux fell within a narrow range (around 10-fold or less). In fact, there was very little correlation between receptor binding affinities and functional potency or efficacy. For example, the correlation coefficients (R) for [^{3}H]-nicotine binding vs EC$_{50}$ or Emax for dopamine release or Rb$^+$ efflux ranged from 0.15 to 0.61. This is not completely unexpected, since high affinity nicotine binding is thought to represent binding to a high affinity desensitized (as opposed to activatable) receptor conformation (Lippiello et al., 1987) and α-bungarotoxin probably recognizes antagonist binding sites at a low affinity nicotinic receptor subtype (Nordberg et al., 1989). With respect to efficacy, anabaseine was the only compound in this group which showed full agonist activity vs nicotine (96%), based on dopamine release. Pyridyl-methyl-pyrrolidine also showed reasonably good dopamine release vs nicotine (88%). All others were partial agonists. The potencies of these six compounds for dopamine release were all several-fold lower than nicotine. However, their potencies for Rb$^+$ efflux were all quite

ASSAY	S-(-)-Nicotine	R-(+)-Nicotine	Anatabine	Anabaseine	PMP	Noranhydroecgonine
Ki Nicotine (nM)	2	113	240	60	49	870
Ki α-bungarotoxin (nM)	600	3100	400	123	1400	22000
EC$_{50}$ Dopamine (nM)	125	1000	1300	700	900	ND
Emax Dopamine (% Nic)	100	76	49	96	88	25
EC$_{50}$ Rb$^+$ Efflux	600	1300	230	1000	700	ND
Emax Rb$^+$ Efflux	100	59	55	78	54	40
Physiological Test Battery (EC$_{50}$ vs Nicotine)						
Body Temperature	6	28	30	>30	15	36 (I)
Y-Maze Rears	7	20	22	14	14	12 (I)
Y-maze Crosses	3	20	20	15	12	12 (I)
Acoustic Startle	6	30	55	30	12	12 (I)
Respiration	3	28	69	5	16	24 (I)

TABLE I. *In vitro* and *in vivo* effects of representative nicotinic agonists. ND = not determined; I = increased; PMP = pyridyl-methyl-pyrrolidine

good relative to nicotine, with anatabine being 2- to -3-fold better. Several compounds demonstrated different effects on neurotransmitter release in striatum and on Rb^+ ion efflux in thalamus, suggesting that these two processes may be mediated by different receptor subtypes. For example, in this particular group of compounds anatabine appears to be the most selective for Rb^+ efflux and anabaseine for dopamine release.

Physiological and Behavioral Effects

All of the compounds were less potent than nicotine with respect to *in vivo* physiological and behavioral effects. The compound which most resembled nicotine *in vivo* was PMP. In general, the *in vitro* results were a crude predictor of rank order potency *in vivo*. However, there was a relatively poor correlation between *in vitro* functional effects and these particular *in vivo* physiological and behavioral endpoints. This may indicate that many of the *in vitro* and *in vivo* effects measured in the present studies are mediated by one or several of the various CNS receptor subtypes which have been proposed (Luetje and Patrick, 1991). Thus, a more accurate matching of *in vitro* functional effects with *in vivo* endpoints will be needed to more effectively evaluate individual compounds.

CONCLUSIONS

Based on what is now known about nicotine's effects on memory and learning, both in animals and humans, nicotinic agonists may offer a novel therapeutic approach for ameliorating some of the cognitive deficits seen in AD and other neurodegenerative diseases. However, more information on the specific nicotinic receptor subtypes which are expressed in the CNS and their relationship to various behavioral endpoints will be needed in order to design and target novel compounds appropriately. Similarly, a greater understanding of receptor activation and desensitization will be valuable for addressing the issues of tolerance and side effects in developing effective agonists for the long term treatment of AD.

ACKNOWLEDGMENTS

The authors wish to thank Drs. M. Bencherif, R. Prince and G. Dull for their expert advice, and Drs. J.D. deBethizy and Ezio Giacobini for their helpful review and comments.

REFERENCES

Becker RE (1991): Therapy of the cognitive deficit in Alzheimer's disease: The cholinergic system. In: *Cholinergic Basis for Alzheimer therapy*, Becker R and Giacobini E, eds. Boston: Birkhauser, pp. 1-22.

Grady S, Marks MJ, Wonnacott S and Collins AC (1992): Characterization of nicotinic receptor mediated [^{3}H]dopamine release from synaptosomes prepared from mouse striatum. *J Neurochem* 59:848-856.

Hodges H, Sinden J, Turner JJ, Netto CA, Sowinski P and Gray, JA (1992): Nicotine as a tool to characterize the role of the forebrain cholinergic projection system in cognition. In: *The Biology of Nicotine: Current Research Issues*, Lippiello PM et al., eds. New York: Raven Press, pp. 157-182.

Jones GMM, Sahakian BJ, Levy R, Warburton DM and Gray JA (1992): Effects of subcutaneous nicotine on attention, information processing and short-term memory in Alzheimer's disease. *Psychopharmacology* 108:485-494.

Lippiello PM and Fernandes KG (1986): The binding of L-[^{3}H] nicotine to a single class of high affinity sites in rat brain membranes. *Mol Pharmacol* 29:448-454.

Lippiello PM, Sears SB and Fernandes KG (1987): Kinetics and mechanism of L-[^{3}H] nicotine binding to putative high affinity receptor sites in brain. *Mol Pharmacol* 31:392-400.

Luetje CW and Patrick J (1991): Both α- and β-subunits contribute to the agonist sensitivity of neuronal nicotinic ACh receptors. *J Neurosci* 11:837-845.

Marks MJ, Stitzel JA and Collins AC (1987): Influence of kinetics of nicotine administration on tolerance development and receptor levels. *Pharmacol Biochem Behav* 27:505-512.

Marks MJ, Stitzel JA, Romm E, Wehner, JM and Collins AC (1986): Nicotinic binding sites in rat and mouse brain: comparison of acetylcholine, nicotine and α-bungarotoxin. *Mol Pharmacol* 30:427-436.

Marks MJ, Farnham DA, Grady SR and Collins AC (1993): Nicotinic receptor function determined by stimulation of rubidium efflux from mouse brain synaptosomes. *J Pharmacol Exp Ther* 264:542-552.

Newhouse PA, Sunderland T, Tariot PN, Blumhardt CL, Weingartner H, Mellow A and Murphy DL (1988): Intravenous nicotine in Alzheimer's disease: a pilot study. *Psychopharmacology* 95:171-175.

Nordberg A, Nilsson-Hakansson L, Adem A, Hardy J, Alafuzoff I, Lai Z, Herrera-Marschitz P and Winblad B (1989): The role of nicotinic receptors in the pathophysiology of Alzheimer's disease. *Prog Brain Res* 79:353-362.

Rowell PP and Winkler DL (1984): Nicotinic stimulation of [^{3}H]ACh release from mouse cerebral cortical synaptosomes. *J Neurochem* 43:1593-1598.

Sjak-Shie NN, Burks JN and Meyer EM (1990): Long-term actions of nicotinic receptor stimulation in nucleus basalis lesioned rats: blockade of transsynaptic cell loss. In: *Advances in Behavioral Biology*, Nagatsu T, Fisher A and Yoshida M, eds. New York: Plenum Press, pp. 471-475.

Alzheimer Disease: Therapeutic Strategies
edited by E. Giacobini and R. Becker.
© 1994 Birkhäuser Boston

THE ROLE OF NICOTINIC SYSTEMS IN THE COGNITIVE DISORDER OF ALZHEIMER'S DISEASE

Paul A. Newhouse and Alexandra Potter
Clinical Neuroscience Research Unit, Department of Psychiatry, University of Vermont College of Medicine, Burlington, VT

June Corwin
Department of Psychiatry, New York University School of Medicine and Manhattan VA Medical Center, NY, NY

Robert Lenox
Department of Psychiatry, University of Florida College of Medicine, Gainesville, FL

INTRODUCTION

Interest in the role of nicotinic systems in the cognitive disorder of Alzheimer's disease (AD) increased after the development of the ability to image and map central nervous system (CNS) nicotinic receptors (Schwartz, 1986). Subsequently, Whitehouse et al. (1986) and others (e.g. Aubert et al., 1992) have shown that there is a marked reduction in nicotinic receptor density in the brains of AD patients compared to age-matched controls. These results are in contrast to binding studies of muscarinic receptors, which have generally shown little change, unless subtypes are considered (Giacobini, 1990).

However, the demonstration of a decline in receptor number does not in and of itself indicate that these changes are responsible for the cognitive symptomatology of the disorder. It is necessary to show functional or cognitive consequences from the loss of these receptors or their associated cell processes *in vivo*. There are a number of possible approaches to verifying that receptor changes produce significant changes in cognitive abilities during the course of the illness. We focus here on reviewing a series of studies of the effects of nicotinic antagonists on cognitive functioning in young and older normal humans and present some preliminary results on studies in AD patients.

This strategy has been used successfully in the past to evaluate the role of muscarinic cholinergic systems in cognition by using antagonists such as scopolamine (Sunderland et al., 1989). The use of antagonists allows the identification of cognitive operations affected by the interruption of agonist neurotransmission. Further, cognitive deficits that follow drug administration of antagonists can be compared to those of specific disease states to evaluate the clinical significance of certain neurochemical defects. The effects may indicate which cognitive domains are affected by lesions to the system of interest (Weingartner et al., 1987).

These studies examined the effects of a temporary blockade of central nicotinic receptors by the drug mecamylamine on aspects of cognition. Mecamylamine is a centrally active non-competitive antagonist of nicotine (and presumably acetylcholine) at C6 (ganglionic) type nicotinic receptors (Martin et al., 1989). We have previously presented data showing that mecamylamine administered acutely to young and older healthy volunteers produces dose and age-related impairment of several cognitive processes (Newhouse et al., 1992, 1994).

METHODS

A detailed description of experimental methodology is provided in Newhouse et al. (1994). In general, all normal subjects were healthy and cognitively intact as verified by physical exam, laboratory, and cognitive tests. Alzheimer disease subjects fulfilled diagnostic criteria for probable AD.

Cognitive testing consisted of a computer battery, one oral memory test and, and behavioral ratings. Tests included: the Repeated Acquisition Test (RAT), which tests a subject's ability to retrieve previously acquired information as well as the ability to learn new information (Thompson, 1973); the High-Low Imagery Test, a recognition memory test with high and low imagery words (Corwin et al., 1987); a choice reaction time test and a manikin spatial rotation test, both from the Walter Reed PAB (Thorne et al., 1985); and the Selective Reminding Test.

All drugs were administered double-blind. The doses administered were 5, 10, and 20 mg of mecamylamine and placebo. Drug was administered at 09:00. Cognitive testing was conducted at +60 and +120 minutes.

RESULTS

Mecamylamine administration produced dose-related impairment of the acquisition of new information with group differences in sensitivity. This was most clearly demonstrated by the RAT task in which subjects learn a button-pushing sequence. The young normals showed a significant increase in errors after the 20 mg dose. By contrast, the elderly normals showed significant impairment after the 10 and 20 mg dose, and the AD subjects showed impairment after all three active doses (5, 10, and 20 mg). In the retrieval condition (old learning), there were no significant dose-related impairments in any group.

The selective reminding task, which involves verbal learning, demonstrated a similar pattern. Here, the young normals showed a small dose-related decline in total recall, but no change in recall failure. The old normals showed a significant and substantial increase in recall failure however, after the 20 mg dose, and the AD patients showed increased recall failure after the 10 and 20 mg doses.

For the High-Low Imagery task, a test of recognition memory, there was a dose-related decline in discrimination for both normal groups with the elderly normals showing a greater effect than the young. Perhaps more interestingly, in the old normals, mecamylamine produced a dose-related change in response bias with a significant liberal shift after the 20 mg dose.

Regarding psychomotor speed, mecamylamine produced dose-related slowing in a number of tasks that measured reaction time. These included increases in mean reaction time for the CRT and manikin tasks. Although there were no significant dose by group interactions for the speed measures, older subjects tended to show proportionately greater increases in reaction time than the younger subjects did.

Physiological effects were consistent with peripheral ganglionic blockade. By contrast, there were minimal behavioral effects. Although there were small changes in the scores of some observer rating scales, these were clinically nonsignificant. No changes were seen in subject mood or physical side-effects ratings.

DISCUSSION

In this investigation, the nicotinic antagonist mecamylamine produced cognitive impairment on several tasks. These effects included impairment of acquisition on the RAT task, impaired recall on the Selective Reminding task, slowing of reaction time, and impairment of discrimination and liberalization of response bias on the Hi-Low Imagery task. Further, there was evidence that elderly normals were proportionately more sensitive to the effects of mecamylamine and AD patients were still more responsive suggesting a continuum of increasing sensitivity with increasing receptor loss. The lack of clinically significant behavioral changes and physical side-effects suggests that the cognitive effects were secondary to specific blockade of nicotinic receptors and not due to non-specific effects on arousal or overall well-being. These results suggest that the loss of central nicotinic receptors seen in normal aging (Court et al., 1992) and in AD and Parkinson's Disease (PD) (Aubert et al., 1992) have functional consequences. The deficits produced by mecamylamine resemble in several respects those seen in AD and to a lesser extent PD. Deficits in short- and long-term memory, impaired attention, liberal response bias, and decreases in reaction time are hallmarks of the dementing picture seen in these disorders. The age-related nature of some of the findings suggest that the decline in nicotinic receptors with age produces increased vulnerability to the effects of nicotinic blockade. This model of experimental nicotinic deficits appears to have some power to explain the derivation of some of the deficits in AD and PD, particularly as the cognitive deficits are not contaminated by gross behavioral or physical effects.

These results suggest that nicotinic modulation may be of benefit for the alleviation or improvement of cognitive impairments in various dementing disorders which show a loss of nicotinic receptors (Newhouse et al., 1988). Nicotine is unlikely to be an ideal candidate for this task, due to its low therapeutic index, but other, more selective agonists may be more useful.

ACKNOWLEDGEMENTS

This work was supported by NIMH grant R29-46625 to P.N. and by GCRC M01-00109.

REFERENCES

Aubert I, Araujo DM, Cécyre D, Robitaille Y, Gauthier S and Quirion R (1992): Comparative alterations of nicotinic and muscarinic binding sites in Alzheimer and Parkinson diseases. *J Neurochem* 58:529-541.

Corwin J, Peselow E, Fieve R and Rotrosen J (1987): Memory in untreated depression: severity and task requirement effects. *Abstract, ACNP Annual Meeting (December, San Juan)*.

Court JA, Piggott MA, Perry EK, Barlow RB and Perry RH (1992): Age associated decline in high-affinity nicotine binding in human brain frontal-cortex does not correlate with the changes in choline-acetyltransferase activity. *Neurosci Res Comm* 10:125-133.

Giacobini E (1990): Cholinergic receptors in human brain: effects of aging and Alzheimer's disease. *J Neurosci Res* 27:548-560.

Martin BR, Onaivi ES and Martin TJ (1989): What is the nature of mecamylamine's antagonism of the central effects of nicotine? *Biochemical Pharmacology* 38:3391-3397.

Newhouse P, Potter A, Corwin J and Lenox R (1992): Acute nicotinic blockade produces cognitive impairment in normal humans. *Psychopharmacology* 108:480-484.

Newhouse P, Potter A, Corwin J and Lenox R (1994): Age-related effects of the nicotinic antagonist mecamylamine on cognition and behavior. *Neuropsychopharmacology* 10:93-107.

Newhouse P, Sunderland T, Tariot P, Blumhardt CL, Weingartner H, Mellow A and Murphy DL (1988): Intravenous nicotine in Alzheimer's disease: a pilot study. *Psychopharmacology* 95, 171-175.

Schwartz R (1986): Autoradiographic distribution of high affinity muscarinic and nicotinic cholinergic receptors labeled with [^{3}H]acetylcholine in rat brain. *Life Sciences* 38:2111-2119.

Sunderland T, Tariot PN and Newhouse PA (1989): Differential responsivity of mood, behavior, and cognition to cholinergic agents in elderly neuropsychiatric populations. *Brain Res Rev* 13:371-389.

Thompson D (1973): Repeated acquisition as a behavioral base line for studying drug effects. *J Pharmacol Exp Ther* 184:506-514.

Thorne D, Genser S, Sing H and Hegge F (1985): The Walter Reed performance assessment battery. *Neurobehav Toxicol Teratol* 7:415-418.

Weingartner H, Cohen R, Sunderland T, Tariot P, Thompson K and Newhouse P (1987): Diagnosis and assessment of cognitive dysfunctions in the elderly. In: *Psychopharmacology, the Third Generation of Progress*, Melzer H, ed. New York: Raven Press, pp. 909-919.

Whitehouse P, Martino A, Antuono P and Kellar K (1986): Nicotinic acetylcholine binding sites in Alzheimer's disease. *Brain Res* 371,146-151.

Alzheimer Disease: Therapeutic Strategies
edited by E. Giacobini and R. Becker.
© 1994 Birkhäuser Boston

ABT-418: A NOVEL CHOLINERGIC CHANNEL ACTIVATOR (ChCA) FOR THE POTENTIAL TREATMENT OF ALZHEIMER'S DISEASE

Stephen P. Arneric, James P. Sullivan, Michael W. Decker,
Jorge D. Brioni, Clark A. Briggs, Diana Donnelly-Roberts,
Kennan C. Marsh, A. David Rodrigues, David S. Garvey and
Michael Williams
Abbott Laboratories, Neuroscience, D-47W, Pharmaceutical Products
Division, Abbott Park, IL 60064-3500 USA

Jerry J. Buccafusco
Department of Pharmacology and Toxicology, Medical College of Georgia,
Augusta, GA 30912-2300 USA

Evidence is accumulating to suggest that compounds which activate neuronal nicotinic acetylcholine receptors (nAChRs) may have potential benefit in the treatment of dementia, especially Alzheimer's disease (AD) (for review: Arneric and Williams, 1994). The focus of this chapter is to summarize the preclinical pharmacology of ABT-418 [(S)-3-methyl-5-(1-methyl-2-pyrrolidinyl)isoxazole], a novel analog of (-)-nicotine that is in clinical development for the treatment of AD. ABT-418 is a cholinergic channel activator (ChCA) with cognitive enhancement and anxiolytic-like activity possessing a substantially reduced side-effect profile compared to (-)-nicotine (Arneric et al., 1994; Decker et al., 1994a). The enhanced preclinical safety profile and excellent transdermal delivery across species are consistent with the early Phase I clinical studies (Sebree et al., 1993).

SELECTIVE ChCAs FOR THE TREATMENT OF AD

Recent evidence suggests the existence of a diversity of neuronal nAChRs subtypes with a wide distribution in brain, that each subtype may be involved in mediating specific functions/behaviors, and that these subtypes have a defined pharmacology that may be selectively targeted (Arneric et al., 1995).

The negative connotations associated with the recreational use of (-)-nicotine in tobacco products and the consequent impact on the health of individuals has tended to limit the medicinal chemistry research in this area (Arneric and Williams, 1994). However, the plethora of receptor targets revealed by nAChR cloning have enhanced the possibility that new molecular entities can be developed which are free of the side effect liabilities associated with (-)-nicotine.

Classical nAChR agonists (e.g. (-)-nicotine) bind to the acetylcholine binding site on the α subunit, whereas recent evidence suggests that neuronal nAChR function can be enhanced via sites distinct from (-)-nicotine. These sites are not subject to the same desensitization mechanisms described for (-)-nicotine (Arneric et al., 1995). A broader class of agents can be termed cholinergic channel activators (ChCAs) since they would include nAChR agonists as well allosteric modulators. The actions of these agents may occur via the selective interaction with central nAChRs subtypes or some may act by positive allosteric modulation. Functionally, ChCAs selective for nAChR subtypes could enhance central neuronal nAChR mediated transmission without having the side-effect liabilities normally associated with (-)-nicotine. In particular, ChCAs lacking cardiovascular or other CNS side effects associated with (-)-nicotine may represent a potential therapeutic strategy to ameliorate many of the CNS deficits accompanying AD or other related disorders.

At the last Springfield Symposium the question was raised whether it was possible to develop functionally selective compounds for subtypes of nAChRs (Arneric, 1991). ABT-418 is the first of a new class of compounds that has fewer of the *in vivo* liabilities associated with (-)-nicotine, a profile that may result from the selective activation of putative nAChR subtypes. What follows is a synopsis of the *in vitro* and *in vivo* preclinical pharmacology of ABT-418.

PRECLINICAL PHARMACOLOGY OF ABT-418

ABT-418 potently (K_i = 3 $\pm$ 0.4 nM) interacts with the $\alpha 4\beta 2$ subtype of nAChRs, the major subtype in rodent brain (Arneric et al., 1994). ABT-418 was significantly less potent (K_i > 10,000 nM) against the nicotinic receptors labeled by $[^{125}I]\alpha$-bungarotoxin in brain and neuromuscular junction. In 34 other receptor/uptake/enzyme binding assays the K_i values for ABT-418 were greater than 10,000 nM (Arneric et al., 1994).

Functionally, ABT-418 is as potent (estimated EC_{50} = 0.5 μM) and efficacious as (-)-nicotine (estimated EC_{50} = 0.7 μM) to stimulate $^{86}Rb^+$ efflux from mouse thalamus synaptosomes. This assay has been proposed to reflect the activation of nAChRs channel containing an $\alpha 4\beta 2$ configuration (Marks et al., 1993). In addition, ABT-418 activates nAChR channel currents in PC12 cells as evaluated by whole-cell patch clamp studies -- an effect prevented by the nAChR channel blocker mecamylamine (Arneric et al., 1994). PC12 cells express ganglion-like nAChRs distinct from the $\alpha 4\beta b2$ subtype, and in this preparation ABT-418 was four fold less potent than (-)-nicotine (EC_{50} 214 $\pm$ 30 μM vs 52 $\pm$ 4 μM) in eliciting a functional response, which is consistent with the absence of cardiovascular liabilities seen in dog and monkeys. ABT-418 and (-)-nicotine stimulated the evoked release of $[^3H]$dopamine from rat striatal slices with EC_{50} values of 380 $\pm$ 50 nM and

40 ± 10 nM, respectively (Arneric et al., 1994). The decreased potency of ABT-418 on dopamine release compared to (-)-nicotine agrees with *in vivo* drug discrimination studies suggesting that ABT-418 has less abuse potential than (-)-nicotine (Brioni et al., 1994b). Thus, ABT-418 demonstrated functional selectivity for the major subtype of brain nAChR.

ABT-418 has been evaluated in a series of animal test paradigms to assess cognition enhancement. ABT-418 had a positive effect at 0.062 μmol/kg on the retention of inhibitory avoidance with pre-training injections in mice and at 0.62 μmol/kg with post-training injection in rats, i.p. (-)-Nicotine produced similar effects at 3- to 10-fold higher doses (Decker et al., 1994a). The cognition enhancing activity of ABT-418 in this model in mice was prevented by mecamylamine (5 μmol/kg, i.p.). The effects were stereoselective since the (R)-enantiomer of ABT-418 was without effect. Enhancement of performance was maintained in aged rats (20 months) following continuous infusion with osmotic minipumps over an 11-day treatment period without altering the total number of binding sites measured with [^{3}H]-(-)-cytisine (unpublished). The *Morris water maze* paradigm was used to measure reference spatial memory in the medial septal lesioned rat. ABT-418, given i.p. (0.19 and 1.9 μmol/kg) restored performance in a dose-related manner back to control levels (Decker et al., 1994b). The *delayed matching-to-sample task* assesses short term memory as well as attentive aspects of memory in primates. ABT-418 enhanced performance of this task in normal, young monkeys at an average maximally effective dose of 15 nmol/kg, i.m., whereas (-)-nicotine was effective at 19 nmol/kg, i.m. No adverse events were observed with ABT-418 at doses up to 500 nmol/kg following i.m. administration (Buccafusco et al., unpublished).

While ABT-418 had approximately the same potency as (-)-nicotine in memory tasks, the compound was remarkably less potent than (-)-nicotine in producing EEG activation, hypothermia, seizures, death, and reduction of locomotor activity in rodents. ABT-418 had significantly less emetic (Decker et al., 1994a) and pressor liability in dog as compared to (-)-nicotine (unpublished observation). In rodent, dog and monkey ABT-418 demonstrated substantial transdermal bioavailability, yet poor oral bioavailability due to rapid metabolism (Rodrigues et al., 1994). Levels of ABT-418 within the range that elicited cognitive enhancement in the *Morris water maze* paradigm were maintained for up to 48 hours.

ABT-418 demonstrated anxiolytic-like activity in both mice and rats in the *elevated plus maze* model of anxiety at doses of 0.19 and 0.62 μmol/kg, i.p., respectively. ABT-418 was approximately 15-fold more potent than diazepam in mice, but was less efficacious in eliciting anxiolytic-like activity. Nonetheless, in contrast to diazepam, ABT-418 did not potentiate ethanol-induced narcosis, nor did it impair rotorod performance in the effective dose range (Brioni et al., 1994a; Decker et al., 1994a). Transdermal application of ABT-418 to rats via a Hill Top™ chamber elicited anxiolytic-like activity for at least 4 hours. The anxiolytic-like effect of ABT-418 in rats was blocked by mecamylamine (15 μmol/kg) (Brioni et al., 1994a). ABT-418 (0.62 μmol/kg, i.p.) also reduced the anxiety elicited by withdrawal from 14 days of (-)-nicotine treatment by continuous minipump infusion (Brioni et al., 1994a).

Assay Procedure	ABT-418	(-)-Nicotine
Mouse Inhibitory Avoidance[1]	0.062	0.62
(ED_{min}, μmol/kg, i.p.)		
Mouse Elevated Plus Maze[1]	0.19	0.62
(ED_{min}, μmol/kg, i.p.)		
Rat Cerebral Circulation[1]	0.002	0.43
Enhancement of Basal Forebrain		
Vasodilation (ED_{max}, μmol/kg, i.v.)		
Monkey Delayed Matching-to-Sample Task	15	19
"Best Dose" (nmol/kg, i.m.)		
Toxicity (μmol/kg, i.p. mice)[1]		
- ALD	138 ± 5	70 ± 4
- Seizure (ED_{50}; 95% C.I.)	62 [51-75]	41 [34-49]
- hypothermia	19	6.2
Therapeutic index[1]		
(inhibitory avoidance versus ALD)	2225	113
Emetic Liability in Dog[1]	0/3	3/3
(dogs responding to 500 nmol/kg, i.v.)		
Pharmacokinetics		
RAT[1] $t_{1/2}$	23 min.	44 min.
p.o. bioavailability	27%	18%
DOG $t_{1/2}$	12	55
MONKEY $t_{1/2}$	35	45

TABLE I. *In Vivo* Pharmacology of ABT-418 and (-)-Nicotine. ED_{min} is defined as the minimum dose of the drug that elicited a statistically significant response. [1]Modified from Decker et al., 1994a.

ABT-418 is a prototype of a new class of compounds that selectively activate neuronal nAChRs without eliciting the dose-limiting side effects typically observed with (-)-nicotine. ABT-418 may be a safe and effective ChCA for the potential treatment of the cognitive and emotional impairments of AD.

ACKNOWLEDGEMENTS

The authors thank D.J. Anderson, M.J. Buckley, D. Cox, P. Curzon, M.L. Hughes, C-H Kang, D.J.B. Kim, M. Piattonni-Kaplan, M.J. Majchrzak, A.B. O'Neill, J.R. Pauly, S. Quigley, R.J. Radek, J.L. Raszkiewicz, A.V. Terry, J.W. Turek, and J.T. Wasicak for their contributions.

REFERENCES

Arneric SP (1991): New nicotinic agonists and cerebral blood flow. In: *Second International Springfield Alzheimer Symposium*, Giacobini E and Becker R, eds., Boston: Birkhauser, pp. 386-394.

Arneric SP, Sullivan JP and Williams M (1995): Neuronal nicotinic acetylcholine receptors: novel targets for CNS therapeutics. In: *Psychopharmacology: 4th Generation of Progress*, Bloom FE and Kupfer DJ, eds. New York: Raven Press (In Press).

Arneric SP and Williams M (1994): Nicotinic agonists in Alzheimer's disease: does the molecular diversity of nicotine receptors offer the opportunity for developing CNS selective cholinergic channel activators? In: *Recent Advances In The Treatment Of Neurodegenerative Disorders and Cognitive Function, Int Acad Biomed Drug Res,* Racagni G, Brunello N and Langer SZ, eds. Basel: Karger, Vol. 7 pp. 58-70.

Arneric SP, Sullivan JP, Briggs CA, Donnelly-Roberts D, Anderson DJ, Raszkiewicz JL, Hughes M, Cadman ED, Adams P, Garvey DS, Wasicak J and Williams M (1994): ABT-418: A novel cholinergic ligand with cognition enhancing and anxiolytic activities I. *In vitro* characterization. *J Pharmacol Exp Ther* 270:(In Press).

Brioni JD, O'Neill AB, Kim DJB, Decker MW, Sullivan JP and Arneric SP (1994a): Anxiolytic-like effects of the novel cholinergic channel activator, ABT-418. *J Pharmacol Exp Ther* (In Press).

Brioni JD, Kim DJB, Brodie MS, Decker MW and Arneric SP (1994b): ABT-418: Discriminative stimulus properties and effect on ventral tegmental cell activity. *Psychopharmacol* (Submitted).

Decker MW, Brioni J, Sullivan JP, Buckley M, Radek R, Raszkiewicz JL, Hughes M, Giardina W, Wasicak JT, Williams M and Arneric SP (1994a): ABT-418: A novel cholinergic ligand with cognition enhancing and anxiolytic activites: II. *In vivo* characterization. *J Pharmacol Exp Ther* 270:(In Press).

Decker MW, Curzon P, Brioni JD and Arneric SP (1994b): Effects of ABT- 418, a novel cholinergic channel ligand, on place learning in septal-lesioned rats. *Eur J Pharmacol* (Submitted).

Marks MJ, Garnham DA, Grady SR, Collins AC (1993): Nicotinic receptor function determined by stimulation of rubidium efflux from mouse brain synaptosomes. *J Pharmacol Exp Ther* 264:542-552.

Rodrigues AD, Ferrero JL, Amann MT, Rotert GA, Cepa SP, Surber BW, Machinist JM, Sullivan JP, Garvey DS, Fitzgerald M and Arneric SP (1994): The *in vitro* hepatic metabolism of ABT-418, a cholinergic channel activator, in rat, dog, cynomolgus monkey and human. *Drug Metabolism & Disposition* (In Press).

Sebree TS, Grebb JA, Kittle C and Kashkin KB (1993): A phase I, single, rising-dose study of A-81418, a novel cholinergic channel activator (ChCA). *American College of Neuropsychopharmacology, 32nd Annual Meeting, Dec. 13-17.*

Alzheimer Disease: Therapeutic Strategies
edited by E. Giacobini and R. Becker.
© 1994 Birkhäuser Boston

NICOTINE, CATECHOLAMINES AND COGNITIVE ENHANCEMENT

Jeffrey A. Gray, Grigory A. Grigoryan, Chuly Lee,
Stephen N. Mitchell and Helen Hodges
Department of Psychology, Institute of Psychiatry, De Crespigny Park,
London SE5 8AF, UK

Our group has for some time been studying the effects of nicotine upon performance in rats that have sustained damage to the brain (Hodges et al., 1992). This damage was made with the intention of producing partial animal models of two conditions which involve major cognitive decline in human beings, dementia of the Alzheimer type (DAT) and alcoholic dementia, attributed in some degree to degeneration in the forebrain cholinergic projection system (FCPS), which carries afferents from nucleus basalis magnocellularis (NBM) (in human, nucleus basalis of Meynert) to the neocortex, and from the medial septal area (MSA) and nucleus of the diagonal band of Broca (DBB) to the hippocampal formation.

The first of these models consists of lesions made by local injection of excitotoxins (initially ibotenate, with subsequent replication of major findings using quisqualate and (s)-alpha-amino-3-hydroxy-5-methyl-4-isoxazoleproprionic acid, AMPA) into the nuclei of origin of both branches of the FCPS, i.e., the MSA/DBB (deafferenting the hippocampal formation) and the NBM (deafferenting frontal, temporal and parietal neocortex) (Arendt et al., 1989; Hodges et al., 1991a; Turner et al., 1992). The second model involves chronic (c. 6 months) administration of ethanol in the drinking water, causing widespread loss of cortical and hippocampal cholinergic, noradrenergic, serotonergic and (less markedly) dopaminergic markers, as well as actual loss of cells in the NBM and MSA/DBB (Arendt et al., 1988, 1989; Hodges et al., 1991c). In both models, cognitive performance in the radial-arm maze, measuring both reference and working memory in both spatial and non-spatial or 'cue' (largely visual and tactile) modalities, is severely impaired. The impairment is enduring (up to 1 year) and affects all 4 components of performance (i.e., working and reference memory in both the spatial and cue tasks). The latter observation suggests that the central cognitive deficit caused by the two treatments lies in a general and pervasive difficulty in handling information of many kinds, rather than a specific problem, e.g. in a particular form of memory or perception. In human experimental psychology, this type of capacity is often termed 'vigilance'.

Although both models involve substantial non-cholinergic damage (neurons of other classes destroyed by injection of excitotoxins into the NBM and MSA/DBB; loss of other neurochemical markers throughout the brain after chronic alcohol), it is possible substantially to reverse the behavioral impairments by transplants into the denervated hippocampus and neocortex of embryonic neural tissue containing cholinergic precursor cells, but not by non-cholinergic transplants; and this behavioral recovery is paralleled by recovery in cholinergic but not in non-cholinergic neurochemical markers (Arendt et al., 1989; Hodges et al., 1991a,c). Furthermore, the cognitive deficits observed in both models are sensitive to cholinergic agents, both agonists (improving performance) and antagonists (further impairing performance), at doses which do not influence performance in intact animals (Hodges et al., 1991b,c; Turner et al., 1992). Thus there is considerable reason to suppose that, in both models, an essential substrate of the observed cognitive change lies in damage to the FCPS. Evidence that the two types of brain damage do indeed relate to the human conditions that they are intended to model comes from the observation (Hodges et al., 1990) that, in both cases, the impaired performance in the radial-arm maze is reversed by systemic administration of the cholinesterase inhibitor, tetrahydroaminoacridine (Tacrine), which has been reported to ameliorate cognitive impairment in patients with DAT (Eagger et al., 1991).

Post-mortem studies of patients with DAT have demonstrated large reductions of nicotinic receptors in both neocortex and hippocampus. Among the cholinergic agonists with which we were able to reverse the radial-arm maze deficits caused by either excitotoxic lesions of the FCPS or chronic alcohol was nicotine, given intraperitoneally (i.p.) at quite low doses (0.05 and 0.1 mg/kg); while the nicotinic antagonist, mecamylamine (1 and 2 mg/kg i.p.), exacerbated these deficits (Hodges et al., 1991b,c; Turner et al., 1992). These effects of nicotinic agonists and antagonists are not limited to performance in the radial-arm maze. In other experiments (Hodges et al., 1992) animals with lesions of the nuclei of origin of the FCPS, induced by injection of ibotenate or AMPA, were tested in both reference and working memory versions of Morris' water maze, in which the rat has to swim to a submerged, invisible platform. In these experiments, nicotine improved learning in intact animals. In addition, the deficits caused by the lesions in acquisition and retention of the path to a fixed platform position, in reversal of this position, and in repeated acquisition to a series of new platform positions were substantially reversed by 0.1 mg/kg nicotine. Both the ubiquity and the pattern of lesion effects in these experiments were consistent with the inference drawn from the effects observed in the radial-arm maze that the FCPS subserves a very general function, such as vigilance, in cognitive performance; and the reversal by nicotine of these effects was similarly consistent with the hypothesis that this compound increases vigilance.

On the basis of these findings it might be expected that nicotine would have beneficial effects upon cognitive performance in the relevant patient groups. In agreement with this prediction, we have shown that nicotine improved performance on a vigilance task (detection of series of odd digits in a sequential visual display of single digits), at doses that had no effect on normal controls, with a linear relation to dose over the range 0.4-0.8 mg subcutaneous (s.c.) (Jones et al., 1992). Consistent with the results of our experiments with rats (see above), and also with a report on DAT patients by Newhouse et al. (1988), there was no effect of nicotine on a memory task (delayed matching to location on a visual display).

There is evidence that some behavioral effects of nicotine are mediated by interactions with catecholamine (CA) systems. We have shown, for example, in the rat that blockade of latent inhibition (giving rise to a broadening of selective attention) by systemic nicotine is mediated by dopamine (DA) release (Joseph et al., 1993), most probably in the nucleus accumbens. In other experiments, we have demonstrated that systemic nicotine induces tyrosine hydroxylase (the rate-limiting enzyme in CA synthesis) in the locus coeruleus and elicits noradrenaline (NA) release in the hippocampus (Mitchell et al., 1993); these effects, too, may be related to changes in cognitive function. We have therefore begun to investigate the possibility that CAs are involved in the improved vigilance caused by systemic nicotine. Our results so far tend to negate this possibility.

The improvement caused by nicotine in the radial-arm maze performance of animals with ibotenate- and quisqualate-induced lesions of the FCPS is not mimicked by the CA-releasing drug, d-amphetamine, 0.5 and 2 mg/kg i.p. (Turner et al., 1992). Nor was it possible to block the improvement caused by nicotine (0.1 mg/kg s.c.) in animals with AMPA-induced FCPS lesions by concomitant administration of the beta-adrenoceptor blocker, propranolol (0.5 and 5 mg/kg i.p.), although at the higher dose this drug itself increased errors in both control and lesioned rats. In order to test the role of the noradrenergic system further, we assessed the effects of nicotine in animals with lesions (produced by local injection of the CA-specific neurotoxin, 6-OHDA) of the dorsal noradrenergic bundle (DNAB), which carries noradrenergic afferents from the locus coeruleus to the whole of the forebrain. Animals with *both* 6-OHDA lesions to the DNAB *and* excitotoxic lesions to the FCPS were tested on repeated acquisition of navigation to the submerged platform in the working-memory version of Morris' water maze, in which the platform position is varied for successive blocks of 5 trials. The animals with lesions to either the FCPS alone or the FCPS plus DNAB were equally impaired relative to intact controls, and both showed improvement in response to systemic nicotine. Critically, the extent of this improvement did not differ between the two lesion groups. These findings essentially rule out mediation by forebrain noradrenergic systems of the beneficial effect of nicotine on cognitive performance in FCPS-lesioned animals.

To test the hypothesis that the enhancing effects of nicotine in FCPS-lesioned animals are mediated by interaction with dopaminergic systems, we initially studied whether pretreatment with the DA receptor antagonist, haloperidol (0.25 mg/kg s.c.), could counter the action of nicotine (0.1 mg/kg s.c.), using the water-maze task described above. Although haloperidol alone failed to alter water-maze performance, it markedly reversed the effects of nicotine. However, in a parallel experiment with human subjects, we failed to observe any interaction between nicotine and haloperidol. In this experiment overnight deprived smokers were tested on the vigilance task in a double-blind design combining s.c. nicotine (0.8 mg) or placebo with oral haloperidol (5 mg) or placebo. The beneficial effect of nicotine on rate of signal detection was unchanged by concomitant administration of haloperidol. Since we have shown that the dose of haloperidol used is sufficient to increase nicotine intake in such smokers (Dawe et al., 1994), this result weakens the hypothesis that the beneficial effects of nicotine upon human vigilance performance are due to an interaction with the dopaminergic system.

Given the positive results obtained in the haloperidol-nicotine interaction study with rats, we next investigated the possible role played by nucleus accumbens. The dopaminergic afferentation of this structure appears to be critical in mediating the effects of nicotine upon selective attention in the latent inhibition (LI) paradigm (Joseph et al., 1993). Rats were therefore prepared with excitotoxic lesions of the FCPS either alone or with this lesion together with 6-OHDA injections (destroying dopaminergic terminals) into nucleus accumbens. These animals were tested in the water maze. Nicotine improved performance significantly and equally in both these groups, while having no effects on performance in animals with only accumbal lesions. These findings indicate that, although some cognitive effects of nicotine can be prevented by haloperidol administration, nucleus accumbens is not the site for this interaction.

We have obtained little evidence, then, that interaction with CAs underlies the beneficial effects of nicotine on vigilance in patients with DAT, or in animal models of this condition or of alcoholic dementia; the most likely mode of nicotine's action in such subjects is by substitution for ACh at denervated post-synaptic nicotinic synapses in the hippocampus and/or neocortex.

ACKNOWLEDGEMENTS

Supported by the Wellcome Trust, R J Reynolds Tobacco Company, the Council for Tobacco Research, BAT and Schering AG, Berlin.

REFERENCES

Arendt T, Hennig D, Gray JA and Marchbanks R (1988): Loss of neurons in the rat basal forebrain cholinergic projection system after prolonged intake of ethanol. *Brain Research Bulletin* 21:563-570.

Arendt T, Allen Y, Marchbanks RM, Schugens MM, Sinden J, Lantos PL and Gray JA (1989): Cholinergic system and memory in the rat: effects of chronic ethanol, embryonic basal forebrain brain transplants and excitotoxic lesions of cholinergic basal forebrain projection system. *Neuroscience* 33:435-462.

Dawe S, Gerada C, Russell MAH and Gray JA (1994): Nicotine intake in smokers increases following a single dose of haloperidol. *Psychopharmacology* (In Press).

Eagger SA, Levy R and Sahakian BJ (1991): Tacrine in Alzheimer's disease. *Lancet* 337:989-992.

Hodges H, Ribeiro A, Gray JA and Marchbanks RM (1990): Low dose tetrahydroaminoacridine (THA) improves cognitive function in lesioned and alcohol-treated rats but does not affect brain acetylcholine. *Pharmacol Biochem Behav* 36:291-298.

Hodges H, Allen Y, Kershaw T, Lantos PL, Gray JA and Sinden JD (1991a): Effects of cholinergic-rich neural grafts on radial maze performance of rats after excitotoxic lesions of the forebrain cholinergic projection system: 1. Amelioration of cognitive deficits by transplants into cortex and hippocampus but not into basal forebrain. *Neuroscience* 45:587-607.

Hodges H, Allen Y, Sinden J, Lantos PL and Gray JA (1991b): The effects of cholinergic-rich neural grafts on radial maze performance of rats after excitotoxic lesions of the forebrain cholinergic projection system: 2. Cholinergic drugs as probes to investigate lesion-induced deficits and transplant-induced functional recovery. *Neuroscience* 45:609-623.

Hodges H, Allen Y, Sinden J, Mitchell SN, Arendt T, Lantos PL and Gray JA (1991c): The effects of cholinergic drugs and cholinergic-rich fetal neural transplants on alcohol-induced deficits in radial maze performance in rats. *Behav Brain Res* 43:7-28.

Hodges H, Sinden J, Turner JD, Netto CA, Sowinski P and Gray JA (1992): Nicotine as a tool to characterize the role of the forebrain cholinergic projection system in cognition. In: *The Biology of Nicotine*, Lippiello PM, Collins AC, Gray JA, Robinson JH, eds. New York: Raven Press, pp. 157-180.

Jones GMM, Sahakian BJ, Levy R, Warburton DM and Gray JA (1992): Effects of acute subcutaneous nicotine on attention, information processing and short-term memory in Alzheimer's disease. *Psychopharmacology* 198:485-494.

Joseph MH, Peters SL and Gray JA (1993): Nicotine blocks latent inhibition in rats: evidence for a critical role of increased functional activity of dopamine in the mesolimbic system at conditioning rather than pre-exposure. *Psychopharmacology* 110:187-192.

Mitchell SN, Smith KM, Grigoryan GA, Sinden JD, Joseph MH and Gray JA (1993): Increases in tyrosine hydroxylase mRNA in the locus coeruleus after a single dose of nicotine are followed by time-dependent increases in enzyme activity, noradrenaline release and behavioral function. *Neuroscience* 56:989-997.

Newhouse P, Sunderland T, Tariot P, Blumhardt C, Weingartner H and Mellow W (1988): Intravenous nicotine in Alzheimer's disease: a pilot study. *Psychopharmacology* 95:171-175.

Turner JJ, Hodges H, Sinden JD and Gray JA (1992): Comparison of radial maze performance of rats after ibotenate and quisqualate lesions of the forebrain cholinergic projection system: effects of pharmacological challenge and changes in training regime. *Behavioral Pharmacology* 3:359-373.

Alzheimer Disease: Therapeutic Strategies
edited by E. Giacobini and R. Becker.
© 1994 Birkhäuser Boston

THE SUBUNIT SPECIFIC EFFECTS OF NOVEL ANABASEINE-DERIVED NICOTINIC AGENTS

Roger L. Papke, Christopher M. de Fiebre, William Kem and Edwin M. Meyer
Department of Pharmacology and Therapeutics, University of Florida
College of Medicine, Gainesville, FL 32610

INTRODUCTION

Nicotinic Receptor Involvement in Learning and Memory
Nicotine readily crosses the blood-brain barrier and elicits a variety of behavioral and physiological actions. Generally, nicotine improves a variety of spatial-memory and avoidance tasks in animals, while enhancing delayed recall, information manipulation, focused attention and other memory-related behaviors in humans. Nicotine also alters mood and reaction time, which can be difficult to distinguish from changes in memory-related behaviors. One characteristic of nicotine-induced improvements in memory-related behaviors is that these are generally seen over narrow dose-ranges, with higher doses causing a variety of side effects that interfere with performance (Warburton, 1990). This narrow dose-response range may be due in part to the nicotinic activation of a multiplicity of receptors in the brain and periphery, which is a powerful impetus for targeting drugs to those nicotinic receptor subtypes selectively involved in learning and memory in order to treat conditions such as Alzheimer's disease (AD).

In recent years the cloning of genes coding for neuronal nicotinic acetylcholine receptor (nAChR) subunits (for review see Papke, 1993) has made possible new approaches to the study of nicotinic function in the nervous system. *In situ* hybridization analysis of the patterns of nicotinic receptor subunit RNA expression (Sequela et al., 1993; Wada et al., 1989) suggests the existence of specific subunit combinations in different parts of the brain. This hypothesis has been supported by immunoprecipitation studies (Flores et al., 1992). The ectopic expression of the cloned subunits in defined cell systems makes it possible to study the physiological properties of those specific subunit combinations. Ligand binding studies reveal two main classes of brain nicotinic receptors: one labeled with high affinity by $[^3H]$nicotine or $[^3H]ACh$; the other by $[^{125}I]\alpha$-bungarotoxin (Clarke et al., 1985). Approximately 90% of the former binding sites appear to be associated with the $\alpha4\beta2$ subtype, based on precipitation with a specific antibody (Flores et al., 1992). Binding sites for α-bungarotoxin are found to be predominantly associated with $\alpha 7$ subunits.

In these experiments, the *Xenopus* oocyte receptor expression system was utilized in order to compare the intrinsic nicotinic receptor activities of anabaseine (ANA) and the anabaseine-related compound (Zoltewicz et al., 1993), 2,4-dimethoxybenzylidene-anabaseine (DMXB), to the endogenous activator, acetylcholine (ACh). DMXB has been shown to have cytoprotective (Martin et al., 1994) and behavioral efficacy (Meyer et al., 1994; Woodruff-Pak et al., 1994). We have focused on $\alpha 4\beta 2$ and $\alpha 7$-type receptors, as these gene products may represent the major receptor subtypes in the cortex and hippocampus, respectively (Wada et al., 1989; Sequela et al., 1993).

METHODS

RNA was transcribed *in vitro* from cDNA clones and injected into *Xenopus* oocytes (Boulter et al., 1987). Data were then obtained by means of two electrode voltage clamp recordings. Recordings were made at room temperature (21-24°C) in Frog Ringer (115 mM NaCl, 10 mM HEPES, 2.5 mM KCl, and 1.8 mM $CaCl_2$, pH 7.3) with 1 μM atropine. Voltage electrodes were filled with 3M KCl, and to reduce Ca^{+2} dependent chloride currents, current electrodes were filled with 250 mM CsCl, 250 mM CsF, and 100 mM EGTA (pH 7.3). Recordings were made at a holding potential of -50 mV, and current responses were recorded on a Macintosh computer using National Instruments analog-to-digital conversion system with Labview software.

RESULTS

Agonist Effects of the Anabaseine Compounds
Unsubstituted anabaseine had considerable partial agonist activity at $\alpha 4\beta 2$ receptors and was a full agonist at $\alpha 7$ receptors (Fig. 1). DMXB was found to be a strong partial agonist ($\approx 30\%$ ACh activity) for $\alpha 7$ receptors (Fig. 1A), but a very weak partial agonist ($< 1\%$ ACh maximal activity) for $\alpha 4\beta 2$ receptors (Fig. 1B).

Noncompetitive Effects on Neuronal Nicotinic Receptors
In addition to agonist or partial agonist activity, these compounds appeared to have inhibitory effects on nicotinic receptors, such that they reduced the response to subsequent applications of ACh. This effect for DMXB is illustrated in Fig. 2A. In the case of the $\alpha 7$-type receptors, high concentrations (100-500 μM) were required to observe inhibitory effects, and therefore they are likely to be less important than the agonist effects which are obtained at lower concentrations.

It was observed that the anabaseine-stimulated currents of $\alpha 4\beta 2$ injected oocytes became protracted in time. In order to measure this effect, total currents were calculated as the area under the curve for 5 min following an anabaseine application, and these were normalized to the oocyte's total (5 min) 10 μM ACh current. While the plot of the peak values of the anabaseine-stimulated currents reached a plateau at about 2 μM, a plot of the total current anabaseine-stimulated current (Fig. 1B) continued to increase up to the highest concentration of anabaseine tested (500 μM).

Agents which are open-channel blockers have been reported to prolong the duration of ACh-induced bursts (Neher and Steinbach, 1978). This suggests that the failure of the anabaseine concentration-response relationship to obtain the same maximum value as the ACh-stimulated currents may be due to a combination of agonist and noncompetitive antagonist effects. Responses to nicotine but not to ACh (de Fiebre et al., submitted) have concentration-response relationships for peak and total currents that are like the anabaseine responses. The fact that nicotine has this effect suggests that a confusion might arise between desensitization and residual noncompetitive inhibition by nicotine.

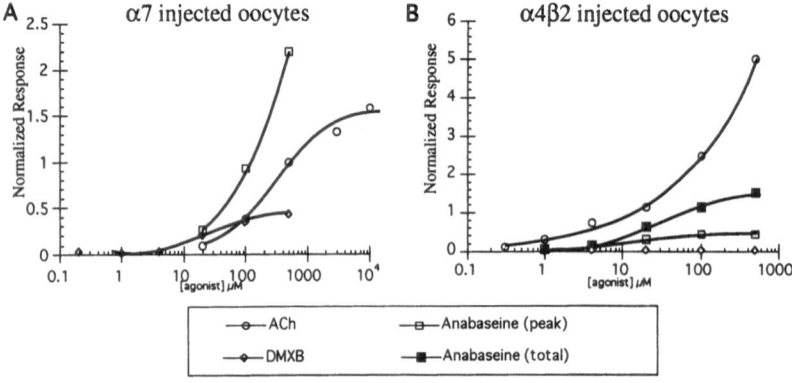

FIGURE 1. Concentration-response relationships of $\alpha 7$ (**A**) or $\alpha 4\beta 2$ (**B**) injected oocytes for ACh, anabaseine, and DMXB. The responses were normalized to the oocyte's response to either 500 μM or 10 μM ACh (in parts **A** and **B** respectively), applied 5 min before the experimental application. In part **B** the total ANA currents were normalized to the oocytes total (5 min) 10 μM ACh current.

While the derivative compounds have very little direct agonist activity for $\alpha 4\beta 2$ receptors, they still cause concentration-dependent inhibition of subsequent ACh stimulated currents (Fig. 2A). This inhibition can be shown to be noncompetitive with ACh, since the inhibition obtained with relatively low concentrations of the drugs is enhanced if the compounds are co-applied with ACh (Fig. 2A).

Low Concentration Effects of DMXB on the Potentiation of $\alpha 4\beta 2$ Responses
In addition to the agonist and antagonist effects of DMXB described above, we also observed that 10 nM of DMXB applied to $\alpha 4\beta 2$ injected oocytes potentiated subsequent responses to applied ACh (Fig. 2A). The mechanism of this

potentiation appeared to involve the antagonism of an endogenous rundown in current responses, and did not involve the enlistment of previously inactive receptors. Rundown may involve a second messenger-mediated regulation of receptor function and is present at varying degrees in different batches of oocytes. In oocyte lots which did not show rundown, the application of 10 nM DMXB had no effect (Fig. 2B, normal Ca2$^+$ conditions). In the same lot of oocytes, rundown could be induced by making recordings in high calcium Ringers. The mechanism of this effect, and whether it is restricted to $\alpha 4\beta 2$-type receptors is currently under further investigation.

DISCUSSION

It has been proposed that nicotinic agonist be used in the treatment of AD. While the few reports on the efficacy of nicotine in treating AD have indicated that scores on several measures of cognitive function were improved, long-term efficacy was not examined, and toxic effects of nicotine were reported to limit its usefulness (Jones et al., 1992). Because these toxic effects may be due to nicotine's lack of specificity for nicotinic receptor subtypes, selective agonists may be as effective in treating the disease without producing as pronounced a toxicity as nicotine.

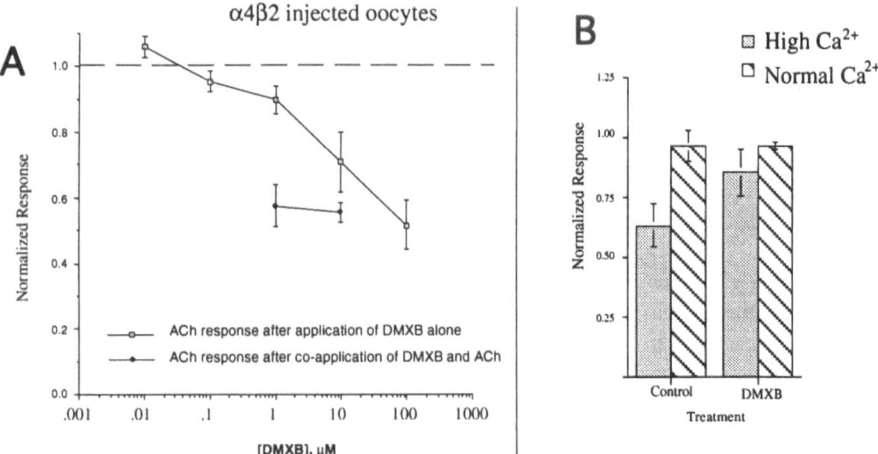

FIGURE 2. **A.** The responses of $\alpha 4\beta 2$ injected oocytes of 10 μM ACh, obtained 5 min after the application of either DMXB or DMXB co-applied with 10 μM ACh. **B.** The effect of 10 nM DMXB on the normalized responses of $\alpha 4\beta 2$ injected oocytes to the application of 10 μM ACh when the recordings were made in either normal (1.8 mM) calcium, or high (19 mM) calcium.

While DMXB has been shown to facilitate passive avoidance behavior in nucleus basalis-lesioned animals (Meyer et al., 1994), the concentration range for this effect is rather narrow, such that 0.6 μMoles/kg, but not 0.1 μMoles/kg or 6.0 μMoles/kg exerted this action. It is possible that the behavioral effects of DMXB rely on some sort of gating phenomenon which involves inhibition of some receptor subtypes and activation of others. Alternatively, the facilitation of $\alpha 4\beta 2$ responses may be an important effect of these compounds.

The subunit selectivity and complex ensemble of effects described in this report suggests that this family of compounds may have great potential for targeting sites and modes of action, with potential therapeutic usefulness. ANA is a potent displacer of [^{3}H]cytisine, while of the compounds tested, DMXB is the most potent for displacing the binding of [^{125}I]α-bungarotoxin (de Fiebre et al., submitted), so that for these compounds binding may be well correlated to the efficacy for receptor activation. Further study of the correlations between the receptor subtype specificity for physiological effects in *Xenopus* oocyte studies with cytoprotective and behavioral efficacy in whole animal studies may permit the complex threads of the brain to be untangled, so that a model may be developed for the role of nicotinic receptors in AD.

ACKNOWLEDGEMENTS

This work was supported by the Taiho Pharmaceutical Co., NIA P01 AG10485 (Project 2) to EMM. C.M. de F was supported by training grant numbers, AG-00196 and AA-07561. Technical assistance was provided by Wayne Gottlieb. Uwen Dao, Jeffrey C. Henry, and Samuel Muraskin assisted in oocyte recordings.

REFERENCES

Boulter J, Connolly J, Deneris E, Goldman D, Heinemann S and Patrick J (1987): Functional expression of two neural nicotinic acetylcholine receptors from cDNA clones identifies a gene family. *Proc Natl Acad Sci USA* 84:7763-7767.

Clarke PBS, Schwartz RD, Paul SM, Pert CB and Pert A (1985): Nicotinic binding in rat brain: autoradiographic comparison of [^{3}H] acetylcholine [^{3}H] nicotine and [^{125}I]-alpha-bungarotoxin. *J Neurosci* 5:1307-1315.

Flores CM, Rogers SW, Pabreza LA, Wolfe BB and Kellar KJ (1992): A subtype of nicotinic cholinergic receptor in rat brain is composed of $\alpha 4$ and $\beta 2$ subunits and is up-regulated by chronic nicotine treatment. *Molec Pharm* 41:31-37.

Jones GMM, Sahakian BJ, Levy R, Warburton DM and Gray JA (1992): Effects of nicotine on attention, information processing, and short-term memory in patients with dementia of Alzheimer. *Psychopharm* 108:485-494.

Martin EJ, Panikar KS, King MA, Deyrup M, Hunter B, Wang G and Meyer E (1994): Cytoprotective actions of 2,4-dimethoxybenzylidene anabaseine in differentiated PC12 cells and septal cholinergic cells. *Drug Devel Res* 31:134-141.

Meyer E, de Fiebre CM, Hunter B, Simpkins CE, Frauworth N and de Fiebre NC (1994): Effects of anabaseine-related analogs on rat brain nicotinic receptor binding and on avoidance behaviors. *Drug Devel Res* 31:127-134.

Neher E and Steinbach JH (1978): Local anaesthetics transiently block current through single acetylcholine receptor channels. *J Physiol* 277:135-176.

Papke RL (1993): The kinetic properties of neuronal nicotinic receptors: genetic basis of functional diversity. *Prog in Neurobio* 41:509-531.

Sequela P, Wadiche J, Dineley-Miller K, Dani JA and Patrick JW (1993): Molecular cloning, functional properties and distribution of rat brain alpha7: A nicotinic cation channel highly permeable to calcium. *J Neurosci* 13(2):596-604.

Wada E, Wada K, Boulter J, Deneris E, Heinemann S, Patrick J and Swanson LW (1989): Distribution of α2, α3, α4, and ß2 neuronal nicotinic receptor subunit mRNAs in the central nervous system: A hybridization histochemical study in the rat. *J Comp Neurol* 284:314-335.

Warburton DM (1990): Psychopharmacological aspects of nicotine. In: *Nicotine Psychopharmacology, Molecular, Cellular and Behavioral Aspects*, Wonnacott S, Russell MAH and Stolerman IP, eds. New York: Oxford University Press, pp.77-111.

Woodruff-Pak DS, Li Y and Kem WR (1994): A nicotinic agonist (GTS-21), eyeblink classical conditioning, and nicotinic receptor binding in rabbit brain. *Brain Res* 645:309-317.

Zoltewicz JA, Prokai-Tatrai K and Bloom L (1993): Long range transmission of polar effects in cholinergic 3-arylideneanabaseines. Conformations calculated by molecular modelling. *Heterocycles* 35(1):171-179.

Alzheimer Disease: Therapeutic Strategies
edited by E. Giacobini and R. Becker.
© 1994 Birkhäuser Boston

SEROTONIN DEPLETION DECREASES THERAPEUTIC EFFECT OF THA AND NICOTINE

Paavo J. Riekkinen Jr., Minna K. Riekkinen and Jouni S. Sirviö
Department of Neurology, University of Kuopio, Kuopio, Finland

INTRODUCTION

Recently, several studies have elucidated the interactions between the basal forebrain cholinergic and brain stem serotoninergic systems in the regulation of behavioral functions (Jäkälä et al., 1992; Sirviö et al., 1994). Anatomical studies have revealed that the basal forebrain, hippocampus and cortex have cholinergic and serotoninergic afferents. Several behavioral studies have studied the effects of concurrent serotoninergic and cholinergic manipulations (Sirviö et al., 1994). Depletion of forebrain serotonin levels by 5-hydroxytryptamine (5-HT) synthesis inhibitor, p-chlorophenylalanine (PCPA), or 5-HT neurotoxin, 5,7-dihydroxytryptamine, treatment did not impair water maze (WM) or passive avoidance (PA) behavior (Vanderwolf, 1987; Nilsson et al., 1990; Riekkinen et al., 1993; Riekkinen and Riekkinen Jr, 1994). Interestingly, a combination of muscarinic or nicotinic acetylcholine receptor antagonists and 5-HT depletion produced a severe defect of PA and WM (Riekkinen et al., 1993; Riekkinen and Riekkinen Jr, 1994). Indeed, Vanderwolf (1987) proposed that a combined systemic injection of a large muscarinic acetylcholine antagonist (scopolamine 5 mg/kg) dose and serotonin synthesis inhibitor disrupted the animals' behavior and resulted in aimless performance, i.e., environmental sensory stimuli did not regulate animals' motor behavior or behavioral output in an apt way, suggesting a profound dysregulation of behavior, mimicking the symptoms typical of severe dementia of Alzheimer's disease type (Vanderwolf, 1987). The interaction between serotoninergic and cholinergic cells may have significant pharmacological consequences for the transmitter replacement therapy for Alzheimer's disease. Indeed, in Alzheimer's disease the brain stem serotoninergic and basal forebrain cholinergic projection neurons degenerate that renders serotoninergic and nicotinic/muscarinic cholinergic receptors hypostimulated (Reinikainen et al., 1988). Interestingly, in our recent study we found that serotonin synthesis inhibition decreased the antiamnestic effect of anti-cholinesterase drugs, such as THA and physostigmine, and nicotine, a nicotinic acetylcholine receptor agonist (Riekkinen et al., 1993; Riekkinen and Riekkinen Jr, 1994). However, this study examined the behavioral effects of systemically injected acetylcholine receptor antagonists that indiscriminately block the activity of all the central cholinergic systems. Our earlier studies cannot explain the site of action (basal forebrain projection cells, intrinsic striatal cells, brain stem projections' cells) of systemically injected acetylcholine antagonists and the cholinergic systems that interact with serotonin cells to regulate behavioral functions. This issue is an important one because during Alzheimer's disease the cholinergic cells of basal forebrain degenerate severely, whereas the striatal and the brain stem cholinergic systems do not severely degenerate (Reinikainen et al., 1988). We designed the present study to elucidate the pharmacological interaction between the 5-HT cells of brain stem and the cholinergic cells of basal forebrain. Therefore, we investigated the pharmacological effect of 5-HT synthesis inhibition on WM and PA promoting action of THA and nicotine in medial septal (MS)-lesioned rats.

MATERIALS AND METHODS

Male Kuo:Wistar rats were used in the present study (300-360 g). The local Ethical Committee has accepted our methods and study design. The following groups were used: **GROUP 1:** controls (n=12), MS-lesioned + NaCl 0.9% (n=12), + THA 1 mg/kg (n=6), + THA 3 mg/kg (n=12), + THA 5 mg/kg (n=8); **GROUP 2:** controls (n=12), MS-lesioned + NaCl 0.9% (n=12), + nicotine 0.03 mg/kg (n=5), + nicotine 0.1 mg/kg (n=12), + nicotine 0.3 mg/kg (n=12); **GROUP 3:** controls (n=12), MS-lesioned (n=12), MS + PCPA-lesioned (n=12), + THA 1 mg/kg (n=6), + THA 3 mg/kg (n=12), + THA 5 mg/kg (n=8); **GROUP 4:** controls (n=12), MS+PCPA-lesioned (n=12), + nicotine 0.03 mg/kg (n=6), + nicotine 0.1 mg/kg (n=12), + nicotine 0.3 mg/kg (n=12). THA (1, 3 and 5 mg/kg, 60 min pretesting) and nicotine (0.03, 0.1 and 0.3 mg/kg, 25 min pretesting) were dissolved in physiological saline (NaCl 0.9%) and injected i.p. 2 ml/kg. We used electrolytic MS lesions (Riekkinen Jr and Riekkinen, 1989). PCPA (400 mg/kg/day * 3 day, i.p) was used to deplete 5-HT. The WM testing (Riekkinen Jr and Riekkinen, 1989) consisted of five consecutive days of testing (3 trials per day). The computer calculated escape distance values. The PA testing was conducted 24 hr after training (Riekkinen Jr and Riekkinen, 1989) and retention latencies were measured. 5-HT, 5-hydroxyindoleacetic acid, noradrenaline, dopamine and homovanillic acid levels, and choline acetyltransferase (ChAT) activity were measured from the hippocampus. MS lesioning was located by using cresyl violet staining. The one-way-ANOVA test followed by Duncan's post hoc multiple group comparison was used.

RESULTS

MS- and MS+PCPA-lesioned rats were impaired during the PA retention trial and PCPA treatment aggravated MS lesioning-induced PA failure. In MS-lesioned rats THA 3 mg/kg to some extent alleviated performance failure during the PA retention trial, but the other doses tested (1 and 5 mg/kg) were ineffective. Nicotine 0.1 and 0.3 mg/kg significantly improved performance of MS-lesioned rats, but the smallest dose (0.03 mg/kg) did not facilitate PA behavior. THA 3 mg/kg improved PA retention of MS + PCPA-lesioned rats. Nicotine did not significantly improve PA retention of combined-lesioned rats.

THA at 5 mg/kg produced a severe swimming defect and for that reason the effect of treatment with the highest dose was not tested in WM. A significant overall group effect was observed in the analysis of escape distance values measured during the first three training days of Group 1 and 2 rats. The analysis of escape distance values measured during the fourth and fifth training day did not reveal any significant overall effects. Nicotine 0.1 or 0.3 mg/kg and THA 3 mg/kg treated MS-lesioned rats were not impaired compared with the controls during the first three training days, but the MS-lesioned rats injected with nicotine at 0.03 mg/kg or THA at 1 mg/kg were as impaired as the MS-lesioned rats treated with saline.

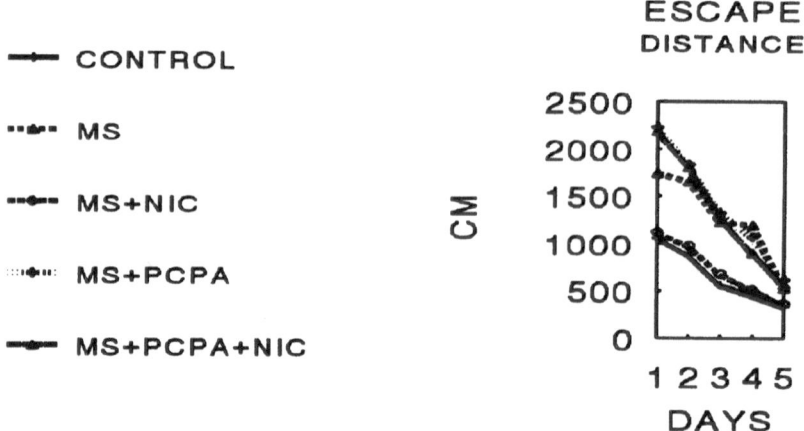

FIGURE 1. Note that treatment with nicotine at 0.3 mg/kg (NIC) nearly completely alleviated medial septal (MS) lesioning-induced water maze navigation failure. The therapeutic effect of nicotine 0.3 mg/kg was completely blocked by PCPA treatment (MS + PCPA = combined-lesioned rats). PCPA treatment aggravated MS lesioning-induced WM failure only during the first day of training. The values on Y-axis represent group means of daily training trials. X-axis: training days 1-5.

An analysis of escape distance values of Group 3 and 4 measured during the first, second and third training day revealed significant overall group effects and showed that MS- and MS + PCPA-lesioned rats had longer escape distance values than the controls. The escape distance values of the combined-lesioned groups were the worst during the first day, but no significant difference was found between single- and combined-lesioned groups during the other days.

Nicotine treated, combined-lesioned rats were as impaired as the vehicle treated combined-lesioned rats during the first three training days. However,

THA 3 mg/kg treated rats performed better than the control solution-treated MS + PCPA-lesioned rats during the first three water maze training days.

PCPA treatment decreased serotonin (-78%) and 5-hydroxyindoleacetic acid (-83%) levels in the hippocampus. The ChAT activity in the hippocampus was decreased by MS and combined MS + PCPA lesionings.

DISCUSSION

The present study shows that combined lesionings of brain stem 5-HT and medial septal systems have important behavioral and pharmacological consequences. Firstly, PCPA treatment aggravated PA defect of MS-lesioned rats. Secondly, PCPA treatment also increased slightly escape distance values of MS-lesioned rats during the first training day. Thirdly, PCPA treatment completely blocked the therapeutic effect of nicotine on WM and PA behavior, but therapeutic effect of THA on PA and spatial navigation was only slightly decreased or not affected at all, respectively.

The present results showing that nicotine and THA improve PA and WM behavior of MS-lesioned rats are in good agreement with the earlier results (Riekkinen Jr and Riekkinen, 1993). A more interesting and novel discovery was that the joined lesioning of MS and 5-HT systems blocked the PA and WM behavior promoting effect of nicotine, but only to some extent decreased the effect of THA on PA. The pretraining injected nicotine dose-dependently (0.03, 0.1 and 0.3 mg/kg, s.c.) facilitated PA performance of MS-lesioned rats, but PCPA treatment completely blocked the therapeutic effect of nicotine at the dose range used. It could be argued that even the highest dose of nicotine was inadequately small and at a greater dose nicotine would have promoted PA behavior of the combined-lesioned rats. However, nicotine at a slightly higher dose than used in this study cause marked peripheral and central side-effects and therefore higher doses were not used (Riekkinen Jr and Riekkinen, 1993). In good agreement with earlier data THA at 3 mg/kg promoted PA behavior of MS-lesioned rats and had a bell-shaped dose-response curve (Riekkinen Jr et al., 1991). Interestingly, in our earlier study THA 3 mg/kg facilitated PA of nucleus basalis-lesioned rats but a dose of 5 mg/kg caused cholinergic side-effects inhibiting performance. Indeed, the side-effects (diarrhea, salivation, lacrimation) of acute THA at 5 mg/kg treatment may have impaired PA behavior and caused the bell-shaped dose-response. Previously we described during a chronic treatment a tolerance to the side-effects of THA treatment and a broadening of the dose window (Riekkinen Jr et al., 1991). A more significant finding, however, was that PCPA treatment differently modulated the effect of THA on PA and WM behavior of MS-lesioned rats; THA promoted WM spatial navigation as effectively in single MS-lesioned as in combined-lesioned rats, but less completely promoted PA behavior of combined- than single-lesioned rats. It is, therefore, possible that intact 5-HT system is not a prerequisite for effective WM navigation but normal functioning of 5-HT cells is important for

PA behavior. Earlier experiments investigating the pharmacological consequences of a combined cholinergic and serotonergic block support the present results showing that a 5-HT depletion decreases the effect of nicotine and THA. Riekkinen et al. (1993) and Riekkinen and Riekkinen Jr (1994) reported that treatment with nicotine, THA and physostigmine less effectively promoted WM and PA behavior of combined nicotinic acetylcholine receptor antagonist (mecamylamine)+PCPA-treated than single mecamylamine treated rats. Interestingly, PCPA treatment more severely blocked PA than WM promoting action of THA and physostigmine. Therefore, it is tempting to suggest that the 5-HT systems may at least partly mediate the therapeutic effect of nicotine, THA and physostigmine on spatial and avoidance behavior.

REFERENCES

Jäkälä PJ, Sirviö J, Jolkkonen J, Riekkinen P Jr and Riekkinen P (1992): The effects of p-chlorophenylalanine induced serotonin synthesis inhibition and muscarinic blockade on the performance of rats in a 5-choice serial reaction time task. *Behav Brain Res* 51:29-40.

Nilsson OG, Brudin P and Björklund A (1990): Amelioration of spatial memory impairment by intra-hippocampal grafts of mixed septal and raphe tissue in rats with combined cholinergic and serotonergic denervation of the forebrain. *Brain Res* 515:193-206.

Reinikainen KJ, Riekkinen P Jr, Paljärvi L, Soininen H, Helkala E-L, Jolkkonen J and Laakso M (1988): Cholinergic deficit in Alzheimer's disease: a study based on CSF and autopsy data. *Neurochem Res* 13:135-146.

Riekkinen M, Sirviö JS and Riekkinen P Jr (1993): Pharmacological consequences of combined nicotinic and serotonergic manipulations. *Brain Res* 662:139-146.

Riekkinen M and Riekkinen P Jr (1994): Effects of THA and physostigmine on spatial navigation and passive avoidance in mecamylamine+PCPA treated rats. *Exp Neurol* 125:111-118.

Riekkinen P Jr, Sirviö JS, Riekkinen M and Riekkinen P (1991): Effects of THA on passive avoidance retention performance of intact, nucleus basalis, frontal cortex and nucleus basalis + frontal cortex-lesioned rats. *Pharmacol Biochem Behav* 39:841-846.

Riekkinen P Jr and Riekkinen M (1993): Nicotinic cholinergic stimulation in experimental models of behavior. In: *Aspects of Synaptic Transmission 2: Acetylcholine, Sigma Receptors, CCK and Eicosanoids, Neurotoxins.* Stone TW, ed. London: Taylor and Francis, pp. 73-90.

Sirviö JS, Riekkinen P Jr, Jäkälä P and Riekkinen P (1994): Role of serotonin in cognitive functions. *Progress in Neurobiology* (In Press).

Vanderwolf CH (1987): Near total loss of 'learning' and 'memory' as a result of combined cholinergic and serotonergic blockade in the rat. *Behav Brain Res* 23:43-57.

PART VI

MUSCARINIC AGONISTS: PRECLINICAL AND CLINICAL APPROACHES

Alzheimer Disease: Therapeutic Strategies
edited by E. Giacobini and R. Becker.
© 1994 Birkhäuser Boston

SELECTIVE SIGNALING VIA NOVEL MUSCARINIC AGONISTS: IMPLICATIONS FOR ALZHEIMER'S DISEASE TREATMENTS AND CLINICAL UPDATE

Abraham Fisher, Eliahu Heldman, David Gurwitz, Rachel Haring, Yishai Karton, Haim Meshulam, Zippora Pittel, Daniele Marciano, Itzhak Marcovitch and Rachel Brandeis
Israel Institute for Biological Research, Ness-Ziona 70450, Israel

Terese A. Treves, Ruth Verchovsky, Sonia Klimowsky and Amos D. Korczyn
Tel Aviv Medical Center, Department of Neurology, Tel Aviv, Israel

INTRODUCTION

Five human muscarinic acetylcholine receptors (mAChR) (m1-m5), have been cloned and expressed in suitable cell systems (reviewed by Hulme et al., 1990).* mAChRs have two binding domains, a ligand-binding extracellular (and including membrane-spanning) domain and a G-protein binding intracellular domain. This second domain, by interaction with various G-proteins, controls and modulates second messenger systems (Hulme et al., 1990).

Although the "cholinergic hypothesis" in AD indicates the potential of a cholinergic replacement therapy, clinical trials with some muscarinic agonists were disappointing (reviewed by Giacobini, 1990; Potter, 1992). These agonists are either non-selective or more M2 and M3 than M1 selective and thus may produce peripheral and central side-effects mediated by M2 or M3 AChR. (Potter, 1992). M1-type mAChRs are predominant in cerebral cortex and hippocampus and may have important roles in cognitive processes in AD, in particular short-term memory (Potter, 1992).

M1 AChRs are preserved in AD (Potter, 1992). Therefore a rational treatment in AD can be M1 (or m1) agonists, or a combination of M1 (or m1) agonism with M2 (or m2), or with M3 (or m3) antagonism in one compound

---

* The m1, m2, m3, m4 AChRs fit the pharmacological definition of the M1, M2, M3 and M4 AChRs, respectively (Hulme et al., 1990). We use the term m1-m5 and M1-M3 agonists (or antagonists) for ligands defined using the cloned m1-m5 and M1-M3 pharmacologically characterized mAChRs, respectively.

(Fisher et al., 1991, 1992, 1993; Potter, 1992). Such selective M1 (or m1) agonists should also activate hypofunctional signals in AD, yet avoid hyperfunctional signaling pathways (Fisher et al., 1993; Gurwitz et al., 1994). Notably, abnormalities in AD may also occur along various signal transduction pathways (Harrison et al., 1991). Mismetabolism of amyloid precursor proteins (APPs) may induce AD (Matson et al., 1993). Interestingly, activation of m1 and m3 mAChRs enhances secretion of APPs *in vitro* (Nitsch et al., 1992).

To address some of these recent findings, we describe new properties of rigid analogs of acetylcholine (ACh) (Fisher et al., 1990, 1991, 1992, 1993) (Fig. 1). Among these, the best characterized is AF102B (reviewed by Fisher et al., 1993). This paper also surveys a recent study on AF102B in Israeli AD patients.

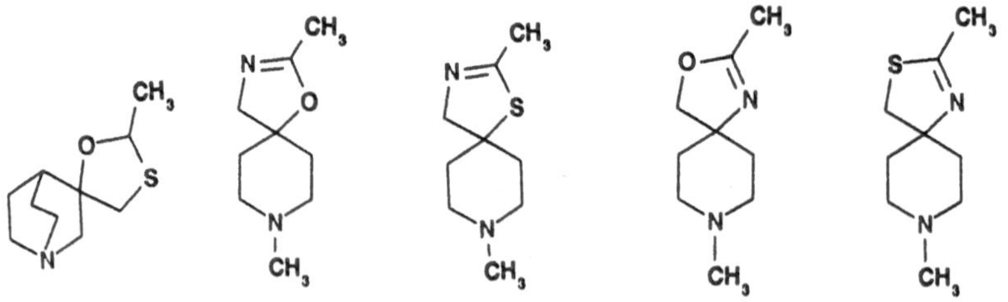

AF102B   AF150   AF150(S)   AF151   AF151(S)

FIGURE 1

RESULTS AND DISCUSSION

AF102B is a selective M1 agonist. AF102B can act as a full agonist, a partial agonist, or an antagonist depending on the tissue, the mAChR subtype and the functional assays studied. Thus, AF102B can be considered as a selective M1 (or m1) agonist when defined through functional assays (Fisher et al., 1993). Selectivity and efficacy was tested first in binding studies using rat brain regions rich in M1 AChRs, e.g., cerebral cortex *vs* brain regions rich in M2 AChRs, e.g., cerebellum. The results showed that AF150, AF151, AF150(S) and AF151(S) are more efficacious agonists than AF102B for M1 AChRs in rat cortex *vs* cerebellum (Fisher et al., 1992, 1993).

Studies in Cell Cultures on Second Messengers
The compounds in Fig. 1 are full agonists in elevating $[Ca^{2+}]_i$ in Chinese hamster ovary (CHO) cells stably transfected with cloned m1AChR. In CHO and in rat pheochromocytoma (PC12) cells stably transfected with m1AChR (PC12M1) (re: Pinkas-Kramarski et al., 1992), AF102B and AF150(S) are partial agonists [30-50% *vs* carbachol (CCh)] but AF150, AF151, and AF151(S) are full agonists in stimulating phosphoinositides (PI) hydrolysis or arachidonic acid release. Yet, all the compounds behaved as antagonists

when compared with CCh in elevating cAMP levels (Fisher et al., 1992; Gurwitz et al., 1994).

Neurotrophic-like Effects in PC12M1 Cells

Oxotremorine induced extensive neurite outgrowth, which synergized with nerve growth factor (NGF)-mediated neurites in PC12M1 cells (Pinkas-Kramarski et al., 1992). AF102B (up to 100 μM) induced only minimal to moderate neurite outgrowth. Yet, AF102B synergized strongly (ED_{50} = 5 μM) with 2 nM NGF, which by itself mediated only a mild response. Preliminary studies showed that AF150(S) and AF151(S) were also synergistic (EC_{50} ~ 1 μM) with NGF (2 nM). The synergism of AF102B and NGF was not observed in non-transfected PC12 cells, and was completely blocked in PC12M1 cells by 10 μM atropine, showing involvement of m1AChRs. In addition, atropine retracted neurites which were previously extended by co-incubation of PC12M1 cells with AF102B and NGF. Neurites extended by a combined treatment with NGF and AF102B were stable for long periods (> 10 days). This shows that the continued presence of AF102B did not desensitize the signaling mechanism(s) responsible for maintenance of neurites (Gurwitz et al., 1993).

m1 AChR-Stimulated APPs Secretion from PC12M1 Cells

In PC12M1 cells, stimulation of m1AChRs by AF102B enhances secretion of APPs to the culture medium, and lowers the level of membrane associated APPs. Notably, while being a partial agonist (30% vs. CCh) in stimulating PI hydrolysis, AF102B is as powerful as the full agonist CCh for stimulating APPs secretion in PC12M1 cells, as judged from the decline in membrane-associated APPs. The enhanced APPs secretion induced by AF102B is potentiated by NGF. This was also evident from the increased disappearance of membrane-bound APPs following m1AChR stimulation in NGF-differentiated cells (Haring et al., unpublished results).

Studies in Animal Models that Mimic the Cholinergic Hypofunction in AD

AF102B, AF150, AF150(S) and AF151 improved memory and learning deficits in a variety of animal models for AD. These agonists were without adverse central or peripheral side-effects at the effective doses and showed a relatively wide safety margin (Fisher et al., 1991; Fisher et al., 1993).

Clinical Update for AF102B in AD Patients

Phase I and II clinical trials were already done on AF102B in Japan and USA. In Israel, we have evaluated AF102B during 10 weeks, in a single-blind placebo-controlled, parallel-group study in patients of both sexes diagnosed with probable AD. We tested the safety and efficacy of AF102B in escalating doses of 20, 40, 60 mg, t.i.d., p.o., each dose for two weeks, together with two weeks placebo *lead in* and two weeks placebo *lead out*. Of 43 AD patients mildly, moderately, and moderately-severely demented who enrolled in the study, we could calculate data of efficacy for 24 patients on AF102B and eight on placebo. The primary outcome efficacy measure used to evaluate AF102B vs placebo was the Alzheimer's Disease Assessment Scale (ADAS), in particular its cognitive subscale, the ADAS-*cognitive* (re also Farlow et al., 1992).

We showed a significant effect in favor of AF102B vs placebo at the dose of 40 mg and especially at 60 mg, t.i.d., in ADAS, in ADAS-*cognitive* scale, and in some additional cognitive measures like ADAS-*word recognition*. In these subscales we detected a dose-related improvement since the dose of 60 mg, t.i.d., p.o. was more effective than 40 mg, and 20 mg, t.i.d. Better efficacy was noted in the mildly demented patients, in particular at the dose of 40 and 60 mg, t.i.d. The dose of 60 mg, t.i.d., was also efficacious in moderately and more severely demented patients. The caregiver(s) noted also improvement vs placebo at 40 and 60 mg, t.i.d. The compound was well tolerated by the patients with only one dropout due to adverse effects as compared with more dropouts in the placebo group. Adverse effects were of cholinergic nature and included diaphoresis (20% of the patients) and excessive salivation (7%). No other significant adverse effects were noted.

CONCLUSIONS

The functionally selective m1 agonists shown in Fig. 1 can be candidates for the treatment of AD. The *"ligand-mediated selective signaling"* (Gurwitz et al., 1994), e.g., activation of only distinct G-protein subset(s) (e.g., Gq, Gp but not Gs), might be of clinical significance, since altered signal transduction via Gs might be relevant in the pathophysiology of AD (Harrison et al., 1991). These findings can be linked with the enhanced secretion of APPs, *in vitro*, following stimulation of m1AChRs by m1 agonists like AF102B. Consequently, m1 agonists may prevent β-amyloid formation by promoting selectively and positively the secretase processing pathway in AD. Such agonists may also enhance the action of NGF in AD, due to their synergistic effect with NGF. Thus, M1 (or m1) agonists may be useful in a cholinergic replacement treatment and also in delaying the progression of AD. Hence, m1 agonists might have a more important role in the treatment of AD than originally envisaged. The favorable results with AF102B in AD patients certainly encourage further clinical trials to evaluate its full therapeutic potential in this disease.

ACKNOWLEDGEMENT

Supported in part by Snow Brand Milk Products, Japan.

REFERENCES

Farlow M, Gracon SI, Hershey A, Lewis KW, Sadowsky, CH and Dolan-Ureno, J for the Tacrine Study Group (1992): A controlled trial of tacrine in Alzheimer's disease. *JAMA* 268:2523-2529.

Fisher A, Brandeis R, Karton I, Pittel Z, Gurwitz D, Haring R, Sapir M, Levy A and Heldman E (1991) *Cis*-2-methyl-spiro(1,3-oxathiolane-5,3') quinuclidine an M1 selective cholinergic agonist attenuates cognitive dysfunctions in an animal model of Alzheimer's disease. *J Pharmacol Exptl Ther* 257:392-403.

Fisher A, Segall Y, Shirin E, Meshulam H and Karton Y (1990) Spiro-nitrogen-bridged and unbridged heterocyclic compounds. *US Pat Appl Apr 10; (CIP)*.

Fisher A, Karton Y, Heldman E, Gurwitz D, Haring R, Meshulam H, Brandeis R, Pittel Z, Segall Y, Marciano D, Markovitch I, Samocha Z, Shirin E, Sapir M, Green B, Shoham G and Barak D (1993): Progress in medicinal chemistry of novel selective muscarinic agonists. *Drug Design and Discovery* 9:221-235.

Fisher A, Gurwitz D, Barak D, Haring R, Karton Y, Brandeis R, Pittel Z, Marciano D, Meshulam H, Vogel Z and Heldman E (1992): Rigid analogs of acetylcholine can be M1-selective agonists: implications for a rational treatment strategy in Alzheimer's disease. *Biorg Med Chem Lett* 2:839-844.

Giacobini E (1990): The cholinergic system in Alzheimer disease In: *Progress Brain Res*, Aquilonius SM and Gillberg P, eds. Amsterdam: Elsevier, Vol. 84, pp. 321-332.

Gurwitz D, Haring R, Heldman E, Fraser C M, Manor D and Fisher A (1994) Discrete activation of transduction pathways associated with acetylcholine m1 receptor by several muscarinic ligands. *Eur J Pharmacol* 267:21-31.

Gurwitz D, Haring R, Pinkas-Kramarski R, Stein R and Fisher A (1993): Neurotrophic-like effects of AF102B, an M1-selective muscarinic agonist, in PC12 cells transfected with M1 muscarinic receptors. *Soc Neurosci Abs* 19:1767.

Harrison PJ, Barton AJL, McDonald B and Pearson RCA (1991): Alzheimer's disease: specific increases in a G-protein subunit (Gsα) mRNA in hippocampal and cortical neurons. *Mol Brain Res* 10:71-81.

Hulme EC, Birdsall NJM and Buckley NJ (1990): Muscarinic receptor subtypes. *Ann Rev Pharmacol Toxicol* 30:633-673.

Mattson MP, Barger SW, Cheng B, Lieberburg I, Smith-Swintosky VL and Russell ER (1993): β-Amyloid precursor protein metabolites and loss of neuronal Ca^{2+} homeostasis in Alzheimer's disease. *TINS* 16:409-414.

Nitsch RN, Slack BE, Wurtman RJ and Growdon JH (1992): Release of Alzheimer amyloid precursor derivatives stimulated by activation of muscarinic acetylcholine receptors. *Science* 258:304-307.

Pinkas-Kramarski R, Stein R, Lindenboim L and Sokolovsky M (1992): Growth factor-like effects mediated by muscarinic receptors in PC12M1 cells. *J Neurochem* 59:2158-2166.

Potter LT (1992): Strategies for the treatment of Alzheimer's disease - cholinergic agonist. In: *Alzheimer's Disease: New Treatment Strategies*, Khachaturian ZS and Blass JP, eds. New York: Marcel Dekker, pp. 57-66.

Alzheimer Disease: Therapeutic Strategies
edited by E. Giacobini and R. Becker.
© 1994 Birkhäuser Boston

SELECTIVE MUSCARINIC AGONISTS FOR ALZHEIMER DISEASE TREATMENT

Roy D. Schwarz, Michael J. Callahan, Robert E. Davis,
Juan C. Jaen, William Lipinski, Charlotte Raby,
Carolyn J. Spencer and Haile Tecle
Parke-Davis Pharmaceutical Research, Division of Warner-Lambert Co.,
Ann Arbor, MI 48105 USA

INTRODUCTION

Replacement therapy in Alzheimer Disease (AD) with muscarinic agonists may be of therapeutic benefit in alleviating certain cognitive deficits associated with the disorder. Based upon this "cholinergic hypothesis" (Bartus et al., 1982), a number of clinical trials were conducted over the last decade with a variety of agonists (Table I). The overall results with these compounds were equivocal with some patients reporting positive responses, some showing no responses, and others unable to complete the trials due to troublesome cholinergic side effects. Two conclusions from these studies were that either the design (e.g. outcome measures) of the trials were insufficient to determine efficacy or that the compounds themselves had major deficiencies which prevented the cholinergic hypothesis from being adequately tested.

Second generation muscarinic agonists have been synthesized in order to overcome the problems of limited oral activity, poor bioavailability, short duration of action, or lack of central nervous system (CNS) penetration seen with classical agonists (Schwarz et al., 1991). Clinical results are forthcoming, but it may still be difficult to adequately separate efficacious doses from those which produce dose-limiting peripheral side effects with non-selective agonists.

Five subtypes of muscarinic receptors (m1-m5) have now been characterized on the basis of cloning, sequencing, and expression studies (Kubo et al., 1986; Bonner et al., 1987; Peralta et al., 1987). Anatomical receptor distribution studies, in combination with results from functional experiments, have led to the idea that selective agonists of the m1 subtype may possess the best profile for AD therapy when comparing efficacy versus propensity to produce adverse side effects (Davis et al., 1993).

Agonist	Investigators	Reference	Date
Arecoline	Christie et al.	Br J Psychiatry 138:46	1981
	Tariot et al.	Arch Gen Psychiatry 45:901	1988
	Raffaele et al.	Prog Neuropsychopharmacol	
		Biol Psychiatry 15:643	1991
	Soncrant et al.	Psychopharmacol 112:421	1993
Bethanechol	Harbaugh et al.	Neurosurgery 15:514	1984
	Gauthier et al.	Can J Neurol Sci 13:394	1986
	Penn et al.	Neurology 38:219	1988
	Harbaugh et al.	J Neurosurgery 71:481	1989
	Read et al.	Arch Neurol 47:1025	1990
Oxotremorine	Davis et al.	Am J Psychiatry 144:468	1987
Pilocarpine	Caine	New Engl J Med 303:585	1980
RS-86	Wettstein et al.	Psychopharmacol 845:572	1984
	Bruno et al.	Arch Neurol 43:659	1986
	Hollander et al.	Biol Psychiatry 22:1067	1989
	Mouradian et al.	Neurology 38:606	1988

TABLE I. Human clinical trials with muscarinic agonists.

Recently, a novel series of 1-azabicyclo[2.2.1]-hexan-3-one oximes have been synthesized which appear to be functionally selective *in vitro* and show few cholinergic side effects *in vivo* (Tecle et al., 1993). Of these, PD142505 is considered as a prototypic compound and the following results summarize both *in vitro* and *in vivo* findings with this agent.

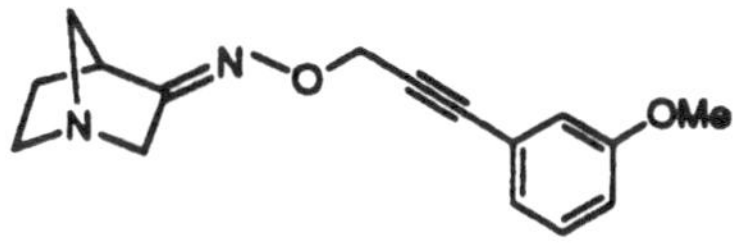

FIGURE 1. Structure of PD142505.

PHARMACOLOGICAL CHARACTERIZATION OF PD142505

Measurement of In Vitro Activity
Previous whole cell receptor binding studies using CHO cells stably transfected with the five receptor subtypes had shown that agonists fell into two general categories (Schwarz et al., 1993). Group I compounds (AF-102B, arecoline, BM-5, CI-979 and RS-86) showed no difference in affinity between any of the subtypes while Group II compounds (carbachol, L-670,207, McN-A-343, oxotremorine, and pilocarpine) showed some selectivity among subtypes (selectivity defined as being greater than a 3-fold difference in affinity). Table

II shows that PD142505 was like Group II compounds when using [^{3}H]-QNB as the ligand (having a 3-fold selectivity between m1 and m2 receptors) but it possessed no selectivity when [^{3}H]-NMS was used as the ligand. Thus, determination of subtype selectivity using receptor binding is highly ligand- (and assay condition-) specific.

	IC$_{50}$ (μM)			
Ligand	m1	m2	m3	m4
[^{3}H]-QNB	9.2	24.8	6.2	7.4
[^{3}H]-NMS	4.5	6.6	5.2	5.2

TABLE II. Subtype selectivity of PD142505 determined by receptor binding.

In general, m1, m3, and m5 receptors are linked to phospholipase C and are involved in the production of diacylglycerol and inositol trisphosphate which in turn liberates free intracellular Ca^{++} while m2 and m4 receptors are negatively coupled to adenylyl cyclase (Kubo et al., 1986; Bonner et al., 1987).

Using transfected m1, m3, and m5 CHO cells, muscarinic agonists stimulate the production of total [^{3}H]-inositol phosphates (IPs). In all three cell lines full agonists, such as carbachol or muscarine, produce maximal responses, while partial agonists (e.g. arecoline, pilocarpine) yield lesser effects. PD142505 produced a partial response in m1 cells (67% of carbachol), but much weaker effects in m3 (7%) and m5 (11%) cells (Fig. 2A). While the m5 response could be the result of a low receptor reserve, the small effect in m3 cells cannot be similarly explained since m1 and m3 cell lines both contain about the same number of receptors. (For a discussion of receptor reserve in transfected cells, see Schwarz et al., 1993.)

In m2 and m4 CHO cells, muscarinic agonists decrease forskolin-stimulated cAMP accumulation with a maximal inhibition of approximately 50%. Unlike the effects observed on PI hydrolysis, there is no differentiation among agonists as to full versus partial effects since all agonists examined show the same maximal response. In marked contrast, PD142505 showed no significant effect at concentrations of 1-100 μM and even at a concentration of 1 mM inhibited forskolin stimulation by only about 28% in Hm2 cells (Fig. 2B).

All known muscarinic agonists decrease K$^+$-stimulated release of [^{3}H]-ACh from rat brain slices *in vitro* through the activation of autoreceptors. Based upon pharmacological characterization, it is believed that receptors of the M$_2$ subtype predominate presynaptically and control release (Starke et al., 1989). From the functional results described in the previous section, it was anticipated that PD142505 would not decrease release since it had little or no m2 activity. However, the compound decreased K$^+$-stimulated [^{3}H]-ACh release in a concentration-dependent manner (30% maximal effect) similar to other agonists with the effect being reversed by scopolamine. It may be that the characterization of all presynaptic muscarinic receptors as being only of the M_2 subtype is an oversimplification.

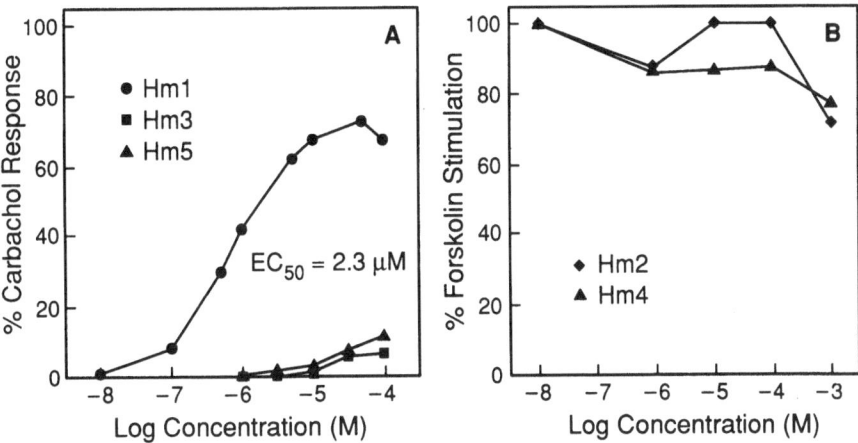

FIGURE 2. The effect of PD142505 on (**A**) PI hydrolysis in Hm1, Hm3 and Hm5 CHO cells and (**B**) forskolin-stimulated cAMP accumulation in Hm2 and Hm4 CHO cells.

In Vivo Activity

Several animal models show that PD142505 is well tolerated and can gain access to the CNS. Using C57BL/10SnJ mice in a modified water-maze model, PD142505 significantly decreased the mean latency to find a hidden platform at doses of 1.0 and 3.2 mg/kg (PO) compared to vehicle treated animals. The magnitude of this effect was similar to that seen with an optimal dose (10 mg/kg) of tacrine, an acetylcholinesterase inhibitor (AChEI). Additionally, like other muscarinic agonists, PD142505 decreased body temperature in rats. However, this occurred at 178 mg/kg (PO) and at this high dose, m1 receptors may not be involved and the effect could be an indication of the activation of other muscarinic subtypes.

Classical muscarinic agonists and AChEIs produce marked GI disturbances via the activation of the parasympathetic nervous system. In a peripheral model of GI motility and stomach emptying, PD142505 failed to produce any significant effects at doses up to 178 mg/kg (PO). Further, other cholinergic symptoms such as salivation, lacrimation, and diarrhea were not observed up to doses of 320 mg/kg (PO). If translatable to humans, these results suggest that this agent may produce fewer peripheral cholinergic side effects.

SUMMARY

In summary, PD142505 appears to possess a unique pharmacological profile consistent with m1 selectivity. While receptor binding results showed only a small difference in affinity between m1 and m2 receptors, the functional measures (PI hydrolysis and cAMP accumulation) revealed a marked selectivity among receptor subtypes. Further, this *in vitro* functional selectivity appeared to translate as a clear separation between *in vivo* cholinergic central effects and peripheral side effects.

ACKNOWLEDGEMENTS

The authors would like to acknowledge the following individuals who also contributed to this work: D. Lauffer, L. Lauffer, and C. Nelson.

REFERENCES

Bartus RT, Dean RL, Beer B and Lippa AS (1982): The cholinergic hypothesis of geriatric memory dysfunction. *Science* 217:408-416.

Bonner TI, Buckley NJ, Young AC and Brann MR (1987): Identification of a family of muscarinic acetylcholine receptor genes. *Science* 237:527-532.

Davis R, Raby C, Callahan MJ, Lipinski W, Schwarz RD, Dudley DT, Lauffer D, Reece P, Jaen J and Tecle H (1993): Subtype selective muscarinic agonists: potential therapeutic agents for Alzheimer's disease. In: *Cholinergic Function and Dysfunction*, Cuello A, ed. New York, Elsevier, pp. 439-445.

Kubo T, Fukuda K, Mikami A, Maeda A, Takahashi M, Mishina M, Haga T, Haga K, Ichiyama A, Kangawa K, Tojima M, Matsuo H, Hirose T and Numa S (1986): Cloning, sequencing, and expression of complementary DNA encoding the muscarinic acetylcholine receptor. *Nature* 323:411-416.

Peralta EG, Ashkenazi A, Winslow JW, Smith DH, Ramachandran J and Capon DJ (1987): Distinct primary structures, ligand-binding properties and tissue-specific expression of four human muscarinic acetylcholine receptors. *EMBO J* 6:3923-3929.

Schwarz RD, Coughenour LL, Davis RE, Dudley DT, Moos WH, Pavia MR and Tecle H (1991): Novel muscarinic agonists for the treatment of Alzheimer's disease. In: *Cholinergic Basis for Alzheimer Therapy*, Becker R and Giacobini E, eds. Boston: Birkhauser, pp. 347-353.

Schwarz RD, Davis RE, Jaen JC, Spencer CJ, Tecle H and Thomas AJ (1993): Characterization of muscarinic agonists in recombinant cell lines. *Life Sci* 52:465-472.

Starke K, Gothert M and Kilbinger H (1989): Modulation of neurotransmitter release by presynaptic autoreceptors. *Physiol Reviews* 69:865-962.

Tecle H, Lauffer DJ, Mirzadegan T, Moos WH, Moreland DW, Pavia MR, Schwarz RD and Davis RE (1993): Synthesis and SAR of bulky 1-azabicyclo[2.2.1]-3-one oximes as muscarinic receptor subtype selective agonists. *Life Sci* 52:505-511.

Alzheimer Disease: Therapeutic Strategies
edited by E. Giacobini and R. Becker.
© 1994 Birkhäuser Boston

XANOMELINE: AN EFFICACIOUS AND SPECIFIC M1 RECEPTOR AGONIST - PRECLINICAL UPDATE

Harlan E. Shannon, Frank P. Bymaster, David O. Calligaro,
Beverley Greenwood, Charles H. Mitch and John S. Ward
Lilly Research Laboratories, Eli Lilly & Co., Indianapolis, IN

Per Sauerberg, Preben Olesen, Malcolm Sheardown,
Michael D.B. Swedberg and Peter D. Suzdak
Novo Nordisk CNS Division, Måløv, Denmark

INTRODUCTION

Although neurochemical deficits in Alzheimer's disease (AD) are varied and complex (e.g., Katzman, 1986), the earliest, most marked and consistent neurochemical changes in AD result from the degeneration of the basal forebrain cholinergic neurons which project to the hippocampus and cortex (Davies and Maloney, 1976; Whitehouse et al., 1982; Coyle et al., 1983). Accordingly, cholinergic receptor agonists and acetylcholinesterase inhibitors have been proposed by numerous investigators as neurotransmitter replacement therapy and potential treatment for the cognitive and other symptoms in AD. Muscarinic receptor agonists which have thus far been tested in AD (oxotremorine, arecoline, pilocarpine, RS86 and bethanechol) (Palacios and Spiegel, 1986; Pomara et al., 1986; Whitehouse, 1988) have not proven to be therapeutically useful (but see Soncrant et al., 1993). One reason for the lack of efficacy of these compounds in AD may be their lack of efficacy at M1 receptors (e.g., Potter and Ferendelli, 1989; Shannon et al., 1993). An efficacious and selective M1 agonist might be expected to provide a more appropriate test of the cholinergic hypothesis of dementia.

Xanomeline is an efficacious and selective muscarinic cholinergic M1 receptor agonist which crosses the blood-brain barrier and is orally bioavailable (Sauerberg et al., 1992; Mitch et al., 1993; Bymaster et al., 1994; Shannon et al., 1994). As such, xanomeline may have therapeutic utility in the treatment of AD. The present report summarizes the preclinical pharmacology of xanomeline demonstrating its efficacy and selectivity as an M1 muscarinic receptor agonist.

RECEPTOR BINDING

Xanomeline has high affinity for M1 receptors (IC_{50} = 5-10 nM) as measured by inhibition of [^{3}H]-pirenzepine binding in brain hippocampal and cortical membranes. Xanomeline also has high affinity for inhibiting the binding of the muscarinic agonist [^{3}H]-oxotremorine-M (IC_{50} = 3-10 nM), consistent with xanomeline being an agonist. Xanomeline is 10- to 20-fold less potent in inhibiting [^{3}H]-QNB binding (IC_{50} = 70 nM) at M2 receptors in brain stem and forebrain membranes. Xanomeline has modest affinity for serotonin-1C receptors (IC_{50} = 120 nM). Xanomeline did not interact appreciably with a number of other receptors and neurotransmitter uptake sites at concentrations well in excess of those required for M1 receptor occupancy. Thus, in receptor binding studies, xanomeline shows a high degree of selectivity for muscarinic M1 receptors.

ISOLATED TISSUES AND TISSUE CULTURE

Results in isolated tissue preparations support the specificity of xanomeline for M1 receptors in functional assays. At M1 receptors in the rabbit vas deferens, xanomeline had an EC_{50} of 0.006 nM. The selective M1 antagonist pirenzepine blocked the effects of xanomeline in the rabbit vas deferens with a dissociation constant of approximately 4 nM. In the guinea pig atria, which contains only M2 receptors, xanomeline produced a negative inotropic response, but with an EC_{50} of approximately 3 μM. The effects of xanomeline in the atria were blocked by the nonselective muscarinic antagonist atropine, but not by pirenzepine. At M3 receptors in the guinea pig bladder, xanomeline was without appreciable agonist or antagonist activity at concentrations up to 10 μM. Thus, xanomeline exhibited a very high degree of specificity for M1 muscarinic receptors in isolated tissue preparations.

Xanomeline increased phosphoinositol (PI) hydrolysis in three cell lines transfected with m1 receptors: CHO, A9L and BHK. The cell lines differed with respect to number of receptors per cell (CHO > A9L $\geq$ BHK) and, presumably, in cellular content of G proteins. The EC_{50} values for xanomeline for stimulating PI hydrolysis were 0.004 μM, 0.2 μM and 21 μM in CHO, A9L and BHK cells, respectively. In comparison, the EC_{50} values for the nonselective agonist carbachol for increasing PI hydrolysis were 2.3, 5.8 and 80 μM in CHO, A9L and BHK cells, respectively. The maximal stimulation of PI hydrolysis produced by xanomeline, expressed as percent of the effect produced by the nonselective agonist carbachol, was 100%, 55% and 72% in CHO, A9L and BHK cells, respectively. In contrast, in cells expressing human m3 receptors, the maximal stimulation of PI hydrolysis produced by xanomeline was 40%, 20% and 35% of carbachol in CHO, A9L and BHK cells, respectively. In BHK cells expressing the human m5 receptor, xanomeline stimulated phospholipid hydrolysis to 57% of carbachol with an EC_{50} of 10 μM.

Further, in CHO cells expressing human m2 receptors, xanomeline inhibited forskolin-stimulated cyclic AMP production to 51% of carbachol with an EC_{50} of 2.5 μM. In NG108-15 cells expressing the human m4 receptor, xanomeline inhibited forskolin-stimulated cyclic AMP production to 54% of carbachol with an EC_{50} of 0.015 μM. Thus, these data in cultured cells expressing human muscarinic receptors demonstrate that xanomeline is a potent agonist at human m1 receptors. In addition, while xanomeline also is an agonist at other muscarinic receptors, its rank order of efficacies is m1 > m5 $\geq$ m4 $\geq$ m2 > m3.

NEUROCHEMICAL EFFECTS *IN VIVO*

The effects of xanomeline on neurochemical parameters in rat brain provide *in vivo* evidence for its M1 specificity and oral bioavailability. M1 receptors are located postsynaptically in cortex and hippocampus, as well as presynaptically on dopamine neurons in striatum (the latter termed M1 heteroreceptors). Stimulation of M1 heteroreceptors increases dopamine release and thereby increases brain levels of dopamine metabolites such as DOPAC. Nonselective, centrally acting muscarinic agonists such as oxotremorine increase DOPAC levels *in vivo* to approximately 150% of vehicle control. M2 receptors, on the other hand, are located presynaptically in areas such as striatum, and stimulation of these autoreceptors decreases acetylcholine release, thereby increasing brain tissue levels of acetylcholine. Agonists such as oxotremorine produce large increases (200-300% of control) in acetylcholine levels which are sustained for the duration of action of the drug. Xanomeline, after s.c. administration to rats, increased DOPAC levels in striatum to as much as 165% of control over the dose range of 0.1-10 mg/kg. After oral administration, xanomeline increased DOPAC levels to as much as 155% of control over the dose range of 3-60 mg/kg. Xanomeline significantly increased DOPAC levels in striatum for as long as 3 hrs. Moreover, the *ex vivo* inhibition of [^{3}H]-pirenzepine binding in brain tissue after oral administration of xanomeline closely paralleled the changes in DOPAC levels. In contrast, xanomeline increased acetylcholine levels in striatum to only approximately 170% and 150% of control after s.c. and oral administration, respectively. Moreover, the increases in acetylcholine peaked at 20 min and were of short duration (< 1 hr). Furthermore, xanomeline did not block the increases in tissue levels of acetylcholine produced by oxotremorine. Thus, as measured by neurochemical parameters, xanomeline is a selective, orally available M1 agonist *in vivo*.

OTHER EFFECTS

Nonselective muscarinic agonists produce a number of undesirable parasympathomimetic effects in animals and humans including hypothermia, copious salivation and tremor. In contrast to nonselective muscarinic agonists such as oxotremorine, pilocarpine and RS86, xanomeline did not produce hypothermia, salivation or tremors in rats or mice at doses up to 100 mg/kg. Furthermore, xanomeline was not an antagonist of oxotremorine on these parameters. Thus, *in vivo*, xanomeline is neither an agonist nor an antagonist at receptors which mediate hypothermia, salivation and tremor.

Considerable evidence supports the existence of M1 receptors in rat sympathetic ganglia which enhance sympathetic outflow. Xanomeline produced depolarization of isolated rat superior cervical ganglia, and this effect was blocked by the M1 antagonist pirenzepine. *In vivo*, xanomeline increased heart rate in a dose-dependent manner after s.c. administration to conscious rats. The increases in heart rate produced by xanomeline were blocked by the β-adrenergic blocker propranolol, as well as by the M1 selective antagonists trihexyphenidyl and pirenzepine. These data indicate that xanomeline is an agonist at M1 receptors in sympathetic ganglia of rats.

In mice, xanomeline (0.3-10 mg/kg) reversed deficits in passive avoidance behavior produced by the relatively selective M1 antagonist trihexyphenidyl. Over this same dose-range, xanomeline also decreased locomotor activity in mice and rats.

Since nonselective muscarinic agonists enhance gastric and intestinal secretions and increase GI motility, particularly through actions at M2 and M3 receptors, xanomeline was examined also for its effects on the gastrointestinal system. After s.c. administration, xanomeline (1.0-10 mg/kg) did not induce or inhibit gastric acid secretion in rats. In anesthetized ferrets, xanomeline produced dose-related inhibition of jejunal, ileal and colonic motility at doses of 0.3-1000 mg/kg administered intra-arterially. At these doses, xanomeline increased transmural potential difference across the small intestine which is indicative of a Cl⁻ movement into the lumen and a resulting water secretion. Salivation or significant changes in heart rate or blood pressure were not observed at any of the doses tested by the intra-arterial route of administration in the anesthetized ferret. These data indicate xanomeline does not produce abdominal cramping as can occur with nonselective muscarinic agonists.

CONCLUSION

These data, taken in concert, support the contention that xanomeline is an orally-active, potent and selective M1 receptor agonist with a wide margin of safety. Xanomeline, therefore, may be useful in the treatment of AD.

REFERENCES

Bymaster FP, Wong DT, Mitch CH, Ward JS, Calligaro DO, Schoepp DD, Shannon HE, Sheardown MJ, Olesen PH, Suzdak PD, Swedberg MDB and Sauerberg P (1994): Neurochemical effects of the M1 muscarinic agonist xanomeline (LY246708/NNC11-0232). *J Pharmacol Exp Ther* (In Press).
Coyle JT, Price DL and Delong MR (1983): Alzheimer's disease: a disorder of cortical cholinergic innervation. *Science* 219:1184-1190.

Davies P and Maloney AJF (1976): Selective loss of central cholinergic neurons of the Alzheimer's type. *Lancet* 2:1403.

Katzman R (1986): Alzheimer's disease. *New Engl J Med* 314:964-973.

Mitch CH, Bymaster FP, Calligaro DO, Quimby SJ, Sawyer BD, Shannon HE, Ward JS, Olesen PH, Sauerberg P, Sheardown MJ and Suzdak PD (1993): Xanomeline: a potent and selective M1 agonist *in vitro*. *Life Sci* 52:550.

Palacios JM and Spiegel R (1986): Muscarinic cholinergic agonists: Pharmacological and clinical perspectives. In: *Progress in Brain Research,* Swaab DE, Ehers E, Mirmiran M, van Gool WA and van Haaren E, eds. Amsterdam: Elsevier BV, Vol. 70.

Pomara N, Bagne CS, Stanley M and Yarbrough GC (1986): Prospective strategies for cholinergic interventions in Alzheimer's disease. *Prog Neuropsychopharmacol* 10:553-569.

Potter LT and Ferrendelli CA (1989): Affinities of different cholinergic agonists for the high and low affinity states of hippocampal M1 muscarinic receptors. *J Pharmacol Exp Ther* 248:974-978.

Sauerberg P, Olesen PH, Nielsen S, Treppendahl S, Sheardown M, Honoré T, Mitch CH, Ward JS, Pike AJ, Bymaster FP, Sawyer BD and Shannon HE (1992): Novel functional M1 selective muscarinic agonists. Synthesis and structure-activity relationships of 3-(1,2,5-thiadiazolyl)-1,2,5,6-tetrahydro-1-methylpyridines. *J Med Chem* 35:2274-2283.

Shannon HE, Sawyer BD, Bemis KG, Bymaster FP, Heath I, Mitch CH and Ward JS (1993): Muscarinic M1 receptor agonist actions of muscarinic receptor agonists in rabbit vas deferens. *Eur J Pharmacol* 232:47-57.

Shannon HE, Bymaster FP, Calligaro DO, Greenwood B, Mitch CH, Sawyer BD, Ward JS, Wong DT, Olesen PH, Sheardown MJ, Swedberg MDB, Suzdak PD and Sauerberg P (1994): Xanomeline: A novel muscarinic receptor agonist with functional selectivity for M1 receptors. *J Pharmacol Exp Ther* (In Press).

Soncrant TT, Raffaele KC, Asthana S, Berardi A, Morris PP and Haxby JV (1993): Memory improvement without toxicity during chronic, low dose intravenous arecoline in Alzheimer disease. *Psychopharmacology* 112:421-427.

Whitehouse PJ, Price DL, Struble RG et al. (1982): Alzheimer's disease and senile dementia: loss of neurons in the basal forebrain. *Science* 215:1237-1239.

Whitehouse PJ (1988): Intraventricular bethanechol in Alzheimer's disease: A continuing controversy. *Neurobiology* 38:307-308.

Alzheimer Disease: Therapeutic Strategies
edited by E. Giacobini and R. Becker.
© 1994 Birkhäuser Boston

XANOMELINE, A SPECIFIC M1 AGONIST: EARLY CLINICAL STUDIES

N.C. Bodick, A.F. DeLong, P.L. Bonate, T. Gillespie, D.P. Henry, J.H. Satterwhite, R.A. Lucas, J. Heaton and G.V. Carter
Lilly Research Laboratories, Eli Lilly and Company, Indianapolis, IN 46202; and Lilly Research Centre, Erl Wood Manor Windlesham, Surrey, GU20 6PH

L. Farde
Department of Clinical Neuroscience, Psychiatry Section, Karolinska Hospital, S-10401 Stockholm, Sweden

N.R. Cutler, J.J. Sramek, R.D. Seifert, J.J. Conrad and T.S. Wardle
California Clinical Trials, Beverly Hills, CA 90211

INTRODUCTION

Xanomeline tartrate is a specific M1 Agonist which is currently in Phase 2 clinical development for mild and moderate Alzheimer's disease. Presented below are the early clinical studies which provided rationale to proceed to the study of efficacy in Alzheimer's. Preclinical studies with xanomeline are presented elsewhere in this volume.

SINGLE AND MULTIPLE DOSE SAFETY, PHARMACODYNAMICS AND PHARMACOKINETICS

A single blind (subject) oral dose-escalation study was conducted in 36 healthy male volunteers. Doses ranged from 1 to 150 mg (base). Pharmacodynamic signs of cholinergic activity (pulse rate, blood pressure, pupillometry, salivary flow, respiratory function, ECG, and urinary frequency) were measured. Single dose escalation and one week multiple dose regiments were followed.

In the single dose, dose escalation design, 4 groups of 9 subjects were studied. Each subject received 2 doses of xanomeline tartrate and 1 random placebo. For single doses up to 75 mg, no significant events were recorded. At 100 mg, 2/9 and at 150 mg 4/9 subjects reported several episodes of watery diarrhea lasting a few hours without abdominal pain or nausea. At 100/150 mg, mean supine resting heart rate was increased (14.5 bpm, $p = .001$) between 2-4 hrs post-dose, as was diastolic (10.5 mm, p=.001) and systolic (12.0 mm, p=.02) blood pressure. Some evidence of postural hypotension was also apparent. Mean pharmacokinetic parameters (± SD) were as follows:

Dose (mg)	N	Cmax (ng/mL)	Tmax (hr)	AUC(0-t) (ng/mL * hr)	t 1/2 (hr)
100	5	8.95 (5.8)	2.4 (0.9)	42.8 (27.8)	2.96 (0.8)
150	7	13.81 (11.5)	2.5 (1.0)	65.8 (45.8)	4.56 (2.2)

Blood samples collected on Days 1, 4, and 7 indicated a slight increase in plasma concentrations over the 7-day dosing period with Cmax values of 2.11 (0.3), 3.09 (0.4), and 4.13 (1.8) ng/mL, respectively, following the 75 mg dose.

In the multiple dose regiment, 4 groups of three subjects were studied. Following multiple doses (twice daily x 13 doses) of 40 mg (2 subjects) or 75 mg (6 subjects) with 4 placebo subject controls, xanomeline tartrate was well tolerated. No GI side effects occurred and supine resting heart rate/blood pressure remained normal. Catecholamine and cortisol turnover was not altered at these doses. No significant alterations in clinical biochemistry or hematology were experienced in these studies. No treatment effects on hematology/biochemistry were evident after single doses. Daily enzymes (AST, ALT, g-GT) showed no clinically significant changes after multiple doses, and ECG's showed no change in conduction parameters. Following 75 mg bid multiple doses (n = 6) profiles were taken on day 1, 4 and 7. Plasma concentrations for xanomeline were measured by HPLC/UV (with LOQ 1.5 ng/ml) and showed a slight increase over the course of the week with Cmax values of 2.11 (0.3), 3.09 (0.4), and 4.13 (1.8) ng/ml, respectively.

The general safety profile and tolerability of xanomeline tartrate was thought to warrant further clinical study.

ABSORPTION, DISTRIBUTION, METABOLISM, AND ELIMINATION OF RADIOLABELED XANOMELINE IN HEALTHY MALE SUBJECTS

To study the disposition of xanomeline in humans, four healthy male subjects received an oral 75 mg dose of radioactive (100 mCi) xanomeline tartrate. Using liquid scintillation spectroscopy, isocratic/gradient high performance liquid chromatography (HPLC) with radioactivity, ultraviolet (UV) and mass spectrometric (MS/MS) detection, we monitored radioactivity, parent drug, and metabolites in biological fluids.

Radioactivity in plasma attained a maximal concentration of 860 +/- 90 ng-eq - 14C/mL at 2 hrs after a 75 mg oral dose of radiolabeled xanomeline. Elimination of radioactivity from plasma proceeded in two distinct phases. A rapid initial elimination phase was apparent between 2 to 12 hrs and a slower terminal elimination phase of radioactivity predominated after 12 hrs.

Approximately 75% of the radiolabel was recovered in urine within 24 hrs. Overall, 95% of the radiolabeled dose was recovered in urine and feces. Recovery of radiolabel in excreta was quantitative and within the limits of experimental error associated with metabolic balance studies.

Xanomeline plasma concentrations were a fraction of the total circulating plasma radioactivity. A maximum plasma concentration of approximately 2 +/- 1 ng/mL was attained at about 1.6 hrs after dosing. The area under the plasma concentration curve averaged 12.4 ng hr/mL. Xanomeline was eliminated from plasma with an apparent elimination half life of 3.6 hrs.

Plasma Xanomeline Concentration and Radioactivity

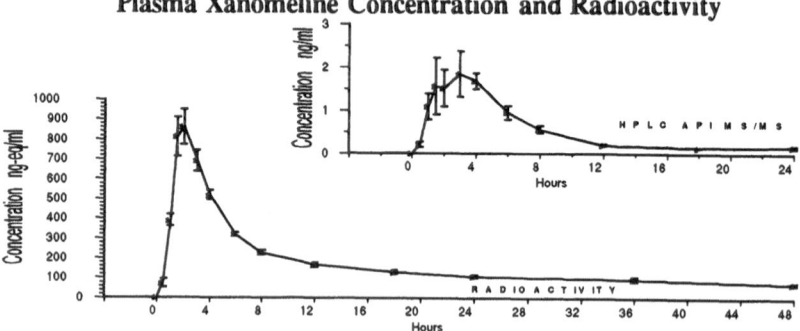

HPLC gradient analysis of plasma and urine indicated that xanomeline is biotransformed into a number of metabolite analogs. Only trace levels of parent drug were present. The majority of the metabolites have been tentatively identified by mass spectrometric techniques and by comparison of chromatographic retention times to authentic reference compounds. Biotransformation occurs on both the side chain and ring structure moieties of the molecule. None of the metabolites tested so far have shown significant pharmacologic activity. However, the existence of a metabolite which contributes to drug pharmacology and or side effects cannot be ruled out.

SAFETY, TOLERANCE, AND PHARMACOKINETICS IN HEALTHY ELDERLY SUBJECTS

Xanomeline tartrate was given to 16 healthy elderly subjects (8 men, 8 women) mean age 70.4 years (range 65-81), for continuous periods of 8 days. Subjects were studied in groups of 4, with one subject allocated placebo in each group. In group 1, the dose was given fasted (bid). A dose escalation in the range of 30-75 mg bid was allowed. Groups 2 and 3 were dosed with food t.i.d. (8 am/1 pm/6 pm) in an escalation algorithm from 15-50 mg t.i.d. Group 4 was dosed without dose escalation at 40 mg t.i.d. for 8 days.

All subjects completed the study except one, allocated to receive placebo in group 1, who had episodic atrial fibrillation. GI symptoms (nausea, vomiting, and watery diarrhea) occurred in the fasting group (2 subjects). Continuation or reduction of dose ameliorated these symptoms. Two subjects on xanomeline had mildly increased AST/ALT at study termination that returned to normal within a week. Both were taking total daily doses of 150 mg. Mild and transitory cardiovascular events were reported (dizziness, hypotension) but did not require termination of treatment. Urinary frequency and sleep quality were not different between treatments. Plasma samples were taken on Days 1, 4, and 8 for pharmacokinetic analysis. Although the variability was too great to characterize the pharmacokinetics within individuals, maximum and pre-dose plasma concentrations exhibited an increasing trend over the 8-day dosing period (group 4), suggesting the drug may accumulate in elderly subjects.

Mean Plasma Concentrations in Elderly Volunteers Following Doses of 40 mg t.i.d.

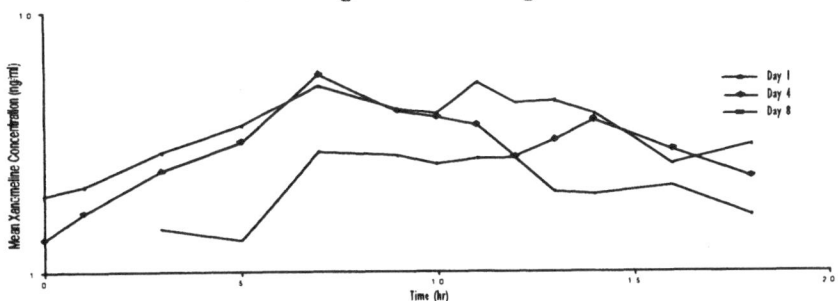

Xanomeline was generally well tolerated in these elderly subjects with a similar profile of events seen in young healthy subjects. Further studies in patients with Alzheimer's disease were warranted.

SAFETY AND TOLERANCE OF XANOMELINE TARTRATE IN PATIENTS WITH ALZHEIMER'S DISEASE

Clinical trials of other cholinergic compounds have shown that the AD patient population frequently tolerates drugs quite differently from healthy volunteers. "Bridging studies" which determine the safety and tolerance of a drug in the target population aid in the selection of appropriate doses for phase II efficacy tests.

Study 1 consisted of 25, 35, 50, 60, and 75 mg t.i.d. with food. Study 2 consisted of 90, 100, and 115 mg t.i.d. with food. Both studies were over a 7-day inpatient treatment administration period. In each study each of 4 treatment panels consisted of 6 patients (4 on xanomeline tartrate and 2 on placebo). In Study 1, of the 20 patients randomized to xanomeline tartrate, 2 discontinued due to severe adverse events. One patient on 60 mg t.i.d. experienced severe diarrhea and discontinued on Day 1, and 1 patient on 75 mg t.i.d. suffered severe nausea and vomiting and discontinued on Day 2.

In Study 2, of the 12 patients randomized to xanomeline tartrate, 4 discontinued due to severe adverse events: 2 from the 100 mg t.i.d. panel (1 due to severe vomiting, and the other patient due to abdominal pain, although the investigators did not feel this patient had reached an intolerable dose), and 2 from the 115 mg t.i.d. panel (1 due to vomiting and 1, although he had numerous gastrointestinal events, discontinued primarily due to hypotension).

Maximally tolerated dose (MTD) was defined as the largest dose tested prior to reaching a minimally intolerable dose at which 50% of the patients on xanomeline tartrate (2 of 4 in a panel) experienced severe adverse events or at which the seriousness of a single event warranted discontinuation of the patients from the study. By this criterion, xanomeline tartrate appears to be safe and well tolerated at higher dosages in patients with probable AD than in healthy elderly volunteers. The 100 mg t.i.d. dose with food, therefore, was defined as the maximally tolerated dose in probable AD patients.

SPECIFIC BINDING TO CENTRAL MUSCARINIC RECEPTORS AS DEMONSTRATED WITH PET

Xanomeline was labeled with ^{11}C and the brain uptake was examined by positron emission tomography (PET) in cynomolgus monkey and man. In the experiments on monkeys, more than 5% of the radioactivity was in brain 15 minutes after intravenous injection of unlabeled xanomeline (6 mg/kg). Pretreatment with scopolamine (0.2 mg/kg) or biperiden (1 mg/kg) markedly reduced the brain uptake of $[^{11}C]$ xanomeline. This reduction indicates specific binding in vivo to muscarinic receptors in the primate brain. In human subjects about 4% of the radioactivity injected was in brain 15 minutes after intravenous injection. Consistent with the monkey studies the highest uptake of radioactivity was in the cortex and the striatum. The PET examinations indicate that xanomeline passes the blood brain barrier and binds to muscarinic receptors in the living brain.

EFFICACY STUDIES

The first efficacy study in mild and moderate Alzheimer's Disease will be complete in the summer of 1994. Approximately 300 patients have been enrolled in a parallel, 4 arm protocol of 6 months duration. Effects on clinical impression, cognition and behavior will be assessed.

Alzheimer Disease: Therapeutic Strategies
edited by E. Giacobini and R. Becker.
© 1994 Birkhäuser Boston

CI-979/RU 35926: A NOVEL MUSCARINIC AGONIST FOR THE TREATMENT OF ALZHEIMER'S DISEASE

Toni M. Hoover
CNS Clinical Research, Parke-Davis Pharmaceutical Research, Division of
Warner-Lambert Company, Ann Arbor, MI

INTRODUCTION

The etiologies of Alzheimer's disease (AD) remain unknown. However, several biochemical deficits have been identified with the most prominent involving the central cholinergic system (Bartus et al., 1982; McGeer et al, 1984). Facilitating the activity of remaining intact neurons to compensate for the losses in the cholinergic system is one strategy for therapeutic interventions. The evaluations of potential cholinomimetic interventions have focused on precursors of acetylcholine (ACh), acetylcholinesterase inhibitors, cholinergic releasing agents, and cholinergic receptor agonists (Becker and Giacobini, 1988; DeFeudis, 1988).

Numerous trials have been conducted using precursor loading with choline or lecithin (phosphatidylcholine) and have generally failed to reveal significant improvements in cognitive performance of patients with AD (Etienne et al., 1981; Thal et al., 1981; Little et al., 1985). Some intriguing but inconclusive results have been seen with the cholinesterase inhibitor physostigmine in that there has been evidence of effects on verbal memory and picture recognition in some patients; however, the effects have not been considered clinically meaningful (Thal et al., 1983; Mohs et al., 1985). These findings encouraged further investigations of other cholinesterase inhibitors. Studies of tacrine (Cognex®, tacrine hydrochloride) have unequivocally demonstrated clinically meaningful effects on measures of cognitive performance and global assessments that are recognizable by clinicians and caregivers (Davis et al., 1992; Farlow et al., 1992; Knapp et al., 1994). The therapeutic effects of tacrine presumably depend upon the availability of functioning presynaptic neurons to produce ACh. Therefore, it is possible that the utility of this therapy and similar interventions will be limited with continued neuronal degeneration.

Postsynaptic muscarinic receptors in the neocortex and hippocampus are largely spared in AD, suggesting that agents active at these sites could enhance cholinergic function (Caulfield et al., 1982; Quirion et al., 1986). This finding has resulted in the investigation of muscarinic receptor agonists, such as arecoline, oxotremorine, RS-86, and intraventricular bethanechol. This therapeutic approach has an advantage relative to the aforementioned approaches in that intact presynaptic neurons are not a prerequisite. It is therefore conceivable that effective muscarinic agonists might be useful therapeutics throughout the course of AD. However, the muscarinic agonists investigated thus far have not demonstrated consistent patterns of improved cognitive performance and have revealed prominent peripheral cholinergic side effects (Wettstein and Spiegel, 1984; Bruno et al., 1986; Davis et al., 1987; Penn et al, 1988; Tariot et al., 1988). The disappointing clinical results from these agents may have been related to an inadequate separation of efficacy and safety; i.e., cognitive effects seen within the same dose range as intolerable cholinomimetic effects.

CI-979/RU 35926 (hereafter referred to as CI-979) is an orally active muscarinic receptor agonist being jointly developed by Parke-Davis and Roussel-Uclaf (Toja et al., 1991). The following is a brief summary of the preclinical and clinical studies conducted to support the development of this agent as an antidementia drug.

PRECLINICAL STUDIES

CI-979 is an orally active muscarinic agonist that is representative of a series of tetrahydropyridine ketoximes related to arecoline. *In vitro* studies have demonstrated that CI-979 binds with agonist-like affinities at sites labeled with cis-methyldioxolane (CMD) and quinuclidinylbenzylate (QNB). The compound exhibits receptor-binding selectivity for the m1 receptor subtype (genetically defined) when compared to its activity at M2 receptor subtype sites (pharmacologically defined). Unlike most known muscarinic agonists, CI-979 binds with equal affinity at m1, m2, m3 and m4 human muscarinic receptor sites (Parke-Davis, unpublished data).

In vivo studies of CI-979 have demonstrated enhanced central cholinergic effects in rodents and monkeys in several animal models of cognitive dysfunction. CI-979 reduced spontaneous swimming activity and reversed scopolamine-induced increases in the swimming activity of rats. It significantly reduces the body temperature in rodents. Quantitative electroencephalographic (QEEG) studies in rats and monkeys have revealed the ability to decrease total power (i.e., increase cortical arousal). CI-979 increased local cerebral blood flow (LCBF) in rats. The effects of CI-979 were evident in studies of nucleus basalis Magnocellularis-lesioned rats. The performance of the lesioned rats treated with CI-979 was consistent with that of control animals (Parke-Davis, unpublished data).

Studies of CI-979 have been conducted to define the potential for side effects that may result from stimulation of the peripheral cholinergic system. Studies of motor activity, cardiovascular, gastrointestinal, and pulmonary effects have demonstrated that central cholinomimetic activity is produced at doses that have minimal or no effects on the peripheral cholinergic system (Parke-Davis, unpublished data). These studies have been useful in establishing an adequate separation between the predicted effective dose in humans and the dose-range producing intolerable peripheral effects, which is necessary in order to proceed to clinical investigations of this agent.

CLINICAL STUDIES

Eight clinical pharmacology studies of CI-979 have been completed using double-blind and open-label study designs. A total of 149 normal volunteers and 10 patients with AD have been exposed in these studies. The range of doses evaluated included 0.002-4 mg in single-dose studies and 0.5-3 mg in multiple-dose studies.

A double-blind, placebo-controlled, rising, single-dose tolerance study of CI-979 in 28 healthy male subjects revealed a linear dose relationship for plasma concentration (Cmax) and area under the curve (AUC) values for single doses ranging from 0.1-4 mg. The mean elimination half-life (t½) ranged between 2 and 5 hours with very little of the dose excreted as unchanged drug in the urine due to extensive metabolism. Single doses less than 2 mg were well tolerated. Higher doses were associated with cholinergic symptoms such as hypersalivation, diaphoresis, and postural hypotension (Parke-Davis, unpublished data).

Multiple doses of 0.5 mg, 1 and 2 mg CI-979 were evaluated in a double-blind, placebo-controlled, parallel-group, single- and multiple-dose tolerance study in 24 normal volunteers. The pharmacokinetic profile for multiple dosing was consistent with the results from the single-dose study. Steady-state concentrations were achieved within 24 hours following the initiation of the multiple-dose administration. The maximum tolerated dose was determined to be 1 mg q6h. Higher doses were associated with gastrointestinal symptoms (e.g., vomiting, diarrhea, and abdominal pain) and diaphoresis (Parke-Davis, unpublished data).

Prior to initiating studies of CI-979 in the targeted patient population, a double-blind, parallel-group, multiple-dose tolerance study was conducted in 10 male patients with probable AD. The dose was titrated over 20 days from 0.5 mg q6h to 3 mg q6h. This study confirmed that doses of 0.5 mg q6h and 1 mg q6h were well-tolerated. Furthermore, there was evidence that 2 mg q6h was better tolerated in this study than in the previous studies. Dose-limiting effects were evident at 2.5 mg q6h and 3 mg q6h (Cutler et al., 1994). This study suggested that either patients with AD handled this compound differently than normal volunteers or the titration regimen appeared to improve tolerance to cholinergic symptoms or both.

To further investigate this issue a double-blind, placebo-controlled, parallel-group study in 33 normal volunteers was conducted to evaluate the utility of the titration schedule to improve the profile of the compound in healthy elderly

242   T. M. Hoover

subjects. Three treatment arms included placebo, a fixed dose of 2 mg q6h, and
titration to 2 mg q6h. The percentage of early withdrawals was greatest in the
fixed dose group, followed by the placebo group. The treatment group
incorporating a gradual dose escalation had the lowest proportion of withdrawals
due to adverse effects. The adverse effects were consistent with findings from
prior studies (Parke-Davis, unpublished data).

The results from the clinical pharmacology studies suggested that the
maximum dose of CI-979 to be evaluated during Phase 2 studies should be 2 mg
q6h using a titration scheme. A 12-week, double-blind, placebo-controlled,
parallel-group, multicenter study in patients with probable AD is underway and
is designed to evaluate the efficacy, safety and dose-response of CI-979. This
study will define the size of the treatment effect on a variety of well-established
efficacy parameters over a range of doses.

ACKNOWLEDGEMENTS

The author wishes to acknowledge the contributions of Robert Davis, Ph.D. and
the numerous colleagues at Parke-Davis Pharmaceutical Research
(Neurodegenerative Disorders Group, Pharmacokinetic and Drug Metabolism
Department, Pathology and Experimental Toxicology Department, Clinical
Pharmacology Department, and CNS Antidementia Group) and Roussel-Uclaf.

REFERENCES

Bartus RT, Dean RL, Beer B and Lippa AS (1982): The cholinergic hypothesis of
geriatric memory dysfunction. *Science* 217:408-417.
Becker RE and Giacobini E (1988): Mechanisms of cholinesterase inhibition in senile
dementia of the Alzheimer type: Clinical, pharmacological, and therapeutic aspects.
Drug Development Research 12:163-195.
Bruno G, Mohr E, Gillespie M et al. (1986): Clinical trials with the cholinergic drug
RS86 in Alzheimer's disease. *Arch Neurol* 43:659-661.
Caulfield MP, Straughan DW, Cross AJ et al. (1982): Cortical muscarinic subtypes and
Alzheimer's disease. *Lancet* 2:1277.
Cutler NR, Sramek JJ, Seifert RD et al. (1994): Safety and tolerance of the muscarinic
agonist CI-979. *Clinical Pharmacology and Therapeutics*: 174:(In Press).
Davis KL, Thal LJ, Gamzu ER et al. (1992): A double-blind, placebo-controlled,
multicenter study of tacrine for Alzheimer's disease. *N Engl J Med* 327:1253-1259.
DeFeudis FV (1988): Central cholinergic systems, cholinergic drugs and Alzheimer's
disease - an overview. *Drugs of Today* 24:473-490.
Etienne P, Dastoor D, Gauthier S et al. (1981): Alzheimer's disease: Lack of effect of
lecithin treatment for 3 months. *Neurology* 31:1552-1554.
Farlow M, Gracon SI, Hershey LA et al. (1992): A controlled trial of tacrine in
Alzheimer's disease. *JAMA* 268:2523-2529.
Knapp MJ, Knopman DX, Solomon PR, et al. (1994): A 30-week randomized controlled
trial of high-dose tacrine in patients with Alzheimer's disease. *JAMA* 271:985-991.

Little A, Levy R, Chuaqui-Kidd P, and Hand D (1985): A double-blind, placebo-controlled trial of high-dose lecithin in Alzheimer's disease. *J Neurology, Neurosurgery, and Psychiatry* 48:736-742.

McGeer PL, McGeer EG, Suzuki J et al. (1984): Aging, Alzheimer's disease, and the cholinergic system of the basal forebrain. *Neurology*:741-745.

Mohs R, Davis K, Johns C et al. (1985): Oral physostigmine treatment of patients with Alzheimer's disease. *Am J Psychiatry* 142:28-33.

Penn RD, Martin EM, Wilson RS et al. (1988): Intraventricular bethanechol infusion for Alzheimer's disease: results of double-blind and escalating-dose trials. *Neurology* 38:219-222.

Quirion R, Martel JC, Robitaille Y et al. (1986): Neurotransmitter and receptor deficits in senile dementia of the Alzheimer's type. *Canadian J Neurological Sci* 13:503-510.

Tariot P, Cohen R, Welkowitz et al. (1988): Arecholine in Alzheimer's disease. *J Am Geriatric Society* 36:582.

Thal LJ, Fuld P et al. (1983): Oral physostigmine and lecithin improve memory in Alzheimer's disease. *Annals Neurology* 13:491-496.

Thal LJ, Rosen W, Sharpless S and Crystal H (1981): Choline chloride fails to improve cognition in Alzheimer's disease. *Neurobiology of Aging* 2:205-208.

Toja E, Bonetti C, Butti A et al. (1991): 1-alkyl-1,2,5,6-tetrahydropyridine-3-carboxaldehyde-O-alkyl-oximes: a new class of potent orally active muscarinic agonists related to arecoline. *Eur J Med Chem* 26:853-868.

Wettstein A and Spiegel R (1984): Clinical trials with the cholinergic drug RS86 in Alzheimer's disease (AD) and senile dementia of the Alzheimer type (SDAT). *Psychopharmacology* 84:572-573.

PART VII

DRUGS TO ENHANCE ACETYLCHOLINE SYNTHESIS AND RELEASE

Alzheimer Disease: Therapeutic Strategies
edited by E. Giacobini and R. Becker.
© 1994 Birkhäuser Boston

CHOLINE METABOLISM, MEMBRANE PHOSPHOLIPIDS, AND ALZHEIMER'S DISEASE

Steven A. Farber, Barbara E. Slack, Enrico DeMicheli and Richard J. Wurtman
Department of Brain and Cognitive Sciences, Massachusetts Institute of Technology, Cambridge, MA

Roger M. Nitsch and John H. Growdon
Department of Neurology, Massachusetts General Hospital, Harvard Medical School, Boston, MA

Bruce M. Cohen, Andrew L. Stoll and Perry F. Renshaw
Brain Imaging Center, McLean Hospital, Harvard Medical School, Belmont, MA

INTRODUCTION

Alzheimer's Disease (AD) and even apparently-normal aging are associated with defects in brain choline metabolism. This chapter describes these abnormalities as well as some of the experimental systems used to study their mechanisms and effects. Cell culture, superfused brain slices, *in vivo* microdialysis, postmortem tissue analysis, and *in vivo* magnetic resonance spectroscopy (MRS) studies have been employed. Available data suggest that these defects provide a biochemical basis for the special vulnerability of cholinergic neurons in AD.

Studies of Postmortem Brain Tissue from Alzheimer's Disease Patients
Levels of phosphatidylcholine (PC) and phosphatidylethanolamine (PE), both major components of cell membranes, are decreased by 12-15 % ($p < 0.05$) in brain cortex obtained from AD patients. The PC breakdown product glycerophosphocholine (GPC) is increased by 68% in all brain regions studied. Glycerophosphocholine levels are not elevated in individuals with Huntington's disease, Parkinson's disease or Down's syndrome. Brain levels of choline (Ch), a precursor of both PC and acetylcholine (ACh), are decreased by 40-50% in frontal and parietal cortex, and the GPC-to-Ch ratio is 3-fold higher in these neurons in AD than in control brains (Nitsch et al., 1992). The abnormality in brain PC metabolism in AD may reflect increased PC turnover, as suggested by the reduction in PC levels and, elevation in the PC metabolite GPC. The

reduction in Ch reflects impaired utilization of Ch from GPC, or a primary defect which leads to the increase in PC turnover (Fig. 1).

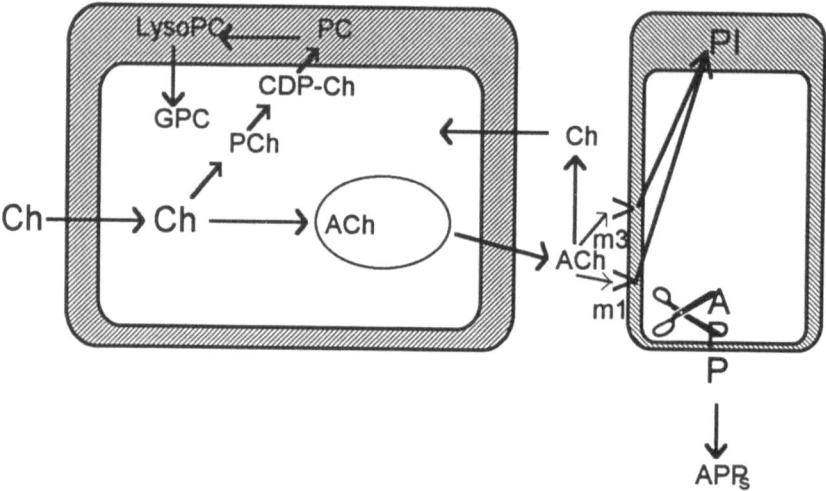

FIGURE 1. Pathways of choline metabolism. Abbreviations: acetylcholine (ACh), amyloid precursor protein (APP), secreted form of the amyloid precursor protein (APPs), choline (Ch), cytidine diphosphate - choline (CDP-Ch), glycerophosphocholine (GPC), lysophosphatidycholine (LysoPC), phosphatidylcholine (PC), phosphatidylinositol (PI) and phosphocholine (PCh).

Despite the degeneration of cholinergic terminals in AD, the activity of the high-affinity choline uptake process - a unique feature of these cholinergic terminals - appears to be increased in postmortem AD brain (Slotkin et al., 1990). This observation is consistent with the possibility that the remaining cholinergic cells increase their firing rates which might accelerate membrane phospholipid turnover and increase the demand for already-scarce Ch even more.

In Vivo Magnetic Resonance Spectroscopy of Ch Uptake in Young and Older Humans

In vivo Ch uptake into human brain was measured by using MRS. A single dose of Ch (50 mg/kg free base, p.o.) was given to young (37 ± 3 years) or older (72 ± 7 years) healthy volunteers. Three hours after Ch administration brain Ch levels were measured by MRS and expressed as ratios normalized to the creatine resonance. Plasma choline levels, determined by HPLC, were compared to baseline levels prior to Ch intake. In both young and older patients Ch ingestion increased plasma Ch levels (young; 211%; older; 170% of baseline). In contrast, brain Ch levels increased in young subjects [(187 ± 34% of baseline (p < 0.001)])] but not in the older subjects (Cohen et al., 1994). These data suggest that the transport of Ch across the blood-brain barrier is impaired in aging and raise the possibility that this impairment might contribute to the low brain Ch levels and, ultimately, special vulnerability of cholinergic cells in AD.

Choline (mg/kg)	Release/10 min Resting (pmols)	(% basal)	Evoked (pmols)	(% basal)
		Choline		
0	10.9± 1.2	75 ± 5	11.4 ± 1.0	76 ± 3
30	15.0 ± 4.2	141 ± 26*	13.9 ± 4.1	139 ± 22*
60	17.0 ± 2.6	135 ± 14*	16.1 ± 2.4	125 ± 13*
120	20.9 ± 4.0	152 ± 16**	17.4 ± 3.2	126 ± 11*
		Acetylcholine		
0	2.76 ± .18	113 ± 7	10.7 ± 1.0	357 ± 30
30	2.92 ± .42	116 ± 5	10.2 ± 0.9	427 ± 30
60	2.20 ± .52	110 ± 5	13.2 ± 1.5	502 ± 49*
120	3.54 ± .26	141 ± 5**	15.2 ± 1.4	600 ± 34**

TABLE I. Baseline levels of ACh and Ch were determined during the initial 30 min of collection (3 hr after probe implantation) after which rats received either isotonic saline (n = 10) or choline chloride-30 mg/kg (n=6), 60 mg/kg (n=10) or 120 mg/kg (n=11) i.p. Three additional 10 min samples were collected and then microdialysis probes were stimulated for 10 min (current 200 μA; pulse duration, 0.6 ms; frequency, 20 Hz). Resting levels represent the release immediately prior to stimulation. Data (means ± S.E.M.) are expressed as both pmol/10 min and percents of basal levels. The normalized data were analyzed using ANOVA with a post-hoc Newman-Keuls test (* $p < 0.05$, ** $p < 0.01$).

Choline Increases Brain Acetylcholine Release

We developed a novel microdialysis probe containing a tungsten electrode which enables the local stimulation of brain tissue *in vivo* (Farber et al., 1993). The probe was placed in the striatum of anesthetized rats. Stimulation induced ACh release was found to be dependent on the current, pulse duration and the frequency of stimulation. To assess the effect of multiple stimulations, ACh release was assayed at 10 min intervals and stimulation applied for 10 min every 30 min. Acetylcholine release was not diminished by repeated stimulation and was blocked by tetrodotoxin. Basal unstimulated ACh release was increased by the highest dose of Ch (120 mg/kg) 30 min after injection (i.p.). In contrast, electrically stimulated ACh release was increased in a dose dependent fashion with much lower doses of Ch (Table I).

Phospholipid Metabolism in Superfused Brain Slices

Ulus et al. (1988) had shown that striatal slices continue to release large amounts of ACh when stimulated electrically for 1 hr; PC levels decrease during the same interval. The reduction in membrane lipid could be blocked by stimulating the slices in the presence of Ch. To determine whether the reduction in PC resulted in part from impaired synthesis of the phospholipid, we exposed superfused slices to [^{14}C]Ch and measured it and its metabolites with and without stimulation. Levels of radioactive Ch and ACh were unchanged by stimulation, however PCh and PC labeling were markedly reduced [from 2315 $\pm$ 236 to 971 $\pm$ 256 dpm/mg (p < 0.001) and from 876 $\pm$ 161 to 416 $\pm$ 85 dpm/mg (p < 0.03])]. Stimulation increased the radioactivity recovered in released ACh by 899% (p < 0.01). These data suggest that PC synthesis is inhibited and ACh synthesis enhanced when slices containing cholinergic neurons are continuously stimulated (Farber et al., 1994). This phenomenon could make cholinergic neurons vulnerable to a prolonged increase in firing rate, in that transmitter synthesis is maintained while membrane integrity is sacrificed.

Partial Uncoupling of ATP Synthesis Increases PC Turnover

Defects in energy metabolism have been reported to be associated with AD. Biopsy samples of neocortex removed from patients with AD show alterations consistent with a partial uncoupling of oxidative phosphorylation (Sims et al., 1983). Differentiated PC12 cells prelabeled with [^{14}C]Ch were treated with a partial mitochondrial uncoupler, carbonyl cyanide m-chlorophenylhydrozone (CCCP). This treatment did not cause any visible changes in the cells and did not increase lactate dehydrogenase activity in the medium. CCCP (30 μM) treatment for 4 hrs increased radioactive GPC levels in the cells to 184 $\pm$ 10% of control (p < 0.01) while ACh and Ch radioactivity were reduced (to 66 $\pm$ 11% of control (p < 0.05) and to 42 $\pm$ 5% of control (p < 0.01). Phosphocholine radioactivity was unchanged. The evidence that PC metabolism in PC12 cells is enhanced in response to CCCP was further supported by a large increase in CDP-Ch radioactivity (546 $\pm$ 98% of control (p < 0.02). The changes in GPC, PCh, Ch and ACh seen in PC12 cells are similar to the profile of changes observed in post-mortem AD brain and are consistent with an increase in PC turnover. Hence, impaired energy metabolism might, by increasing PC turnover, provide another factor that puts cholinergic neurons at risk in AD.

ACKNOWLEDGEMENTS

This research was supported by a National Institutes of Health Grant MH-28783 and the Center for Brain Sciences and Metabolism Charitable Trust.

REFERENCES

Cohen BM, Stoll AI, Renshaw PF, DeMicheli E and Wurtman RJ (1994): Differences in choline uptake in brain measured in vivo by proton MRS in young and elderly adults. *Abstract to the Society of Magnetic Resonance* (In Press).

Farber SA, Kischka U, Marshall DL and Wurtman RJ (1993): Potentiation by choline of basal and electrically evoked acetylcholine release, as studied using a novel device which both stimulates and perfuses rat corpus striatum. *Brain Res* 607:177-184.

Farber SA, Savci V, Wei A, Slack BE and Wurtman RJ (1994): Neuronal activity inhibits choline phosphorylation while enhancing its acetylation in superfused rat brain slices. (Submitted).

Nitsch RM, Blusztajn JK, Pittas AG, Slack BE, Growdon JH and Wurtman RJ (1992): Evidence for a membrane defect in Alzheimer disease brain. *Proc Natl Acad Sci USA* 89:1671-1675.

Sims NR, Bowen DM, Neary D and Davison AN (1983): Metabolic processes in Alzheimer's disease: Adenine nucleotide content and production of $^{14}CO_2$ from [U-^{14}C]glucose *in vitro* in human neocortex. *J Neurochem* 41:1329-1334.

Slotkin TA, Seidler FJ, Crain BJ, Bell JM, Bissette G and Nemeroff CB (1990): Regulatory changes in presynaptic cholinergic function assessed in rapid autopsy material from patients with Alzheimer's disease: Implications for etiology and therapy. *Proc Natl Acad Sci USA* 87:2452-2455.

Ulus IH, Wurtman RJ, Mauron C and Blusztajn JK (1989): Choline increases acetylcholine release and protects against the stimulation-induced decrease in phosphatide levels within membranes of rat corpus striatum. *Brain Res* 484:217-227.

Alzheimer Disease: Therapeutic Strategies
edited by E. Giacobini and R. Becker.
© 1994 Birkhäuser Boston

NEUROTRANSMITTER RELEASE ENHANCEMENT AS A POSSIBLE THERAPY FOR NEURODEGENERATIVE DISEASES: UPDATE ON LINOPIRDINE (DUP996)

Robert Zaczek, Robert J. Chorvat, Richard A. Earl and S. William Tam
Central Nervous System Diseases Research, The DuPont Merck Research
Laboratories, Wilmington, DE

Cholinergic approaches to palliate the symptoms of Alzheimer's disease (AD) have focussed on the discovery and development of direct cholinergic agonists or cholinesterase inhibitors. As an alternative approach to develop drugs that bolster compromised cognitive processes, increasing presynaptic release of acetylcholine (ACh) offers another means of enhancing cholinergic activity. The aminopyridines have long been known to increase neurotransmitter release, but these compounds increase release under basal as well as stimulated conditions. Nickolson et al. (1990) hypothesized, however, that compounds which specifically enhance stimulated ACh release would prove to be superior therapeutic agents. Their efforts to identify compounds which enhance K^+-stimulated and not basal release of ACh led to the discovery of linopirdine (DuP996), an agent which has undergone clinical evaluation for its efficacy in AD patients.

The unique release enhancing properties of linopirdine and related compounds are shown in Fig. 1. Linopirdine has no effect on basal efflux of [^{3}H]ACh. However, upon stimulating the brain slices by increasing the extracellular K^+ concentration to 25 mM, an approximate 3-fold increase in [^{3}H]ACh release occurs in the presence of the drug. This is in contrast to the effects of 3,4-diaminopyridine (3,4-DAP) which does increase basal release (Fig. 1). Similar stimulus-induced release enhancing effects of linopirdine are also observed in a paradigm used to measure the release of endogenous ACh *in vitro* (Saydoff and Zaczek, 1993a).

The release enhancing effects of linopirdine are not limited to ACh. The stimulated-release of dopamine (DA), serotonin and glutamate from rat brain slices are also enhanced in the presence of linopirdine (Nickolson et al., 1990; Zaczek et al., 1993b). However, there appears to be some level of neurotransmitter selectivity for the action of the compound. While the apparent release of ACh and DA are enhanced to levels of 200% or greater over control, the release of [^{3}H]-d-aspartate, a marker of glutamate release, is increased to only 60% over control (Zaczek et al., 1993b) and [^{3}H]norepinephrine release from neocortical or hippocampal slices is not enhanced at all (Nickolson, et al., 1990, Zaczek et al., 1993b,c). The capacity of linopirdine to modulate the release of several neurotransmitters may be beneficial in the treatment of AD since the disease produces deficits in a number of neurotransmitter systems.

In addition to the ability of linopirdine to enhance ACh release stimulated by increased extracellular K^+, it also enhances the release of ACh evoked by the Na^+ channel opener veratridine and the K^+ channel blocker 3,4-DAP (Zaczek et al., 1993a). Moreover this agent also increases the release of ACh in freely moving animals as demonstrated in microdialysis studies (Marynowski et al., 1993; Smith et al., 1993a,b; see Fig. 2). It does not, however, enhance the *in vitro* ACh release stimulated by n-methyl-D-aspartate (NMDA) or direct current application (Smith et al., 1993a,b; Zaczek et al., 1993a).

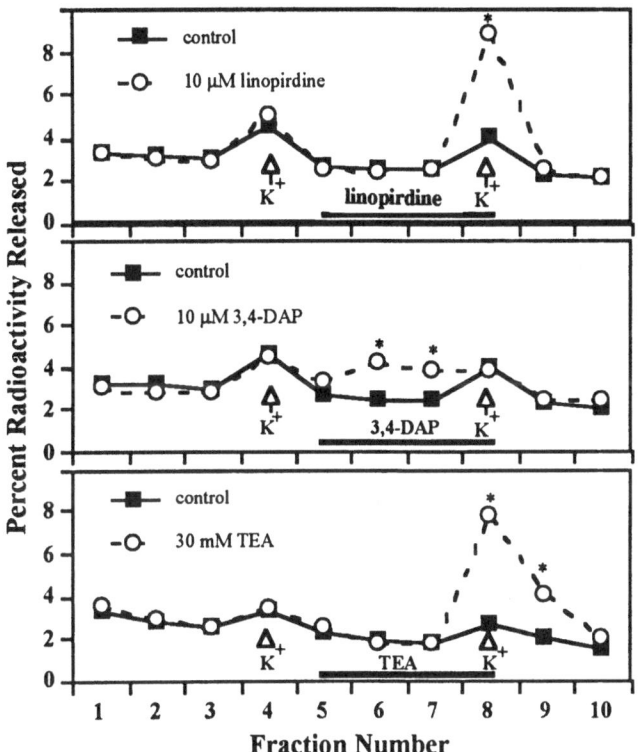

FIGURE 1. Effects of linopirdine, 3,4-DAP and TEA on [³H]ACh release from rat neocortical slices. Linopirdine enhances release only in the presence of the K^+ stimulus. Note that 3,4-DAP increases basal efflux before K^+ stimulation. Like linopirdine, TEA does not increase basal release before the introduction of the K^+ stimulus at fraction 8. TEA does, however, robustly enhance K^+-stimulated release at fraction 8. Statistically significant differences between control and drug treated slices at the level of $p < .05$ are indicated by * .

The mechanism of action of linopirdine is unclear. Recent studies indicate that linopirdine does not interact with numerous sites associated with the control of neurotransmitter release, including N, P or L type Ca^{++} channels, Cl^- channels, tetrodotoxin-sensitive Na^+ channels, aminopyridine-sensitive K^+ channels, intracellular Ca^{++} pools, muscarinic or purinergic receptors (Saydoff and Zaczek, 1993b; Vickroy, 1993; Maciag et al., 1994). However, supporting a role of K^+ channels in linopirdine actions are reports demonstrating the attenuation of K^+ currents in hippocampal slices (Lampe and Brown, 1991; Aiken and Brown, 1993). We have recently found that tetraethylammonium (TEA), an agent which blocks several voltage-activated K^+ channels, has linopirdine-like effects on K^+-stimulated [³H]ACh release (Maciag et al., 1994). As shown in Fig. 1, at physiologically relevant concentrations (30 mM), TEA enhances K^+-stimulated [³H]ACh release without affecting basal efflux . Thus far, data are consistent with linopirdine acting at a subset of TEA-sensitive K^+ channels to enhance release, but further work is required to corroborate these preliminary observations.

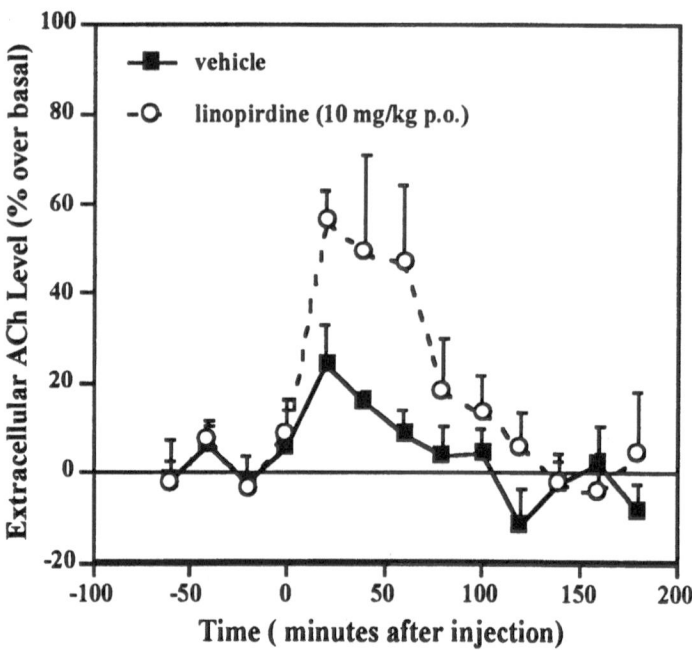

FIGURE 2. Effects of linopirdine on extracellular hippocampal ACh levels in freely moving rats. Dialysis probes were placed into ventral hippocampi and perfused with artificial CSF containing 100 μM physostigmine. After an equilibration period, 20 min fractions were collected and injected on-line onto an HPLC-EC system for ACh measurement.

In summary, linopirdine enhances stimulated, but not basal, release of ACh in rat brain slices. This profile contrasts that of other release enhancers such as the aminopyridines which also increase basal efflux of ACh. In addition to its effects on ACh release, linopirdine enhances the release of other neurotransmitters which are also decreased in AD. *In vivo*, the drug increases the extracellular levels of ACh in the brains of freely moving rats. While the mechanism of linopirdine-induced release enhancement remains uncertain, recent data are consistent with the involvement of the blockade of a subset of TEA-sensitive K^+channels.

REFERENCES

Aiken SP and Brown BS (1993): Linopirdine (DuP996), a neurotransmitter release enhancer, blocks M-current in rat CA1 hippocampal neurons. *Biophys J* 66:A210.

Lampe BW and Brown BS (1991): Electrophysiological effects of DuP996 on hippocampal CA1 neurons. *Soc Neurosci Abstr* 21:632.19.

Maciag CM, Logue AR, Tinker WJ, Saydoff JA, Tam SW and Zaczek R (1994): Studies on the role of K+, Cl- and Na+ ion permeabilities on the acetylcholine release enhancing effects of linopirdine (DuP996) in rat cerebral cortical slices. *J Pharmacol Exp Ther* (In Press).

Marynowski M, Maciag C, Rominger CM, Tam SW and Zaczek R (1993): Effects of linopirdine (DuP996) on hippocampal extracellular levels of acetylcholine in freely moving animals. *Soc Neurosci Abstr* 23:423.8.

Nickolson VJ, Tam SW, Meyers MJ and Cook L (1990): DuP996 (3,3(4-pyrindylmethyl)1-phenylindolin-2-one) enhances the stimulus evoked release of acetylcholine from rat brain *in vitro* and *in vivo*. *Drug Dev Res* 19:285-300.

Saydoff JA and Zaczek R (1993a): Linopirdine enhances KCl evoked release, but not basal release, of endogenous dopamine in superfused rat striatum. *FASEB Abstr:*1521.

Saydoff JA and Zaczek R (1993b): The role of Ca^{2+} channels, adenosine, and Ca^{2+} stores on KCl evoked acetylcholine release and linopirdine (DuP996) release enhancement in rat hippocampal slices. *Soc Neurosci Abstr* 23:423.9.

Smith CP, Broughm, LR and Vargus HM (1993a): Linopirdine (DuP996) selectively enhances acetylcholine release induced by high potassium but not electrical stimulation in rat brain slices and guinea-pig ileum. *Drug Dev Res* 29:262-270.

Smith TM, Ramirez AD, Heck SD, Jasys VJ, Volkmann RA, Forman JT and Liston DR (1993b): *In vivo* microdialysis and pharmacokinetic studies with DuP996. *Soc Neurosci Abstr* 19:423.11.

Vickroy TW (1993): Presynaptic cholinergic actions by the putative cognitive enhancing agent DuP996. *J Pharmacol Exp Ther* 264:910-917.

Zaczek R, Maciag C and Tinker, WJ (1993a): Effects of linopirdine (DuP996) on the KCl, veratridine, NMDA and electrically induced release of [³H] acetylcholine from superfused brain slices. *Soc Neurosci Abstr* 23:423.7.

Zaczek R, Tinker WJ, Logue AR, Cain GA, Teleha CA and Tam SW (1993b): Effects of linopirdine, HP 749, and glycyl-prolyl-glutamate on transmitter release and uptake. *Drug Dev Res* 29:203-208.

Zaczek R, Tinker WJ, and Tam SW (1993c): Unique properties of norepinephrine release from terminals arising from the locus coeruleus: high potassium sensitivity and lack of linopirdine (DuP996) enhancement. *Neurosci Letts* 155:107-111.

PART VIII

NOOTROPIC DRUGS IN AD TREATMENT

Alzheimer Disease: Therapeutic Strategies
edited by E. Giacobini and R. Becker.
© 1994 Birkhäuser Boston

NOOTROPIC DRUGS: THE GAP BETWEEN PRECLINICAL AND CLINICAL RESULTS

Giancarlo Pepeu, Maria Grazia Giovannini, Ileana Marconcini Pepeu and Luciano Bartolini
Department of Preclinical and Clinical Pharmacology, University of Florence, Viale Morgagni 65, 50134 Florence, Italy

INTRODUCTION

In this presentation the term "nootropic drugs" indicates a group of cognition enhancers with different chemical structures, but mostly pyrrolidinone derivatives (Merlini and Pinza, 1989), which enhance information acquisition, protect against learning and memory impairment induced by age, drugs and brain lesions, and have a low toxicity (Schindler et al., 1984). Interest in the potential usefulness of these drugs for treatment of cognitive disorders has resulted in recent years in a better understanding of their pharmacological properties. However, so far the clinical results have not matched the expectations borne out by the pharmacological experiments. This paper is a short overview of the state of the art of the pharmacology and clinical trials on the nootropics.

The first issue in the preclinical studies on cognition enhancers is the adequacy of animal models to mimic the complexity of human cognitive processes and their pathological modifications. This issue has been addressed repeatedly in recent time (Pepeu et al., 1990; Sarter et al., 1992a,b). The discrepancy between the large number of drugs which show cognition enhancing properties in animal tests involving working and spatial memory and the small number of drugs actually tested with some results in man (Sarter, 1991) calls for the use of selective screening aimed at investigating in animals forms of memory as complex as possible in order to limit the number of false positives.

Here we report only some recent observations demonstrating the effectiveness of nootropic drugs in improving learning and memory in normal and impaired animals, and the result of a study on object recognition in the rat.

OBJECT RECOGNITION TEST

The object recognition test assesses a form of episodic memory similar to that measured in subhuman primates by visual recognition and is neuroanatomically different from spatial and working memory (Rothblat and Kromer, 1991). The data presented in Table I were obtained in male Wistar rats according to the procedure of Ennaceur and Delacour (1988) and Scali et al. (1994). The objects to be discriminated were cubes, pyramids and cylinders made of gray plastic. On the day of the test, a session of two trials separated by an intertrial period of 1 or 4 hr was carried out. In the first trial two identical objects were presented in the two opposite corners of a box. During the second trial, one of the objects presented was replaced by a new object and the times spent in exploration of the familiar and new objects were recorded separately.

NORMAL ANIMALS

In normal adult rats, piracetam has been shown to enhance Y-maze learning (Soerensen and Smith, 1993). Both piracetam and pramiracetam produced a significant improvement in retention in an object recognition test when the intertrial interval was 24 hr (Ennaceur et al., 1989). Table I shows that aniracetam also prolongs the duration of object recognition in normal rats as demonstrated by a discrimination index larger than that of saline treated controls. The demonstrations that cognitive processes in normal animals can be improved by nootropics are not matched by comparable findings in normal men since only one report seems to exist demonstrating improved verbal learning after piracetam in students (see ref. in Vernon and Sorkin, 1991). The lack of studies on normal subjects is not surprising, since drugs are usually meant for treating pathological conditions and are tested on patients. Nevertheless controlled studies on normal subjects could have heuristic value and either support or definitively disprove the claims that nootropics "may increase your intelligence" (Dean et al., 1993).

AGING ANIMALS

Age-associated impairment in learning and memory has been demonstrated in non-human primates and rodents (see ref. in Pepeu et al., 1990). The impairment can be restored by nerve growth factor (NGF) (Fischer et al., 1991; Scali et al., 1994) and several cognition enhancers. Table I shows that aniracetam restores object recognition in aging rats. Oxiracetam has a similar effect (data not shown). Other nootropics, such as piracetam (Yamada et al., 1985), phosphatidylserine and acetylcarnitine, have been shown to improve learning and memory in aging rats (Pepeu et al., 1990). On the other hand, it has long been known that physostigmine and tacrine improve memory deficits in old animals (Bartus et al., 1980).

A few controlled studies demonstrate that nootropic drugs improve some cognitive processes in normal aging men. Piracetam has been shown to improve the responses to learning and memory tests in normally aging individuals (Mindus et al., 1976) and performance in elderly motorists (Schmidt et al.,

1991). However, a definite answer to the question whether these treatments improve the daily life of the elderly to such an extent as to justify long-term medication and its cost, needs more extensive, controlled studies.

Conditions	Intertrial Time (hr)	N° rats	Exploration Time in sec Mean ± SEM		Discrimination Index
			Familiar Object	Novel Object	
4-mo-old rats					
Saline	1	18	5.0 ± 1.4	12.2 ± 1.3 ◆	0.40
Saline	4	6	6.2 ± 1.2	6.5 ± 1.1	0.02*
Aniracetam 50 mg/kg os	4	7	4.2 ± 0.9	7.0 ± 1.3 ◆	0.25#
NBM lesion + saline	1	10	5.1 ± 0.6	7.2 ± 1.0	0.16◇
NBM lesion + Aniracetam 50 mg/kg os	1	12	5.7 ± 0.9	11.7 ± 1.2 ◆	0.33
22-24-mo-old-rats					
Saline	1	7	7.6 ± 1.4	8.3 ± 1.5	0.04*
Aniracetam 50 mg/kg os	1	8	7.0 ± 1.3	13.8 ± 1.4 ◆	0.38

TABLE I. Effect of Aniracetam on Object Recognition. The discrimination index is calculated as N-F/N+F (F = time spent exploring the familiar object; N = time spent exploring the novel object); aniracetam was administered 90 min before the training trial. NBM = nucleus basalis magnocellularis. Bilateral lesions were placed 21 days before testing. ◆ p < 0.01 vs familiar (two-tailed t-test); * p < 0.01 vs 4-mo-old saline-treated rats, 1 hr intertrial time; ◇ p < 0.05 vs NBM + aniracetam; # p < 0.05 vs saline 4 hr intertrial time.

ANIMALS WITH IMPAIRED COGNITIVE PROCESSES

Nootropic activity has been demonstrated mostly in animals with an impairment of the cognitive processes induced by brain lesions, hypoxia, inhibition of protein synthesis, amnesic treatments such as anticholinergics, benzodiazepines, ethanol, or electroshock. Most of the data available have been reviewed by Sarter et al. (1992a,b). In rats with bilateral lesions of the nucleus basalis magnocellularis (NBM) aniracetam is able to restore object recognition, as shown in Table I, and oxiracetam has been shown to increase the retest latencies in a one-trial passive avoidance experience (Pepeu et al., 1990). It has been demonstrated that both piracetam and aniracetam improve the performance of several behavioral tests in rats subjected to ischemic and hypoxic insult (Chleide et al., 1991; Himori and Mishima, 1994). Nucleus basalis magnocellularis lesions and ischemic-hypoxic insults are meant to mimic the cholinergic hypofunction occurring in Alzheimer's disease (AD), and the pathogenetic events leading to multi-infarct dementia, respectively. Tacrine has been shown to improve spatial and working memory in rats with NBM lesions, to attenuate scopolamine amnesia and even to improve cognition in normal animals, under some experimental conditions (see ref. in Sarter et al., 1992a). These preclinical effects are matched by a therapeutic efficacy, demonstrated by controlled clinical trials in a small part of the AD patients treated (Farlow et al., 1992; Davis et al., 1992).

On the basis of the findings which demonstrate that the effectiveness of nootropic drugs on animal models is comparable to that of tacrine and physostigmine, piracetam, aniracetam and other nootropics should also be clinically effective. However, this assumption has not yet been supported by clinical trials as large as those which gave statistical strength to the results obtained with tacrine (Wilcock et al., 1994). Nevertheless, therapeutic activity in AD patients has been repeatedly demonstrated with aniracetam, piracetam, oxiracetam, nebracetam (Vernon and Sorkin, 1991; Lee and Benfield, 1994; Bottini et al., 1992; Urakami et al., 1993).

MECHANISMS OF ACTION

While the therapeutic activity of tacrine is attributed mainly to its anticholinesterase activity, no definite mechanism has been yet established for the nootropic drugs of the pyrrolidinone series. It has been demonstrated that they enhance the activity of the forebrain cholinergic system (Pepeu and Spignoli, 1990). Recently, we reported (Giovannini et al., 1993) that aniracetam and oxiracetam increase extracellular ACh levels in the hippocampus. On the other hand, it has been shown that aniracetam is a positive modulator of AMPA-sensitive inotropic glutamate receptors (Ito et al., 1990; Copani et al., 1992), and it is believed that facilitation of glutamate receptors enhances memory (Staubly et al., 1994). Whether the activation of the cholinergic system may be a consequence of the effect on glutamate receptors is a matter for future investigation.

ACKNOWLEDGEMENTS

The research from our laboratory was supported by grants from CNR, Target Project on Aging.

REFERENCES

Bartus RT, Dean RL and Beer B (1980): Memory deficits in aged Cebus monkeys and facilitation with central cholinomimetics. *Neurobiol Aging* 1:145-152.

Bottini G, Vallar G, Cappa S, Monza GC, Scarpini E, Baron P, Cheldi A and Scarlato G (1992): Oxiracetam in dementia: a double-blind, placebo-controlled study. *Acta Neurol Scand* 86:237-241.

Chleide E, Bruhwyler J and Mercier M (1991): Enhanced resistance effect of piracetam upon hypoxia-induced impaired retention of fixed-interval responding in rats. *Pharmacol Biochem Behav* 40:1-6.

Copani A, Genazzani A, Aleppo G, Casabona G, Canonico PL, Scapagnini and Nicoletti F (1992): Nootropic drugs positively modulate α-amino-3-hydroxy-5-methyl-4-isoxazolepropionic acid-sensitive glutamate receptors in neuronal cultures. *J Neurochem* 58:1199-1204.

Davis KL, Thal LJ, Gamze ER, Davis CS, Woolson RF, Gracon SI, Drachman DA, Schneider LS, Whitehouse PJ, Hoover TM, Morris JC, Kawas CH, Knopman DS, Earl NL, Kumar and Doody RS (1992): A double-blind, placebo-controlled multicenter study of tacrine for Alzheimer's disease. *New Engl J Med* 327:1253-1259.

Dean W, Morgenthaler J and Fowkes SW (1993): *Smart Drugs II, The Next Generation.* Menlo Park, CA., Health Freedom Publications, pp. 1-287.

Ennaceur A, Cavoy A, Costa J and Delacour J (1989): A new one-trial test for neurobiological studies of memory in rats. II: effects of piracetam and pramiracetam. *Behav Brain Res* 33:197-207.

Ennaceur A and Delacour J (1988): A new one trial test for neurobiological studies of memory in rats. 1: Behavioral data. *Behav Brain Res* 31:47-59.

Farlow M, Gracon SI, Hershey LA, Lewis KW, Sadowsky CH and Dolan-Ureno J (1992): A controlled trial of tacrine in Alzheimer's disease. *J Amer Med Assoc* 268:2523-2529.

Fischer W, Björklund A, Chen K and Gage FH (1991): NGF improves spatial memory in aged rodents as a function of age. *J Neurosci* 11:1889-1906.

Giovannini MG, Rodinò P, Mutolo D and Pepeu G (1993): Oxiracetam and aniracetam increase acetylcholine release from the rat hippocampus *in vivo*. *Drug Dev Res* 28:503-509.

Himori N and Mishima K (1994): Amelioration by aniracetam of abnormalities as revealed in choice reaction performance and shuttle behavior. *Pharmacol Biochem Behav* 47:219-225.

Ito I, Tanabe S, Kohda A and Sugiyama H (1990): Allosteric potentiation of quisqualate receptors by a nootropic drug aniracetam. *J Physiol* 424:533-543.

Lee CR and Benfield P (1994): Aniracetam: an overview of its pharmacodynamic and pharmakinetic properties and a review of its therapeutic potential in senile cognitive disorders. *Drugs and Aging* 3:257-273.

Merlini L and Pinza M (1989): Trends in searching for new cognition enhancing drugs. *Progr Neuropsychopharmacol Biol Psychiat* 13:S61-S75.

Mindus P, Cronholm B, Levander SE and Schalling D (1976): Piracetam-induced improvement of mental performance: a controlled study in normally aging individuals. *Acta Psych Scand* 54:150-160.

Pepeu G, Marconcini Pepeu I and Casamenti F (1990): The validity of animal models in the search for drugs for the aging brain. *Drug Des Deliv* 7:1-10.

Pepeu G and Spignoli G (1990): Neurochemical actions of "nootropic drugs". In: *Alzheimer's Disease - Advances in Neurology*, Wurtman RJ, Corkin S, Growdon JH, Ritter-Walker E, eds. New York: Raven Press, Vol 51:247-252.

Rothblat LA and Kromer LF (1991): Object recognition memory in the rat: the role of hippocampus. *Behav Brain Res* 42:25-32.

Sarter M (1991): Taking stock of cognition enhancers. *TIPS* 12:456-461.

Sarter M, Hagan J and Dudchenko P (1992a): Behavioral screening for cognition enhancers: from indiscriminate to valid testing: Part I. *Psychopharmacol* 107:144-159.

Sarter M, Hagan J and Dudchenko P (1992b): Behavioral screening for cognition enhancers: from indiscriminate to valid testing: Part II. *Psychopharmacol* 107:461-473.

Scali C, Casamenti F, Pazzagli M, Bartolini L and Pepeu G (1994): Nerve growth factor increases extracellular acetylcholine levels in the parietal cortex and hippocampus of aged rats and restores object recognition. *Neurosci Lett* 170:117-120.

Schindler U, Rush DK and Fielding S (1984): Animal models for studying effects on cognition. *Drug Dev Res* 4:567-576.

Schmidt U, Brendemuehl D, Engels K, Schenk N and Ludemann E (1991): Piracetam in elderly motorists. *Pharmacopsychiat* 24:121-126.

Soerensen JB and Smith DF (1993): Enhancement of Y-maze learning by piracetam, 2-thio-1-pyrrolidine-acetamide and 2-thio-1-pyrrolidine-thioacetamide in rats. *J Neural Transm [P-D Sect]* 6:139-144.

Staubly U, Rogers G and Lynch G (1994): Facilitation of glutamate receptors enhances memory. *Proc Natl Acad Sci USA* 91:777-781.

Urakami K, Shimomura T, Ohshima T, Okada A, Adachi Y, Takahashi K, Asakura M and Matsumura R (1993): Clinical effect of WEB 1881 (Nebracetam fumarate) on patients with dementia of the Alzheimer type and study of its clinical pharmacology. *Clin Neuropharmacol* 16:347-358.

Vernon MW and Sorkin EM (1991): Piracetam: an overview of its pharmacological properties and a review of its therapeutic use in senile cognitive disorders. *Drugs and Aging* 1:17-35.

Wilcock GK, Scott M and Pearsall T (1994): Long-term use of tacrine. *Lancet* 343:294.

Yamada K, Inoue T, Tanaka M and Furukava T (1985): Prolongation of latencies for passive avoidance responses in rats treated with aniracetam and piracetam. *Pharmacol Biochem Behav* 22:645-648.

Alzheimer Disease: Therapeutic Strategies
edited by E. Giacobini and R. Becker.
© 1994 Birkhäuser Boston

NOOTROPIC DRUGS IN ALZHEIMER DISEASE TREATMENT. NEW PHARMACOLOGICAL STRATEGIES

Tatiana A. Voronina
Institute of Pharmacology Russian Academy of Medical Sciences, Moscow, Russia

INTRODUCTION

Various pharmacological strategies have been employed in the treatment of Alzheimer's disease (AD): cholinergic enhancers, psychostimulants, vasodilators, neuropeptides, opiate antagonists, nootropics and others (Court and Perry, 1992; Miller et al., 1992). Nootropics (NT) constitute a relatively new group of drugs, which are able to facilitate cognitive functions and prevent impairment of memory, induced by natural and pathological aging, brain insult, trauma, disease and intoxication. These actions are demonstrated in experimental animal models and in human (Vernon and Sorkin, 1991; Voronina, 1992). Piracetam was the first drug presented of this group. At present there has appeared a whole range of new NT in the series of pyrrolidone derivatives (oxiracetam, aniracetam, etiracetam, pramiracetam, nebracetam and etc.) and new substances of nonpyrrolidone structure. The pyrrolidone NT are often recognized as cognitive enhancing agents or "true" NT, because they proved to have none of sedative, stimulant, analeptic, anticonvulsive, myorelaxant properties. Nootropics are used for the treatment of age-related mental decline [normal aging, senile dementia, AD, mental retardation in children, psychoorganic syndromes, cerebrovascular disorders, brain trauma, post stroke, multiple sclerosis, drug abuse (alcohol, cocaine etc.), cerebral ischemia, hypoxic coma, Parkinson's disease and etc.].

To date, the multifaceted study of the new NT among the novel class of heteroaromatic antioxidants - derivatives of 3-hydroxypyridine, structurally close to the group of vitamin B6 is under progress. Mexidol (MXD), the 2-ethyl-6-methyl-3-hydroxypyridine succinate, due to scavenger effect and activation of superoxide dismutase is able to inhibit lipid peroxidation, stabilize membrane structures of brain and vascular wall, improve energetic cell exchange and to change membrane phospholipid composition (Smirnov and Dyumayev, 1982; Voronina, 1992).

The next step in the development of new NT was the introduction of amino acid residues into position 5 of the 3-hydroxypyridine molecule. Nooglutil (NGT) is N-(5-hydroxynicotinoyl)-L-glutamic acid. Some studies suggest that NGT might improve cognitive function via regulative effect on subtypes of N-methyl-D-aspartate (NMDA) receptors (Voronina et al., 1988b). This review focus on our studies of MXD, NGT and NT known as promising drugs to treat age and AD related memory impairments.

RESULTS

It has been established that NT of the pyrrolidone series: piracetam (PRT), aniracetam (ART), and NT of the nonpyrrolidone group : demanol aceglumate (DA), meclofenoxate (MF), pyrithinol (PT), nicergoline (NG), physostigmine, acetyl-L-carnitine, MXD and NGT possess a pronounced antiamnestic effect, preventing and removing amnesia caused in rats or mice by scopolamine (Table I), maximal electroshock, proline, hypoxia, or deprivation of paradoxical sleep phase when testing passive-avoidance reflex in double compartment box (equipment Lafayette and Co, USA) and active-avoidance reflex in shuttle-box (Voronina et al., 1988a,b; Voronina, 1992). At the same time, substances belonging to other classes of psychotropic drugs (imipramine, amitriptyline, chlorpromazine, haloperidol, diazepam) do not possess any antiamnestic effect. It was demonstrated on rats in free behavior test that PRT, PT, DA, MXD, NGT increase the amplitude of the positive and negative evoked transcallosal potential in brain (Voronina, 1992). An important component in the spectrum of NT activity is their antihypoxic effect. It has been demonstrated that PRT, ART, DA, PT, NG, MXD and NGT increase mice survival rate as compared to the controls under conditions of hypobaric hypoxia, acute hypoxia with hypercapnia and acute hemic hypoxia (Voronina et al., 1988b). It was shown that mechanism of antihypoxic effect of MXD is accounted for succinate oxidation in mitochondrial respiratory chain. Activation of succinate oxidase pathway in that situation may be regarded as compensatory trigger mechanism starting since NADH-oxidase pathway is limited and promoting the increase of tissue resistance to oxygen deficiency (Lukianova et al., 1993).

Thus NT possess a clear-cut antiamnestic and antihypoxic effects and when evaluating their potentials for in AD management the improvement of mental performance after scopolamine treatment, the antihypoxic effects and the increase of the resistance to various extreme factors are the major actions to be considered. The mechanism of pyrrolidone NT action is poorly understood yet, but there is an impression that NT effects in AD can be attributed to the action of its cholinergic mechanisms (Vernon and Sorkin, 1991)

Mexidol has substantial distinctions from the typical NT. In contrast to NT MXD possesses some additional anxiolytic, anticonvulsive and antistress properties. As in case of diazepam the treatment with MXD resulted in increased number of punished responses in Vogel's conflict situation test.

Bicuculline, picrotoxin but not Ro 15-1788 were able to decrease MXD anxiolytic effect. The study of MXD action on benzodiazepine receptors in mice brain revealed a significant increase in ^{3}H-diazepam specific binding. Additionally MXD was shown to prevent convulsions caused by bicuculline, thiosemicarbazide, pentylenetetrazol. All these results suggest that MXD anxiolytic and anticonvulsive effects may be mediated through the modulation of GABA-benzodiazepine receptor complex (Voronina and Seredenin, 1988).

Compound	Dose in mg/kg	I. Retention in sec	Dose in mg/kg/day	II. Retention in sec
Control I	saline	87.1 ± 10.3	-	-
Control II	saline	33.7 ± 5.8	saline	233.7 ± 8.1
Mexidol	50	62.3 ± 8.8*	50	295.3 ± 7.3*
Nooglutil	50	67.1 ± 7.3*	50	319.3 ± 9.3*
Piracetam	400	47.3 ± 6.2*	300	307.2 ± 5.6*
Meclofenoxate	50	65.2 ± 9.3*	50	291.7 ± 6.3*

TABLE I. Effect of nootropic on two kinds of amnesia in passive avoidance test with one-trial learning procedure. Control I - without amnesia; Control II -with amnesia. I - scopolamine (2.5 mg/kg subcutaneously, 30 min before learning) - induced amnesia on outbred 3 month old mice with registration of retention 24 hours after learning. II - amnesia of (CBA x $C_{57}Bl_6$)F_1, 27 month old mice with registration of amnesia 14 days after learning. The time spending in light compartment of the camera was taken as the index of retention. * p < 0.05 in comparison with control II.

The free radical hypothesis, one of most widely accepted theories of aging, proposes that free radicals and/or peroxides are involved in subcellular enzymes, membranes and nucleic acids damaging and phospholipid levels and turnover changing (Harman et al., 1976). It was shown, that membrane phospholipid metabolism of the brain is altered in AD (Nitsch et al., 1991).

Effects of the antioxidants MXD and NGT on behaviorally-impaired aged rats were studied in more detail. Experiments were performed on CBA male mice and outbred male rats (3, 5, 16, 24, 29 and 31 months old). Two critical ages were established based on the following indices: appearing of age-related impairments memory, learning and neurological insufficiency and maximum display of disturbances. Age related differences in cholesterol and triglycerides levels, in peptidase activity and in the lipid peroxidation processes were shown (Zolotov et al., 1989; Voronina et al., 1990a). Although, aged rats do not mimic all of neurochemical and pathological processes associated with AD, they demonstrate progressive loss of mental functions and may be used when studying the new substances. Rats 3, 18 and 24 months old and mice 27 months old were treated with MXD (50 mg/kg), NGT (50 mg/kg), PRT (300 mg/kg), meclofenoxate (50 mg/kg) for 1 month in drinking water (Table I). It was found that MXD and NGT improved behavioral disorders caused by aging including learning, memory (passive and active avoidance tests) and motor functions (Voronina and Kutepova, 1988; Voronina et al., 1990b). It was also revealed that 3-hydroxypyridine derivative intake with food prolonged the mean and maximum life expectancy in mice of different strains (Obukhova, 1985).

Thus MXD and NGT are able to produce an excellent antihypoxic and antiamnestic action on different kinds of amnesia, including scopolamine amnesia, to improve the general health status, learning and memory performance in both young and aging animals, they exert positive effects on cerebral circulation, increase transcallosal evoked potentials, MXD show antistress and anxiolytic properties.

Mexidol (ampules 5%) undergoes phase I of the clinical trials. Mexidol appears capable of improving memory function, general mental state in aged patients, as well as in patients with atherosclerotic dementia. Mexidol is also effective in ischemic cerebral hemisphere insult, discirculative encephalopathy and vegetovascular dystonia and alcohol abstinent syndrome.

Molecular mechanisms of action of MXD are determined by its antioxidant, membrane-protective properties and by bioenergetic metabolic facilitation.

Mexidol increases concentration of polar fraction of phospholipids - phophatidylserine and phosphatidylinositide, decreases cholesterol/phospholipid ratio, demonstrates a potent hypocholesterinemic action, decreases concentration of low-density lipoproteins and increases high-density lipoproteins (Smirnov and Dyumayev, 1982). It was shown that the main metabolite of MXD (phosphorylated on hydroxyl group) inhibits prolyl endopeptidase, dipeptidyl aminopeptidase IV, kininase II and enkephalinase which are responsible to control regulatory neuropeptides (substance P, thyroliberin, vasopressin, angiotensins), influencing behavioral reactions (Zolotov et al., 1989).

Mexidol and NGT may be regarded as the drugs showing promises to be applied in medical practice in the field dealing with management of age-related disorders and AD.

REFERENCES

Court JA and Perry EK (1991): Dementia - The neurochemical basis of putative transmitter orientated therapy. *Pharmac Ther* 52:423-443.

Harman D, Eddy DE and Noffsinger J (1976): Free radical theory of aging: inhibition of amyloidosis in mice by antioxidants; possible mechanisms. *J Am Geriatr Soc* 24(5):203-210.

Lukianova LD, Atabaeva RE and Shepeleva SG (1993): Study of bioenergetic mechanisms of antihypoxic effect of succinate containing derivative of 3-hydroxypyridine (Mexidol). *Bull Exper Biol Med* (Moscow) 3:259-260.

Miller SW, Mahoney JM and Jann MW (1992): Therapeutic frontiers in Alzheimer's disease. *Pharmacotherapy* 12(3):217-231.

Nitsch R, Puttas A, Bluszain JK, Slak BE, Growdon JH, and Wurtman RJ (1991): Alterations of phospholipid metabolites in postmortem brain from patients with Alzheimer's disease. In: *Aging and Alzheimer's Disease - Annals of New York Academy of Sciences.* Growdon JH, Corkin S, Ritter-Walker J and Wurtman RJ, eds. New York: Elsevier 640:110-113.

Obukhova LK (1985): Molecular mechanisms inhibition of the aging by synthetical antioxidants. In: *Physical chemistry and biology base of function living system. Nauka Gen Biol* (Moscow) 2:150-154.

Smirnov LD and Dyumayev KM (1982): β-hydroxy derivatives of six-ring nitrogen heterocycles. Synthesis, inhibitory activity and biological properties. *Chem Farm J* (Moscow) 4:28-44.

Vernon MW and Sorkin EM (1991): Piracetam overview of its pharmacological properties and review of its therapeutic use in senile cognitive disorders. *Drug and Aging* 1(1):17-35.

Voronina TA and Kutepova OA (1988): Experimentally established gerontopsychotropic properties of 3-hydroxypyridine antioxidant. *Drug Dev Res* 14:353-358.

Voronina TA and Seredenin SB (1988): Analysis of the mechanism of psychotropic action of 3-hydroxypyridine derivative. *Ann Ist Super Sanita* 24(3):461-466.

Voronina TA, Nerobkova LN, Garibova TL, Dikova M and Nikolov R (1988a): Effect of Nicergoline on learning and memory. *Meth and Find Exptl Clin Pharmacol* 10(7):431-435.

Voronina TA, Smirnov LD, Stolijrova LG and Garibova TL (1988b): N-nicotinoyl amino acids with antihypoxic and antiamnestic activity. *Patent of USSR* Nr. 1368314.

Voronina TA, Kutepova OA and Zolotov NN (1990a): Age-dependent impairments of learning and memory and their pharmacological correction. *Europ J Pharmacol* 183(6):2369.

Voronina TA, Nerobkova LN, Kutepova OA and Gugutcidse DA (1990b): Pharmacological correction of CNS functional disorders and parkinsonian syndrome in old animals. *Ann Inst Super Sanita* 26(1):55-60.

Voronina TA (1992): Present-day problems in experimental psychopharmacology of nootropic drugs. In: *Sov Med Rev J Neuropharmacology,* Valdman AB, ed. Harwood Academic Publisher GmbH. 2:51-106.

Zolotov NN, Voronina TA and Smirnov LD (1989): Psychotropic activity of synthetic antioxidants on the basis of 3-hydroxypyridine. A possible relationship with regulatory protease system. *Regulation of the free radical reactions.* Varna, Abstr. 193.

Alzheimer Disease: Therapeutic Strategies
edited by E. Giacobini and R. Becker.
© 1994 Birkhäuser Boston

THERAPEUTIC EFFICACY OF NOOTROPIC DRUGS IN ALZHEIMER'S DISEASE AND AGE RELATED COGNITIVE DYSFUNCTION

Julian A. Gray, Jennifer A. Nagel and Roman Amrein
CNS Clinical Research, F. Hoffmann-La Roche Ltd., 4002 Basel, Switzerland

Giorgio Marini
International Clinical Research, Roche SpA, 20131 Milan, Italy

Umberto Senin
Istituto di Gerontologia e Geriatric,
Università degli Studi di Perugia, 06122 Perugia, Italy

The therapeutic efficacy of nootropic drugs in dementia and age-related cognitive decline has been the object of numerous studies. Most trials have been of short duration, i.e. up to three months. Within this time period cognitive improvement has been reported in some but not all studies of nootropic drugs, including among others piracetam (Vernon and Sorkin, 1991), aniracetam (Marini and Bonavita et al., 1992), oxiracetam (Villardita et al., 1992) and pramiracetam (Marini and Caratti et al., 1992). The clinical significance of the short term effects reported is not clear. Furthermore, in many cases the inclusion criteria differ significantly from those currently accepted for dementia studies. In particular, many studies were performed in mixed population of patients with mental decline of varying etiology, rather than with clearly defined dementia of the Alzheimer type or other specific disorders. Similarly, the sample sizes involved were often low compared to current standards, and in some instances may have been determined based more on practical than on statistical considerations.

In summary, although there is evidence for some acute efficacy of the nootropic drugs in dementia it is difficult to draw firm conclusions concerning the clinical size and significance of these effects based on the current evidence.

More intriguing than the acute effects described above are the recent preliminary data suggesting that long term administration of the nootropic drugs aniracetam and piracetam may lead to a sustained and increased improvement compared to placebo.

The data on piracetam stem from a recent publication (Croisile et al., 1993) concerning the effects of "long term and high dose piracetam treatment of Alzheimer's disease". Results were reported of a one-year, double-blind, parallel group study employing a high dose of piracetam (8 g/day orally) versus placebo in thirty-three ambulant patients with early probable Alzheimer's disease. A wide battery of tests were used to assess cognition and behavior. Repeated measures, single-factor ANOVA at the 12 month time point, revealed a significant difference between piracetam and placebo groups only for one test, Rey 3 (recall of the names of figures). However, analysis of the regression slopes for the two groups indicated a slowing of decline in performance under piracetam treatment in four subtests: Aphasia battery, Logical Story, Rey 2, and Recent Memory. Fisher's discriminant analysis supported this conclusion, and indicated that the main effect of piracetam was on memory performance.

Although the number of patients involved in this study was small, the results point towards the possibility that nootropic drugs could have a long-term effect on decline of symptoms in Alzheimer patients. This hypothesis is further supported by recent published and unpublished data concerning aniracetam, as described below.

In an already published double-blind study of longer-term administration of aniracetam versus placebo (Senin et al., 1991), one hundred nine patients were randomized to receive 750 mg aniracetam twice daily or placebo for six months, after a two-week placebo run-in phase. Tolerability was generally very good, consistent with the known pharmacological profile of the pyrrolidinone drugs.

A significant time-related deterioration in psychometric performance and behavior was observed in the patients receiving placebo over the six months of the main study. In contrast, significant improvement with time was observed in patients receiving aniracetam, this being reflected in all the tests employed, including the Sandoz Clinical Assessment Geriatric Scale (SCAG), the Blessed Dementia Scale part 1 and part 2 (Blessed information-memory-concentration test), the Rey 15-Word Test (short and long-term recall), the Corsi Cube Test (visuo-spatial memory), the Toulouse-Piéron Test (attention), the Gibson Spiral Maze (psychomotricity) and the Raven Colored Progressive Matrices (perception and abstract reasoning). The changes after aniracetam were significantly different from placebo at the $p < 0.001$ level in all cases after six months, at the $p < 0.001$ level for most measures.

Three of the six centers involved in the study opted to enter their patients into an extension phase, in which the same medication was taken for a further five months. Altogether sixteen patients on aniracetam and sixteen patients on placebo entered the extension phase. These data are reported here for the first time.

Baseline demographic and psychometric variables did not differ significantly between the groups with the exception of the mean Hamilton depression score which was higher in the aniracetam patients than in the control group (mean 10.6 ± 0.7 vs 8.6 ± 0.7, $p < 0.05$).

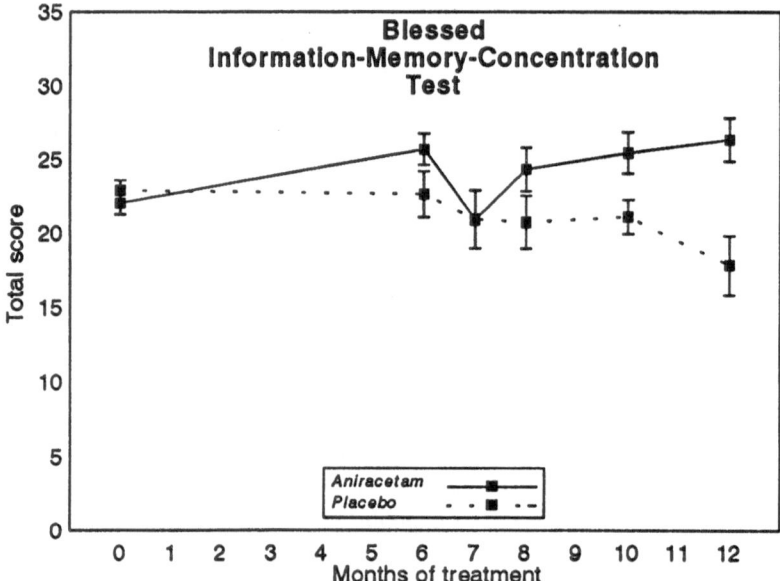

FIGURE 1.

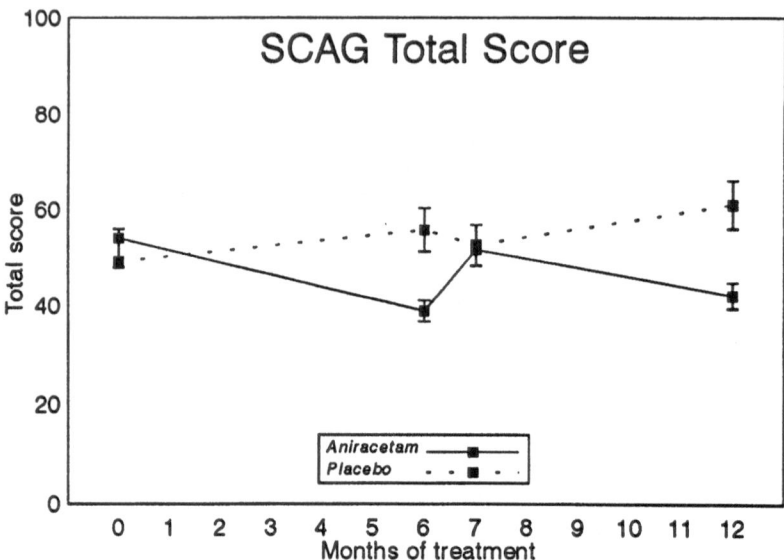

FIGURE 2.

FIGURES 1 and 2. Total scores (mean ± SEM) for the Blessed Information Memory Concentration Test (Figure 1) and SCAG (Figure 2). Patients were treated with placebo (N = 16) or aniracetam (N = 16) (750 mg twice daily) for 6 months. After a one month washout, patients were treated for a further 5 months (months 8-12).

During the one month washout phase, performance declined in the patients on aniracetam, but remained unchanged in the patients who had received placebo (Figs. 1 and 2).

During the remaining five months of the study (months 8 to 12) patients receiving aniracetam continued to show improvement in the SCAG and Blessed Dementia Scale, while placebo patients continued to decline (Figs. 1 and 2). The mean rate of decline of Blessed Dementia scores (information-memory-concentration test) in patients who received placebo was approximately 5 points over 1 year, similar to that reported in the literature (Katzman et al., 1988).

A similar pattern of improvement on aniracetam and decline on placebo was observed in the other tests, including the Rey test, Corsi Cube test, Toulouse-Piéron test, Gibson spiral maze and Raven Colored Progressive Matrices.

The improvement in cognition and behavior after aniracetam compared to placebo in the subgroup of patients in the extension phase was more marked at the twelve month evaluation than at the six month time point. These data, while preliminary and based on a very small sample size, suggest the possibility of an effect of aniracetam on the underlying disease process, with prevention of mental decline, as suggested in the 12-month piracetam study already described.

If confirmed in a larger population, these data would suggest that it is in long-term use that nootropic compounds may find their optimal role in Alzheimer's disease and other states of mental decline. Their excellent tolerability would make such use clinically practicable.

The mechanism of action of such an effect on mental decline is not clear, but could involve attenuation of excitatory amino acid toxicity (Pizzi et al., 1993). Recently aniracetam has been shown to reduce free radical generation in a mouse ischemic model (unpublished data, Nippon Roche), adding another possible neuroprotective mechanism.

ACKNOWLEDGEMENT

We thank Elliot Schwam and James Martin for reviewing the manuscript.

REFERENCES

Croisile B, Trillet M, Fondarai J, Laurent B, Mauguiere F and Billardon M (1993): Long-term and high-dose piracetam treatment of Alzheimer's disease. *Neurology* 43:301-305.

Katzman R, Brown T, Thal LJ, Fuld PA, Aronson M, Butters N, Klauber MR, Wiederholt W, Pay M, Renbing X, Ooi WL, Hofstler R and Terry RD (1988): Comparison of rate of annual change of mental status score in four independent studies of patients with Alzheimer's disease. *Annals of Neurology* 24:384-389.

Marini G, Bonavita F, Carapezzi C, Cirillo G, Diana R, Forte PL, Ponari O, Renzi G, Sartoni PP, Senin U, Tammaro AE, Criscuolo D and Cucinotta D (1992): Farmacoterapia dei sintomi del declino funzionale cerebrale nell'anziano: confronto aniracetam vs oxiracetam. *Giornale di Gerontologia* 40:97-104.

Marini G, Caratti C, Peluffo F, Celasco G and Gasparro MG (1992): Placebo-controlled double-blind study of pramiracetam (C1-879) in the treatment of elderly subjects with memory impairment. *Advances in Therapy* 9(3):136-146.

Pizzi M, Fallacara C, Arrighi V, Memo M and Spano P-F (1993): Attenuation of excitatory amino acid toxicity by metabotropic glutamate receptor agonists and aniracetam in primary cultures of cerebellar granule cells. *Journal of Neurochemistry* 61(2):683-689.

Senin U, Abate G, Fieschi C, Gori G, Guala A, Marini G, Villardita C, Parnetti L (1991): Aniracetam (Ro 13-5057) in the treatment of senile dementia of Alzheimer type (SDAT): Results of a placebo controlled multicenter clinical study. *European Neuropsychopharmacology* 1:511-517.

Vernon MW and Sorkin EM (1991): Piracetam. An overview of its pharmacological properties and a review of its therapeutic use in senile cognitive disorders. *Drugs and Aging* 1(1):17-35.

Villardita C, Grioli S, Lomeo C, Cattaneo C and Parini J (1992): Clinical studies with oxiracetam in patients with dementia of Alzheimer type and multi-infarct dementia of mild to moderate degree. *Neuropsychobiology* 25(1):24-28.

PART IX

NEUROTROPHINS, GROWTH FACTORS, AND NEUROPROTECTION IN THE TREATMENT OF ALZHEIMER'S DISEASE

Alzheimer Disease: Therapeutic Strategies
edited by E. Giacobini and R. Becker.
© 1994 Birkhäuser Boston

TOWARD THE REPAIR OF CORTICAL SYNAPSES IN ALZHEIMER'S DISEASE

A. Claudio Cuello
McGill University, Department of Pharmacology and Therapeutics, 3655
Drummond Street, Suite 1325, Montreal, Quebec, Canada H3G 1Y6

In this short review I would like to put forward the concept that trophic factor induced synaptogenesis in the cerebral cortex of Alzheimer's sufferers should be a desirable therapeutical objective. This review deals with the experimental, clinical, and histopathological data which gives credence to this idea.

LOSS OF SYNAPSES IN ALZHEIMER'S DISEASE

The most obvious components of Alzheimer's pathology are, unquestionably, the plaques and tangles. Therefore, a great deal of attention has been paid to the crucial proteins involved in the generation of these pathological elements: the β-amyloid protein (as the proteinaceous nucleus of plaques) and tau (as the core protein of paired helical filaments). Concomitantly with the plaques and tangles, it is becoming clearly evident that in Alzheimer's Disease (AD) there is a very significant loss of synaptic profiles in the neuropile of the neocortical tissue. In ultrastructural studies of the frontal cortex (from biopsies and autopsies), DeKosky and Scheff (1990) demonstrated a significant loss in the prevalence of synaptic profiles in AD as compared with age matched controls; the loss correlated to cognitive deficits. The synaptic attrition is perhaps more readily apparent in the entorhinal cortex-hippocampal complex. Hamos et al. (1989) showed that the density of synapsin I immunoreactivity (IR) is severely depleted in the AD hippocampus, particularly in the molecular layer. Furthermore, while age-related loss in neuronal cell bodies and synapses density are observed in the entorhinal cortex, these depletions become more marked in AD with a loss of synapsin I-IR of about 90% from age matched cortices (Lippa et al., 1992). The marked depletion of synaptic markers in the hippocampus has been further stressed by Honer et al. (1992) by applying ELISA for the quantification of synaptophysin IR. Terry et al. (1991) have performed very exhaustive studies on the profiles which react to synaptophysin antibodies in AD cortices by applying immunohistochemical techniques in combination with image analysis (Masliah et al., 1990a). Notably, they have shown a lack of correlation between the appearance of β-amyloid proteins in the neuropile (as judged by the appearance of diffuse plaques), and the occurrence of synaptophysin IR profiles (Masliah et al, 1990b). More importantly, Terry et al. (1991) have formally proposed that the "physical basis" of cognitive alterations in AD is the synaptic loss observed in the neocortex, particularly for the mid-frontal regions. High correlations were found between the diminution of synapses (synaptophysin positive profiles) and the degree of deterioration of higher mental functions, according to three widely used tests in the assessment of the disease: the Blessed IMC, Minimental State Examination and the total Dementia Rating Scale (Terry et al., 1991). No striking correlations were found for other factors such as plaques, tangles, or particular neurotransmitter markers, including choline acetyltransferase (ChAT). Using the monoclonal antibody 6-243 (Wischik et al., 1988), which recognizes the core epitopes of paired helical filaments (phf), we observed that there was a relationship between the abundance of intra- and extracellular phf epitopes in perikarya and dystrophic neurites and the duration of the clinically diagnosed dementia (Mena et al., 1991). In other words, the cognitive alterations and dementia states are much more likely to be produced by the neuronal loss and synaptic disconnections than merely by β-amyloid accumulation. The unresolved relationship among β-amyloid deposition, tangle formation, and synaptic losses remain crucial to our understanding of AD pathophysiology.

THE SYNAPTIC TRANSMITTER DEFICITS IN ALZHEIMER'S DISEASE

Alzheimer is obviously a disease brought about by the "disengagement" of neurons and synapses from the CNS circuitry mainly in the neuropile of the entorhinal, hippocampal, frontal, parietal and temporal cortices. A good number of cortical transmitter systems are affected by the disease (for review see Francis et al., 1993). At advanced stages the levels of somatostatin are diminished and the depletion of monoamines are apparently accompanied by an increased turnover. Due to the important involvement of pyramidal neurons in the AD pathology, it is reasonable to expect a severe reduction in glutamatergic transmission. This, however, is not obvious due to technical difficulties in assessing the depletion of excitatory neurotransmitters in post-mortem tissue (Francis et al., 1993). Because the synaptic attrition is widespread, the functional deficits and AD pathology can not be ascribed to a single neurotransmitter system. However, it is of considerable interest that terminals which do not originate from perikarya located in cortical structures, such as the projecting fibers from forebrain cholinergic neurons of the nucleus basalis of Meynert, are characteristically involved in the disease (Bowen et al., 1976; Davies and Maloney, 1976; Whitehouse et al., 1982). The "cholinergic link" has found a rather interesting twist with the observation that the activation of muscarinic receptors (m_1 and m_3) in cell culture systems promote the production non-amyloidogenic residues of the amyloid precursor protein (APP) (Nitsch et al., 1992) from which it can be extrapolated so that a cholinergic deficit might accelerate the production and accumulation of the A4, amyloidogenic fragment. Electrical stimulation of hippocampal slices *in vitro* also provoke non-amyloidogenic processing of APP, via an atropine sensitive mechanism (Nitsch et al., 1993). Whether or not the permanent depletion of cholinergic synapses plays a role in the cognitive deficit remains an issue of academic and clinical interest. A great deal of effort has been concentrated in devising a "cholinergic therapy", with modest success. The "cure" of AD, might be years ahead of us, pending the understanding of the molecular relationship of the many factors involved. However, before such time arrives, it is reasonable to propose a therapy which will stabilize the neuronal attrition and promote synaptogenesis.

THE PLASTICITY OF CNS SYNAPSES

The number of CNS synaptic complexes probably varies in adult animals, including man. For example, it is known that deafferentation of major pathways produce "vacated synaptic sites" in CNS nuclei. This was early realized by Raisman in his electron microscopical studies in the septum, when he described the occupancy of the vacated sites by new synapses from neighboring inputs (Raisman, 1969). Similar studies have been extended to several CNS regions and the phenomenon is generally referred to as "reactive synaptogenesis" (Raisman and Field, 1973; Cotman and Nadler, 1978; Steward, 1986). The number of synapses also changes during ontogeny, including in the human species.

Furthermore, in experimental mammals, long-term potentiation (LTP) in the hippocampus revealed ultrastructural evidence for modifications in both pre- and post-synaptic elements (e.g. see Van Herreveld and Fifkova, 1975; Applegate et al., 1987; Geinisman et al., 1993).

We are still unaware of the fine molecular mechanisms governing the elimination, the recruitment, or the reshaping of synaptic complexes on the adult CNS. Nevertheless, these observations, taken together, would support the notion that the architecture of synapses in the CNS, including the cerebral cortex, could possibly be manipulated pharmacologically.

TROPHIC FACTOR INDUCED SYNAPTOGENESIS

There is now compelling evidence for nerve growth factor (NGF) effectiveness in the rescue of degenerating perikarya of cholinergic cell bodies of the medial septum (for review see Hefti et al., 1989), and the nucleus basalis (for review see Cuello, 1993). The demonstration of NGF efficacy on primate CNS lesions is very important when considering its clinical application. Thus, short-term NGF (both mouse and human recombinant) administration, and short survival times (2 and 4 weeks), have shown prevention of cholinergic cell losses in the medial septum after axotomy in *Macaca fascicularis* (Tuszynski et al., 1990, 1991; Koliatsos et al, 1990, 1991). Furthermore, short-term administration of human-recombinant NGF and long-term survival (6 months) have shown protection from injury-induced atrophy of cholinergic neurons of the nucleus basalis magnocellularis of Meynert in *Cercopithecus aethiops* (Liberini et al., 1993).

In both experimental models of CNS cholinergic lesions in rodents, axotomy of septo-hippocampal fibers and unilateral infarction of neocortex, the administration of NGF leads to biochemical changes (activity of ChAT, high affinity choline uptake, turnover of ACh) indicative of improvement of presynaptic functions of cholinergic projections in the hippocampus (Lapchak and Hefti, 1991) and cerebral cortex (Cuello et al., 1989, DiPatre et al., 1989, Garofalo and Cuello, 1990, 1994), respectively. Considering that animals lacking NGF genes develop relatively normal basal forebrain cholinergic cells (Crowley et al., 1994), it is likely that NGF is only one trophic factor for these neurons and, thus, probably other neurotrophic factors might provoke similar effects, as does NGF; however, comprehensive information is not yet available. Are these NGF-induced changes on presynaptic markers of cholinergic activity purely reflecting activation of biosynthesis of enzymes and transporters or the expression of actual reshaping of synaptic elements? In the cerebral cortex of adult rats bearing partial cortical infarctions our group (Garofalo et al., 1992, 1993) has shown that they represent a trophic factor-induced remodelling of cholinergic terminals, presynaptic boutons, and their synaptic membrane differentiations. NGF not only prevents the retraction of cholinergic terminals in the cerebral cortex, but even expands their extensions and there is a net increase above control levels in the number of cholinergic varicosities as determined by light microscopy and automated image analysis (Garofalo et al., 1992). Furthermore, when studying analogous material under electron microscopy the individual presynaptic boutons of cortically-lesioned and NGF-treated rats are moderately *hypertrophic* (Garofalo et al., 1992); while there is a net increment in the incidence of membrane synaptic differentiations (Garofalo et al., 1992). Taking into account the tri-dimensional reconstructions, the actual enlargement of cholinergic synaptic boutons is in the order of 100% (Garofalo et al., 1993). Are these changes beneficial for cortical functions? These cortically lesioned animals show deficits in retaining learned tasks such as passive avoidance, or finding the hidden platform in the Morris water maze (Garofalo and Cuello, 1990, 1994). The NGF administration fully corrects these deficits to the point that in their behavior they become indistinguishable from sham-operated, or naive animals (Garofalo and Cuello, 1994). It is, therefore, possible that these changes are not restricted to remodelling of the one neurotransmitter-specific synapses in the cerebral cortex, but very likely, of several transmitter systems. Thus, with Drs. Kolb and Ribeiro-da-Silva we found evidence for post-synaptic changes in pyramidal neurons which utilize glutamate as a transmitter, a neuronal system which apparently lacks trkA, the high affinity receptor for NGF.

Whether trophic factor therapy could be effective in recovering degenerating synapses in AD is a most important issue. The shown efficacy of NGF in primate cholinergic perikarya (see above), and the fact that compensatory synaptic plasticity has been proposed to occur in the hippocampus of AD (Geddes et al., 1985) would suggest that possibility. Preliminary clinical attempts reporting temporary improvements of verbal episodic memory give credibility to this possibility (Seiger et al., 1993). However, if neurotrophic therapy remains an objective, there will be many unresolved issues regarding the selection of patients, pharmaceutical formulations, possible collateral, unwanted effects, etc. This we hope to learn in the coming years.

ACKNOWLEDGMENTS

The author would like to thank the MRC Canada for support, collaborators, particularly Drs. L. Garofalo and A. Ribeiro-da-Silva, as well as Drs. R. Capek and B. Collier for critical review of the manuscript, and Mrs. O. Mackprang and D. Torsein for editorial work.

REFERENCES

Applegate MD, Kerr DS and Landfield PW (1987): Redistribution of synaptic vesicles during long-term potentiation in the hippocampus. Brain Res 401:401-406.

Bowen DM, Smith CB, White P and Davison AN (1976): Neurotransmitter-related enzymes and indices of hypoxia in senile dementia and other abiotrophies. Brain 99:459-496.

Cotman CW and Nadler JV (1978): Reactive synaptogenesis in hippocampus. Neuronal Plasticity, Cotman CW, ed. New York: Plenum Press, pp. 227-271.

Crowley C, Spencer SD, Nishimura MC, Chen KS, Pitts-Meek S, Armanini MP, Ling LH, McMahon SB, Shelton DL, Levinson AD and Phillips HS (1994): Mice lacking nerve growth factor display perinatal loss of sensory and sympathetic neurons yet develop basal forebrain cholinergic neurons. Cell 76:1001-1011.

Cuello AC (1993): Trophic responses of forebrain cholinergic neurons: a discussion. In: Cholinergic Function and Dysfunction, Cuello AC, ed. Amsterdam: Elsevier Science Publishers BV, pp. 265-277.

Cuello AC, Garofalo L, Kenigsberg RL and Maysinger D (1989): Ganglioside potentiate in vivo and in vitro effects of nerve growth factor on central cholinergic neurons. Proc Natl Acad Sci USA 86:2056-2060.

Davies P and Maloney AJF (1976): Selective loss of central cholinergic neurons in Alzheimer's disease. Lancet 2:1403.

DeKosky ST and Scheff SW (1990): Synapse loss in frontal cortex biopsies in Alzheimer's disease: correlation with cognitive severity. Ann Neurol 27:457-464.

DiPatre PL, Casamenti F, Cenni A and Pepeu G (1989): Interaction between nerve growth factor and GM1 monosialoganglioside in preventing cortical choline acetyltransferase and high affinity choline uptake decrease after lesion of the nucleus basalis. Brain Res 480:219-224.

Francis PT, Sims NR, Procter AW and Bowen DM (1993): Cortical pyramidal neurone loss may cause glutamatergic hypoactivity and cognitive impairment in Alzheimer's disease: investigative and therapeutic perspectives. *J Neurochem* 60(5):1589-1604.

Garofalo L and Cuello AC (1990): Nerve growth factor and the monosialoganglioside GM1 modulate cholinergic markers and affect behavior of decorticated adult rats. *Eur J Pharmacol* 183:934-935.

Garofalo L and Cuello AC (1994): Nerve Growth Factor and the Monosialoganglioside GM1: analogous and different in vivo effects on biochemical, morphological and behavioral parameters of adult cortically lesioned rats. *Exp Neurol* 125:195-217.

Garofalo L, Ribeiro-da-Silva A and Cuello AC (1992): Nerve growth factor induced synaptogenesis and hypertrophy of cortical cholinergic terminals. *Proc Natl Acad Sci USA* 89:2639-2643.

Garofalo L, Ribeiro-da-Silva A and Cuello AC (1993): Potentiation of nerve growth factor-induced alterations in cholinergic fibre length and presynaptic terminal size in cortex of lesioned rats by the monosialoganglioside GM1. *Neuroscience* 57(1):21-40.

Geddes JW, Monaghan DT, Cotman CW, Lott IT, Kim RC and Chang-Chui H (1985): Plasticity of hippocampal circuitry in Alzheimer's disease. *Science* 230:1179-1181.

Geinisman Y, de Toledo-Morrell L, Morrell F, Heller RE, Rossi M and Parshall RF (1993): Structural synaptic correlate of long-term potentiation: formation of Axospinous synapses with multiple, completely partitioned transmission zones. *Hippocampus* 3(4):435-446.

Hamos JE, DeGennaro LJ and Drachman DA (1989): Synaptic loss in Alzheimer's disease and other dementias. *Neurology* 39:355-361.

Hefti F, Hartikka J and Knusel B (1989): Function of neurotrophic factors in the adult and aging brain and their possible use in the treatment of neurodegenerative diseases. *Neurobiol Aging* 10:515-533.

Honer WG, Dickson DW, Gleeson J and Davies P (1992): Regional synaptic pathology in Alzheimer's disease. *Neurobiol Aging* 13:375-382.

Koliatsos VE, Nauta HJW, Clatterbuck RE, Holtzman DM, Mobley WC and Price DL (1990): Mouse nerve growth factor prevents degeneration of axotomized basal forebrain cholinergic neurons in the monkey. *J Neurosci* 10:3801-3813.

Koliatsos VE, Clatterbuck RE, Nauta HJW, Knüsel B, Burton LE, Hefti FF, Mobley WC and Price DL (1991): Human nerve growth factor prevents degeneration of basal forebrain cholinergic neurons in primates. *Ann Neurol* 30:831-840.

Lapchak PA and Hefti F (1991): Effect of recombinant human nerve growth factor on Presynaptic cholinergic function in rat hippocampal slices following partial septohippocampal lesions: measures of [^{3}H]acetylcholine synthesis, [^{3}H]acetylcholine release a choline acetyltransferase activity. *Neuroscience* 42:639-649.

Liberini P, Pioro EP, Maysinger D, Ervin FR and Cuello AC (1993): Long-term protective effects of human recombinant nerve growth factor and monosialoganglioside GM1 treatment on primate nucleus basalis cholinergic neurons after neocortical infarction. *Neuroscience* 53(3):625-637.

Lippa CF, Hamos JE, Pulaski-Salo D, Degennaro LJ and Drachman DA (1992): Alzheimer's disease and aging: effects on perforant pathway perikarya and synapses. *Neurobiol Aging* 13:405-411.

Masliah E, Terry RD, Alford M and DeTeresa RM (1990a): Quantitative immuno-histochemistry of synaptophysin in human neocortex: an alternative method to estimate density of presynaptic terminals in paraffin sections. *H Histochem Cytochem* 38:837-844.

Masliah E, Terry RD, Mallory M, Alford M and Hansen LA (1990b): Diffuse plaques do not accentuate synapse loss in Alzheimer's disease. *Am J Pathol* 137(6):1293-1297.

Mena R, Wischik CM, Novak M, Milstein C and Cuello AC (1991): A progressive deposition of paired helical filaments (PHF) in the brain characterizes the evolution of dementia in Alzheimer's disease. *J Neuropathol Exp Neurol* 50(4):474-490.

Nitsch RM, Slack BE, Wurtman RJ and Growdon JH (1992): Release of Alzheimer amyloid precursor derivatives stimulated by activation of muscarinic acetylcholine receptors. *Science* 258:304-307.

Nitsch RM, Farber SA, Growdon JH and Wurtman RJ (1993): Release of amyloid beta-protein precursor derivatives by electrical depolarization of rat hippocampal slices. *PNAS USA* 90(11):5191-5193.

Raisman G (1969): Neuronal plasticity in the septal nuclei of the adult rat. *Brain Res* 14: 25-48.

Raisman G and Field PM (1973): A quantitative investigation of the development of collateral reinnervation after partial deafferentation of the septal nucleus. *Brain Res* 50:241-264.

Seiger Å, Nordberg A, von Holst H, Bäckman L, Ebendal T, Alafuzoff I, Amberla K, Hartvig P, Herlitz A, Lilja A, Lundqvist H, Långström B, Meyerson B, Persson A, Viitanen M, Winblad B and Olson L (1993): Intracranial infusion of purified nerve growth factor to an Alzheimer patient: the first attempt of a possible future treatment strategy. *Behav Brain Res* 57:255-261.

Steward O (1986): Lesion induced synapse growth in the hippocampus. In search of cellular and molecular mechanisms. In: *The Hippocampus*, Isaacson RL and Pribram KH, eds. New York: Plennum Press, pp. 65-111.

Terry RD, Masliah E, Salomon DP, Butters N, DeTeresa R, Hill R, Hansen LA and Katzman R (1991): Physical basis of cognitive alterations in Alzheimer's disease: synapse loss is the major correlate of cognitive impairment. *Ann Neurol* 30:572-580.

Tutzynski MH, Sang UH, Amaral DG and Gage F (1990): Nerve growth factor infusion in the primate brain reduces lesion-induced neural degeneration. *J Neurosci* 10:6304-3614.

Tutzynski MH, Sang UH, Yoshida K and Gage FH (1991): Recombinant human growth factor infusions prevent cholinergic neural degeneration in the adult primate brain. *Ann Neurol* 30:625-636.

Van Herreveld A and Fifkova E (1975): Swelling of dendritic spines in the fascia dentata after stimulation of the performant fibers as a mechanism of post-tetanic potentiation. *Exp Neurol* 49:736-749.

Whitehouse PJ, Price DL, Struble RG, Clark AW, Coyle JT and De Long Mr (1982): Alzheimer's disease and senile dementia: loss of neurons in basal forebrain. *Science* 215:1237-1239.

Wischik CM, Novak M, Thøgersen HC, Edwards PC, Runswick MJ, Jakes R, Walker JE, Milstein C, Roth M and Klug A (1988): Isolation of a fragment of tau derived from the core of the paired helical filament of Alzheimer disease. *PNAS USA* 85:4506-4510.

Alzheimer Disease: Therapeutic Strategies
edited by E. Giacobini and R. Becker.
© 1994 Birkhäuser Boston

GANGLIOSIDES IN ALZHEIMER'S DISEASE: EXPERIMENTAL AND CLINICAL DATA

Lars Svennerholm
Department of Clinical Neuroscience, University of Göteborg, Sweden

Gino Toffano
Fidia Research Laboratories, Abano Terme (Pd), Italy

NEUROBIOLOGY OF GANGLIOSIDES

Gangliosides are glycosphingolipids which consist of a carbohydrate chain comprising one or more sialic acid residues, attached to a double lipophilic tail formed by the amino alcohol sphingosine and a fatty acid (Fig. 1). They are characteristic compounds of the outer surface of the plasma membrane of eukaryotic cells being restricted to vertebrates and certain higher invertebrates. In vertebrates they occur in virtually all tissues and are particularly abundant in the central nervous system. The gangliosides lie embedded with their hydrophobic tail in the plasma membranes; their carbohydrate moieties are spread over the cell surface. In each species and each tissue the molecular patterns of gangliosides differ and undergo changes during development and under various forms of physiological influences. The most consistent ganglioside composition is found in the mammalian brain in which four gangliosides, GM1, GD1a, GD1b and GT1b, dominate in all species. These gangliosides belong to the gangliotetraose family and can be considered to be derivatives of GM1-ganglioside. The biosynthesis of gangliosides occurs in the endoplasmic reticulum-Golgi apparatus. In the brain the gangliosides are then transported by fast axonal flow to the nerve terminals. Gangliosides can also be transferred to the plasma membrane from the outside. Exogenously administered gangliosides are rapidly taken up by the cells and inserted in their plasma membrane. The membrane incorporation of GM1 is associated with a corresponding increase in the cholera binding capacity and the ATPase activity of the cells (reviewed by Svennerholm, 1984). Gangliosides have also been shown to be taken up by the neurons, by which the functional dynamics of the cellular membranes are influenced in several ways.

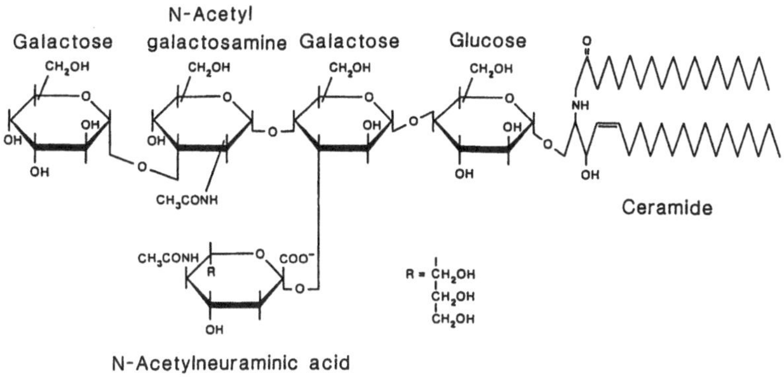

N-Acetylneuraminic acid

FIGURE 1. Structure formula of GM1-ganglioside.

NEUROPLASTICITY IN CNS REPAIR

Research into CNS repair has been held back by the widely accepted view that no regeneration could take place in the injured CNS. During the last 10-15 years a number of animal experiments have shown that, under the appropriate experimental conditions, the brain can indeed reorganize and repair itself. Neuroscientists have coined the term "neuroplasticity" to indicate the adaptive mechanism by which the nervous system recovers normal function following injury. An understanding of the concept of neuroplasticity as a repair mechanism for the damaged CNS is essential for the interpretation of experimental results obtained by the exogenous administration of GM1. This ganglioside acts on the molecular mechanism used by neurons to adapt to the changed environment that exists, for example, after injury, when the neurons are deprived of their normal pattern of connections.

PHARMACOLOGY OF GM1 STUDIED *IN VITRO*

The studies which demonstrated a trophic effect of gangliosides *in vitro* and also *in vivo* (for review see Ledeen, 1984; Consolazione and Toffano, 1988) are of special importance. Differentiation and neurite outgrowth were also shown to be enhanced by gangliosides (Ledeen, 1984). Another aspect of ganglioside effect *in vitro* emerged from studies utilizing PC12 pheochromocytoma cells, which failed to respond to gangliosides alone. These cells, however, do become responsive to gangliosides in the presence of nerve growth factor (NGF) (Consolazione and Toffano, 1988). The synergistic relationship of gangliosides-neuronotrophic factors has also been demonstrated in primary neuronal systems which require NGF or other trophic compounds for survival and/or neurite elongation (Consolazione and Toffano, 1988). The fact that a broad spectrum of sialoglycolipids, including naturally occurring gangliosides and synthetic analogues, produced similar results in neuroblastoma cells suggests that this effect is pharmacological rather than physiological in nature.

IN VIVO LESION MODELS

The first evidence that gangliosides may accelerate nervous system repair was given by Ceccarelli et al. (1976), who demonstrated that parenteral administration of a ganglioside mixture, isolated from bovine brain, was capable of enhancing recovery of denervated nictating membrane in the cat. In several concomitant independent studies a number of different brain lesion models have been used to investigate the action of GM1-ganglioside. These have included unilateral hemitransection of the nigrostriatal pathway and experimentally induced injury to the entorhinal cortex, caudate nucleus, magnocellular forebrain and basal nucleus. Significant benefit was observed in treated animals and this was judged by improvements in tyrosine hydroxylase immunoreactivity, number of dopamine-positive terminals and a range of behavior tests. GM1 has shown a constant protective and reparative effect when lesions were induced by chemical agents including 1-methyl-4-phenyl-1,2,3,6-tetrahydropyridine. Mice made severely Parkinsonian by MPTP showed accelerated biochemical and behavioral recovery by GM1-treatment (Schneider, 1992) and GM1 also promoted the recovery of surviving dopaminergic neurons in MPTP-treated monkeys (Herrero et al., 1993). These last two studies showed that GM1 did not protect against cell death but exerted a neurotrophic effect on surviving dopaminergic neurons. Cuello and his collaborators have been particularly interested in testing whether exogenously applied gangliosides could prevent the retrograde and anterograde atrophy of CNS cholinergic neurons of nucleus basalis magnocellularis or cortex secondary to cortical damage (for review see Cuello et al., 1994). GM1-treatment applied alone or in combination with NGF was found to reduce the degeneration, result in total protection from shrinkage of the neuron and increase the choline acetyltransferase activity in the rat and in nonhuman primate. Their results suggested that a relatively short treatment period may be sufficient to protect cholinergic neurons after a cortical infarction. Ischemic injury provides another relevant model for the study of the protective effect of GM1 since it induces a series of well recognized pathophysiological processes including oedema, hypoxia, ionic imbalance, membrane dysfunction and cell death. Karpiak et al. (1988) demonstrated reduced mortality, preserved membrane function and reduced edema for rats receiving GM1.

GANGLIOSIDE TREATMENT OF PATIENTS

Stroke
The animal studies suggested that gangliosides might have a significant beneficial effect on stroke patients. A number of pilot studies suggested that gangliosides led to significant improvement, and a large randomized placebo-controlled,

double masked multicenter study was performed to assess the safety and efficacy of GM1 in stroke patients. Only patients treated within 5 hours after the onset of stroke were enrolled. Significant improvement of the treatment groups of patients was shown for the subgroups of patients treated within 3 hours.

Spinal Cord Injury
In a prospective, randomized, placebo-controlled double-blind trial the GM1 treated patients had significantly greater improvements in motor score, attributable to regained useful motor strength in initially paralyzed muscles (Geisler et al., 1991).

GANGLIOSIDE TREATMENT OF ALZHEIMER PATIENTS

In a study of the biochemical changes in brains from deceased Alzheimer patients we found a strongly significant loss of gangliosides - the optimum biochemical marker for neuronal membranes. Our original finding in caudate nuclei has recently been confirmed by the demonstration of equally large losses of gangliosides in frontal and temporal cortices and hippocampus as in caudate nuclei (Svennerholm and Gottfries, 1994) in patients with the early onset form of Alzheimer disease (AD Type I). The biochemical studies demonstrated that the ganglioside loss was not combined with any significant demyelination. Therefore we assumed that the marked loss of gangliosides depended mainly on a loss of dendrite and axonal arborization from preserved neurons. It was thus evident that AD Type I patients fulfilled the criteria for an intervention with a growth promoting drug. In collaboration with Professor Carl-Gerhard Gottfries and several members of Department of Clinical Neuroscience, 16 patients with AD Type I received 100 mg GM1 daily for three months by intramuscular or subcutaneous injection; the latter injection route led to higher plasma level and less discomfort for the patients. The patients, examined after three and six months, did not show any sign of clinical improvement but only a continuous deterioration. Brain biopsies performed after treatment for seven days with a tritium labelled GM1 showed that less than 0.1% of the given dose had reached the brain tissue. In order to achieve the higher dose of GM1 which had shown a morphological, biochemical and behavioral effect in treated aged animals it was necessary to give GM1 intracerebrally. When fine catheters were placed directly in the brain tissue of the animals there was an extremely slow perfusion out to the surrounding tissue. The catheters were instead inserted in the frontal portion of each of the two lateral ventricles and connected with a Rickham reservoir implanted under the scalp. This device gives continuous access to the ventricular portion of the cerebrospinal fluid. The Rickham reservoir is also connected with a fine teflon tubing which is tunnelated under the skin to a micropump (Synchromed) implanted under the skin of the belly. The pump is programmed to deliver the drug at a constant rate and can be easily reprogrammed from the outside. Five patients with AD Type I have been treated intracerebroventricularly for a year with a daily dose of 20-30 mg GM1. After one year, the ganglioside has been omitted and the patient has only received physiological saline for three months. The dose was originally varied between 10 and 50 mg, but all five patients required at least 20 mg GM1 daily for optimum activity. Some patients showed signs of confusion when the GM1 dose was higher than 30 mg. All five patients have tolerated GM1 with no adverse effects. The pump has been refilled with GM1 every 30-45 days, and on these occasions the remaining fluid has been sent to microbiological laboratory for culturing during 14 days and endotoxin determinations. All tests have been normal during the whole period. The patients have been examined by neurologist, psychiatrist, psychologist and nurse with regular intervals.

In all the five patients the disease process has been halted, the psychometric tests have shown unchanged or in the two patients with the highest Mini-Mental Test and the lowest GBS score at the beginning of the study improved results. The patients have shown increased activity and more syntonous mood. When the ganglioside administration was replaced by placebo the patients started to deteriorate after 2-3 weeks. A final evaluation of the clinical results will first be performed when 10 patients have undergone the treatment schedule (12 months of GM1 + 3 months of placebo).

REFERENCES

Ceccarelli B, Apoli F and Finesso M (1976): Effects of brain gangliosides on functional recovery in experimental regeneration and reinnervation. In: *Ganglioside Function*, Porcelatti G, Ceccarelli B and Tettamanti G, eds. Plenum: New York, pp. 275-293.

Consolazione A and Toffano G (1988): Ganglioside role in functional recovery of damaged nervous system. In: *New Trends in Ganglioside Research: Neurochemical and Neuroregenerative Aspects*, Ledeen RW, Hogan EL, Tettamanti G, Yates AJ and Yu RK, eds. Fidia Research Series Vol 14. Padova: Liviana Press, pp. 523-529.

Cuello CA, Garofalo L, Liberini P and Maysinger D (1994): Cooperative effects of gangliosides on trophic factor-induced neuronal cell recovery and synaptogenesis: studies in rodarts and subhuman primates. *Progr Brain Research* 101:337-355.

Geisler FH, Dorsey FC and Coleman WP (1991): Recovery of motor function after spinal cord injury - a randomized placebo-controlled trial with GM1 ganglioside. *N Engl J Med* 324:1829-1838.

Herrero M-T, Kastner A, Perez-Otaño I, Hirsch EC. Luquin M-R, Javoy-Aqid F, Del Rio J, Obeso JA and Aqid Y (1993): Gangliosides and parkinsonism. *Neurology* 43:2132-2134.

Karpiak SE, Li YS and Mahadik SP (1988): Ischemic injury reduced by GM1 ganglioside. In: *New Trends in Ganglioside Research*, Ledeen RW, Hogan EL, Tettamanti G, Yates AJ and Yu RK, eds. Fidia Research Series Vol 14. Padova: Liviana Press, pp. 549-556.

Ledeen RW (1984): Biology of gangliosides: Neurotigenic and neuronotrophic properties. *J Neurosci Res* 12:147-159.

Schneider JS (1992):   Effects of age on GM1 ganglioside induced recovery of concentrations of dopamine in the striatum in 1-methyl-4-phenyl-1,2,3,6-tetrahydropyridine-treated mice. *Neuropharmacology* 31:185-192.

Svennerholm L (1984):   Biological significance of gangliosides. In: *Cellular and Pathological Aspects of Glycoconjugate Metabolism*, Dreyfus H, Massarelli R, Freysz L and Rebel G, eds. Paris: INSERM, pp. 21-24.

Svennerholm L and Gottfries CG (1994): Membrane lipids selectively diminished in Alzheimer brains suggest synapse loss as a primary event in early-onset form (Type I) and demyelination in late-onset form (Type II). *J Neurochem* 62:1039-1047.

PART X

EXCITATORY AMINO ACIDS, CA⁺⁺ CELLULAR HOMEOSTASIS, NITRIC OXIDE, AND AD TREATMENT

Alzheimer Disease: Therapeutic Strategies
edited by E. Giacobini and R. Becker.
© 1994 Birkhäuser Boston

EXCITATORY TRANSMITTER NEUROTOXICITY AND ALZHEIMER'S DISEASE

John W. Olney and Nuri B. Farber
Washington University Medical School, St. Louis, MO 63110

INTRODUCTION

Both of the predominant excitatory transmitters in the mammalian central nervous system (CNS), glutamate (Glu) and acetylcholine (ACh), harbor neurotoxic potential which we postulate may contribute to the pathophysiology of Alzheimer's disease (AD). Surprisingly, either hyperactivation or suppression of Glu receptors can cause excitotoxic degeneration of CNS neurons. Evidence supporting this paradoxical conclusion and the relevance of such evidence to AD will be discussed.

CLASSICAL EXCITOTOXICITY AND AD

It is well recognized that Glu, aspartate (Asp) and related excitatory amino acids (EAA) have the Jekyll-Hyde properties of stimulating CNS neurons for beneficial purposes or stimulating them to death when mechanisms for controlling such stimulation fail. Evidence summarized below suggests a possible role for either endogenous or exogenous (or both) excitotoxins in the neuropathology of AD.

Increased Extracellular Glu, Dementia Pugilistica and AD
One set of observations suggesting a link between EAA and AD is as follows: 1) exposing cultured human neurons to increased extracellular concentrations of Glu reportedly stimulates the production of paired helical filaments resembling those that form neurofibrillary tangles (NFT) in AD (De Boni and McLachlan, 1985); 2) head trauma in experimental animals causes endogenous excitotoxins (Glu and Asp) to leak out of cells and accumulate in the extracellular compartment of brain (Faden et al., 1989) where they can exert excitotoxic action at external membrane receptors; 3) the sport of boxing subjects the human head to repeated trauma, which presumably entails repeated exposure of CNS neurons to abnormally elevated concentrations of extracellular Glu, and the outcome is a high incidence of dementia pugilistica, a dementing disorder in which the brain has numerous NFT and abnormal increases in ß-amyloid

protein. Dementia pugilistica provides a unique opportunity to learn what happens to the human brain when it is subjected to repeated trauma, an opportunity made possible by the fact that modern society considers it entertaining to watch men hit one another in the head. Without condoning this barbaric practice, medical science can learn from it that there is a strong association between repetitive exposure of neurons in the young adult human brain to increased extracellular concentrations of excitotoxins and early onset of a dementing process characterized by some of the major neuropathological stigmata of AD.

If elevated extracellular concentrations of excitotoxins were involved in the pathophysiology of AD, one might be able to detect this aberration by measuring the concentrations of Glu and Asp in CSF of AD patients. Such measurements have been performed in several studies with confusing results showing either an increase, a decrease or no change from normal. A major flaw in most of these studies which renders the results uninterpretable is that the measurements were made on patient samples that were heterogeneous for stage of illness. A very recent study (Csernansky et al., 1994) performed on well characterized AD patients stratified into groups according to stage of illness revealed a significant elevation in the CSF Asp and a large but not quite significant elevation in CSF Glu. These changes were confined to patients in the late stages of the illness.

Normal Glu Concentrations, Abnormal Energy Metabolism and AD
A major advance in understanding how endogenous Glu might play a role in neurodegenerative diseases was provided by evidence (Benveniste et al., 1984) that under energy deficient conditions (hypoxia/ischemia and hypoglycemia) Glu and Asp escape from the intracellular compartment and accumulate in excitotoxic concentrations extracellularly. Evidence that EAA antagonists protect against neuronal degeneration associated with these conditions served to confirm the role of endogenous Glu.

Henneberry and colleagues (1989) have developed evidence for an alternate mechanism by which energy impairment might trigger an excitotoxic process. Based on *in vitro* studies on cultured neurons, they proposed that when energy resources are reduced below a certain critical level, energy-dependent mechanisms responsible for maintaining the normal resting potential of neural membranes fail, leading to a partial membrane depolarization that relieves the voltage-dependent $Mg++$ block which, under ordinary physiological conditions, obstructs ion flow through the n-methyl-D-aspartate (NMDA) receptor channel. In the absence of the $Mg++$ block, even normal physiological amounts of Glu being released for transmitter purposes would be enough to trigger abnormal increases in current flow and excitotoxic cell death. Such a mechanism might take days, weeks or months to run its excitotoxic course.

Evidence of abnormal energy metabolism (reviewed by Beal et al., 1993) has been reported in both Down's Syndrome and AD. In fibroblasts from individuals with Down's syndrome, impairment of pyruvate dehydrogenase complex has been reported. In brain biopsies from AD patients evidence has been found for uncoupling of oxidative phosphorylation such that oxidation of glucose to CO_2 occurs without achieving phosphorylation of ADP to ATP. In addition, abnormal oxidation of glucose has been found in cultured fibroblasts from AD patients and mitochondrial gene mutations have recently been reported in patients with AD.

Cysteine, BMAA and Guamanian APD

Cysteine (Cys) is a common sulfur-containing amino acid which has devastating brain damaging actions when fed or administered subcutaneously to immature rodents.   Cysteine destroys neurons by a Glu-type excitotoxic mechanism involving activation of both the NMDA and AMPA subtypes of Glu receptor (Olney et al., 1990).   There are several interesting parallels between Cys and ß-methyl-amino-L-alanine (BMAA), an excitotoxin found in the seeds of a cycad plant which has been identified as a putative causal factor in three neurological disorders (amyotrophic lateral sclerosis/parkinsonism/dementia) (APD) that have occurred endemically as a triadic complex in Guam and related western Pacific islands. Both Cys and BMAA lack the ω acidic terminal group that is shared by all other straight-chain excitotoxic molecules, a feature that may facilitate their penetration of blood-brain barriers, and both molecules have excitotoxic potential that is markedly enhanced in the presence of bicarbonate (Olney et al., 1990; Weiss and Choi, 1988), which promotes conversion of either agent to an α-aminocarbamate that stereochemically resembles potent excitotoxic molecules (Nunn et al., 1991). The excitotoxic activity of BMAA, like that of Cys, is exerted through both NMDA and AMPA receptors (Olney et al., unpublished). Thus, Cys and BMAA represent interesting molecules present in foods which are taken into the body as seemingly innocuous substances that penetrate blood-brain barriers, then after entering the brain can convert, in the presence of bicarbonate, to potentially powerful excitotoxins.

The above similarities between Cys and BMAA fuel suspicion that they could contribute to the same disease processes.   However, a more direct basis for considering this possibility is that Heafield et al. (1990) recently reported that patients in England with motor neuron disease, parkinsonism or Alzheimer's dementia have an apparent metabolic abnormality in common. All three patient samples were found to have ratios of Cys to sulfate in the blood five-fold higher than is found in normal controls.   It will be important to obtain second laboratory confirmation of this finding with respect to AD; Perry et al. (1991) have reported nonconfirmation with respect to motor neuron disease.

GLU HYPOFUNCTION, CHOLINERGIC EXCITOTOXICITY AND AD

In this section we will advance a novel hypothesis that major aspects of the neuropathology of AD might be understood in terms of a complex Glu/ACh combined excitotoxic syndrome that is initially triggered by inactivation of

NMDA receptors. Recently we found (Olney et al., 1989, 1991) that experimental induction of NMDA receptor hypofunction (NRH) causes neurons in several neocortical and limbic brain regions to degenerate, either reversibly or irreversibly, depending on severity and duration of the NRH. We induce NRH by administration of NMDA receptor antagonists to adult rats. We interpret our results as follows: the NMDA antagonist blocks NMDA receptors that tonically drive GABAergic neurons which maintain inhibitory control over the release of ACh at m1 and/or m3 receptors and Glu at kainate receptors (Price et al., 1994) on primary neurons in the neocortex, hippocampus and related limbic brain regions. The net effect of NMDA receptor blockade is disinhibition of ACh and Glu release, hyperactivation of both m1/m3 and kainate receptors and excitotoxic degeneration of neurons, especially those endowed with both m1/m3 and kainate receptors.

How might this relate to AD? There is evidence from *in vitro* studies that over-expression of ß-amyloid precursor protein (ß-APP) alters ß-APP processing and results in fragments that are neurotoxic. It has also been shown that activation of m1 or m3 receptors stimulates secretion of ß-APP derivatives via a PKC mechanism (Nitsch et al., 1992; Buxbaum et al., 1992). The interpretation currently embraced regarding the latter evidence is that m1/m3 activation may increase processing and secretion of non-amyloidogenic products and reduce ß/A4 production. However, these are relatively acute *in vitro* experiments on cultured non-neural cells and it is not clear how persistent chronic hyperactivation of m1/m3 receptors in the *in vivo* adult brain might affect expression of ß-APP or production of ß/A4. Moreover, NRH involves not only persistent *in vivo* hyperactivation of m3 receptors, but simultaneous hyperactivation of KA and sigma receptors on the same neurons (Price et al., 1994). We propose that neurons being simultaneously hyperstimulated through three receptor systems, including m3 cholinergic receptors linked to phosphoinositide/PKC second messengers, might perform protein phosphorylation functions in a deranged manner, and this might be conducive to either neurofibrillary tangle (NFT) formation or to ß amyloidosis (or both). Neurons that degenerate following NRH, like neurons that develop NFT in AD, show abnormal expression of 72 Kd heat shock protein (Olney et al., 1991; Hamos et al., 1991). Whether these degenerating neurons express other abnormal products relevant to AD remains to be studied. NRH induces neuronal degeneration only in adult animals (Farber et al., 1992) just as the ravages of AD affect only the adult CNS. The suggestion that cholinergic hyperactivity might be an important triggering mechanism underlying pathomorphological stigmata of AD seemingly contradicts evidence that cholinergic neurons degenerate and die in AD. However, recent neuroimaging studies on subjects with *early* AD document loss of non-cholinergic neurons, preservation of cholinergic neurons and abnormal increases in phosphoinositide metabolites (Ross et al., 1993). Thus, death of cholinergic neurons in AD may occur as a late event after hyperactivity of these neurons has wreaked havoc upon many other neurons which they innervate. It is reasonable to invoke NRH as an operative mechanism in AD in that the NMDA receptor system becomes hypofunctional in old age (Wenk et al., 1991), a phenomenon that may be exaggerated in AD.

SUMMARY

Here we have reviewed several ways in which excitatory transmitter systems might contribute to the neuropathology of AD.

REFERENCES

Beal MF, Hyman BT and Koroshetz W (1993): Do defects in mitochondrial energy metabolism underlie the pathology of neurodegenerative diseases? *TINS* 16:125-131.

Benveniste H, Drejer J, Schousboe A and Diemer NM (1984): Elevation of the extracellular concentrations of glutamate and aspartate in rat hippocampus during transient cerebral ischemia. *J Neurochem* 43:1369-1374.

Buxbaum JD, Oishi M and Greengard P (1992): Cholinergic agonists and interleukin 1 regulate processing and secretion of the Alzheimer ß/A4 amyloid protein precursor. *Proc Natl Acad Sci USA* 89:10075-10078.

Csernansky JG, Bardgett ME, Sheline YI and Olney JW (1994): Stage-specific increases in CSF excitatory amino acids in Alzheimer's disease. *Soc Neurosci Abstr* (In Press).

DeBoni U and McLachlan DRC (1985): Controlled induction of paired helical filaments of the Alzheimer type in cultured human neurons by glutamate and aspartate. *J Neurol Sci* 68:105-118.

Faden AI, Panter S and Vink R (1989): The role of excitatory amino acids and NMDA receptors in traumatic brain injury. *Science* 244:798-800.

Farber NB, Price MT, Labruyere J and Olney JW (1992): Age dependency of NMDA antagonist neurotoxicity. *Soc Neurosci Abst* 18:1148.

Hamos JE, Oblas B, Welch WJ, Bole DG and Drachman DA (1991): Expression of heat shock proteins in Alzheimer's disease. *Neurology* 41:345-350.

Heafield MT, Fearn S, Steventon GB, Williams AD and Sturman SG (1990): Plasma cysteine and sulphate levels in patients with motor neurone, Parkinson's and Alzheimer's disease. *Neurosci Lett* 110:216-220.

Henneberry RL, Novelli A, Cox JA and Lysko PG (1989): Neurotoxicity at the NMDA receptor in energy-compromised neurons. An hypothesis for cell death in aging and disease. *Ann NY Acad Sci* 568:225-233.

Nitsch RM, Slack BE, Wurtman RJ and Growdon JH (1992): Release of Alzheimer amyloid precursor derivatives stimulated by activation of muscarinic acetylcholine receptors. *Science* 258:304-307.

Nunn PB, Davis AJ and O'Brien P (1991): Carbamate formation and the neurotoxicity of L-a amino acids. *Science* 251:1619-1620.

Olney JW, Labruyere J and Price MT (1989): Pathological changes induced in cerebrocortical neurons by phencyclidine. *Science* 244:1360-1362.

Olney JW, Labruyere J, Wang G, Sesma MA, Wozniak DF and Price MT (1991): NMDA antagonist neurotoxicity: mechanism and protection. *Science* 254:1515-1518.

Olney JW, Zorumski C, Price MT and Labruyere J (1990):   L-Cysteine, a bicarbonate-sensitive endogenous excitotoxin. *Science* 248:596-599.

Perry TL, Krieger C, Hansen S and Tabatabaei A (1991): ALS: fasting plasma levels of cysteine and inorganic sulfate are normal, as are brain contents of cysteine. *Neurology* 41:487-490.

Price MT, Farber NB, Foster J and Olney JW (1994):   Tracing the circuitry that mediates NMDA antagonist neurotoxicity. *Soc Neurosci Abstr* (In Press).

Ross BD, Miller BL and Moats RA (1993): Alzheimer disease: Depiction of increased cerebral myo-inositol with proton MR spectroscopy. *Radiology* 187:433-437.

Weiss JH and Choi DW (1988):   Beta-N-methylamino-L-alanine neurotoxicity: Requirement for bicarbonate as a cofactor. *Science* 241:973-975.

Wenk GL, Walker LC, Price DL and Cork LC (1991): Loss of NMDA, but not GABA-A, binding in the brains of aged rats and monkeys. *Neurobiol Aging* 12:93-98.

Alzheimer Disease: Therapeutic Strategies
edited by E. Giacobini and R. Becker.
© 1994 Birkhäuser Boston

FREE INTRACELLULAR CALCIUM IN AGING AND ALZHEIMER'S DISEASE

Walter Müller, Anne Eckert, Henrike Hartmann and Hans Förstl
Departments of Psychopharmacology and Psychiatry,
Central Institute of Mental Health, D-68159 Mannheim, Germany

INTRODUCTION

According to the calcium hypothesis of brain aging, abnormal intracellular calcium homeostasis has been proposed to be involved in the pathology of Alzheimer's disease (AD) and multifarct dementia (MID). Since free intracellular calcium plays a key role in many cellular functions, imbalances in calcium regulation could finally lead to degeneration of neurons during aging and disease. Thus, pharmacological mechanisms controlling neuronal calcium homeostasis represent a major strategy for the development of new treatments of AD or other age-related disturbances of cognitive functions.

In man, the limitations of current *in vivo* neurochemical techniques, as well as ethical considerations, confine much of the research to the use of brain tissue obtained at autopsy. However, postmortem tissue can not be used for measurements of the free intracellular calcium concentration, $[Ca^{2+}]_i$. Therefore, the presence of a peripheral model that could reflect comparable changes in the central nervous system (CNS) and that would allow the study of disturbances of $[Ca^{2+}]_i$ in man would be highly desirable. Therefore, non-neuronal cells like lymphocytes or fibroblasts have been used to study directly alterations in cellular calcium regulation, because it is widely accepted that calcium also acts as second messenger of transmembrane signalling in these cell types.

AGE-RELATED CHANGES IN $[Ca^{2+}]_i$ IN PERIPHERAL CELLS

Only few data are presently available giving detailed information about specific characteristics of age-related changes in calcium homeostasis in peripheral cells (for reviews: Eckert et al., 1994a; Gibson and Peterson, 1987). In most cases, unaltered basal $[Ca^{2+}]_i$ in lymphocytes of aged humans was found. In contrast, Peterson et al. (1986) found a reduction of $[Ca^{2+}]_i$ in fibroblasts of old controls confirming findings of Toth et al. (1989) in lymphocytes. Stimulation of lymphocytes with mitogens or antibodies gave inconclusive results, since increase, decrease, and no alterations of $[Ca^{2+}]_i$ were found. The results from this small number of studies do not give a final answer about the possible direction of $[Ca^{2+}]_i$ changes in aged humans. Accordingly, based on our initial observations on specific age-related changes of Ca^{2+} homeostasis in dissociated neurons of the mouse brain (Hartmann and Müller, 1993; Hartmann et al., 1993a), our present strategy aims at demonstrating corresponding changes of intracellular Ca^{2+} regulation in mouse lymphocytes and even more important in human lymphocytes.

In intact brain cells of adult mice depolarization with KCl induced a fast increase in $[Ca^{2+}]_i$, which was significantly lower in brain cells of aged animals (Hartmann et al., 1993a).

In contrast to the results obtained in neurons, basal $[Ca^{2+}]_i$ in T-lymphocytes isolated from spleens of the aged mice was significantly increased (Hartmann et al., 1994a). Activation of T-cells with the mitogen phytohemagglutinin (PHA) resulted in a Ca^{2+} rise, which was reduced by aging similar to the significantly lower increase of $[Ca^{2+}]_i$ after activation of neurons. Measurements of basal $[Ca^{2+}]_i$ in human lymphocytes revealed no age difference. However, parallel to our findings in mouse lymphocytes, the PHA-induced Ca^{2+} rise was significantly lower in cells of aged subjects (Hartmann et al., 1994a). Similar to the reduced depolarization-induced Ca^{2+} influx in aged brain cells, age-related impairment of PHA-induced Ca^{2+} elevation in lymphocytes mainly affects the signal maintenance in the plateau phase dominated by Ca^{2+} influx.

AGE-RELATED CHANGES IN $[Ca^{2+}]_i$ IN AD

The available data in respect to AD are similarly controversial (for reviews: Eckert et al., 1994a, Gibson and Peterson, 1987). Findings about reduced $[Ca^{2+}]_i$ in fibroblasts of AD-patients by Peterson et al. (1986) could not be confirmed by Huang et al. (1991). However, Etcheberrigaray et al. (1993) reported that tetraethylammonium (TEA)-depolarization-induced elevation of $[Ca^{2+}]_i$ was reduced in fibroblasts of AD-patients.

Therefore, we compared $[Ca^{2+}]_i$ in lymphocytes of AD-patients and of age-matched controls. PHA-induced Ca^{2+} rise was not different (Hartmann et al., 1994a, Eckert et al., 1993b). Consistent with findings of Bondy et al. (1994) after stimulation with high concentration of PHA (100 μg/ml), no AD-specific alterations of $[Ca^{2+}]_i$ could be found. This is in contrast to experiments of Adunsky et al. (1991) who described a dramatically increased response in lymphocytes of AD-patients under these conditions. Taken together, our data do not suggest general alterations of Ca^{2+} homeostasis in AD.

DESTABILIZATION OF THE NEURONAL Ca²⁺ HOMEOSTASIS BY ß-AMYLOID

One of the most important markers of AD is the deposition of ß-amyloid. ß-Amyloid has recently been shown to possess neurotoxic properties, probably by destabilizing the cellular Ca^{2+} homeostasis (Mattson et al., 1992). Most previous findings have been obtained with neuronal cell cultures usually established from embryonic or fetal cells which differ in some respect from mature fully differentiated cells. Therefore, we investigated the effect of ß-amyloid on the neuronal Ca^{2+} homeostasis in fully differentiated brain cells from adult mice (Hartmann et al., 1993b).

A short preincubation of the cells with ß-amyloid in a concentration of 1 μM resulted in an amplification of the K^+-induced rise in $[Ca^{2+}]_i$ and led to higher levels in the plateau phase. ß-Amyloid alone did not influence basal $[Ca^{2+}]_i$. The effect of ß-amyloid on the Ca^{2+} homeostasis was specific for the biologically active fragment 25-35 (ßA25-35) and was also seen with the entire peptide 1-40. Preincubation with the fragments 1-28 or 12-28 resulted only in a slight, not significant amplification of the Ca^{2+}-response.

ß-AMYLOID ENHANCES THE PHA-INDUCED Ca²⁺ RESPONSE IN LYMPHOCYTES. SPECIFIC CHANGES IN ALZHEIMER'S DISEASE

Confirming our findings using dissociated neurons from the adult mouse, the Ca^{2+} regulation in human lymphocytes is affected by ß-amyloid in a similar fashion (Eckert et al., 1993a). Accordingly, the lymphocyte seems to be a suitable model to study ß-amyloid's effects on calcium signalling in man and especially in AD patients.

In a preliminary study, we used this model to examine the Ca^{2+}-amplifying effect of ß-amyloid on lymphocytes in AD. Surprisingly, the ß-amyloid sensitivity was strongly reduced in the AD group (Eckert et al., 1993b). In the meantime, we have confirmed this observation for a much larger group of AD patients (Eckert et al., 1994b). This observation is not merely an effect of aging, since the ß-amyloid effect is not different between young and aged non-demented controls. There is, however, some overlap between groups. While only very few AD patients had normal responses, several of the non-demented controls showed low responses to the Ca^{2+} amplifying effect of ßA25-35. The difference between patients and controls is highly significant, which suggests that the lymphocyte response to the Ca^{2+} amplifying effect of ßA25-35 may represent a potential marker for AD.

If one accepts the ßA25-35 effect on lymphocyte $[Ca^{2+}]_i$ as a model for its neurotoxic properties on central neurons, the present observation of a highly significant reduction of this effect in AD is unexpected. It suggests that the assumption of a direct relationship between ßA4 formation, neurotoxicity, and *neurodegeneration* may be an oversimplification. Obviously, additional mechanisms need to be considered. Our preliminary data strongly suggest ApoE ε4 allele frequency as one possible factor leading to low ßA25-35 responses, since reduced sensitivity to ßA25-35 is significantly more pronounced in patients heterozygotic or homozygotic for ApoE ε4 (Eckert et al., 1994b). Obviously, ApoE ε4 allele dose but also other not yet identified factors are similarly associated with low Ca^{2+} responses to ßA25-35 as well as with the disease.

In the periphery, ApoE ε4 allele frequency seems to be associated with higher plasma cholesterol levels, but lower ApoE plasma levels. However, we did not see significant differences of plasma cholesterol between patients and controls or correlations between plasma cholesterol and the Ca^{2+} responses to ßA25-35. Moreover, ApoE is the only lipoprotein present in the brain, where it is involved in the mobilization and redistribution of cholesterol in growth, maintenance, and repair of myelin and neuronal membranes during development but also after injury. Preincubation with cholesterol significantly decreases the Ca^{2+} amplifying effect of ßA25-35 on central neurons of the mouse and human lymphocytes (Hartmann et al., 1994b). Specific changes of the structure of neuronal membranes in AD affected brain areas are well documented. Some of these changes can be explained by a specific reduction of the cholesterol content and can be normalized by experimentally elevating the cholesterol levels (Mason et al., 1992). Based on our findings we would like to formulate the hypothesis of an enhanced ßA4 neurotoxicity in cholesterol low areas like cortical grey matter. In conclusion, our data suggest the modulation of ß-amyloid neurotoxicity by cholesterol as a possible link between AD pathology and ApoE polymorphism. If this hypothesis can be further experimentally supported, it will have important implications for the development of future treatments of AD.

ACKNOWLEDGEMENTS

This study was supported by grants of the Deutsche Forschungsgemeinschaft, SFB 258, projects K2 and A3, and by the Forschungsfond Fakultät Mannheim.

REFERENCES

Adunsky A, Baram D, Hershkowitz M and Mekori YA (1991): Increased cytosolic free calcium in lymphocytes of Alzheimer patients. *J Neuroimmunol* 33:167-172.

Bondy B, Klages U, Müller-Spahn F and Hock C (1994): Cytosolic free $[Ca^{2+}]$ in mononuclear blood cells from demented patients and healthy controls. *Eur Arch Psychiatry Clin Neurosci* 243:224-228.

Eckert A, Hartmann H and Müller WE (1993a): ß-Amyloid protein enhances the mitogen-induced calcium response in circulating human lymphocytes. *FEBS Lett* 330:49-52.

Eckert A, Förstl H, Hartmann H and Müller WE (1993b): Decreased ß-amyloid sensitivity in Alzheimer's disease. *Lancet* 342:805-806.

Eckert A, Hartmann H, Förstl H and Müller WE (1994a): Alterations of intracellular calcium regulation during aging and Alzheimer's disease in non-neuronal cells. *Life Sci* (In Press).

Eckert A, Förstl H, Hartmann H, Czech C, Mönning U, Beyreuther K and Müller WE (1994b): The amplifying effect of ß-amyloid on cellular calcium signalling is reduced in Alzheimer's disease: possible relationship to apolipoprotein E polymorphism (Submitted).

Etcheberrigaray R, Ito E, Oka K, Tofel-Grehl B, Gibson GE and Alkon DL (1993): Potassium channel dysfunction in fibroblasts identifies patients with Alzheimer's disease. *Proc Natl Aca Sci USA* 90:8209-8213.

Gibson GE and Peterson C (1987): Calcium and the aging nervous system. *Neurobiol Aging* 8:329-343.

Hartmann H and Müller WE (1993): Age-related changes in receptor-mediated and depolarization-induced phosphatidylinositol turnover in mouse brain. *Brain Res* 622:86-92.

Hartmann H, Eckert A and Müller WE (1993a): Aging enhances the calcium sensitivity of central neurons of the mouse as an adaptive response to reduced free intracellular calcium. *Neurosci Lett* 152:181-184.

Hartmann H, Eckert A and Müller WE (1993b): ß-amyloid protein amplifies calcium signalling in central neurons from the adult mouse. *Biochem Biophys Res Commun* 194:1216-1220.

Hartmann H, Eckert A and Müller WE (1994a): Similar age-related changes of free intracellular calcium in lymphocytes and central neurons: effects of Alzheimer's disease. *Eur Arch Psychiatry Clin Neurosci* 243:218-223.

Hartmann H, Eckert A and Müller WE (1994b): Apolipoprotein E and cholesterol affect neuronal calcium signalling. The possible relationship to ß-amyloid neurotoxicity. *Biochem Biophys Res Comm* 200:1185-1192.

Huang HM, Toral-Borza L, Thaler H, Tofel-Grehl B and Gibson GE (1991): Inositol phosphates and intracellular calcium after bradykinin stimulation in fibroblasts from young, aged and Alzheimer's donors. *Neurobiol Aging* 2:469-473.

Mason RP, Shopemaker WJ, Shajenko L, Chambers TE and Herbette LG (1992): Evidence for changes in the Alzheimer's disease brain cortical membrane structure mediated by cholesterol. *Neurobiol Aging* 13:413-419.

Mattson MP, Cheng B, Davies D, Bryant K, Lieberburg I and Rydel RE (1992): ß-amyloid peptides destabilize calcium homeostasis and render human cortical neurons vulnerable to exocitotoxicity. *J Neurosci* 12:376-389.

Peterson C, Rattan RR, Shelanski ML and Goldman JE (1986): Cytosolic free calcium and cell spreading decrease in fibroblasts from aged and Alzheimer donors. *Proc Natl Acad Sci USA* 83:7999-8001.

Toth S, Csermely P, Beregi E, Szkladanyi and Szabo LD (1989): Decreased cytosolic free calcium concentration of aged human lymphocytes in resting state. *Compr Gerontol Suppl Issue A + B* 3:16-22.

Alzheimer Disease: Therapeutic Strategies
edited by E. Giacobini and R. Becker.
© 1994 Birkhäuser Boston

NITRIC OXIDE SYNTHASE IN A
LESION MODEL OF ALZHEIMER'S DISEASE

Kiminobu Sugaya and Michael McKinney
Mayo Clinic Jacksonville, Jacksonville, FL

INTRODUCTION

Basal forebrain cholinergic neurons degenerate in Alzheimer's disease (AD), but the prominent cholinergic groups of the upper brainstem have been reported to be preserved in this disease (Woolf et al., 1989). While the etiology of cell death in AD is unknown, excitotoxic and/or oxidative mechanisms may explain part of it (Jeandel et al., 1989; Pappolla et al., 1992). Although such mechanisms themselves may not be part of the initiating event(s) in neurodegeneration of AD, they may contribute significantly. It seems possible that the observed differential vulnerability of rostral and caudal cholinergic cells in AD may be explained by differential tolerance for oxidative stress, and that this might relate to their differential expression of protection mechanisms against free radicals. Degeneration of neurons in AD may not be due to a sudden release of glutamate or radicals; more likely it is the involvement of a slowly evolving process that would stress more vulnerable neuronal populations. One possibility is that an on-going activation of neuroglia could secondarily lead to slow neuronal death. Neuroglia are known to release both growth promoting factors and cytotoxic agents after injury to the brain. One of these toxic agents may be nitric oxide (NO).

Nitric oxide is a free radical postulated to act as a neurotransmitter, neuromodulator, or second messenger molecule in many physiological systems (Moncada et al., 1991). However, the NO radical can react with the superoxide anion, to eventually produce the hydroxyl anion, which may be the immediate cause of protein and lipid damage in free radical toxicity (Carley-Usmar et al., 1992). Two major types of NO-generating enzymes have been described thus far, distinguished by dependency of their activity on calcium ion and calmodulin. The Ca^{2+}-independent, cytokine-inducible enzyme (i-NOS) is found in macrophages and other nonneuronal cells while the Ca^{2+}/calmodulin-regulated enzyme (c-NOS) is constitutively expressed in brain neurons and several types of non-neural cells. c-NOS is considered to be represented by NADPH-diaphorase histochemical activity (Hope et al., 1991) and it is known that some classes of NADPH-diaphorase neurons survive in AD (Hyman et al., 1992) or after lesion (Boegman and Parent, 1988).   The resistance of c-NOS-expressing neurons to degeneration may be because they contain biochemical protective mechanisms, perhaps higher amounts of superoxide dismutase or other oxygen metabolizing enzymes, to protect themselves against self-induced damage by this free radical or a metabolite of it (cf. Dawson et al., 1993).   Alternatively, neurons with less robust expression of such protective systems might be more vulnerable to free radical toxicity.

In this study, we examined the expression levels of c-NOS, superoxide dismutase (SOD) and beta-amyloid precursor protein (BAPP) mRNAs after an excitotoxic lesion of rat brain using ibotenic acid.   The expression of these mRNAs were examined using a method combining *in situ* hybridization histochemistry (ISHH) with immunocytochemistry for choline acetyltransferase (ChAT) and NADPH-diaphorase in the same sections.

MATERIALS AND METHODS

Small (100-500 bp) fragments of cDNA unique for each of the genes, were amplified by PCR, ligated into vectors, and transformed into competent cells. Inserts were verified by sequencing (fmol DNA Sequencing System, Promega). [^{35}S]-riboprobes were transcribed from recombinant vectors using RNA polymerases and [^{35}S]-UTP (DuPont/New England Nuclear), after linearizing the plasmid.

Coronal rat brain sections (25 μm) were incubated with 2.5 μg/ml of anti-ChAT monoclonal antibody (Boehringer-Mannheim).   Visualization of the antibody was performed with a Vectastain kit (Vector Laboratories) according to the manufacturer's instructions, using diaminobenzidine as the substrate. NADPH diaphorase staining was performed after ChAT immunostaining by incubating sections with 1 mg/ml beta-NADPH and 0.1 mg/ml nitroblue tetrazolium in 0.1 M phosphate buffer (pH 7.4) containing 0.3% Triton X-100 for 60 min at room temperature (RT).

Choline acetyltransferase immuno- and NADPH-diaphorase-stained brain sections were treated with proteinase K followed by acetylation.   The sections were prehybridized with 50% formamide, 1X Denhardt's Solution, 10% dextran sulfate, 4X SSC, 0.25 mg/ml yeast tRNA, 0.3 mg/ml herring sperm DNA and 100 mM dithiothreitol for 1 hr at 60°C.   Hybridization was in the same buffer with 10^7 cpm/ml [^{35}S]-riboprobe for 18 hr at 60°C in a sealed humidified container.   After hybridization the sections were washed and treated with RNase to reduce background.   Sections were mounted onto glass slides and juxtaposed to Amersham Hyperfilm Beta-Max X-ray film for 3 days.   For emulsion coating, the brain sections were defatted, dipped in Kodak NTB-2 (diluted 1:1 with 0.6 M ammonium acetate) and stored in sealed boxes at 4°C for 1 week. After development, the sections were lightly counter-stained with cresyl violet. Both macro- and micro-autoradiograph images were analyzed by NIH image on a Quadra 840AV (Apple).

RESULTS AND DISCUSSION

In the cholinergic cell groups of basal forebrain, ChAT-immunostained cells expressed varying levels of c-NOS mRNA. Most of c-NOS-positive neurons were in the vertical limbs of diagonal band (DBV), the medial septum (MS), and the substantia innominata (SI). Notably, c-NOS-positive cells were essentially absent in nucleus basalis magnocellularis (NBM). Figure 1 is a composite of population distribution plots of frequencies of cells expressing differing levels of NOS grain densities in the five subgroups of the basal forebrain cholinergic complex. Very low fractions of the populations of ChAT-positive neurons in the NBM and horizontal limbs of diagonal band (DBH) possessed c-NOS mRNA. However, the DBV, MS and SI contained fractions of ChAT-positive cells expressing moderate levels of c-NOS mRNA. The two major cholinergic groups of the upper brainstem, the laterodorsal tegmental nucleus (LDTN) and the pedunculopontine tegmental nucleus (PPTN) exhibited the most intense expression of c-NOS mRNA in the brain (Fig. 2). Less than 5% of the ChAT-positive cells in NBM and DBH, but about 30% of the ChAT-positive cells in DBV and MS, and 56% of the ChAT-positive cells in SI expressed c-NOS mRNA at least five times background levels (20 grains/cell) while, all the ChAT stained cells in LDTN and PPTN expressed more than this level of c-NOS mRNA (Fig. 3).

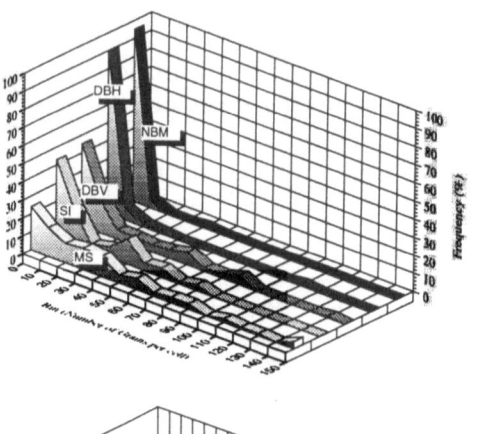

FIGURE 1. Histogram of the population of silver grain on rostral ChAT immuno-satined neurons in brain NOS mRNA micro-autoradiography ISHH. Reprinted with permission of Elsevier Science B.V. from Sugaya K (1994): Molecular Brain Research, Vol. 23, 111-125.

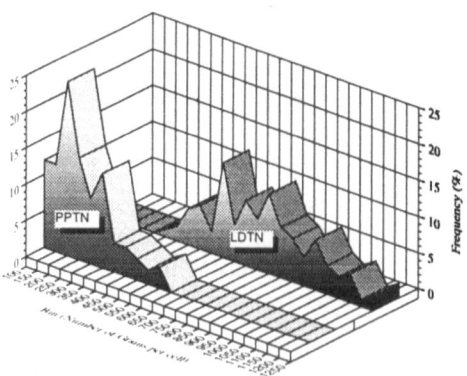

FIGURE 2. Histogram of the population of silver grain on upper brainstem ChAT immuno-satined neurons in brain NOS mRNA micro-autoradiography ISHH. Reprinted with permission of Elsevier Science B.V. from Sugaya K (1994): Molecular Brain Research, Vol. 23, 111-125.

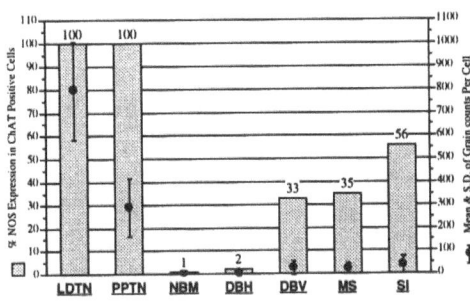

FIGURE 3. The percentage of NOS mRNA expression cells among cholinergic(ChAT-positive) neurons in different nuclei (Bar graph, left Y-axis). We set the threshold of silver grain counts at a level of 5 times background. Also plotted are the average ± standard deviations of NOS mRNA silver grain counts per cell in each nucleus (Line Graph, right Y-axis). Reprinted with permission of Elsevier Science B.V. from Sugaya K (1994): Molecular Brain Research, Vol. 23, 111-125.

Many data support a hypothesis of involvement of free radicals in the aging process (Cutler, 1991), and given the fact that NO has been shown under some conditions to be neurotoxic, some neurodegenerative aspects of brain disease or biological aging may be linked to aberrant NO production. However, paradoxically, NADPH diaphorase-positive neurons have been shown to be more resistant to lesioning with excitatory amino acids (Boegman and Parent, 1988) and to the degeneration in AD (Hyman et al., 1992). These results support the speculation that NOS-expressed neurons may possess robust protection systems against free radicals. This hypothesis holds that, if NO is involved in cell loss in AD, those cholinergic neurons that are NOS-positive should be relatively preserved. The biochemical protective mechanism(s) postulated to exist in NOS-positive neurons are undefined at this time, but candidates would include systems for trapping or disposing of superoxide and/or NO.

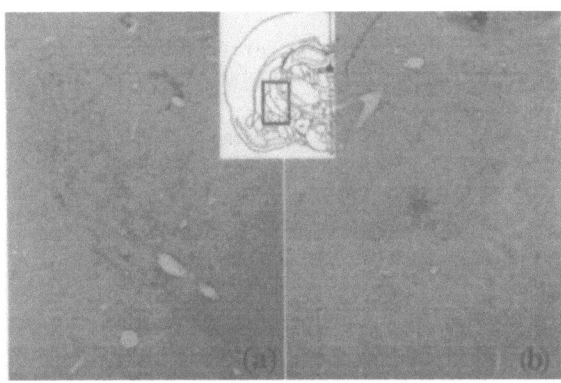

FIGURE 4. NADPH-diaphorase activity after NBM lesion. (a) lesion hemisphere. (b) intact hemisphere. The Box in upper panel shows the pictured area.

After an ibotenic lesion of the rat NBM, we observed an increase in NADPH diaphorase activity without a corresponding increase c-NOS mRNA expression (Fig. 4). Cu/Zn-SOD and BAPP mRNA were also expressed at higher levels in the cerebral cortex of the lesion hemisphere than in the contralateral site (data not shown).   SOD activity is elevated after ischemia (Sutherland et al., 1991) and in aging brain (DeHaan et al., 1992), and BAPP immunoreactivity has been shown to elevate in reactive astrocytes following neuronal damage (Siman et al., 1989).   Thus, our results may indicate the expression of i-NOS, the induction of protective systems and the activation of glia.

Activated microglia can kill neurons in co-culture by their formation of NO (Chao et al., 1992).   The delayed neuronal death after ischemia has also been ascribed to NO production by microglia and macrophages (Lees, 1993).   Thus, delayed cell death after ibotenic acid lesion may relate to the induction of i-NOS in activated glia.   The activation of glia is presumably a part of self-defense responses that probably has some beneficial consequences, e.g. the production of growth factors.   However, chronic glial activation may produce detrimental effects which could involve NO production.

CONCLUSION

The neuropathology of cholinergic neurons in AD parallels the NOS phenotype: the NBM and other rostral cholinergic groups degenerate, while the NOS-rich brainstem groups are preserved.   We hypothesize that certain NOS-negative cholinergic neurons may be vulnerable in AD and that part of neurodegeneration may be caused by induction of i-NOS in the activated microglia in AD.

ACKNOWLEDGMENTS

We thank Dr. S.H. Snyder for the gift of rat brain NOS cDNA.   This work was supported by the Mayo Foundation and by NIA grant AG09973.

REFERENCES

Boegman RJ and Parent A (1988):   Differential sensitivity of neuropeptide Y, somatostatin and NADPH-diaphorase containing neurons in rat cortex and striatum to quinolinic acid. *Brain Res* 445:358-362.

Carley-Usmar V, Hogg N, O'Leary V, Wilson M and Moncada S (1992):   The simultaneous generation of superoxide and nitric oxide can initiate lipid peroxidation in human low density lipoprotein. *Free Rad Res Comms* 17:9-20.

Chao C, Hu S, Molitor T, Shaskan E and Peterson P (1992):   Activated microglia mediate neuronal cell injury via a nitric oxide mechanism. *J Immunol* 149:2736-2741.

Cutler RG (1991):   Antioxidants and aging. *Am J Clin Nutr* 53:373S-379S.

Dawson VL, Dawson TM, Bartley DA, Uhl GR and Snyder SH (1993):   Mechanisms of nitric oxide-mediated neurotoxicity in primary brain cultures. *J Neuroscience* 13:2651-2661.

DeHaan JB, Newman JD and Kola I (1992):   Cu/Zn superoxide dismutase mRNA and enzyme activity, and susceptibility to lipid peroxidation, increases with aging in murine brains. *Mol Brain Res* 13:179-187.

Hope BT, Michael GJ, Knigge KM and Vincent SR (1991):   Neuronal NADPH diaphorase is a nitric oxide synthase. *Proc Natl Acad Sci USA* 88:2811-2814.

Hyman B, Marzloff K, Wenniger J, Dawson T, Bredt D and Snyder S (1992): Relative sparing of nitric oxide synthase-containing neurons in the hippocampal formation in Alzheimer's disease. *Ann Neurol* 32:818-820.

Jeandel C, Nicolas MB, Dubois F, Nabet-Belleville F, Penin F and Cuny G (1989): Lipid peroxidation and free radical scavengers in Alzheimer's disease. *Gerontology* 35:275-282.

Lees G (1993): The possible contribution of microglia and macrophages to delayed neuronal death after ischemia. *J Neurol Sci* 114:119-122.

Moncada S, Palmer RMJ and Higgs EA (1991): Nitric oxide: physiology, pathophysiology, and pharmacology. *Pharmacol Rev* 43:109-142.

Pappolla MA, Omar RA, Kim KS and Robakis NK (1992): Immunohistochemical evidence of antioxidant stress in Alzheimer's disease. *Amer J Pathol* 140:621-628.

Siman R, Card JP, Nelson RB and Davis LG (1989): Expression of beta-amyloid precursor protein in reactive astrocytes following neuronal damage. *Neuron* 3:275-85.

Sutherland G, Bose R, Louw D and Pinsky C (1991): Global elevation of brain superoxide dismutase activity following forebrain ischemia in rat. *Neurosci Lett* 128:169-172.

Woolf NJ, Jacobs RW and Butcher LL (1989): The pontomesencephalotegmental cholinergic system does not degenerate in Alzheimer's disease. *Neurosci Lett* 96:277-282.

PART XI

ANTIOXIDANT, PROTECTIVE, AND ANTI-INFLAMMATORY AGENTS IN AD THERAPY

Alzheimer Disease: Therapeutic Strategies
edited by E. Giacobini and R. Becker.
© 1994 Birkhäuser Boston

ANTIOXIDANT DRUGS AS NEUROPROTECTIVE AGENTS

Elena B. Burlakova
Department of Kinetics of Chemical and Biological Processes, Institute of
Chemical Physics, Moscow, Russia

Antioxidants [AO] administered into the animal inhibit lipid peroxidation [LPO] and decrease the concentration of peroxides and other oxidation products. The LPO rate, in its turn, is related to the rate of membrane lipid exchange and affects both lipid content and fluidity of the membrane lipid bilayer.

Thus, the LPO increase accelerates the removal of easily oxidizable unsaturated lipids resulting in a higher resistance of lipids to oxidation and a lower lipid fluidity.

These changes lead to a lower consumption of AO with a subsequent rise of their concentration and a decreased LPO rate which returns to normal. Hence, the relation between LPO rate and change in lipid content serves as a regulatory function and maintains the LPO rate at a stationary level.

Membranous proteins, enzymes, receptors and channel-forming proteins are known to be lipid-dependent. Their activity, sensitivity to regulation, substrate specificity and other properties depend on the lipid bilayer fluidity, peroxide amount, content of lipids acting as cofactors, allosteric activators and inhibitors. In this respect, as confirmed in numerous studies, changes of biochemical and biophysical parameters of a membrane lipid component, AO would also affect the activity of enzymes and receptors and the cellular metabolism in normal and pathological states (Burlakova and Khrapova, 1985).

The AO effect on cellular metabolism doesn't confine itself to inhibit lipid peroxidation processes and change in lipid content but also directly modifies fluidity. Antioxidants administered at doses lower than 10^{-7}M are practically unable to inhibit lipid peroxidation (the constants of interaction between AO and lipid peroxide radicals are 10^6 L/Ms or lower). They directly incorporate into the lipid bilayer and, as a result, affect the functional activity of cellular membranes.

There are some data in the literature (Khokhlov et al., 1989) showing that antioxidants bind to membranous proteins. However, it is still unclear if these proteins serve as AO specific receptors and in which ways signal transduction exists. Studies on this problem are missing. It has been shown that a number of antioxidants can directly activate or inhibit the activity of membranous enzymes. In this case, the AO concentration is substantially higher (10^{-5}-10^{-2}M) (Khokhlov et al., 1989). Thus, there are several ways for AO to affect membranous proteins through either receptors or enzymes.

Antioxidants can exhibit a protective effect when reacting with free radicals (Burlakova and Khrapova, 1985). As a rule, the action of various damaging agents enhances peroxidation of membrane lipids and to a certain extent it is a pathogenetic factor.

Contrary to some other protectors (i.e. the known radioprotectors) AO have an ability not only to protect cells from damaging factors, but also to normalize cellular metabolism disturbed by these agents or affected by pathological processes.

Lets consider some examples illustrating the above mentioned effects in neurons.

Dibunol and phenozan are the compounds most studied by us among antioxidants as neuroprotectors and neuromodulators. These substances belong to the class of screened phenols, the constants of their reactions with peroxide radicals (K7) being 1-3 x 10^{+4} L/Ms.

Due to LPO inhibition, AO at the doses of 10^{-3}-10^{-4}M affect content and fluidity of membrane lipids (see Table I) (Molochkina et al., 1990; Molochkina et al., 1992). The experiments on phenozan show the presence of membranous receptors, the content and activity of which differ for various organs. For brain synaptic membrane a dissociation constant of the phenozan complex with high affinity receptors is 4 x 10^{-10} and with low affinity - 6.8 x 10^{-9}M (Khokhlov et al., 1989). Both phenozan and dibunol produce a direct effect on the viscosity of synaptosome lipids incorporated into the membrane. They start to exhibit this action at doses of 10^{-9}-10^{-10}M.

The protective effect of phenozan and dibunol is determined by their action on biochemical and biophysical parameters of synaptic membranes. These antioxidants protect the rats (KM line) from epileptic seizures caused by sound irritants. The duration of the latency period (the preseizure period) increases by 2-4 times, its intensity decreasing by 1.5-3 times (Burlakova, 1989). These drugs also protect the rats of the same line from insults caused by multiple sound irritation. The efficacy of dibunol and phenozan correlates with their antioxidative activity. Antioxidants are also effective in treatment of insults. Dibunol and phenozan protect animals from brain ischemia, senescence (Burlakova et al., 1976), toxic action of cholinolitics and other disturbance factors (i.e. irradiation) and improve memory (Burlakova, 1989).

The mechanism of protection of dibunol and phenozan at doses of 10^{-4}-10^{-6}M is understandable in terms of the above relationship between rate of lipid peroxidation, content change, lipid fluidity and activity of enzymes and receptors (see Table I). Administration of AO induces simultaneous changes in GABA-, serotonin- and cholinergic-systems. This result can be explained by the fact that the receptor activity depends on lipid surrounding. Content and fluidity and AO are universal modifiers of these membrane properties.

Phospholipid mkg/mg prot	a		b	
	Control	Dibunol	Control	Dibunol
Lisophospha-tidylcholine			1.1 ± 0.1	1.7 ± 0.2
Sphingo myeline	2.2 ± 0.7	4.5 ± 0.4	0.8 ± 0.1	1.1 ± 0.1
Phosphatidyl-choline	6.2 ± 0.9	10.8 ± 1.8	10.1 ± 0.9	16.9 ± 1.7
Phosphatidyl-inositol + Phosphatidyl-serine	2.6 ± 0.7	6.8 ± 0.5	2.8 ± 0.3	5.3 ± 0.4
Phosphatidyl-ethanolamine	5.6 ± 0.3	9.8 ± 0.5	8.7 ± 0.9	13.5 ± 1.4
Cardiolipin + Phosphatidic acid	2.0 ± 0.2	2.2 ± 0.6	0.9 ± 0.1	3.2 ± 0.3
Microviscos-ity $\tau_c \times 10^{10}$ sec	2.5 ± 0.5	1.4 ± 0.3	2.5 ± 0.2	4.4 ± 0.4
Monoamino oxidase K_m	$(4.0 \pm 0.1) \times 10^{-4}$	$(2.8 \pm 0.6) \times 10^{-4}$		
Monoamine oxidase V_m	126 ± 3	85 ± 4		
Acetylcholin-esterase K_m, M			2.5×10^{-5}	5.6×10^{-5}
Acetylcholin-esterase V_m, r.u.			0.5	0.6
Adenylate cyclase (activity bM/mg prot min)			22.2 ± 3.2	79.7 ± 8.5

TABLE I. Changes in lipid phase and activity of membrane-bound enzymes in mice brain mitochondrial outer membrane (a) and in Wistar rat brain synaptosomes (b) 18 hr after intraperitoneal administration of dibunol.

Administration of AO activates the neurotransmitter system if higher values of lipid fluidity are necessary for receptor activity, the effectors of these receptors being easy oxidizable lipids (phosphatidylserine, phosphatidylinositol, phosphatidylethanolamine). When the effectors are hard-oxidizable lipids (sphingomyelin, phosphatidylcholine) and receptors or if a membrane enzyme requires a more rigid state of a lipid bilayer, the system shows a lower activity (Borovok et al., 1988; Chernyavskaya et al., 1989; Molochkina et al., 1990).

Among the new tendencies in AO applications are their usage at ultra-low doses (10^{-13}-10^{-18}M) and creation of antioxidant-based complex "hybrid" molecules containing an antioxidant residue and a specific part of the molecule with a high affinity to a certain receptor.

The mechanism of AO action at ultra-low doses is unknown. It is still impossible to clearly define the critical target for AO at ultra-low doses and the mechanism of signal intensification. It is very important that AO at such ultra-low doses change cell sensitivity to other factors of chemical and physical nature, as well as exogenous and endogenous regulators.

Phenozan administered into rat at 10^{-17}-10^{-15}M changes lipid composition and microviscosity of synaptosome. It increases K_m and V_m of acetylcholinesterase, sensitivity of cholinergic system, improves memory and decreases efficacy of barbiturate action.

Substance	Concentration	Effect of AChE activity
Phenozan	3×10^{-15} - 0.5×10^{-4}M	No significant influence
Acetylcholine	10^{-15}-1.7×10^{-4}M	No significant influence competitive inhibition (1.6-fold increase of K_m) $K1 = 2.8 \times 10^{-4}$M (dissociation constant of substrate-inhibitor complex)
"Hybrid" substance ICHPHAN-10	5×10^{-5}M	Mixed inhibition (1.4-fold increase of K_m, 1.5-fold decrease of V_{max}); $K1 = 5.1 \times 10^{-5}$M; $K1' = 1.1 \times 10^{-4}$M (dissociation constant of enzyme-substrate-inhibitor complex)

TABLE II. Influence of "hybrid" compound (antioxidant phenozan + acetylcholine) on purified water-soluble acetylcholinesterase activity (hydrolysis of acetylcholine)

We can state that according to behavioral tests, older animals are more sensitive to phenozan at 10^{-15}M than younger ones. We suggest that these properties can be used in the treatment of diseases such as Parkinson or Alzheimer.

In conclusion, we present results on a hybrid molecule based on phenozan and an acetylcholine residues (Braginskaya, 1992). Contrary to phenozan, the drug actively inhibits acetylcholinesterase (Table II) and at the same time acts as phenozan by changing membrane content and structure and increasing the sensitivity of the cholinergic system.

We feel that a successful application of AO as neuroprotectors will be achieved by creating hybrid molecules and studying AO action at ultra-low doses.

REFERENCES

Borovok NV, Molochkina EM, Dubinskaya NI, Burlakova EB (1988): Lipid component of mice brain synaptosomes modulates activity of serotoninergic system. *Neirokhimia* 7:178-187.

Braginskaya FI, Zorina OM, Molochkina EM, Nikiforov GA, Burlakova EB (1992): Synthetic antioxidants - inhibitors of acetylcholinesterase activity. *Izvestiya Akademii Nauk Ser Biol* 5:690-698.

Burlakova EB, Khrapova NG (1985): Lipid peroxidation in membrane and natural antioxidants. *Uspekhi Khimii* LIV:1540-1558.

Burlakova EB, Molochkina EM, Palmina NP, Slepukhina LV (1976): Alteration in the antioxidative activity of lipids in scenescence. *Voprosy Medicinskoi Khimii* 22:541-546.

Burlakova EB (1989): Role of membrane lipids in transfer and storage information. *Studia Biophysica* 132:63-68.

Cherniavskaya LI, Arkhipova GV, Burlakova EB (1989): Changes in content and physico-chemical properties of rat brain lipids as reason of different sensitivity of CNS of animals to various factors. *Neirokhimiya* 8:249-258.

Khokhlov AP, Yarygin KN, Burlakova EB (1989): Synthetic phenolic antioxidants as polifunctional modulators of biological membranes. *Biologicheskie membrany* 6:133-142.

Molochkina EM, Borovok NV, Burlakova EB (1990): Changes of mice brain mitochondrial outer membrane lipid phase and kinetic properties of membrane-bound monoamine oxidase (MAO) after the administration of an antioxidant *in vivo*. *Neirokhimiya* 9:57-67.

Molochkina EM, Borovok NV, Burlakova EB (1992): Modification of the neural membrane lipid phase by antioxidants as a method to direct membrane functional activities (by example of synaptosomal acetylcholinesterase and phospholipase A_2). *Biologicheskie membrany* 5:1704-1707.

Alzheimer Disease: Therapeutic Strategies
edited by E. Giacobini and R. Becker.
© 1994 Birkhäuser Boston

IMMUNE MECHANISMS IN SENILE PLAQUE FORMATION

Patrick L. McGeer, Douglas G. Walker, Osamu Yasuhara, Andis Klegeris and Edith G. McGeer
Kinsmen Laboratory of Neurological Research,
University of British Columbia, Vancouver, B.C., Canada

Alzheimer disease (AD) is characterized by the appearance of two very different lesions, senile plaques and neurofibrillary tangles (NFTs). The pathological process which causes the disease must be responsible for both, but how they are linked is still a mystery. Neurofibrillary tangles develop intracellularly and involve the appearance of abnormally phosphorylated forms of tau. Senile plaques develop extracellularly with the deposition of beta-amyloid protein (BAP), a component of the larger amyloid precursor protein (APP). Neurofibrillary tangles are not unique to AD. They appear in a number of degenerative neurological diseases in which senile plaques are absent. This is an argument against NFTs causing the appearance of senile plaques. Conversely, extracellular deposits of BAP occur in areas where NFTs do not develop, indicating that BAP deposits, by themselves, do not cause NFTs. However, when senile plaques "mature", dystrophic neurites which contain abnormally phosphorylated tau are always present. Thus, it is possible that NFTs evolve from developing senile plaques.

Recently (Yasuhara et al., 1994), we have identified in the neocortex of elderly normals a form of senile plaque in which the BAP is consolidated into a thioflavine-S-positive form, but where the dystrophic neurites are globular in shape and do not contain abnormal forms of tau. Tangled neurons are not found in such areas. It is therefore possible to postulate the following sequence of events in the pathogenesis of AD: Diffuse deposits ➡ Benign plaques ➡ Classical plaques ➡ Neuronal death. If this hypothesis is true, then the central pathology of AD must center around those elements which gather in the evolving senile plaques.

Many proteins have already been identified which gather in diffuse BAP deposits and senile plaques and there is reason to believe that many more will be found in the future. Those that have been identified to date already provide the framework of an hypothesis of AD pathogenesis, including possible routes for its prevention and treatment.

Table I lists a few of the many extracellular proteins that have been reported as being associated with senile plaques.   Unfortunately, it is not certain at precisely which stage in plaque evolution many of them appear.

ß-Amyloid protein (BAP)	*Proteases*	*Acute Phase*
	α1-Trypsin	Heat shock protein
Complement Proteins	Cathepsin B & D	Amyloid P
C1q		
C3d*, C3c*	*Protease Inhibitors*	*Proteoglycans*
C4d*	α1-Antichymotrypsin	HSPG
	α1-Antitrypsin	CSPG
Complement Inhibitors	α2-Macroglobulin	DSPG
C1 inhibitor	Protease nexin I	
C4-binding protein		*Growth Factors*
Vitronectin*	*Other Enzymes*	bFGF
Clusterin	AChE	TGFb-1
Protectin	BChE	Midkine
	PKC(a)(bII)	
Coagulation Factors		*Other*
Tissue factor	*Receptors*	Apolipoprotein E
Thrombin*	EGFR	Lactoferrin
Hageman factor	α2-MacroglobulinR	ICAM-1*

TABLE I.   Some Extracellular Molecules Reported in Amyloid Deposits.   * proteins which are ligands for surface receptors on microglia, the resident immune cells of the brain.

Microglia have a resting, ramified appearance in diffuse amyloid deposits, similar to their morphology in normal tissue. In senile plaques, however, they agglomerate and display the enlarged cytoplasm and thickened processes of reactive microglia.

A prominent feature of amyloid deposits is accumulation of complement proteins of the classical pathway, while complement receptors are richly present on microglial surfaces. Thus, stimulation of microglial cells can occur through a ligand-receptor interaction involving complement.

Complement is a complex series of proteins designed to amplify the efferent arm of the immune system.   There are two pathways, but only proteins associated with the classical pathway have been identified in AD lesions. The classical pathway is divided into two parts: the first opsonizes tissue, the second assembles a lipophilic molecule known as the membrane attack complex (MAC). The opsonizing components are designed to identify and fix targets for phagocytosis. The MAC is designed to destroy foreign invaders such as bacteria and certain viruses by damaging their external membrane. It is the complement system which gives effect to antibodies generated by the afferent arm of the immune system. Antibodies attach loosely to their target antigens, but it is the complement system which fixes the target and amplifies the signal. If complement is persistently activated by antibodies against the host's own tissues, or by any other means, then the equivalent of a chronic, incurable infection occurs. It is this situation which appears to exist in AD.

The classical complement pathway is activated when C1q binds to its target, leading to dissociation of the C1 complex and activation of the pathway. The target is normally the Fc chain of IgG molecules conformationally modified by binding to antigen. However, several molecules found in senile plaques are capable of binding to C1q, thus activating the classical pathway. These include BAP itself, amyloid P, thrombin, and the Hageman factor.

All extracellular deposits of BAP, whether diffuse or consolidated, show the presence of C1q. Thus, complement activation must be an early event associated with the appearance of extracellular BAP.

The complement cascade continues through a number of proteolytic steps, which also provide amplification, to the opsonizing molecules C4b and C3b. These bind chemically to tissue at the site of activation through thiol ester bonds, and then degrade, forming ligands for the complement receptors CR3 and CR4, which are found on the surface of microglia. All BAP deposits, whether diffuse or consolidated, are strongly positive for C4d and C3d (McGeer et al., 1989), indicating that amplification of the original C1q signal is occurring, as well as chemical attachment to proteins in the deposits, with consequent opsonization for phagocytosis. The exact molecules to which the complement proteins are attached remain unknown but clearly this would be of great interest to understanding the pathogenesis of AD.

If the complement pathway is strongly activated, the process goes on to form the MAC, a multimolecular complex of C5b-9. Initially, parallel arrays of the highly lipophilic C5b67 seek a viable membrane for attachment. When so attached, C8 can bind, followed by multiple molecules of C9. The membrane does not begin to leak until at least one C9 molecule has been added. Additional C9 molecules sharply enhance the lytic potential of the MAC, with 12-18 C9 molecules arranging in a ring, creating a hole up to 50 μm in diameter. Cells which survive MAC insertion tolerate the molecule in their membrane for only about 3.5 minutes. The damaged membrane must either be internalized or shed. Opsonized structures are not necessarily living cells, but the MAC can only insert into viable membranes. In AD, the MAC is associated with dystrophic neurites in senile plaques (McGeer et al., 1989). At the electron microscopic level, it is seen in intracellular elements suggestive of membrane internalization.

The brain appears to generate its own complement proteins. The mRNAs for C1, C3, C4 have all been detected in bulk mRNA extracts from brain. Cultured neuroblastoma, astrocytoma and microglial cells have been shown variously to produce the mRNAs for C1, C3, C4 and C9 (Walker and McGeer, 1993). *In situ* hybridization has revealed the mRNA for C4 in neurons and that for C1 in glial cells. Much remains to be worked out regarding the precise contribution that various endogenous brain cell types make to the activated complement fragments detected immunohistochemically in AD lesions.

Diffuse amyloid deposits and senile plaques differ with respect to both complement components and glial activity. Only in the latter does one see the MAC, aggregates of highly reactive microglia on the amyloid core, and reactive astrocytes ringing the periphery. It is thus conceivable that C5 through C9 are not generated in areas of diffuse amyloid deposits but only in or near senile plaques where, possibly, the altered states of reactive microglia, reactive astrocytes and dystrophic neuronal processes leads to such generation.

A number of inhibitors are known which control various steps in the complement cascade. Some are upregulated in AD (Table I). It is significant that none of these appears in association with diffuse amyloid deposits. They occur exclusively in association with senile plaques, the dystrophic neurites which are associated with such plaques, some neuropil threads, and intracellular tangles in areas of neuronal degeneration (McGeer et al., 1992). Presumably, their appearance is due to upregulation of synthesis in neurons, either under attack by the MAC or undergoing degeneration.

Clearly it is important for an understanding of AD to learn more about the factors that can activate microglia and the complement system, and those that may prevent such activation. The appearance of amyloid P, thrombin and the Hageman factor in association with amyloid deposits is of particular interest since each of these, like BAP itself, has been shown to be capable of activating complement. We have recently been studying the respiratory burst system of macrophages as a means of screening for further such activators and inhibitors.

The respiratory burst apparatus is an attack system possessed by professional phagocytes. Its function is to protect the body from hostile invaders by generating superoxide radicals. Deficiencies in the system, such as occur in chronic granulomatous disease in humans, typically result in early death from infection (Morel et al., 1991). The ability to produce superoxide radicals is clearly essential to immune system competency, yet these toxic radicals are also capable of harming host cells. They are believed to be a factor in many diseases of unknown etiology where autodestruction of tissue occurs.

The respiratory burst apparatus can be activated in cultured phagocytes in multiple ways (for review see Bellavite, 1988; Morel et al., 1991). Some of these methods reflect circumstances that occur in vivo; others are clearly artifacts of the in vitro environment. Interestingly, we have found that synthetic BAP is capable of activating the respiratory burst (Klegeris et al., 1994). The diversity of triggering agents suggests that multiple pathways must exist through which professional phagocytes can be induced to generate superoxide radicals.

Controlling the respiratory burst may be a useful target for therapeutic intervention in many diseases. Such intervention could be selective, blocking some entries into the final common pathway, but leaving others intact. One method of activation involves complement receptors, and we have examined the ability of various substances to block such activation. The experiments involved testing various agents before and after exposing rat peritoneal macrophages to zymosan particles opsonized by incubation with rat serum (opsonized zymosan, OZ). Complement receptors on phagocytes interact with complement fragments attached to such particles. Agents inhibiting a respiratory burst when introduced before, but not after, exposure to OZ, presumably act by influencing complement receptors. Those acting independently of the time of exposure to OZ must be acting at other sites.

The most powerful inhibitor of OZ activation when added before, but not after OZ, was the antibody OX-42 which interacts with the C3bi receptor on macrophages (Robinson et al., 1986). Even at a concentration of 32 μg/ml (or about 2 nM assuming a molecular weight of 150,000 for the IgG), this antibody reduced OZ activation to 30.2% of control. By contrast, the same dilution, when administered after OZ, reduced the activity only to 81.6% of control. Results which showed a trend in the same direction were given by indomethacin and dapsone, but at much higher concentrations (i.e. at 0.1-1 mM). Other types of agents tested included some lipoxygenase and phospholipase A-2 inhibitors which should modify eicosanoid metabolism, prostaglandin E_2 and prednisone. Some showed activity but none were as potent or selective as OX-42.

Complement activation occurs in a number of chronic degenerative diseases, and is a prominent feature of AD (McGeer et al., 1989). Agents which selectively block complement receptors may reduce any autodestructive action of superoxide radicals, and thus ameliorate the effects of such diseases. It is also possible that agents already known to have antiinflammatory effects, such as indomethacin and dapsone, might work, at least partially, by this mechanism.

REFERENCES

Bellavite P (1988): The superoxide-forming enzymatic system of phagocytes. *Free Radical Biol Med* 4:225-261.

Klegeris A, Walker DG and McGeer PL (1994): Activation of macrophages by Alzheimer ß-amyloid peptide. *Biochem Biophy Res Commun* 199:984-991.

McGeer PL, Akiyama H, Itagaki S and McGeer EG (1989): Immune system response in Alzheimer's disease. *Can J Neurol Sci* 16:516-527.

McGeer PL, Kawamata T and Walker DG (1992): Distribution of clusterin in Alzheimer brain tissue. *Brain Res* 579:337-341.

Morel F, Doussiere J and Vignais PV (1991): The superoxide-generating oxidase of phagocytic cells. *Eur J Biochem* 201:523-546.

Robinson AP, White TM and Mason DW (1986): Macrophage heterogeneity in the rat as delineated by two monoclonal antibodies MRC OX-41 and MRC OX-42. *Immunology* 57:239-247.

Walker DG and McGeer PL (1993): Complement gene expression in neuroblastoma and astrocytoma cell lines of human origin. *Neurosci Lett* 157:99-102.

Yasuhara O, Kawamata T, Aimi Y, McGeer EG and McGeer PL (1994): Two types of dystrophic neurites in senile plaques of Alzheimer disease and elderly non-demented cases. *Neurosci Lett* (In Press).

Alzheimer Disease: Therapeutic Strategies
edited by E. Giacobini and R. Becker.
© 1994 Birkhäuser Boston

INFLAMMATORY PATHOLOGY IN ALZHEIMER'S DISEASE

Scott D. Webster and Joseph Rogers
L.J. Roberts Center for Alzheimer's Research,
Sun Health Research Institute, Sun City, AZ

A large body of evidence suggests that there is an inflammatory component to Alzheimer's disease (AD) pathogenesis. The reactive microglial cells of neuritic plaques are characterized by the presence of a variety of inflammatory markers, including HLA-DR, HLA-DP, HLA-DQ, β-2 integrins and Fc receptors (reviewed by Rogers et al., 1992a). Also evident within plaques are the Aβ associated proteins (Selkoe, 1991), many of which are related to inflammatory processes. Some of the most studied are α_1-antichymotrypsin (ACT) (Abraham et al., 1988), complement proteins (McGeer and McGeer, 1992; McGeer and Rogers, 1992), serum amyloid P (SAP) (Coria et al., 1988) and heparin sulfate proteoglycans (HSPG) (Snow et al., 1988). Furthermore, altered levels of the cytokine interleukin 1 (IL-1) and IL-6 have been demonstrated in AD (reviewed in Wood et al., 1993).

By immunohistochemistry, virtually the full range of classical pathway complement proteins, including C1, C1q, C3, C3b, C3c, C3d, C4, C4d, C7, C8, and C5b-9 (McGeer and McGeer, 1992; McGeer and Rogers, 1992), are found associated with Alzheimer's pathology. The mRNAs for several complement proteins and other inflammatory markers have also been demonstrated in AD brain (cf. Johnson et al., 1992). The alternate complement cascade does not seem to be active, as proteins specific for this pathway such as properdin and factor B are not present (Ishii et al., 1988; McGeer et al., 1989).

Inflammation is an inherently destructive process. The immunohistochemical detection of the membrane attack complex (C5b-9) on dystrophic neurites in AD brain samples (McGeer et al., 1989; Rogers et al., 1992b) explicitly connotes a significant pathological occurrence. In the periphery, cells under such attack can be replaced. In brain, postmitotic neurons cannot. As a result, any occurrence of inflammation in brain carries with it a substantial pathogenic risk and must, by definition, be considered a neurodegenerative mechanism.

The presence of classical complement proteins has historically been taken to indicate activation by immunoglobulin (Ig). Immunoglobulin typically activates complement only when it is bound to antigen via the Fab region and to C1q via the Fc region (Abbas et al., 1991). This interaction imposes the requirement of immunohistochemical colocalization of Ig and C1q in situations where Ig-induced complement activation occurs. Some evidence has been presented for the existence of antibrain antibodies in the CSF of AD patients (reviewed by McRae and Dahlstrom, 1992). However, the presence of Ig immunoreactivity in plaques has been difficult to establish, with most studies showing negative or ambiguous results (Rogers et al., 1992b; Eikelenboom et al., 1992). Cortical IgG staining, when present, occurs on patches of neurons whose distribution bears no discernable relationship to that of senile plaques or C1q (Rogers et al., 1992b). Furthermore, such staining is found equally in AD and nondemented patients and may represent technical artifact resulting from postmortem serum leakage and nonspecific Ig binding (Mori et al., 1991; Loeffler et al., 1992). Alzheimer disease, by these standards, cannot be considered an autoimmune disease. Rather, it is more appropriate to emphasize the functional significance of inflammation to the AD pathogenic process.

The close association of C1q and Aß fibrils shown by electron microscopy (Ishii and Haga, 1984) suggests that in the absence of verifiable plaque-associated Igs, Aß might be capable of binding C1q without mediation of Ig. This is not unprecedented, as certain bacteria and RNA viruses are capable of activating C1 and initiating the classical complement cascade without the intervention of Ig (Cooper, 1987). We have demonstrated that C1q possesses $A\beta$ binding capabilities, that this binding fully activates the classical complement cascade (Rogers et al., 1992b), and that Aß mediated complement activation has functional cytotoxic consequences for mixed neuronal cultures (Schultz et al., 1994).

Recent investigations showing that soluble $A\beta$ may be a normal metabolic product suggest that mechanisms must exist whereby soluble $A\beta$ becomes deposited in the fibrillar form under pathological conditions (Cotman and Pike, 1994). Several lines of evidence suggest that C1q, in addition to initiating the classical complement cascade, may be important in the process of amyloid deposition in AD: 1) C1q binds to $A\beta$ (Rogers et al., 1992b), 2) C1q colocalizes strictly to $A\beta$ deposits in senile plaques (Ishii and Haga, 1984), and 3) elevated levels of C1q are found in high pathology regions of AD brains as compared to control brains (Brachova et al., 1993). Recent work from our laboratory demonstrates that the binding of C1q to $A\beta$ favors the conversion of $A\beta$ into the β-pleated, thioflavine positive configuration (Webster et al., 1994). Because C1q is a large, multimeric molecule, it is reasonable to postulate that multiple $A\beta$ binding sites exist (indeed, six Ig binding sites are contained within one C1q molecule). Our data suggest that the binding of C1q to $A\beta$ favors the formation of amyloid fibrils by bringing multiple $A\beta$ peptides into close proximity. Furthermore, C1q binding of $A\beta$ fibrils confers a resistance to resolubilization, possibly by acting as a cross-linking agent (Webster et al., 1994).

At this point in time a precise mechanism describing the initial event in $A\beta$ deposition has not been convincingly demonstrated. It is conceivable that during the early stages of $A\beta$ deposition multiple compounds might compete for binding to soluble $A\beta$ and to nascent $A\beta$ fibrils. Promotion or inhibition of continued fibrillogenesis would therefore be a function of the relative amounts of the different substances in the immediate area of deposition. Snow et al. (1994) showed that injection of $A\beta$ and HSPG into rat brain results in the formation of Congo red and thioflavine positive $A\beta$ deposits at the infusion site and postulated that the deposits were formed after interactions with endogenous compounds such as SAP, ACT, α_2-macroglobulin, apolipoprotein E and complement.

In addition to these data from basic research, clinical studies also suggest that inflammation may play a significant pathogenic role in AD. Thus, several retrospective analyses have found an inverse association of anti-inflammatory drug use with the frequency of AD diagnoses (cf. McGeer et al., 1990), including a more focused study by Breitner and colleagues (1994) based on a large cohort of elderly identical and fraternal twins. A very small clinical trial of a nonsteroidal anti-inflammatory drug that crosses the blood-brain barrier, indomethacin, has also been conducted with encouraging, but by no means definitive, results (Rogers et al., 1993). The substantial (21%) drop-out rate due to indomethacin-induced gastrointestinal adverse reactions was a particular problem. A better understanding of the basic mechanisms by which inflammation exerts pathogenic actions in AD may lead to more effectively targeted drugs in future.

REFERENCES

Abbas AK, Lichtman AH and Pober JS (1991): *Cellular and Molecular Immunology*. Philadelphia: WB Saunders Company.

Abraham CR, Selkoe DJ and Potter H (1988): Immunochemical identification of the serine protease inhibitor, α_1-antichymotrypsin in the brain amyloid deposits of Alzheimer's disease. *Cell* 52:487-501.

Brachova L, Lue L-F, Schultz J, El Rashidy T and Rogers J (1993): Association cortex, cerebellum, and serum concentrations of C1q and factor B in Alzheimer's disease. *Mol Brain Res* 18:329-334.

Breitner JCS, Gau BA, Welsh KA, Plassman BL, McDonald WM, Helms MJ and Anthony JC (1994): Inverse association of anti-inflammatory treatments and Alzheimer's disease. Initial results of a co-twin control study. *Neurology* 44:227-232.

Cooper N (1987): The complement system. In: *Basic and Clinical Immunology Vol. 6*, Stites DP and Terr AI, eds. Norwalk, CN: Appleton and Lange, pp. 114-127.

Coria F, Castano E, Prelli F, Larrondo-Lillo M, van Duinen S, Shelanski ML and Frangione B (1988): Isolation and characterization of amyloid P component from Alzheimer's disease and other types of cerebral amyloidosis. *Lab Invest* 58:454-458.

Cotman CW and Pike CJ (1994): β-amyloid and its contributions to neurodegeneration in Alzheimer disease. In: *Alzheimer Disease*, Terry RD, Katzman R and Bick KL, eds. New York: Raven Press, Inc., pp. 305-315.

Eikelenboom P, Hack CE, Kamphorst W and Rozemuller JM (1992): Distribution pattern and functional state of complement proteins and α_1-antichymotrypsin in cerebral β/A4 deposits in Alzheimer's disease. *Res Immunol* 143:617-620.

Ishii T and Haga S (1984): Immunoelectron microscopic localization of complements in amyloid fibrils of senile plaques. *Acta Neuropath* 63:296-300.

Ishii T, Haga S and Kametani F (1988): Presence of immunoglobulins and complements in the amyloid plaques in the brain of patients with Alzheimer's disease. In: *Immunology and Alzheimer's Disease*, Pouplard-Barthelaix A, Emile J and Christen Y, eds. Berlin: Springer-Verlag, pp. 17-29.

Johnson SA, Lampert-Etchells M, Pasinetti GM, Rozovsky I and Finch CE (1992): Complement mRNA in the mammalian brain: responses to Alzheimer's disease and experimental brain lesioning. *Neurobiol Aging* 13:641-648.

Loeffler DA, Brickman CM, LeWitt PA, Bannon MJ, KuKuruga MA, Cassin B and Kapatos G (1992): Non-specific binding of normal human IgG, including F(ab')$_2$ and Fc fragments, to embryonic rat brain neurons and human cortex synaptosomes. *J Neuroimmunol* 38:45-52.

McGeer PL, Akiyama H, Itagaki S and McGeer EG (1989): Immune system response in Alzheimer's disease. *Canad J Neurol Sci* 16:516-527.

McGeer PL, McGeer E, Rogers J and Sibley J (1990): Anti-inflammatory drugs and Alzheimer's disease. *Lancet* 335:1037.

McGeer PL and McGeer EG (1992): Complement proteins and complement inhibitors in Alzheimer's disease. *Res Immunol* 143:621-624.

McGeer PL and Rogers J (1992): Anti-inflammatory agents as a therapeutic approach to Alzheimer's disease. *Neurology* 42:447-449.

McRae A and Dahlstrom A (1992): Cerebrospinal fluid antibodies: an indicator for immune responses in Alzheimer's disease. *Res Immunol* 143:663-667.

Mori S, Sternberger NH, Herman MM and Sternberger LA (1991): Leakage and neuronal uptake of serum protein in aged and Alzheimer brains. *Lab Invest* 64:345-351.

Rogers J, Civin WH, Styren SD and McGeer PL (1992a): Immune-related mechanisms of Alzheimer's disease pathogenesis. In: *Alzheimer's Disease: New Treatment Strategies*, Khachaturian ZS and Blass JP, eds. New York: Marcel Dekker, Inc., pp. 147-163.

Rogers J, Cooper NR, Webster S, Schultz J, McGeer PL, Styren SD, Civin WH, Brachova L, Bradt B, Ward P and Lieberburg I (1992b): Complement activation by β-amyloid in Alzheimer disease. *Proc Nat Acad Sci USA* 89:10016-10020.

Rogers J, Kirby LC, Hempelman SR, Berry DL, McGeer PL, Kasczniak AW, Zalinski J, Cofield M, Mansukhani L, Willson P and Kogan F (1993): Clinical trial of indomethacin in Alzheimer's disease. *Neurology* 43:1609-1611.

Schultz J, Schaller J, McKinley M, Bradt B, Cooper N, May P and Rogers J (1994): Enhanced cytotoxicity of amyloid β peptide by a complement dependent mechanism in mixed embryonic rat brain cultures. *Neurosci Lett* (In Press).

Selkoe DJ (1991): The molecular pathology of Alzheimer's disease. *Neuron* 6:487-498.

Snow AD, Mar H, Nochlin D, Kimata K, Kato M, Suzuki S, Hassell J and Wight TN (1988): The presence of heparan sulfate proteoglycans in the neuritic plaques and congophilic angiopathy in Alzheimer's disease. *Am J Pathol* 133:456-463.

Snow AD, Sekiguchi R, Nochlin D, Fraser P, Kimata K, Mizutani A, Arai M, Schreier WA and Morgan DG (1994): An important role of heparan sulfate proteoglycan (perlecan) in a model system for the deposition and persistence of fibrillar Aβ-amyloid in rat brain. *Neuron* 12:219-234.

Webster S, O'Barr S and Rogers J (1994): Enhanced aggregation and β structure of amyloid β peptide after co-incubation with C1q. *J Neurosci Res* (In Press).

Wood JA, Wood PL, Ryan R, Graff-Radford NR, Pilapil C, Robitaille Y and Quirion R (1993): Cytokine indices in Alzheimer's temporal cortex: no changes in mature IL-1β or IL-1RA but increases in the associated acute phase proteins IL-6, α2-macroglobulin and C-reactive protein. *Brain Res* 629:245-252.

Alzheimer Disease: Therapeutic Strategies
edited by E. Giacobini and R. Becker.
© 1994 Birkhäuser Boston

ALUMINUM CHELATION THERAPY OF ALZHEIMER'S DISEASE

Donald R. McLachlan and Theo P.A. Kruck
Centre for Research in Neurodegenerative Diseases,
University of Toronto, Toronto, Ontario, Canada

Wanda L. Smith
Geriatric Outreach Program, Chedoke-McMaster Hospitals,
Hamilton, Ontario, Canada

INTRODUCTION

Although controversial in the past, strong evidence now implicates aluminum in the pathogenesis of Alzheimer's disease (AD). A recent epidemiological study employed autopsy verified AD brain and controls together with residential histories as measures of exposure to aluminum from municipal drinking water supplies in the province of Ontario. The results indicate that in communities consuming drinking water with annual average concentrations greater than 0.1 mg/L Al, the risk of dying with AD was 2.5 times greater than in communities with less than 0.1 mg/L (McLachlan et al., 1994). In communities exposed to greater than 0.175 mg/L, the risk rises to 4.8. Similar findings result from assessment of risk based on final hospital discharge diagnoses (Neri et al., 1992) or impairment in cognitive function in an elderly male population (Forbes et al., 1992).

Brains of renal dialysis patients exposed to low concentrations of blood aluminum (average <30 μg/L; control <10 μg/L) have revealed a four-fold increase in the probability of demonstrating extracellular amyloid deposits compared to age-matched controls (Candy et al., 1992) and a marked increase in post-translational modifications in tau, the principle constituent of AD neurofibrillary tangles. An increase in the truncated and hyperphosphorylated isoforms of tau were observed as well as paired helical filaments, an unusual finding in the age group under study (Harrington et al., 1994). Fraser et al. (1993) have shown the hyperphosphorylated tau extracted from AD temporal cortex has considerable secondary structure which, in the presence of trace amounts of aluminum but not iron, calcium or other physiological metals, will assemble into paired helical filaments similar in appearance, at the electron microscope levels, to those found in AD. Taken together, present evidence indicates that aluminum plays a major role in the pathogenesis of AD and exerts a neurotoxic effect early in the course of the illness, probably at a preclinical stage. Clearly, lowering absorption of aluminum or brain tissue concentrations offers possible therapeutic opportunities for slowing the rate of clinical progression of the disease or possibly delaying or preventing the onset of the disease.

Epidemiological and toxicological studies suggest that co-existing factors such as fluoride, silicon, iron, calcium and water pH may modify body uptake of aluminum. Experiments manipulating these variables have generally not been undertaken and no efficacious oral chelating agent is available. However, desferrioxamine (DFO) is a safe effective aluminum chelating agent of high specificity for trivalent metals. Here we describe the outcome of a single-blind, two-year, oral placebo-controlled clinical trial employing 125 mg DFO intramuscularly at 12 hr intervals for five days each week.

METHODS

The sample for the study consisted of 48 individuals with probable AD utilizing NINCDS-ADRDA criteria (McKhann et al., 1984; Crapper McLachlan et al., 1991). Subjects were excluded who had any medical illness and who were taking any medications. At trial entry, the participants were randomly assigned to one of three groups: drug treatment, oral placebo (lecithin 500 mg b.i.d.), and no treatment. Following initial data analysis at the end of the study, the two latter groups were combined as the no-treatment group. The drug-treatment group consisted of 25 participants, 12 males and 13 females, ranging in age from 51.8 to 76.8 years (mean = 63.7 years) at the time of first assessment. The no-treatment group consisted of 23 participants, 11 males and 12 females (mean age = 63.6 years). All participants were initially living in the community with their spouses or children, and spoke English prior to the onset of the disease.

The assessment of drug efficacy was taken as score results on a videotaped home behavioral (VHB) assessment completed at trial entry and six month intervals thereafter. The test was developed to sample activities which routinely occurred in daily living experiences and were familiar to males and females. The test details are described elsewhere (Crapper McLachlan et al., 1993). The assessments were conducted by a psychometrist in the participants' homes and videotaped. The VHB consisted of 48 test items in which 25 items assessed performance of behaviors such as walking, putting on and taking off gloves, combing hair, and brushing teeth, 18 items assessed left/right orientation and body part recognition, and five items assessed the participant's ability to recognize coins and count change. For the first 25 test items, a systematic hierarchy of prompts was introduced, if the participant failed to respond correctly. The prompt provided the participant with an increasing amount of information to facilitate correct response and permitted a graded score from four for first time correct to zero with complete failure after all prompts. Videotapes were scored in random sequence by trained behavior raters blinded to the study protocol. Rating accuracy was assessed independently by an expert rater.

The London Psychogeriatric Rating Scale (LPRS; Hersch et al., 1978) was completed by the caregiver at trial entry and six month intervals. (The LPRS is a 36 item rating scale of mental and physical disability and behavior problems where increasing scores reflect increased impairment.) Standardized clinical measures were completed at one-year intervals including the Wechsler Adult Intelligence Scale (WAIS-R), the Wechsler Memory Scale (WMS), and the Western Aphasia Battery (WAB). These tests provided estimates of cognitive, memory and language functioning which were utilized as criterion references of cognitive functioning.

RESULTS

The internal reliability of the VHB was examined by using coefficient alpha to analyze test consistency and the contribution of individual subtests to scale cohesion ($\alpha > .6$ reflects high internal reliability). Overall, the standardized alpha coefficients were .94, .89 and .71 respectively for each of the three subtests ($p < .001$). Test-retest reliability of the VHB was computed and yielded relative reliability coefficients for the overall score $r = 0.9962$ ($p < 0.0001$) and for each of the subscores $p < .003$. Inter-examiner reliability was computed and reliability coefficients for overall scores was $r = .9836$ ($p < .0025$). Rater accuracy of the VHB scores was also assessed by examining item by item agreement across independent ratings of the same performance. The mean inter-rater agreement was 95% with a range between 85.5 and 100%. The relationship of the VHB to standardized clinical measures was examined with the WAIS-R full scale I.Q. and verbal and performance I.Q.'s, the WMS and the WAB. The resultant correlation coefficients at entry to the study ranged between .44 and .71, and all correlations were significant at $p < .002$. As shown in Fig. 1, an advantage of the VHB is that as the disease progresses, the percentage of participants able to complete the examination is considerably higher with the VHB than the WAIS-R, the WMS or the WAB. By 24-months, 95% of assessments were completed on the VHB, whereas only 39% were completed on the WAIS-R, 31% on the WMS, and 49% on the WAB.

The VHB results for the DFO treated versus the no-treatment group detected differences in progression of the disease. As shown in Fig. 2, for the placebo and no-treatment group combined, the mean semi-annual rate of deterioration or loss in scores was 5.9% ($\pm$ 3.4 SEM) of the maximum score during the first six months, 11% ($\pm$ 3.9 SEM) by 12 months, 20.2% ($\pm$ 7.2 SEM) between 12 to 18 months, and 29.6% ($\pm$ 9.3 SEM) in the interval between 18 to 24 months. Whereas in the treated group, in the first six months, there was a loss of 1.4% ($\pm$ .7 SEM), in the second six month interval 4.5% ($\pm$ 1.8 SEM), in the third six month interval 9.4% (± 2.5 SEM), and in the interval between 18 and 24 months, the rate of change was only 8.6% (± 2.9 SEM).

The mean scores of the LPRS for the treatment and the no-treatment groups at trial entry were 25 and 28 (p = .56), at six months 30 and 37 (p = .24), at 12 months 37 and 35 (p = .83), at 18 months 31 and 54 (p = .01) and at 24 months 47 and 69 (p = .02), respectively.

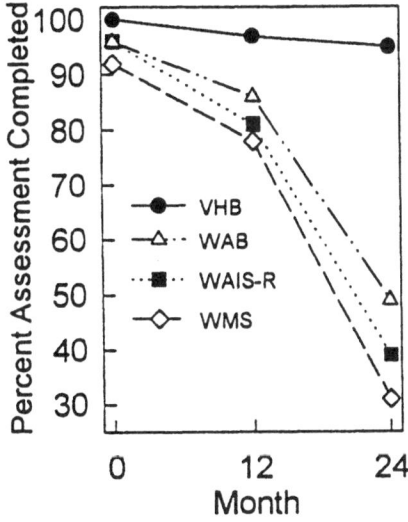

FIGURE 1. Assessment of drug efficacy.

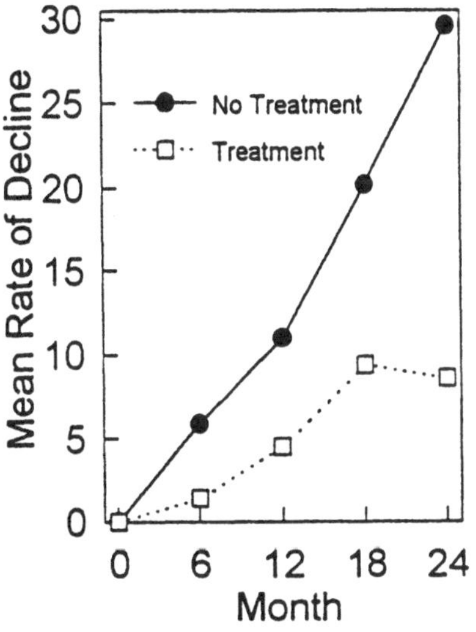

FIGURE 2. Mean semi-annual rate of deterioration for no-treament and treatment (DFO) groups.

DISCUSSION

No patient in the DFO-treated group improved in scores. However, the rate of deterioration was reduced to less than 50% of that of the untreated group, and quality of life, as measured by skills of daily living on the VHB, was preserved for a prolonged period of time. The caregivers' assessment of patient functioning (LPRS) reflected significant differences at 18 and 24 months. In fact, the mean score for the untreated group at two years corresponded to normative values for institutionalized demented patients. Over the five year period encompassing the trial, there were nine deaths in the untreated and only one death in the DFO-treated group. The important critical question of whether DFO removes aluminum from brain tissue could not be addressed in subjects in this trial.

However, in a separate trial in which patients received 500 mg DFO intramuscular twice per day, five days per week, six patients died from causes unrelated to DFO while receiving the drug within 48 hours of death. Three brains (Group A) were from subjects who had received placebo, 2.5 gm and 3.5 gm, respectively, of DFO. Group B was composed of three brains which had received 23.5 gm, 38 gm and 54 gm of DFO total dose. Applying electrothermal atomic absorption spectroscopy to measure bulk tissue neocortical aluminum concentrations, 20 samples from identical loci in each brain were obtained and the mean aluminum concentrations for Group A was 4.04 $\mu g/g$ dry weight and for Group B, 2.67 $\mu g/g$ dry weight. Statistical analysis revealed that each brain within Groups A and B were not statistically significantly different from each other. However, the differences in the mean between Groups A and B are significant at $p < 0.05$. Importantly, iron, manganese and copper were measured in Groups A and B, and on average, were not statistically different.

In summary, DFO therapy lowers brain aluminum concentrations and it significantly alters the course of the disease.

CONCLUSION

Given the weight of epidemiological and toxicological evidence involving aluminum in the pathogenesis of AD, it is likely that the outcome of the clinical trial is related to the removal of brain aluminum. Further clinical trials are warranted to extend the use of this drug, as a palliative treatment, to AD victims who meet less stringent inclusion criteria to those employed in the present trial. Taken together with all information, strategies developed to reduce total body exposure to aluminum in the elderly have the potential for preventing or delaying the onset of the illness.

ACKNOWLEDGEMENTS

Supported by the Extramural Program, National Health and Welfare Canada, and the Ministry of Universities and Colleges of the Province of Ontario. DFO was supplied by CIBA-Geigy, Canada.

REFERENCES

Candy JM, McArthur FK, Oakley AE, Taylor GA, Chen CPL, Mountfort SA, Thompson JE, Chalker PR, Bishop HE, Beyreuther K, Perry G, Ward MK, Martyn CN and Edwardson JA (1992): Aluminum accumulation in relation to senile plaque and neurofibrillary tangle formation in the brains of patients with renal failure. *J Neurol Sci* 107:210-218.
Crapper McLachlan DR, Dalton AJ, Kruck TPA, Bell MY, Smith WL, KalowW and Andrews DF (1991): Intramuscular desferrioxamine in patients with Alzheimer's disease. *Lancet* 337:1304-1308.
Crapper McLachlan DR, Smith WL and Kruck TP (1993): Desferrioxamine and Alzheimer's disease: video home behavior assessment of clinical course and measures of brain aluminum. *Ther Drug Monit* 15:602-607.
Forbes WF, Hayward LM and Agwani N (1992): Geochemical risk factors for mental functioning, based on the Ontario Longitudinal Study of Aging (LSA). I. Results from a preliminary investigation. *Canadian J Aging* (In Press).

Fraser PE, Tam C and McLachlan DR (1993): Aluminum promotes *in vitro* assembly of Alzheimer tau into paired helical filaments. *Abst Soc Neurochemistry (Richmond, Virginia)*.

Harrington CR, Wischik CM, McArthur FK, Taylor GA, Edwardson JA and Candy JM (1994): Alzheimer's-disease-like changes in tau protein processing: Association with aluminium accumulation in brains of renal dialysis patients. *Lancet* 343:993-997.

Hersch EL, Kral VA, and Palmer RB (1978): Clinical value of the London Psychogeriatric Rating Scale. *J Am Geriat Soc* 26:348-354.

McKhann G, Drachman D, Folstein M, Katzman R, Price D and Stadlan EM (1984): Clinical diagnosis of Alzheimer's disease: Report of the NINCDS-ADRDA Work Group under the auspices of Department of Health and Human services Task Force on Alzheimer's Disease. *Neurol* 34:939-944.

McLachlan DR, Rifat S, Bergeron C and Smith JE (1994): Evidence implicating aluminum in neurodegenerative disease: drinking water aluminum content and the risk for autopsy veritifed Alzheimer's disease. *Aluminum Association* (Submitted).

Neri LC, Hewitt D and Rifat SL (1992): Aluminium concentrations in drinking water and population risk for diagnoses of Alzheimer's disease. *Abstract Third International Conference on Alzheimer's Disease and Related Disorders* (Padova, Italy, July).

Alzheimer Disease: Therapeutic Strategies
edited by E. Giacobini and R. Becker.
© 1994 Birkhäuser Boston

IN VITRO EVIDENCE FOR THE USE OF ANTIOXIDANTS IN ALZHEIMER'S DISEASE

J. Steven Richardson, Ujendra Kumar, Subbarao V. Kala, Lihua Chen and Yan Zhou
Department of Pharmacology, College of Medicine,
University of Saskatchewan, Saskatoon, SK, Canada

INTRODUCTION

Any atom or molecule with at least one unpaired electron is a free radical. Substances with an unpaired electron tend to be unstable and so, to attain chemical stability, the free radical will extract an electron from, or donate an electron to, nearby compounds. In biological systems, oxygen based free radicals are generated by a variety of normal metabolic processes such as the activity of oxidase enzymes and microsomal and mitochondrial electron transport. In addition, transitional metals such as iron, copper and zinc will catalyze the formation of free radicals from elemental oxygen and from hydrogen peroxide formed as a by-product of enzyme activity. Also, ionizing radiation will create free radicals when the energized particle collides with water or any other molecule in living tissue. Normally these free radicals are prevented from interacting with molecules crucial for cellular viability by endogenous antioxidant enzymes and free radical scavengers.

However, in situations where the antioxidant defenses are inadequate, free radicals will produce cytotoxic damage to the cell's membrane, enzymes and DNA by altering the electron number, the structure and the function of lipids, proteins, nucleic acids and other cellular constituents. Free radicals have been shown to participate in the lysosomal processing and recycling of polypeptides and other intracellular compounds, to be the agents of destruction in apoptosis and in the bacteriocidal actions of macrophages, and to be responsible for much, if not all, of the neurodegeneration produced by cerebral ischemia and excitatory amino acids. Our studies, and those of other investigators, have produced considerable circumstantial evidence supporting the hypothesis that free radicals initiate and maintain the neurodegenerative cascade in Alzheimer's disease (AD).

METHODS

Autopsy Studies
Comparable samples of frontal cortex (Brodmann's area 47) were taken from donated autopsy brains of people with AD and of neurologically healthy controls. The diagnosis of AD was based on pre-mortem dementia and post-mortem histological analysis of each brain according to the NIA criteria. All brains were removed within 24 hours of the death of the donor and were stored frozen at -86°C. The samples of AD and control tissue, matched on the basis of sex, age at death of the donor and time of post-mortem storage, were homogenized in physiological saline and incubated in room air at 37°C for 15 min with or without the addition of exogenous iron. Peroxidation products (TBAR) formed during the incubation were measured by the thiobarbituric acid method (Subbarao et al., 1990). Free radicals formed during incubation were determined by electron paramagnetic resonance spectroscopy (EPR) with spin trapping (Zhou et al., unpublished). The activities of the antioxidant enzymes superoxide dismutase, catalase and glutathione peroxidase were measured in samples of hippocampus, frontal cortex, entorhinal cortex, temporal cortex, parietal cortex and cerebellum from AD and control brains (Chen et al., 1994). The amount of loosely bound iron in samples of frontal cortex and cerebellum from ADs and controls homogenized in normal saline, was determined in the 40,000 x g supernatant with the bathophenanthroline method (Kala et al., in preparation).

Tissue Culture Studies
These studies used human fibroblasts grown from skin samples taken at autopsy from AD and control brain donors (Kumar et al., 1994), rat hippocampal neurons grown in primary cultures (Kumar et al., unpublished), and a rat PC 12 cell line (Zhou et al., in preparation). The uptake of calcium by mitochondria isolated from AD and control fibroblasts was measured by the ^{45}calcium tracer method. The effect of exposure to iron-induced free radicals on mitochondrial calcium uptake and the actions of the antioxidant drug U-74500A were also determined. Mature cultures of rat hippocampal neurons were exposed to β-amyloid 1 to 40 or β-amyloid 25 to 35 (100 μg/ml of each) with or without the antioxidant drug U-78517F (10 μM) and were examined under a phase contrast microscope 24 hours later. Naive, undifferentiated PC 12 cells were used to study the effects of U-83836E (the L-isomer of U-78517F) on the acute action of β-amyloid 25 to 35 on cytosolic free calcium as determined by the fura-2 AM fluorescent method.

RESULTS

Both under basal conditions and in the presence of exogenous iron, homogenates of AD frontal cortex generate significantly more TBAR ($p < .05$) and oxygen radical spin adducts (p < .05) than do control homogenates. The activity of superoxide dismutase was about 25% lower (p < .05) in AD frontal cortex, hippocampus and cerebellum than in controls. Also, loosely bound iron was over 50% higher (p < .05) in the AD frontal cortex samples than in controls.

Alzheimer disease fibroblast mitochondria take up 45% less (p < .01) calcium than do controls under basal conditions but show a proportionally greater increase (AD 57% vs. Control 42%) in calcium uptake following exposure to iron generated free radicals. Although U-74500A itself has no effect on mitochondrial calcium uptake, it prevents the effect of iron on control mitochondria but only reduces the iron effect on AD mitochondria.

After 24 hours of exposure to 10 μM U-78517F, mature cultures of rat hippocampal neurons do not differ from controls. In both cases, the cell bodies are discrete, dissociated and joined by numerous large diameter and small diameter processes. The small diameter processes show considerable branching. In cultures exposed to either β-amyloid sequence, there is considerable cellular debris, the cell bodies are swollen and clumped together, and there are fewer large diameter processes. There is an increase in small diameter multi-branching processes in cultures given β-amyloid 1 to 40, but there are no small diameter processes at all after β-amyloid 25 to 35. Cultures given both U-78517F and β-amyloid 1 to 40 show little change after 24 hours, other than an increase in the growth of small, multi-branching neurites. U-78517F also reduces the cytotoxic action of β-amyloid 25 to 35. Neurons in these cultures show some swelling and aggregation, some loss of large diameter processes and some cellular debris. Moreover, small diameter branching processes are still present.

Intracellular calcium increases in a dose dependent manner in PC 12 cells exposed acutely to β-amyloid 25 to 35. U-83836E at a concentration of 10 μM has little effect on intracellular calcium itself but produces a 65% reduction in the intracellular calcium response produced by 40 μM β-amyloid 25 to 35.

DISCUSSION

These results are consistent with the hypothesis of an increased free radical burden in AD. In addition to our work (Subbarao et al., 1990; Richardson et al., 1991), increased peroxidation product formation in AD autopsy brain samples has also been reported by Andorn et al. (1990), Hajimohammadreza and Brammer (1990), McIntosh et al. (1991) and Gotz et al. (1992). Elevated iron levels in AD brain samples have also been found by Ehmann et al. (1986), Thompson et al. (1988), Andorn et al. (1990), Basun et al. (1991) and Dedman et al. (1992). The present demonstration that it is the pool of loosely-bound iron that is elevated would provide a source of free iron molecules to catalyze the formation of hydroxyl radicals from the hydrogen peroxide produced by monoamine oxidase and other enzymes in the brain.

The antioxidant drugs used in these studies are members of a family of compounds referred to as the lazaroids. Two of these drugs, U-74500A and U-78517F, have been shown to be free radical scavengers able to bind oxygen-centered and nitrogen-centered radicals (Zhao et al., unpublished). The ability of U-78517F to protect hippocampal neurons from β-amyloid neurotoxicity, indicates that free radicals are at least involved in, if not the sole cause of, β-amyloid cytotoxicity. Behl et al. (1992) reported that the antioxidant vitamin E also protects neurons from β-amyloid toxicity. Our demonstration that U-83836E, the L-isomer of U-78517F, prevents the elevation of intracellular calcium produced by β-amyloid 25-35 in PC 12 cells, is also consistent with the involvement of free radicals in the actions of β-amyloid.

Although elevated free radicals or increased free radical damage have not yet been reported in living patients with probable or confirmed AD, the above results provide considerable circumstantial evidence for excessive free radical activity in AD. Moreover, free radicals have also been implicated in the formation of β-amyloid. It has recently been demonstrated that nerve damage produced by cytotoxic events that are mediated by free radicals, such as excitatory amino acids or ischemia with reperfusion, induces expression of the gene for β-amyloid precursor protein (APP) (Kalaria et al., 1993; Kogure and Kato, 1993; Oostveen and Hall, 1993; Wilmot et al., 1993). This suggests the following general hypothesis for the etiology of AD. Due to various genetic and/or environmental factors, the future AD patient experiences a free radical burden that exceeds the endogenous defenses and produces some neural damage. This activates the formation of APP as part of the repair process, but because of free radical damage to the cellular membrane at the membrane insertion segment of the APP, or due to free radicals acting directly on the APP, the APP is cleaved in such a manner that leads to the formation and deposition of β-amyloid. The ß-amyloid results in the formation of additional free radicals that produce more neurodegeneration that stimulates the formation of more APP. This free radical/APP/β-amyloid cycle continues and maintains the progressive neurodegenerative cascade that eventually destroys sufficient neurons and synapses such that the structures in the limbic system can no longer perform their functions. At this stage, the symptoms of AD appear. Antioxidant therapeutic interventions should disrupt or prevent the free radical/β-amyloid recirculating cascade and the progressive neurodegeneration. Unfortunately, the identification of presymptomatic AD patients is currently impossible, and the selection of a suitable therapeutic end point for clinical trials is problematic.

ACKNOWLEDGEMENTS

Supported in part by grants from the Alzheimer's Association (Chicago, IL), from the Upjohn London Neuroscience Program, and the Alzheimer's Society for Lethbridge (AB) and Area, and by donations from private individuals. The crucial cooperation and assistance of Drs. Nyssen, Ang, George and the staff of the Autopsy Suite, Royal University Hospital, Saskatoon, and Drs. Stevenson and Smith, Pathology, Pasqua Hospital, Regina, are greatly appreciated. The authors would also like to thank Mrs. V. Heffner and Mrs. E. Habbick for their stenographic contributions.

REFERENCES

Andorn AC, Britton RS and Bacon BR (1990): Evidence that lipid peroxidation and total iron are increased in Alzheimer's brain. *Neurobiol Aging* 11:316.

Basun H, Forsell LG, Wetterberg L and Winblad B (1991): Metal and trace elements in plasma and cerebrospinal fluid in normal ageing and Alzheimer's disease. *J Neural Transm [P-D Sect]* 4:231-258.

Behl C, David J, Cole GM and Schubert D (1992): Vitamin E protects nerve cells from amyloid beta protein toxicity. *Biochem Biophys Res Communs* 186:944-950.

Chen L, Richardson JS, Caldwell JE and Ang LC (1994): Regional brain activity of free radical defense enzymes in autopsy samples from patients with Alzheimer's disease and from nondemented controls. *Intern J Neurosci* 75:83-90.

Dedman DJ, Treffry A, Candy JM, Taylor GAA, Morris CM, Bloxham CA, Perry RH, Edwardson JA and Harrison PM (1992): Iron and aluminum in relation to brain ferritin in normal individuals and Alzheimer's disease and renal-dialysis patients. *Biochem J* 287:509-514.

Ehmann WD, Markesbery WR, Alauddin M, Hossian TIM and Brubaker EH (1986): Brain trace elements in Alzheimer's disease. *Neurotoxicol* 7:197-206.

Gotz ME, Freyberger A, Hauer E, Burger R, Sofic E, Gsell W, Heckers S, Jellinger K, Hebenstreit G, Frolich L, Beckmann H and Riederer P (1992): Susceptibility of brains from patients with Alzheimer's disease to oxygen-stimulated lipid peroxidation and differential scanning colorimetry. *Dementia* 3:213-222.

Hajimohammadreza I and Brammer M (1990): Brain membrane fluidity and lipid peroxidation in Alzheimer's disease. *Neurosci Lett* 112:333-337.

Kalaria RN, Bhatti SU, Lust WD and Perry G (1993): The amyloid precursor protein in ischemic brain injury and chronic hypoperfusion. *Ann NY Acad Sci* 695:190-193.

Kogure K and Kato H (1993): Altered gene expression in cerebral ischemia. *Stroke* 24:2121-2127.

Kumar U, Dunlop DM and Richardson JS (1994): Mitochondria from Alzheimer's fibroblasts show decreased uptake of calcium and increased sensitivity to free radicals. *Life Sci* 54:1855-1860.

McIntosh LJ, Trush MA and Troncoso JC (1991): Oxygen free radical mediated processes in Alzheimer's disease. *Soc Neurosci Abst* 17:1071.

Oostveen JA and Hall ED (1993): Regional accumulation of amyloid protein precursor following a bilateral carotid occulsion in the gerbil. *Soc Neurosci Abst* 19:1655.

Richardson JS, Subbarao KV and Ang LC (1991): Autopsy Alzheimer's brains show increased peroxidation to an *in vitro* iron challenge. In: *Alzheimer's Disease: Basic Mechanisms, Diagnosis and Therapeutic Strategies*. Iqbal K, McLachlan DRC, Winblad B and Wisniewski HM, eds. Chichester, UK: John Wiley and Sons, pp. 145-152.

Subbarao KV, Richardson JS and Ang LC (1990): Autopsy samples of Alzheimer's cortex show increased peroxidation *in vitro*. *J Neurochem* 55:342-345.

Thompson CM, Markesbery WR, Ehmann WD, Mao YX and Vance DE (1988): Regional brain trace element studies in Alzheimer's disease. *Neurotoxicol* 9:1-8.

Wilmot CA, Li M, Szczepanik AM and Paul JW (1993): Increased β-amyloid precursor protein expression following intrastriatal infusion of kainic acid or lipopolysaccharide. *Soc Neurosci Abst* 19:186.

PART XII

Treatment of Behavioral and Gait Disturbances

Alzheimer Disease: Therapeutic Strategies
edited by E. Giacobini and R. Becker.
© 1994 Birkhäuser Boston

PHARMACOLOGIC MANAGEMENT OF AGITATION AND DEPRESSION IN DEMENTIA

Lon S. Schneider
Department of Psychiatry and Department of Neurology,
University of Southern California, Los Angeles, CA 90033 USA

Alzheimer's first case is noteworthy not only for its description of the patient's cognitive impairments and neuropathology, but also for the emphasis on her clinical presentation of suspiciousness, paranoid behavior, auditory hallucinations, screaming and apprehension (Alzheimer, 1907). Thus, it illustrates the fact that behavioral symptoms are very common in Alzheimer's dementia, occurring throughout its course, and are often the reasons patients are brought to medical attention. The behavioral signs and symptoms associated with Alzheimer's disease (AD) span a range to include agitation, aggression, psychosis, hallucinations, delusions, depression, wandering, apathy, sleep and appetite disturbances.

Behavior	Frequency (%)	
	Median	Range
Disturbed affect/mood	19.00	0 - 86
Psychotic symptoms		
Delusions	33	
Hallucinations		10 - 73
visual	22	
auditory	13	
Agitation/aggression	44.00	10 - 90
Anxiety	32.00	0 - 50
Withdrawn/passive		40 - 60
Vegetative		
Sleep	27	0 - 47
Appetite	34	12 - 77

TABLE I. Behavioral symptoms in dementia. The table summarizes from selected studies the frequency of symptomatic behaviors. (References are available from the author.)

Table I summarizes the broadly varying frequency of these behaviors (Schneider et al., submitted). Affective disturbances in patients with AD, including major depression, dysthymia and mood lability, are reported in up to 86% of patients. Other mood-related symptoms such as agitation, aggression, anxiety, apathy, passivity and vegetative signs frequently co-exist with affective symptoms, each occurring in from ¼ to ½ of dementia patients, but with great variability.

A reason for the great variability involves the definitions used to describe the behaviors. For example, a "depressed" patient may have depressive *symptoms* or a full depressive syndrome. In 115 consecutive AD patients at one of our clinics, only 12% of our patients fulfilled criteria for major depressive syndrome, not more than would be expected in any geriatric clinic. However, 46% had agitation, 31% had apathy, 19% had insomnia, 12% had delusions and 12% had significant anger. Of course, these may be considered depression-related; and, in another study, they may have been included in the depression category.

It is useful to conceptualize several treatment approaches for the pharmacologic management of dementia in general: (1) treatment of the "primary" cognitive symptoms, (2) treatment of the "secondary" behavioral symptoms, (3) slowing the rate of decline and (4) prolonging the time to disease onset. The last approach is not currently within our ken, although if onset is delayed 5 years the prevalence of AD would be halved (Jorm et al., 1987). The first three have a bearing on the approach to symptomatic behaviors.

Conceptually, improving cognitive symptomatology in dementia may improve behavioral symptomatology, if behaviors such as depression, agitation or hallucinations are modulated by cognitive impairment. For example, delusions may improve with improvement in cognitive functioning. It would not be inappropriate, therefore, to use medications such as cholinesterase inhibitors in studies of patients with both cognitive impairment and symptomatic behaviors.

Another consideration in treating symptomatic behaviors is that of whether the behaviors in a particular patient constitute a stage of illness or a subgroup of the illness. In the latter case, the presence of behavioral symptoms such as depression or psychosis may have prognostic implications. For example, the presence of psychosis in an AD patient may predict more rapid cognitive decline (see Chui et al., 1992 for references).

To assess predictors of cognitive progression in AD, we examined patients admitted to the Rancho Los Amigos Alzheimer's Disease Treatment Center in Downey, California (Chui et al., 1992). Among patients with Mini-Mental State Examinations (MMSE) score of > 15, we assessed whether sex, education, age of onset, initial MMSE score, hallucinations, delusions, agitation, extrapyramidal symptoms or a family history of dementia predicted rate of cognitive decline using two possible endpoints in Cox proportional hazards models: the time to reach either a MMSE endpoint of ≤ 10, or a 5 point drop in MMSE. Of 113 who had baseline MMSE scores > 15, 68% were female;

mean educational level was 12 years; mean age was 72.4 years; mean illness duration was 3.8 years and mean MMSE was 20.2. After classifying according to severity, patients with mild cognitive impairment who had hallucinations, agitation or delusions were 5.1 times, 4.6 times and 3.4 times more likely (all $p > 0.05$), respectively, to reach one of the endpoints compared to patients without these features (see Chui et al., 1992 for details). Although there are several potential reasons for this, including the possibility that these patients represented a distinct subgroup such as diffuse Lewy body disease, the essential point is that patients with symptomatic behaviors are at risk for further cognitive deterioration.

TREATMENT OF PSYCHOSIS, AGITATION, AND DEPRESSION

The consequences of symptomatic behaviors include diminished safety, the inability of the family to care for the patient, earlier institutionalization, inability of the patient to cooperate with the caregiver consequently leading to poor care, and poor quality of life. These behaviors should be treated aggressively when possible.

Depression
Although the efficacy of pharmacological treatment of primary depression in the elderly is established, most of this research has been with noncognitively-impaired, generally physically healthy outpatients (Schneider, 1994). Results from a placebo-controlled clinical trial of nortriptyline demonstrate that frail elderly patients with symptoms of major depression in a residential care setting respond to treatment (Katz et al., 1990), as do elderly and younger adult patients suffering from diseases that are common in late life, such as stroke, pulmonary disease, cancer and arthritis (references are available from author). Many of these patients probably had cognitive impairment and AD but had not been diagnosed.

Treatment response in elderly with both dementia and depression-related symptoms, however, has only recently received limited formal investigation. A randomized trial of imipramine showed no significant advantage over placebo, but both groups improved (Reifler et al., 1989). A placebo-controlled trial of the monoamine oxidase-A (MAO-A) selective inhibitor, moclobemide, however, suggested its efficacy (Hebenstreit et al., 1991). An open nortriptyline trial in inpatients with mixed depression and cognitive impairment, reported 10 of 16 patients improved in both depression and dementia scores, responding similarly to cognitively-intact elderly depressives (Reynolds et al., 1987). Citalopram also may be effective in patients with both dementia and depression (Nyth and Gottfries, 1992).

The NIH Consensus Statement emphasized both the efficacy and potential adverse effects of antidepressant treatment for the elderly in general, stating that nursing home patients, many with dementia, "...respond equally well to standard doses of antidepressant, although their medical fragility can lead to treatment-limiting side effects in as many as one third..." (Friedhoff, 1994).

Agitation

Numerous medications have been advocated for treating agitation including cyclic antidepressants, trazodone, serotonin uptake inhibitors, MAO inhibitors, lithium, buspirone, neuroleptics, and benzodiazepines. Generally, the basis for these recommendations have been case series or reports, and the specific dementia syndrome and target behaviors are not defined but lumped under an "agitation" rubric (Schneider and Sobin, 1994). It is noteworthy that most of these medications have predominant mood effects in cognitively-intact patients.

Trazodone: The evidence suggesting that trazodone may be effective in reducing agitation came from a case series in which 8 of 12 patients with senile dementia or psychosis with cerebral arteriosclerosis who received doses up to 150 mg/day showed improvement in mood, organicity, and arousal. Subsequently, improvement was reported in a number of case reports, with doses from 150 to 500 mg/day (see Schneider and Sobin, 1994 for references).

Serotonin uptake inhibitors: 5 of 12 patients with AD showed reduced irritability, aggressiveness and better tolerance to stress when treated with alaproclate in an open study, but a subsequent placebo-controlled trial in 40 nursing home residents with either AD or multi-infarct dementia showed no significant efficacy (Dehlin et al., 1985). In contrast, a placebo controlled trial involving 98 patients, showed that those with AD, but not vascular dementia, improved in several behavioral symptoms when treated with citalopram (Nyth and Gottfries, 1992). Thus, serotonin uptake inhibitors may be of use in treating symptomatic behaviors in patients with dementia, but more trials are needed.

MAO inhibitors: L-deprenyl (selegiline) may be useful for both cognitive and behavioral symptoms in AD and other dementias. The evidence is derived from several case series in patients with dementia who improved in self-care, cooperativeness, alertness, agitation, anxiety, delusions, anxiety/depression, tension and excitement when they were given 5 mg/day (see Tariot et al., 1993 for citations), although adequate clinical trials have not been done.

Lithium: Most agitated patients with dementia do not respond favorably to lithium although there are occasional exceptions. The elderly may be particularly sensitive to side effects at usual doses (cf. Schneider and Sobin, 1994 for citations).

Buspirone: Despite its recent popularity, the evidence for the effectiveness of buspirone in patients with agitation is meager, consisting of only case reports or series. The time to response for buspirone may be slow, with doses ranging from 10-45 mg/day making case reports difficult to interpret.

Anticonvulsants: Because of its neuromodulatory effects, carbamazepine may be particularly effective in patients with agitation, rage or lability, as suggested by reports in AD patients treated with doses of 400 mg/day. Clinical improvement occurred within 2 to 4 weeks. Lower doses seem to be effective. Valproic acid may be similarly useful.

Neuroleptics: These are by far the most commonly prescribed medications for a variety of behaviors in dementia. As with other medications there are very few controlled trials. Previously, we had examined the efficacy of neuroleptics using meta-analysis (Schneider et al., 1990). We identified seven double-blind, placebo-controlled trials in agitated dementia patients that met minimal methodological standards, and statistically combined them. The magnitude of the neuroleptic effect was significant but small ($r=0.18$), indicating that 18 of 100 subjects benefitted from treatment (beyond that of placebo). Suspiciousness, delusions and hallucinations were most responsive to neuroleptics. A range of symptoms improved, in general only to a modest degree, including assaultiveness, anxiety, overactivity and hostility. Other symptoms such as unsociability, poor self-care, combativeness, agitation and negativism did not.

Methodological problems in most studies include the lack of explicit diagnoses, trial methodology, and validated outcome instruments. In some trials, a prominent placebo effect has been noted averaging about 35-40%. This magnitude emphasizes how uncontrolled trials are difficult to interpret.

REFERENCES

Alzheimer A (1907): Über eine eigenartige Erkrankung der Hirnrinde. *Allgem Zeit Psychiat Psych-Gerich Med* 64:146-148.

Chui HC, Lyness S, Sobel E and Schneider LS (1992): Prognostic implications of symptomatic behaviors in Alzheimer's disease. In: *Heterogeneity of Alzheimer's Disease*, Boller F et al., eds. Berlin: Springer-Verlag, pp. 12-23.

Dehlin O, Hedenrud B, Jansson P and Norgard J (1985): A double-blind comparison of alaproclate and placebo in the treatment of patients with senile dementia. *Acta Psychiatry Scand* 71:190-196.

Friedhoff AJ (1994): Consensus development conference statement. In: *Diagnosis and Treatment of Depression in the Elderly: Proceedings of the NIH Consensus Development Conference*. Schneider LS, Reynolds CF, Lebowitz B and Friedhoff A, eds. Washington: American Psychiatric Press, pp. 491-511.

Hebenstreit GF, Baumhackl U, Chan-Palay V et al. (1991): The treatment of depression in geriatric depressed and demented patients by moclobemide. *Fifth Congress of the International Psychogeriatric Association*. Rome, Italy.

Jorm AF, Korten AE and Henderson AS (1987): The prevalence of dementia: A quantitative integration of the literature. *Acta Psychiatr Scand* 76:465-479.

Katz IR, Simpson GM, Curlik SM et al. (1990): Pharmacologic treatment of major depression for elderly patients in residential care settings. *J Clin Psychiatry* 51(Supp)l:41-47.

Nyth AL and Gottfries CG (1992): The clinical efficacy of citalopram in treatment of emotional disturbances in dementia disorders. A Nordic multicenter study. *Br J Psychiatry* 157:894-901.

Reifler BV, Teri L, Raskind M et al. (1989): Double-blind trial of imipramine in Alzheimer's disease in patients with and without depression. *Am J Psychiatry* 146:45-49.

Reynolds CF, Perel JM, Kupfer DJ, Zimmer B, Stack JA and Hoch CH (1987): Open-trial response to antidepressant treatment in elderly patients with mixed depression and cognitive impairment. *Psychiatry Research* 21:111-122.

Schneider LS, Pollock VE and Lyness SA (1990): A meta-analysis of controlled trials of neuroleptic treatment of dementia. *J Am Geriatr Soc* 38:553-563.

Schneider LS and Sobin P (1994): Treatments for psychiatric symptoms and behavior disturbances in dementia. In: *Dementia*. Burns A and Levy R, eds. London: Chapman and Hall Medical, pp. 519-540.

Schneider LS (1994): Comments on meta-analysis from a clinician's perspective. In: *Diagnosis and Treatment of Depression in the Elderly: Proceedings of the NIH Consensus Development Conference*. Schneider LS, Reynolds CF, Lebowitz B and Friedhoff A, eds. Washington: American Psychiatric Press, pp. 361-373.

Tariot PN, Schneider LS, Patel SV and Goldstein B (1993): Alzheimer's disease and (-)-deprenyl: rationale and findings. In: *Inhibitors of Monoamine Oxidase B Pharmacology and Clinical Use In Neurodegenerative Disorders*. Szelenyi I, ed. Basel: Birkhäuser Verlag AG, pp. 301-317.

Alzheimer Disease: Therapeutic Strategies
edited by E. Giacobini and R. Becker.
© 1994 Birkhäuser Boston

TREATMENT WITH SEROTONERGIC DRUGS OF EMOTIONAL DISTURBANCES IN PATIENTS WITH DEMENTIA DISORDERS

Carl-Gerhard Gottfries

Göteborg University, Department of Clinical Neuroscience, Section of Psychiatry and Neurochemistry, Mölndal, Sweden

Neuropathological and neurochemical postmortem investigations of brains of Alzheimer-afflicted patients have shown that there is a serotonergic deficit, as marked by reduced concentrations of 5-hydroxytryptamine (5-HT, serotonin) and 5-hydroxyindoleacetic acid (5-HIAA) in tissue samples. 5-HIAA is also significantly reduced in the cerebrospinal fluid (CSF) (for review see Cowburn et al., 1989). In vascular dementia (VAD), there are also general neurochemical changes in the brain, as marked by reduced acetylcholine transferase activity and reduced concentrations of 5-HT and 5-HIAA (Gottfries et al., 1994).

In one study (Nyth and Gottfries, 1990), the aim was to examine the effect of citalopram on emotional symptoms and cognitive deficiency in a sample of elderly patients with dementia of the Alzheimer type (AD) or VAD. A total of 98 patients were included in the intention-to-treat analysis. Sixty-one patients completed treatment. The initial dose was 20 mg; in some of the patients the dose was increased to 30 mg during the trial.

GBS ratings (Gottfries et al., 1982) indicated emotional disturbances in most of the patients (87%) at baseline. Four or more disturbances were recorded in each of 39 patients and 1-3 disturbances in each of 46 patients. MADRS ratings indicated no depression at all or only mild depression in most of the patients (mean total MADRS score = 8.1, SD = 6.6). Only two patients were considered to suffer from major depression.

At the end of the double-blind treatment, citalopram-treated patients with AD showed improvement in the GBS items of emotional bluntness, confusion, irritability, anxiety, fear-panic, depressed mood, and restlessness. Improvement in irritability and depressed mood was significantly greater in the citalopram-treated than in the placebo-treated AD patients, and the difference with respect to fear-panic and restlessness bordered on significance. Neither motor performance nor intellectual functions were influenced by the treatment. No changes were recorded for any of the GBS items in the placebo-treated AD patients. The ratings of Clinical Global Impression (CGI) severity of illness showed slight, but significant deterioration in placebo-treated AD patients. The

MADRS mean total score was reduced in the citalopram-treated AD patients, whereas there was no change in the placebo-treated AD patients. No improvement was recorded in the VAD patients during treatment. This group was small, however.

As expected, there was a reduction in the concentration of CSF 5-HIAA after 8-12 weeks of treatment with citalopram. No withdrawal symptoms or rebound phenomena were observed or recorded during the double-blind withdrawal of citalopram.

The results of a global assessment of side-effects did not differ between citalopram- and placebo-treated patients. Concentration difficulties, depression, emotional indifference, dizziness, diminished sexual desire, ejaculatory dysfunction and orgastic dysfunction were recorded only during treatment with citalopram.

In another study, the aim was to further estimate the efficacy of citalopram treatment in elderly depressed patients with or without concomitant dementia. A total of 149 patients were included in the intention-to-treat analysis. Sixteen patients were withdrawn within two weeks, leaving 133 to the efficacy analysis (Nyth et al., 1992).

The HDS mean total score decreased significantly at week two and onwards in the citalopram, as well as the placebo group. At week six, the HDS mean total score was lower in the citalopram than in the placebo group. The difference in improvement was also significant.

In a number of HDS items, namely depressed mood, self-depreciation and guilt feelings, suicidal impulses, agitation, and general somatic symptoms, the citalopram group improved more than the placebo group. This improvement was usually not recorded until week six. The MADRS mean total score was reduced from week two and onwards and, at week six, the MADRS mean total score was significantly lower in the citalopram than in the placebo group. Patients with a HDS total score reduction of $\geq 50\%$ or a MADRS total score reduction of $\geq 50\%$ were defined as responders. At week six, the citalopram group had 53% responders and the placebo group 28% ($p < 0.05$). At week six, the CGI severity of illness mean score had decreased from 3.2 to 1.9 in the citalopram group and from 3.1 to 2.6 in the placebo group. The difference in mean score and in improvement was statistically significant.

In patients with concomitant mild or moderate dementia, treatment with citalopram significantly reduced the mean GBS scores on anxiety, fear-panic, depressed mood, orientation in time, personal orientation, recent memory, distant memory. No improvement was recorded after treatment with placebo. The citalopram-treated patients improved more than the placebo-treated in orientation in time, recent memory, inability to increase tempo, and fear-panic. The difference with respect to depressed mood bordered on significant.

In 63% of the citalopram-treated patients versus 75% of the placebo-treated, no side-effects were recorded during the entire treatment period.

In an open study with citalopram, the effect of long-term treatment of elderly demented individuals with emotional disturbances was investigated (Ragneskog et al., to be published). The sample consisted of 148 patients, 123 of whom were included in the data analysis. There were outpatients as well as inpatients and the mean age was 78 years (variance 58-96). Most of the patients resided in nursing homes. Assessment of efficacy was made using the GBS and CGI scales. Fifty-two patients completed the 12-month treatment. Compared with baseline, this group showed significant improvement in irritability, anxiety, fear-panic, and depression and significant deterioration in motor performance, all according to the GBS scale. According to the CGI ratings, therapeutic efficacy was significantly improved after one month of treatment. Seventy-seven patients (72%) were rated as improved, 26 as unchanged, and four as deteriorated. According to the GBS ratings, the mean values of intellectual and emotional impairment were slightly improved; confusion, irritability, depressed mood, anxiety, fear-panic and restlessness were significantly reduced.

Most of the patients reported no side-effects. Asthenia/tiredness and dizziness were the most common side-effects, reported by 12% and 11%, respectively.

It is clear that citalopram treatment has a beneficial effect on emotional disturbances in patients with dementia and in elderly patients. This effect is broader than that of the traditional tricyclic antidepressants, i.e., it is not confined to mood elevation.

The antidepressant efficacy of paroxetine in the elderly has been evaluated in nine published clinical trials involving a total of 641 patients. The studies primarily included patients who met the criteria for major depression according to DSM-III. All the studies used the HDS and CGI scales as outcome variables. Obviously, paroxetine is associated with fewer anticholinergic and CNS adverse events than tricyclic antidepressants. As with other SSRI drugs, there was an increased incidence of gastrointestinal disorders, particularly nausea, during paroxetine therapy. However, these effects were generally mild and resolved with continued treatment. A marked reduction in anxiety scores compared with baseline were recorded in patients with major depressive disorders (for review, see Holliday and Plosker, 1993).

The new generation of monoamineoxidase (MAO) inhibitors, which selectively inhibit MAO-A or MAO-B, are also of interest in treatment of patients with dementia disorders. Moclobemide, which selectively inhibits MAO-A, may up-regulate activity in the serotonergic and noradrenergic systems. Treatment trials with this drug have been performed in elderly patients and patients with dementia (Chan-Palay, 1991). The results indicate an antidepressant effect, but also enhancement of cognitive functions in patients with dementia disorders. A study in which moclobemide is compared with citalopram and placebo in treatment of patients with AD and emotional disturbances is ongoing in Europe.

Ondansetron is a potent selective and competitive antagonist of 5-HT at the $5-HT_3$ receptor. Activation of $5-HT_3$ receptors in central and peripheral neurons elicits the polarization that results in neurotransmitter release. Within the peripheral nervous system, 5-HT$_3$ receptors have been implicated in the modulation of both sympathetic and parasympathetic neurons. In CNS, 5-HT$_3$ receptors are concentrated in cortical and limbic regions. Evidence from various animal models indicates that ondansetron has therapeutic potential in the treatment of emesis, as well as cognitive and psychiatric disorders, the latter including anxiety, schizophrenia, mania, and drug dependence.

Ondansetron enhances performance in animal models of cognitive function and reverses scopolamine-induced memory deficits. It may exert its effect by blocking 5-HT$_3$ receptor-mediated inhibition of acetylcholine release.

The effect of ondansetron in age-associated memory impairment was tested by Crook and Lakin (1991). The investigators concluded that ondansetron is of considerable interest and merits further study as a putative treatment of age-associated memory impairment and perhaps other adult onset cognitive disorders. At present, ondansetron is being tested in multicenter studies on age-associated memory impairment and AD.

It is obvious that monoaminergic, especially serotonergic, disturbances are found in brains of patients with AD as well as VAD. An age-related decline in monoamines is also found in normal aging. Treatment with serotonergic drugs reduces emotional disturbances in demented patients and in old individuals. It is not adequate to call the new SSRI drugs antidepressants. They should rather be dubbed emotional stabilizers, as they achieve not only increased levels of mood, but also reduced anxiety, fear-panic, and aggressiveness. Some data indicate that this type of drugs, including MAO-inhibitors, also has effect on cognitive impairment. Further studies are needed to confirm this finding. Treatment trials have shown that these drugs have a favorable tolerability among elderly people and demented patients. They should therefore be the first choice in treatment of demented people with emotional disturbances.

REFERENCES

Chan-Palay V (1991): Affective disorder and cognitive disease: basis for therapy. In: *Book of abstracts, 5th Congress of the International Psychogeriatric Association (IPA), Rome, Italy, August 18-23*, p. 31.

Cowburn RF, Hardy JA and Roberts PJ (1989): Neurotransmitter deficits in Alzheimer's disease. In: *Alzheimer's Disease: Towards an Understanding of the Etiology and Pathogenesis*. Davies DC, ed. London: John Libbey, pp. 9-32.

Crook T and Lakin M (1991): Effect of ondansetron in age-associated memory impairment. In: *Proceedings of the 5th World Congress of Biological Psychiatry, Florence, June 9-14*. Racagni G, Brunello N and Fukuda T, eds. *Biol Psychiatry* 2:888-890.

Gottfries CG, Bråne G, Gullberg B and Steen G (1982): A new rating scale for dementia syndromes. *Arch Gerontol Geriatr* 1:311-330.

Gottfries CG, Blennow K, Karlsson I and Wallin A (1994): The neurochemistry of vascular dementia. *Dementia* (In Press).

Holliday SM and Plosker GL (1993): Paroxetine: a review of its pharmacology, therapeutic use in depression and therapeutic potential in diabetic neuropathy. *Drugs and Aging* 3:278-299.

Nyth AL and Gottfries CG (1990): The clinical efficacy of citalopram in treatment of emotional disturbances in dementia disorders. A Nordic multicenter study. *Br J Psychiatry* 157:894-901.

Nyth AL, Gottfries CG, Lyby K, Smedegaard-Andersen L, Gylding-Sabroe JU, Refsum H-E, Öfsti E, Eriksson S and Syversen S (1992): A controlled multicenter clinical study of citalopram and placebo in elderly depressed patients with and without concomitant dementia. *Acta Psychiat Scand* 86:138-145.

Alzheimer Disease: Therapeutic Strategies
edited by E. Giacobini and R. Becker.
© 1994 Birkhäuser Boston

GLUTAMATERGIC HYPOACTIVITY IN ALZHEIMER'S DISEASE: INVESTIGATIVE AND THERAPEUTIC PERSPECTIVES

Paul T. Francis, Iain P. Chessell, Marie-Therese Webster, Andrew W. Procter, Michelle Qume and David M. Bowen
Miriam Marks Department of Neurochemistry, Institute of Neurology, Queen Square, London, U.K.

A substantial presynaptic cholinergic abnormality in the brains of patients with Alzheimer's disease (AD) suggested a basis for rational pharmacological treatments. An additional effect of such neurotransmitter replacement is now emerging as processing pathways for ß-amyloid precursor protein (APP) appear to be regulated by transmitter receptors, at least those coupled to the phosphoinositide (PI)/Ca^{2+} second messenger system such as the acetylcholine muscarinic (M^1) receptor (Nitsch et al., 1992). Activation of this receptor favors the non-amyloidogenic pathway (α-secretase) that leads to a decrease in the intracellular amyloidogenic fragments generated from APP (Fukushima et al., 1993).

Postmortem biochemical studies of AD, where extensive transmitter deficits may be seen, has led some workers to the pessimistic conclusion that a transmitter-based therapy cannot be successful. However, such studies almost invariably examine the end-stage of this slowly progressing disease and this is rarely acknowledged in the interpretation. It has been possible to study samples removed earlier in the disease as neocortical tissue from AD patients has been occasionally removed surgically for diagnostic purposes. Transmitter changes in neurosurgical (biopsy) samples have been emphasized in this chapter.

Neurotransmitters and Receptors
Neurosurgical samples showed a severe deficiency in acetylcholine synthesis by the mid-point of AD which correlated with the rating of dementia (Francis et al., 1993). Cortical inputs using the catecholamines, noradrenaline and dopamine, are relatively unaffected. The situation regarding inputs using 5-HT is complex. Even in autopsy AD brain, half of the many cortical areas assayed showed no evidence of a selective reduction in presynaptic 5-HT activity. Hence, deficiency of presynaptic serotonergic activity is probably never widespread, a feature consistent with the preservation of 5-HIAA concentration in ventricular CSF (VCSF) from living AD patients. Indeed the turnover rate in those 5-HT

nerve endings remaining appears to be enhanced in AD patients, based on the increased ratio of 5-HIAA to 5-HT in cortical tissue and the nucleus basalis. Furthermore, 5-HIAA concentration in lumbar CSF was positively correlated with dementia rating in a series of histologically verified living AD patients, and in another series the mean 5-HIAA value was significantly higher than control (Francis et al., 1994). Recently we have found that for AD subjects dying in the community the concentrations of 5-HT and 5-HIAA were not significantly reduced in the areas studied. Indeed in the temporal cortex the ratio of 5-HIAA to 5-HT was increased in AD compared to controls (Chen et al., 1994). This extends earlier work as long-stay psychiatric hospitals were the probable source of almost all previously studied autopsy material and these are likely to represent a skewed population due to the inadvertent selection of subjects with non-cognitive behavioral problems.

The balance of evidence indicates that GABA and somatostatin are not critically depleted in AD consistent with a maintained inhibitory tone on cortical pyramidal neurones.

Three studies indicated that severity of dementia correlated with degeneration of glutamatergic corticocortical pyramidal neurones in association areas (as reviewed, Francis et al., 1992). Psychological test scores correlated with both the positron emission tomography data, the pyramidal cell counts in cortical layer III and number of synapses in layer III. Thus, a clinically relevant shrinkage or loss of association fibres probably occurred from circumscribed (i.e., parietotemporal) areas and this contributed to the overall reduction observed in glucose metabolism.

Studies on postmortem AD samples have demonstrated that binding sites for most transmitters are unaltered in the cerebral cortex (as reviewed, Francis et al., 1992). The main postsynaptic muscarinic receptor (M_1) seemed to be preserved, which should provide a suitable target for acetylcholine. Nicotinic and M_2 muscarinic receptors (at least the latter may be primarily presynaptic) were reduced. Binding sites for 5-HT were not consistently abnormal. Altered populations of binding sites for glutamate have been reported in the hippocampus but little change was seen in the neocortex, although reduced glutamate binding in cortical layers 1 and 11 has been reported. Apart from reduced sensitivity to modulation by glycine, the properties of the NMDA receptor complex seem to be normal but the number of complexes may be reduced, probably due to pyramidal cell loss. Moreover, $5-HT_{1A}$ receptor-G protein interactions were preserved in AD patients as was found for the M_1 receptor by Pearce and Potter (but not by Flynn and colleagues). However, the groups studying M_1 did not consider factors such as patients' immediate preterminal state (as reviewed, Francis et al., 1992).

Receptor Regulation of Cortical Pyramidal Neurones

It is well established that volkensin, a retrogradely transported toxic lectin, can be used to selectively destroy sub-populations of cortical and hippocampal pyramidal neurones distant from the site of injection. We have used receptor autoradiography with sections of rat brain from volkensin-injected animals to establish the receptor repertoire of cortical pyramidal cells. These studies have emphasized the importance of M_1 receptors for regulating the activity of both corticofugal and corticocortical pyramidal neurones. However, from this work the most selective marker of a subpopulation of corticofugal neurones is the $5HT_{1A}$ receptor. Although this does not appear to be true for corticocortical neurones in the rat, an important species difference should be emphasized. In rats $5\text{-}HT_{1A}$ receptors are found in the lower cortical layers whilst in primates (including man) there is an additional high density in upper layers. This observation suggests that the receptor is enriched on ipsilateral projecting corticocortical pyramidal neurones (Francis et al., 1993). Receptors that are present in the greatest numbers are obvious targets for drugs to normalize activity of these neurones. The most suitable receptors by other criteria are those that are PLC-linked and may avoid the possibility of excitotoxicity. Hence, positive modulation of impulse flow by the M_1 receptor, perhaps in combination with an antagonist of the $5\text{-}HT_{1A}$ receptor induced hyperpolarization, is considered to represent a most promising therapeutic strategy. A further approach suggested by others is the use of nicotinic agonists. This is supported by the present study as these receptors appear to be enriched on pyramidal neurones. Acetylcholinesterase inhibitors are well known to be under development for the treatment of AD and these should stimulate both nicotinic and M_1 receptors.

Amyloid Precursor Protein-Like Immunoreactivity Can Be Altered in Humans by Drugs Affecting Neurotransmitter Function

There are no drugs presently in routine clinical use which would be expected to *increase* APP secretion, in contrast to those used in studies of the cultured cell lines. Yet in affective disorders, lithium is prescribed and our *a priori* hypothesis was that since it is considered to interfere with PIP_2 recycling, such chronic treatment would be associated with lower APP concentrations in VCSF. APP secretion may also be decreased by drugs with anticholinergic or other neuronal activity inhibiting properties such as antidepressants. Therefore, we examined the effect of therapy with these and other drugs, on indices of APP secretion in rare samples of human VCSF (Clarke et al., 1993). On the basis of the *a priori* hypothesis (above) patients were divided into 4 groups according to treatment with lithium or antidepressants.

The mean VCSF APP_{KPI} value determined with antibody 22C11 for patients receiving both lithium and antidepressants was significantly lower than that of patients receiving neither. Results with the other antibodies confirmed the direction of change seen with 22C11. However, the reduction in immunoreactivity was most obvious with the other antibodies, including antibody, 10D5, indicating reduced α-secretase activity. This suggests that either activating PIP$_2$ hydrolysis or stimulating neuronal activity will reduce secretion of ß-amyloid protein.

CONCLUSIONS

The cost of AD is estimated at over £1.4 and £17.8 billion per year (1992/93 prices) for UK and USA respectively, determined without allowance for either informal care not recognized with payment (UK figure) or loss of earnings (Gray and Fenn, 1993; A.M. Gray, personal communication). Many articles have been published on the illness during the past few years. Almost all have considered the ß-amyloid peptide and precursor APP, reflecting the international bias of research. However, such studies are directly relevant to only one aspect of the neuropathology of this dementia, senile plaque formation. Moreover, the articles have not considered plaques in relation to neurotransmission.

Promising transmitter-related drugs for treating cognitive symptoms of the illness are under development by several pharmaceutical companies. This approach is based on another neuropathological feature, selective degeneration of sub-populations of cortical glutamatergic pyramidal neurones, and the well-known cholinergic deficit. In combination, these two features are considered to cause hypoactivity of other glutamatergic pyramidal neurones involved in cognition. The drugs, cholinomimetics and serotonin 1A receptor antagonists, should also beneficially affect metabolism of APP by favoring the non-amyloidogenic pathway, as this is stimulated by depolarization and receptor-linked phosphorylation.

It is important to discover any effect of the drugs on signal-transduction-dependent phosphorylation and dephosphorylation of tau protein. In particular, on the aberrant mechanism that leads to hyperphosphorylation of tau and almost certainly underlies neurofibrillary tangle formation, the other pathological hallmark of AD. Such hyperphosphorylation characteristically occurs in the pyramidal neurones and has been linked by Strittmatter and Roses to the diminished or lack of apolipoprotein E4 binding to tau relative to E3 (Bowen et al., 1994). At least one additional factor, hypoactivity of glutamatergic neurones, may be implicated in the aberrant mechanism, a proposal based on our working hypothesis that such hypoactivity underlies the symptoms of the disease. This is supported by the observation that when treated with a high (1 mM) concentration of glutamate, primary cultures of fetal rat cortical neurones contained much lower amounts of hyperphosphorylated tau (Davis et al., 1994) characteristic of AD, as identified with antibody AT8.

This experiment did not mimic normal relationships of transmitter glutamate to synapses and the cells studied may not have the metabolic processes found in AD brain (Francis et al., 1993) that affect tau. Nevertheless it is hoped that the *observation* will prompt further research to provide more compelling support for the theory that the number of tangles, like plaques and cognitive impairment, will be reduced by a drug designed to improve the state of pyramidal neurone activation. Of course, it is not certain that such a drug will attain therapeutic goals (e.g. delay in onset of care in hospital and residential/nursing homes). However, a positive outcome is now not inconceivable given the recent discoveries (described above). Thus the drug proposed could have a favorable impact on the burden of the illness.

REFERENCES

Bowen DM, Francis PT, Chessell IP and Webster M-T (1994): Neurotransmission-the link integrating Alzheimer research? *Trends Neurosci* 17:149-150.

Chen CPL-H, Alder JT, Hope RA, Francis PT, McDonald B, Esiri MM and Bowen DM (1994): The 5-hydroxytryptaminergic system in Alzheimer's disease exhibits plasticity and is affected by neuroleptic medication. *Br J Pharmacol* (In Press).

Clarke NA, Webster M-T, Francis PT, Procter AW, Hodgkiss AD and Bowen DM (1993): β-Amyloid precursor protein-like immunoreactivity can be altered in humans by drugs affecting neurotransmitter function. *Neurodegeneration* 2:243-248.

Davis DR, Brion J-P, Couck A-M, Gallo J-M, Hanger DP, Ladhani K, Lewis C, Miller CCJ, Rupniak T, Smith C and Anderton BH (1994): Glutamate and colchicine cause dephosphorylation of the microtubule associated protein tau and a change in perikaryal tau-immunoreactivity in rat cortical neurones in primary culture. *Brain Res Assoc* 11:38.

Francis PT, Pangalos MN and Bowen DM (1992): Animal and drug modelling for Alzheimer synaptic pathology. *Prog Neurobiol* 39:517-545.

Francis PT, Sims NR, Procter AW and Bowen DM (1993): Cortical pyramidal neurone loss may cause glutamatergic hypoactivity and cognitive impairment in Alzheimer's disease: investigative and therapeutic perspectives. *J Neurochem* 60:1589-1604.

Francis PT, Cross AJ and Bowen DM (1994): Neurotransmitters and Neuropeptides. In: *Alzheimer Disease*, Terry RD, Katzman R and Bick KL, eds. New York: Raven Press, pp. 247-261.

Fukushima D, Konishi M, Maruyama K, Miyamoto T, Ishiura S and Suzuki K (1993): Activation of the secretory pathway leads to a decrease in the intracellular amyloidogenic fragments generated from the amyloid protein precursor. *Biochem Biophys Res Comm* 194:202-207.

Gray A and Fenn P (1993): Alzheimer disease: the burden of illness in England. *Health Trends* 25:31-37.

Nitsch RM, Slack BE, Wurtman RJ and Growdon JH (1992): Release of Alzheimer amyloid precursor stimulated by activation of muscarinic acetylcholine receptors. *Science* 258:304-307.

Alzheimer Disease: Therapeutic Strategies
edited by E. Giacobini and R. Becker.
© 1994 Birkhäuser Boston

DISTURBANCES OF GAIT IN PATIENTS WITH DEMENTIA

Rodger J. Elble
Department of Neurology and The Center for Alzheimer Disease and Related
Disorders, Southern Illinois Univ. Sch. Med., Springfield, IL 62794-9230

Effective locomotion requires the integration and control of posture, balance and movement. Rudimentary locomotor behaviors emerge from spinal neuronal networks, which function as locomotor pattern generators (Grillner, 1981). The capacity of these pattern generators to produce effective locomotion is inversely proportional to the sophistication of an animal's nervous system. The function of spinal pattern generators in humans (Holmes, 1915) and laboratory primates (Eidelberg et al., 1981a,b) depends critically on descending input from higher centers.

The cerebellum mediates the rhythmicity of locomotion and the phasic coordination of the limbs through rubrospinal, lateral pontomedullary reticulospinal, and vestibulospinal (Dieter's nucleus) pathways (Armstrong, 1988; Kawahara et al., 1985; Mori, 1987). The ventral spinocerebellar pathway carries output from the spinal pattern generators to the cerebellum. This "efference copy" of generator output is integrated with somatosensory feedback via the dorsal spinocerebellar pathway, with visual feedback via the pontine nuclei and inferior olive, with vestibular feedback and, in some instances, with auditory feedback via the pontine nuclei. The cerebellum also receives cerebral inputs by way of the pontine and olivary nuclei. These transcerebellar pathways facilitate the adjustment of motor programs to environmental constraints and use sensory information in the context of prior experience to formulate motor commands. This feedforward control of movement is a critical aspect of effective locomotion and involves neuronal circuits that are affected by many dementing diseases.

Locomotor regions in the mesencephalon and diencephalon are involved in the initiation of locomotion. The anatomical characterization of both regions is incomplete. The diencephalic locomotor region (DLR) is located in the lateral hypothalamic area (Marciello and Sinnamon, 1990). Stimulation of DLR in cats produces stealthy locomotion, as though the animal were in pursuit of prey. The mesencephalic locomotor region (MLR) is located in the dorsolateral midbrain in the region of the pedunculopontine nucleus and the neighboring noncholinergic midbrain extrapyramidal area (Rye et al., 1987, 1988). Brief stimulation of the MLR induces rapid walking or running, depending upon the strength of stimulation. The MLR has reciprocal connections with the ipsilateral basal ganglia (Garcia-Rill, 1986; Rye et al., 1987, 1988). The substantia nigra pars reticulata (SNr) and the globus pallidus interna (GPi) provide GABAergic inputs to the MLR, which have an inhibitory influence on locomotion (Garcia-Rill, 1986). Neuronal activity in SNr and GPi is increased in Parkinson disease, possibly explaining the locomotor problems (e.g., freezing) in these patients (DeLong and Wichmann, 1993). The MLR receives excitatory glutaminergic inputs from the subthalamus and motor cortex, which promote locomotion (Garcia-Rill, 1986). A neural circuit consisting of the nucleus accumbens - ventral pallidum - MLR - ventral tegmental area (dopaminergic) links locomotor pathways with the limbic system (Austin and Kalivas, 1991). Stimulation of the ventral pallidum produces behavioral hyperactivity in rats and dogs (Austin and Kalivas, 1991. Malfunction of this limbic pathway could underlie the behavioral hyperactivity in some patients with dementia.

The MLR and DLR connect with the ventral tegmental field (VTF) and the dorsal tegmental field (DTF) of the caudal midline pons (Mori, 1987). The VTF corresponds to the rostral nucleus raphe magnus, and stimulation of the VTF increases antigravity muscle tone (Mori, 1987). The DTF corresponds to the caudal nucleus raphe centralis superior. Stimulation of the DTF suppresses antigravity muscle tone and can prevent walking when the DLR or MLR is stimulated. Cholinergic agonists, excitatory amino acid agonists, GABAergic antagonists, and substance P facilitate locomotion when injected into the VTF (Kinjo et al., 1990) and inhibit locomotion when injected into the DTF.

Sensorimotor and premotor cortex influence locomotion through direct or indirect connections with MLR, DLR, basal ganglia, cerebellum and spinal cord. These anatomical levels of motor control comprise a highly integrated motor system that is influenced by higher cortical functions, including memory, executive function, attention, motivation, visuospatial function, and praxis. Diencephalic cats are capable of seemingly normal locomotion, but the cerebral hemispheres are needed for precise modifications to suit environmental and cognitive demands (Grillner et al., 1990). The influence of higher cortical functions on locomotion has obvious relevance to the care of demented patients and has received little investigation.

GAIT DISTURBANCES IN DEMENTING DISEASES

Walking is a complex motor behavior, which emerges from neuronal networks that are integrated and distributed at virtually all levels of the neuraxis. Dementing diseases affect multiple regions of the nervous system, and similarities in the sites of pathology exist among common dementing diseases. Consequently, no dementing illness produces a diagnostic disturbance of gait. The primary and compensatory characteristics of gait are relatively specific when there is isolated damage to the peripheral nerves, pyramidal tracts, cerebellum, and substantia nigra pars compacta. Dementing diseases may affect these areas of the motor system, but they also affect those areas of the nervous system involved in the highest levels of motor control.[1] The compensatory changes in gait are least specific when the highest levels of locomotor control are impaired. The most general compensatory change is a reduction in gait velocity, produced by reductions in cadence and stride length.

Many characteristics of gait are a function of stride length and are therefore altered by compensatory reductions in stride. Increased time in double-limb stance, reduced arm swing, reduced toe-floor clearance, a slightly widened base, and reduced rotation of the hip and knee occur when stride (velocity) is reduced. This pattern of walking may be exhibited by anyone walking in a hazardous environment (e.g., an icy surface), and this cautious pattern of walking resembles the caricature of an older person's gait ("senile" gait). Many age-related differences in gait are attributable to the reduced strides of the elderly (Elble et al., 1991b), and the characteristics of cautious gait dominate the patterns of walking that are produced by a variety of neurological illnesses, particularly when these illnesses are mild. Elble and coworkers (1991a) compared the gait characteristics of 19 healthy older people with those of 10 elderly patients with a mixture of neurological conditions, including vascular dementia, shunt-responsive normal pressure hydrocephalus (NPH), dementia of Alzheimer type (DAT), levodopa-resistant parkinsonism, and sensorimotor polyneuropathy. Quantitatively, their kinematic characteristics of gait differed greatly from those of elderly controls, but an analysis of covariance revealed that these differences were statistically attributable to reduced stride.

The gait disturbances of dementing illnesses are imbued with characteristics of senile (cautious) gait and therefore resemble an exaggeration of normal aging. Specific diagnoses require the identification of coexistent neurological signs that have greater localizing or diagnostic significance (e.g., pill-rolling rest tremor, Babinski sign, supranuclear ocular palsy). Nevertheless, recognizable syndromes of walking occur in many conditions and provide clues to the underlying site(s) of pathology, as summarized in Table I.

A few items in Table I require clarification and emphasis. The *principal features* are not mutually exclusive, and the list of *clinical conditions* is not comprehensive. Lower-half parkinsonism is an old but still viable clinical concept. Arm swing is not reduced in lower-half parkinsonism and may appear increased when compared to the length of stride. Step width is increased due to a variable degree of coexistent disequilibrium. By contrast, idiopathic Parkinson disease reduces arm swing to a greater extent than stride, and the patient's base is typically narrow. Start hesitation can result from impaired control of posture, movement or their integration (Elble et al., 1994). Rare

---

[1]"Level" is used here in the functional sense, not in the anatomical sense. The locomotor *system is too complex* and integrated to permit a rigid definition of anatomical levels of motor control.

patients exhibit relatively pure start hesitation with little evidence of other motor impairment (Nutt et al., 1993). Patients with start hesitation and short shuffling steps are often described as having an apractic gait. However, posture, balance and movement are rarely if ever sufficiently preserved to justify the term apraxia.

Principal Feature	Related Terminology	Sites of Pathology	Clinical Conditions
Disequilibrium	Frontal ataxia Thalamic ataxia Subcortical disequilibrium	Prefrontal and premotor cortex Ventrolateral thalamus Brainstem motor nuclei Cerebellum	Binswanger disease NPH PSP
Start hesitation	Gait ignition failure Gait apraxia Magnetic gait	Frontal lobes and their connections with basal ganglia and brainstem locomotor regions Basal ganglia	Binswanger disease NPH Parkinson disease
Short, shuffling steps and en bloc turning	Parkinsonian gait Lower-half parkinsonism Marche á petit pas Gait apraxia Magnetic gait	Substantia nigra pars compacta Subcortical white matter and striatum	Parkinson disease Binswanger disease PSP
Cautious gait	Senile gait	Any part of the central or peripheral nervous system involved in locomotion and related higher cortical functions	All of the above and Alzheimer disease

NPH = normal pressure hydrocephalus. PSP = progressive supranuclear palsy

TABLE I. Categorization of gait disturbances in dementing diseases

Most patients with Alzheimer disease exhibit normal gait and balance, but these patients still fall. A strange environment may at times elicit a cautious pattern of walking, but at other times, Alzheimer patients seem to ambulate into a dangerous environment without appropriate caution. This inability to respond appropriately to a threatening environment probably results from impaired visuospatial function, vigilance, judgment and insight. Further research is needed.

ACKNOWLEDGEMENTS

Supported by grants P30 AG08014 and RO1 AG10837 from the NIA.

REFERENCES

Armstrong DM (1988): The supraspinal control of mammalian locomotion. *J Physiol (London)* 405:1-37.

Austin MC and Kalivas PW (1991): Dopaminergic involvement in locomotion elicited from the ventral pallidum/substantia innominata. *Brain Res* 542:123-131.

DeLong MR and Wichmann T (1993): Basal ganglia--thalamocortical circuits in parkinsonian signs. *Clin Neurosci* 1:18-26.

Eidelberg E, Story JL, Walden JG and Meyer BL (1981a): Anatomical correlates of return of locomotor function after partial spinal cord lesions in cats. *Exp Brain Res* 42:81-88.

Eidelberg E, Walden JG and Nguyen LH (1981b): Locomotor control in macaque monkeys. *Brain* 104:647-663.

Elble RJ, Higgins C and Hughes L (1991a): The syndrome of senile gait. *J Neurol* 239:71-75.

Elble RJ, Moody C, Leffler K and Sinha R (1994): The initiation of normal walking. *Mov Disord* 9:139-146.

Elble RJ, Thomas SS, Higgins C and Colliver J (1991b): Stride-dependent changes in gait of older people. *J Neurol* 238:1-5.

Garcia-Rill E (1986): The basal ganglia and the locomotor regions. *Brain Res Reviews* 11:47-63.

Grillner S (1981): Control of locomotion in bipeds, tetrapods, and fish. In *Handbook of Physiology: The Nervous System, Motor Control*, Brooks VB, ed. Baltimore: Williams & Wilkins, pp. 1179-1236.

Grillner S, Wallén P and Viana di Prisco G (1990): Cellular network underlying locomotion as revealed in a lower vertebrate model: transmitters, membrane properties, circuitry, and stimulation. *Cold Spring Harbor Symposium* 55:779-789.

Holmes G (1915): Spinal injuries of warfare. *Br Med J* 2:815-821.

Kawahara K, Mori S, Tomiyama T and Kanaya T (1985): Discharges in neurons in the midpontine dorsal tegmentum of mesencephalic cat during locomotion. *Brain Res* 341:377-380.

Kinjo N, Atsuta Y, Webber M, Kyle R, Skinner RD and Garcia-Rill E (1990): Medioventral medulla-induced locomotion. *Brain Res Bull* 24:509-516.

Marciello M and Sinnamon HM (1990): Locomotor stepping initiated by glutamate injections into the hypothalamus of the anesthetized rat. *Behav Neurosci* 104:980-990.

Mori S (1987): Integration of posture and locomotion in acute decerebrate cats and in awake, freely moving cats. *Prog Neurobiol* 28:161-195.

Nutt JG, Marsden CD and Thompson PD (1993): Human walking and higher-level gait disorders, particularly in the elderly. *Neurology* 43:268-279.

Rye DB, Saper CB, Lee HJ and Wainer BH (1987): Pedunculopontine tegmental nucleus of the rat: cytoarchitecture, cytochemistry, and some extrapyramidal connections of the mesopontine tegmentum. *J Comp Neurol* 259:483-528.

Rye DB, Lee HJ, Saper CB and Wainer BH (1988): Medullary and spinal efferents of the pedunculopontine tegmental nucleus and adjacent mesopontine tegmentum in the rat. *J Comp Neurol* 269:315-341.

PART XIII

NEUROTOXIC DRUGS, TRANSGENIC ANIMALS, AND AGING PRIMATES AS MODELS OF AD TREATMENT

Alzheimer Disease: Therapeutic Strategies
edited by E. Giacobini and R. Becker.
© 1994 Birkhäuser Boston

THE CENTRALLY CHOLINODEFICIENT ANIMAL AS A MODEL OF ALZHEIMER'S DISEASE (AD)

Israel Hanin
Department of Pharmacology and Experimental Therapeutics
Loyola University Chicago, Stritch School of Medicine, Maywood, IL

INTRODUCTION

In the normal animal, any disruption in central cholinergic function is restored swiftly and reversibly. In order to mimic in animals the persistent cholinergic deficiency observed in brains of patients with AD (Davies and Maloney, 1976; Bowen et al., 1976; Boyd et al., 1977; Perry et al., 1977, 1978; Davis and Yamamura, 1978; Sims et al., 1980; Corkin, 1981; Whitehouse et al., 1981; McKinney et al., 1982; Bartus et al., 1982), it is necessary to overcome this efficient regenerative phenomenon.

Several possible target sites exist, at which a permanent cholinodeficiency could be induced (Hörtnagl and Hanin, 1992). These are at the level of: the cell body (excitotoxins); via inhibition of axonal transport (e.g. colchicine); through inhibition of high affinity transport of choline (choline mustard aziridinium analogs, hemicholinium analogs); via inhibition of acetylcholine synthesis within the nerve terminal (cholinergic false transmitters, inhibitors of vesicular acetylcholine uptake); by inhibiting acetylcholine release from the nerve terminal (e.g. botulinum toxin, notexin, etc); or via interaction with nicotinic and muscarinic receptors. In addition, a cholinodeficiency could be induced by well placed lesions (electrolytic, mechanical via aspiration, ablation, or devascularization) in the brain. This report surveys several of these approaches which have been reported in the literature, and analyzes their utility for developing an animal replicate of the cholinergic hypofunction which exists in AD. Selected examples have been chosen in order to illustrate the phenomenon being described, rather than providing an exhaustive overview of the topic. Moreover, this chapter deals only with situations of cholinodeficiency induced *in vivo*.

VARIOUS LESIONING APPROACHES

NON-CHEMICAL LESIONS OF THE BRAIN have been achieved by electrolytic means, aspiration of tissue, surgical ablation of pathways, or devascularization of cortical pia arachnoid vessels (Pedata et al., 1982; Hohmann and Coyle, 1988; Funnell et al., 1990; McGurk et al., 1991). Devascularizing lesions of the cortex, for example, result in complete atrophy of the frontal 1 and 3, parietal 1 and portions of the frontal 2, as well as the parietal 2 and occipital neocortical regions (Garofalo et al., 1992). This procedure results, in rats, in a significant reduction in choline acetyltransferase (ChAT) activity in the ipsilateral (but not contralateral) nucleus basalis of Meynert (nBM) area of the brain. This, in turn, causes a significant reduction in passive avoidance retention as well as in mean escape latency to find a hidden platform in the Morris water maze test, which can be restored to normal in rats following treatment with cholinomimetic agents, such as physostigmine, pilocarpine, arecoline and oxotremorine (Garofalo et al., 1992). As could be expected with such extensive lesions of the brain, other neuronal pathways besides the cholinergic system, for example the dopaminergic system, will also be significantly affected (Elliott et al., 1989). Thus available non-chemical lesions of the brain are not selective for the cholinergic system alone.

Another approach has been one in which chemical agents are employed with the goal of INHIBITING ACETYLCHOLINE STORAGE OR FORMATION IN THE CHOLINERGIC NERVE TERMINAL. Inhibitors of acetylcholine uptake into intraneuronal vesicles have been studied extensively *in vitro* (Marshall, 1970; Marshall and Parsons, 1987; Gandry-Talarmain et al., 1989; Rogers and Parsons, 1989), but their utility *in vivo* has yet to be established. The false cholinergic transmitter rationale involves the use of analogs of choline which would serve as precursors for acetylation *in vivo*, in a manner similar to that which occurs with choline in the cholinergic nerve terminal. The difference would be in the product of this acetylation, which would be less effective than acetylcholine as a cholinergic agonist at the receptor site, hence diminishing the overall cholinergic efficacy of the nerve terminal. Knusel and coinvestigators (1990), for example, report on the use of N-aminodeanol (NADe), a derivative of choline in which one of the N-methyl groups is replaced with an amino moiety, as a precursor for the biosynthesis of a false cholinergic transmitter *in vivo*. Following 120 days of dietary administration of NADe to rats, levels of choline and acetylcholine were greatly reduced in blood, brain, and peripheral organs, and were replaced with NADe and acetyl-NADe, respectively. Choline acetyltransferase levels and QNB binding were also reduced in striatum and myenteric plexus, and in hippocampus, striatum, and myenteric plexus, respectively. Behavioral studies showed that NADe pretreatment for 120 days results in behavioral hyperactivity, habituation of rearing behavior, less efficient learning (conditioned avoidance response), and progressively poorer learning performance in these rats (Russell et al., 1990). While these studies showed a significant reduction in muscarinic cholinergic neurotransmission, there was not a major loss of cholinergic neurons. Moreover, these effects were still declining after 120 days of exposure to the diet, and longer term effects of this treatment have not yet been conducted. Further studies on the reversibility of this phenomenon, the histological consequences of long-term NADe ingestion, and the response of the NADe-exposed animal to pharmacological challenges are yet to be conducted (Russell et al., 1990).

EXCITOTOXINS have enjoyed an extensive exposure in the literature, due to their ability to kill neurons as a result of their prolonged excitatory effects on receptors of the glutamate type (Olney et al., 1971; Coyle, 1987). Their effect is localized at the level of the cell body, and they do not influence axons or nerve terminals. In an attempt to achieve selective cholinotoxicity, investigators have applied various excitotoxins, in particular ibotenic acid and quisqualic acid, to the nBM, with the goal of destroying these cell bodies, and causing a subsequent degeneration of pathways originating in the nBM and projecting to the cortex. Using this approach, a broad spectrum of behavioral tests which are used to study learning and memory in experimental animals were shown to be disrupted; this effect was attributed to a selective damage by this treatment, to cholinergic projections in the brain (see references in Dunnett et al., 1991).

Recently, the validity of employing excitotoxins as selective cholinergic toxins has been subjected to challenge as a result of some conflicting experimental observations. Specifically, the various excitotoxins, when used at doses inducing equivalent reductions in ChAT levels, do not have similar effects on a variety of behavioral tests. For example, quisqualic acid was as effective as ibotenic acid in causing severe deficits in the passive avoidance retention test, yet only ibotenic acid affected water maze acquisition at equivalent cholinodisruptive doses (Dunnett et al., 1987). Furthermore, quisqualic acid treatment is more effective than ibotenic acid in producing forebrain ChAT depletion, yet ibotenic acid induces larger deficits than quisqualic acid in a variety of behavioral tests (Dunnett, 1985; Dunnett et al., 1987, 1989; Etherington et al., 1987; Wenk et al., 1989; Robbins et al., 1989; Markowska et al., 1990; Connor et al., 1991). Some of the discrepancy could be attributable to differences in the anatomical extent of damage induced by the different excitotoxins which are administered in the nBM. For example, while kainic acid, ibotenic acid, and N-methyl-D-aspartate produce incomplete lesions of the nBM, they also have been shown to disrupt ventral and some dorsal efferents from the globus pallidus to the thalamus and the brainstem. On the other hand, quisqualic acid and AMPA have a more focussed effect on the basal forebrain nuclei (Dunnett et al., 1991). Thus, different cholinergic pathways may be differentially affected by these different excitotoxins, hence affecting response in different behavioral paradigms. In fact, it has been suggested (Dunnett et al., 1991; Francis et al., 1992) that, the discrepancies in the above findings would imply that learning and memory may not be entirely related specifically to the nBM system. At least two other cholinergic projections are known to exist in the vicinity of the nBM: the septo-hippocampal, and the diagonal band-cingulate and prefrontal cortex projections. Differences in the disruption of either of these may have a different effect on memory and learning in the affected animal. It is these pathways which may be susceptible to pharmacological manipulation of cholinergic effects on memory and learning, rather than the nBM.

Furthermore, the excitotoxins may also be affecting other neurotransmitter systems besides just cholinergic neurons (Everitt et al., 1987; Murray and Fibiger, 1985; Dunnett et al., 1987; Arbogast and Koslowski, 1988). For example, autoradiographic studies comparing the effect of ibotenic acid and quisqualic acid on distribution of cholinergic ($[^3H]HC$-3), serotonergic ($[^3H]5$-HT) and dopaminergic D1 ($[^3H]SCH$ 23390) binding sites showed considerable reduction in striatal binding of all three neurotransmitters following ibotenic acid administration (Steckler et al., 1993). Similar conclusions were drawn by Lindefors et al. (1992) who showed, using *in situ* hybridization, widespread nonspecific neuronal degeneration of GABA-ergic as well as cholinergic neurons after ibotenic acid administration in the nBM. Based on such observations, Fibiger has concluded that, at least in the case of ibotenic acid, damage to non-cholinergic cells in the vicinity of the nBM must contribute significantly to decrements in acquisition and performance of learned behaviors in rats (Fibiger, 1991).

The availability of a specific neurotoxin for cholinergic neurons, a CHOLINOTOXIN, would thus be of great value for the study of central cholinergic systems. AF64A (ethylcholine aziridinium) was developed with that goal in mind (Hanin et al., 1987; Hanin, 1990). It is structurally similar to choline, and therefore has a strong affinity for the high affinity choline uptake system (Rylett, 1986; Rylett and Colhoun, 1980). It contains a highly reactive aziridinium moiety, which confers to it its cytotoxic properties (Hörtnagl et al., 1988). Since it does not cross the blood brain barrier, it has to be administered topically into the brain. Intracerebroventricular administration of AF64A results in a dose-dependent, long-term attenuation of cholinergic function in the hippocampus (El-Tamer et al., 1992). Recovery eventually occurs, but the time for such recovery is also dependent on the dose used, and ranges between a week and as long as 6 months, following the bilateral administration of doses of 0.5-2 nmol AF64A per ventricle (El Tamer et al., 1992). A broad spectrum of tests used to study learning and memory in experimental animals have been shown to be disrupted in AF64A-treated animals (Bailey et al., 1986; Blaker and Goodwin, 1987; Brandeis et al., 1986; Caulfield et al., 1983; Cherkin et al., 1986; Chrobak et al., 1987; Gower et al., 1989; Mouton et al., 1988; Nakahara et al., 1988; Nakamura et al., 1988; Sandberg et al., 1984; Tateishi et al., 1987; Walsh et al., 1984; Yamazaki et al., 1991). Improvement from such behavioral deficits in AF64A-treated animals has been achieved by treatment with cholinergic agonists (Brandeis et al., 1986; Nakahara et al., 1988, 1989; Ogura et al., 1987), ganglioside AGF2 (Emerich and Walsh, 1990), vitamin E pretreatment (Johnson et al., 1988), and fetal neuronal septal grafts into the hippocampus of AF64A treated animals (Ikegami et al., 1989).

As in the case of the excitotoxins, the cholinospecificity of AF64A has also been challenged, based on papers published in the early phases of AF64A research. Higher than appropriate doses of the compound were used (Levy et al., 1984; Jarrard et al., 1984; McGurk et al., 1987; Allen et al., 1988), and in some cases AF64A was administered in specific brain areas which are highly sensitive to even very low doses of this toxin, resulting in nonspecific damage. More recently, careful and systematic studies have been conducted with this compound, which have delineated the doses and sites of administration which can safely be used in order to achieve the required cholinotoxicity (Hanin, 1990; El-Tamer et al., 1992).   Moreover, recent histochemical and immunocytochemical studies have confirmed the cholinoselectivity of AF64A treatment (Lorens et al., 1991; Dong et al., 1994). It is interesting to note that the cholinodeficiency produced by AF64A treatment triggers a cascade of secondary changes in levels of other neurotransmitters in the same brain (see review by Hanin, 1990). However, this effect is short-lasting and transient, and probably reflects an adaptive response to the initial cholinergic deficit induced by AF64A (Hörtnagl et al., 1987a,b, 1989a,b). Long after this secondary response has disappeared, the cholinodeficiency still persists.

OTHER AZIRIDINIUM ANALOGS have also been studied, but less extensively. Various structural analogs of hemicholinium have been tested as potential *in vivo* active cholinotoxins by Tagari et al. (1986). Of these, the hemicholinium mustard, HcM-9, has been shown to exhibit effects on cholinergic markers which are comparable to those seen with AF64A, with a similar pattern of cholinospecificity.

Several ADDITIONAL CHEMICAL APPROACHES to obtaining selective cholinotoxicity *in vivo* have been reported. Kudo et al. (1989) have employed a nerve growth factor, diphtheria toxin conjugate, injected into the cerebral cortex, to induce significant reduction of cholinergic neurons in the horizontal limb of the diagonal band, and in the nBM of rats.

Rakonczay et al. (1993) have administered murine monoclonal antibodies against acetylcholinesterase to newborn rats and have observed a long lasting but reversible deficiency in cholinergic function in cerebral cortex and basal ganglia of these animals for several days after such treatment. Work by Heckers et al. (1994) has used 192 IgG-saporin, an immunotoxin against the low affinity p75 nerve growth factor receptor, to induce a selective and complete lesion of nerve growth factor receptor - positive cholinergic basal forebrain neurons projecting to the neocortex and hippocampus. Oron et al. (1994) have induced memory impairments and derangement of the spatio-temporal organization of rat behavior, following prolonged immunization of these animals with heavy neurofilament protein, NF-H. Future studies with such approaches should yield informative and important information.

CONCLUDING REMARKS

The advantages of the availability of a centrally cholinodeficient animal are several fold. These include the ability to: 1) study neurochemical and behavioral consequences of long-term cholinergic deficiency; 2) develop approaches to protect the animal from the induction of such a cholinergic deficiency; 3) test pharmacological strategies for the reversal or attenuation of the cholinergic deficiency; and 4) screen for potential agents for the treatment of cholinergically-mediated memory and learning deficiencies in AD.

An animal model is only as good as the feature(s) which it mimics. One cannot, therefore, realistically expect perfection, and has to be tolerant of the limitations of each animal model which is used. With this in mind, it is nevertheless most encouraging to see how far the field has progressed to date, in the development of various animal analogs of cholinergic hypofunction.

REFERENCES

Allen YS, Marchbanks RM and Sinden JD (1988): *Neurosci Lett* 95:69-74.

Arbogast RE and Kozlowski MR (1988): *Neurotoxicology* 9:39-46.

Bartus RT, Dean RL, Beer B and Lippa AS (1982): *Science* 217:408-417.

Bailey EL, Overstreet DH and Croker AD (1986): *Behav Neural Biol* 45:263-274.

Blaker WD and Goodwin SD (1987): *Pharmacol Biochem Behav* 28:157-163.

Bowen D, Smith CB, White P and Davison AN (1976): *Brain* 99:459-496.

Boyd WD, Graham-White J, Blackwood G, Glen I and McQueen J (1977): *Lancet* 2:711.

Brandeis R, Pittel Z, Lachman C, Heldman E, Luz S, Dachir S, Levy A, Hanin I and Fisher A (1986): In: *Alzheimer's and Parkinson's Diseases: Strategies For Research and Development*, Fisher A, Hanin I and Lachman C, eds. New York: Plenum Press, pp. 469-477.

Caulfield MP, May PJ, Pedder EK and Prince AK (1983): *Brit J Pharmacol* 79:287.

Cherkin A, Smith GE and Flood JF (1986): *Soc Neurosci Abstr* 12:711.

Chrobak JJ, Hanin I and Walsh TJ (1987): *Brain Res* 414:15-21.

Connor DJ, Langlais PJ and Thal (1991): *Brain Res* 555:84-90.

Corkin S (1981): *Trends Neurosci* 4:287-290.

Coyle JT (1987): Excitotoxins. In: *Psychopharmacology: The Third Generation of Progress*, Meltzer H, ed. New York: Raven Press, pp. 333-340.

Davies P and Maloney JF (1976): *Lancet* 2:403.

Davis KL and Yamamura HI (1978): *Life Sci* 23:1729-1734.

Dong XW, Lorens SA and Hanin I (1994): *Brain Res Bull* (In Press).

Dunnett SB (1985): *Psychopharmacology* 87:357-363.

Dunnett SB, Whishaw IQ, Jones GH and Bunch ST (1987): *Neuroscience* 20:653-669.

Dunnett SB, Rogers DC and Jones GH (1989): *Eur J Neurosci* 1:395-406.

Dunnett SB, Everitt BJ and Robbins TW (1991): *TINS* 14:494-501.

Elliott PJ, Garofalo L and Cuello AC (1989): *Neuropharmacology* 28:397-400.

El-Tamer A, Corey J, Wülfert E and Hanin I (1992): *Neuropharmacology* 31:397-402.

Emerich DF and Walsh TJ (1990): *Brain Res* 527:299-307.

Etherington R, Mittleman G and Robbins TW (1987): *Neurosci Res Commun* 1:135-143.

Everitt BJ, Robbins TW, Evenden JL, Marston HM, Jones GH and Sirkia TE (1987): *Neuroscience* 22:441-469.

Fibiger HC (1991): *TINS* 14:220-223.

Francis PT, Pangalos MN and Bowen DM (1992): *Prog Neurobiol* 39:517-545.

Funnell WRJ, Maysinger D and Cuello AC (1990): *J Neurosci Meth* 35:147-156.

Gandry-Talarmain YM, Diebler M-F and O'Regan S (1989): *J Neurochem* 52:822-829.

Garofalo L, Elliott PJ and Cuello AC (1992): *Physiol Behav* 52: 971-977.

Gower AJ, Rousseau D, Jamsin P, Gobert J, Hanin I and Wülfert E (1989): *Eur J Pharmacol* 166:271-281.

Hanin I (1990): In: *Progress in Brain Research: Cholinergic Neurotransmission: Functional and Clinical Aspects*, Vol 84, Aquilonius S-M and Gilberg P-G, eds. Amsterdam: Elsevier, pp. 289-299.

Hanin I, Fisher A, Hörtnagl H, Leventer SM, Potter PE and Walsh TJ (1987): In: *Psychopharmacology: The Third Generation of Progress*, Meltzer H, ed. New York: Raven Press, pp. 341-349.

Heckers S, Ohtaka T, Wiley RG, Lappi DA, Geula G and Mesulam M-M (1994): *J Neurosci* 14:1271-1289.

Hohmann CF and Coyle JT (1988): *Brain Res Bull* 21: 13-20.

Hörtnagl H, Potter PE and Hanin I (1987a): *Brain Res* 421:75-84.

Hörtnagl H, Potter PE and Hanin I (1987b): *Neuroscience* 22:203-213.

Hörtnagl H, Potter PE and Hanin I (1989a): *J Neurochem* 52: 853-858.

Hörtnagl H, Potter PE, Kindel G and Hanin I (1989b): *J Neurosci Methods* 27:103-108.

Hörtnagl H and Hanin I (1992): In: *Handbook of Experimental Pharmacology: Selective Neurotoxicity*, Vol 12, Herken H and Hucho F, eds. Berlin: Springer-Verlag, pp. 293-332.

Hörtnagl H, Potter PE, Happe K, Goldstein S, Leventer S, Wülfert E and Hanin I (1988): *J Neurosci Methods* 23:107-113.

Ikegami S, Nihonmatsu I, Hatanaka H, Takei N and Kawamura H (1989): *Neurosci Lett* 101:17-22.

Jarrard LE, Kent GJ, Meyerhoff JL and Levy A (1984): *Pharmacol Biochem Behav* 21: 273-280.

Johnson GVW, Simonato M and Jope RS (1988): *Neurochem Res* 8:685-692.

Knusel B, Jenden DJ, Lauretz SD, Booth RA, Rice KM, Roch M and Waite JJ (1990): *Pharmacol Biochem Behav* 37:799-809.

Kudo Y, Shiosaka S, Matsuda M and Tohyama M (1989): *Neurosci Lett* 102:125-130.

Levy A, Kant GJ, Meyerhoff JL and Jarrard LE (1984): *Brain Res* 305:169-172.

Lindefors N, Boatell ML, Mahy N and Persson H (1992): *Neurosci Lett* 135: 262-264.

Lorens SA, Kindel G, Dong XW, Lee JM and Hanin I (1991): *Brain Res Bull* 26:965-971.

Markowska AL, Wenk GL and Olton DS (1990): *Behav Neural Biol* 54:13-26.

Marshall IG (1970): *Br J Pharmacol* 38:503-516.

Marshall IG and Parsons SM (1987): *Trends Neurosci* 10:174-177.

McGurk SR, Hartgraves SL, Kelly PH, Gordon MN and Butcher LL (1987): *Neuroscience* 22:215-224.

McGurk S, Levin ED and Butcher LL (1991): *Neuroscience* 44:137-147.

McKinney M, Hedreen L and Coyle JT (1982): In: *Alzheimer's Disease: A Report of Progress in Research*, Corkin S, Davis KL, Growdon JH, Usdin E and Wurtman RJ, eds. New York, Raven Press, pp. 259-265.

Mouton PR, Meyer EM, Dunn AJ, Millard W and Arendash GW (1988): *Brain Res* 444:104-118.

Murray CL and Fibiger HC (1985): *Neuroscience* 14:1025-1032.

Nakahara N, Iga Y, Mizobe F and Kawanishi G (1988): *Jpn J Pharmacol* 48:121-130.

Nakahara N, Iga Y, Saito Y, Mizobe and Kawanishi G (1989): *Jpn J Pharmacol* 51:539-547.

Nakamura S, Nakagawa Y, Kawai M, Tohyama M and Ishihara T (1988): *Behav Brain Res* 29:119-126.

Ogura H, Yamanishi Y and Yamatsu K (1987): *Jpn J Pharmacol* 44:498-501.

Olney JW, Ho OL and Rhee V (1971): *Exp Brain Res* 14:61-76.

Oron L, Dubovik V, Perlman M, Novitsy L and Michaelson M (1994): In: *Alzheimer Disease: Therapeutic Strategies*, Giacobini E and Becke R, eds. Boston: Birkhauser (In Press).

Pedata F, Lo Conte G, Sorbi S, Marconcini-Pepeu I and G Pepeu (1982): *Brain Res* 233:359-367.

Perry EK, Perry RH, Blessed G and Tomlinson E (1977): *Lancet* 1:189-191.

Perry EK, Tomlinson BE, Blessed G, Bergman K, Gibson PH and Perry RH (1978): *Br Med J* 2:1447-1459.

Rakonczay Z, Hammond P and Brimijoin S(1993): *Neuroscience* 54:225-238.

Robbins TW, Everitt BJ, Marston HM, Jones GH and Page KJ (1989): *Neuroscience* 28:337-352.

Rogers GA and Parsons SM (1989): *Mol Pharmacol* 36:333-341.

Russell RW, Jenden DJ, Booth RA, Lauretz SD, Rice KM and Roch M (1990): *Pharmacol Biochem Behav* 37:811-820.

Rylett RJ (1986): *Can J Physiol Pharmacol* 64:334-340.

Rylett RJ and Colhoun EH (1980): *J Neurochem* 34:713-719.

Sandberg K, Sanberg PR, Hanin I, Fisher A and Coyle JT (1984): *Behav Neurosci* 98:162-165.

Sims NR, Smith CCT, Davison AM, Bowen DM, Flack RHA, Snowden JS and Neary D (1980): *Lancet* 1:333-336.

Steckler T, Andrews JS, Marten P and Turner JD (1993): *Pharmacol Biochem Behav* 44:877-889.

Tagari PC, Maysinger D and Cuello CC (1986): *Neurochem Res* 11:1091-1102.

Tateishi N, Takano Y, Honda K, Yamada K, Kamiya Y and Kamiya H-O (1987): *Clin Exp Pharmacol Physiol* 14:611-618.

Walsh TJ, Tilson HA, DeHaven DL, Mailman RB, Fisher A and Hanin I (1984): *Brain Res* 321:91-102.

Wenk GL, Markowska AL and Olton DS (1989): *Behav Neurosci* 103:765-769.

Whitehouse PJ, Price DL, Clark AW, Coyle JT and DeLong MR (1981): *Ann Neurol* 10:122-126.

Yamazaki N, Kato K, Kurihara E and Nagaoka A (1991): *Psychopharmacology* 103:215-221.

Alzheimer Disease: Therapeutic Strategies
edited by E. Giacobini and R. Becker.
© 1994 Birkhäuser Boston

ROLE OF THE CARBOXYTERMINUS OF THE ALZHEIMER AMYLOID PROTEIN PRECURSOR IN ALZHEIMER'S DISEASE NEURODEGENERATION

Rachael L. Neve
Department of Genetics, Harvard Medical School and McLean Hospital, Belmont, MA

Michael R. Kozlowski
Geron Corporation, Menlo Park, CA

INTRODUCTION

Our laboratory has focused on a specific aspect of the β-amyloid protein precursor (β-APP) and its connection with the neuronal destruction of Alzheimer's Disease (AD). Most of this work evolved from our observation several years ago that the carboxyterminal 100 amino acids of the amyloid precursor protein (βAPP-C100; previously termed AB1 or βAPP-C104) is neurotoxic (Yankner et al., 1989). Other laboratories subsequently revealed that βAPP-C100, or more simply C100, was itself amyloidogenic (Maruyama et al., 1990; Wolf et al., 1990). The neurotoxicity of βAPP-C100 has since been confirmed by other laboratories (Martin et al., 1991; Fukuchi et al., 1993).

We hypothesized on the basis of these data that C100 or a similar β/A4-containing fragment of β-APP may be centrally involved in the amyloidogenesis and neurodegeneration of AD. To test this latter hypothesis, we designed and generated two *in vivo* models for the action of βAPP-C100, one based on transplantation of C100-producing cells into mouse brains (Neve et al., 1992), the second transgenic mice expressing C100 in the brain (Kammesheidt et al., 1992). Both animal models, in particular the transgenic mice, displayed neuropathology that resembles features of Alzheimer's disease neuropathology, lending strength to our hypothesis that βAPP-C100, or a βAPP fragment very much like it, may be the perpetrator of neurodegeneration in AD. We subsequently discovered on neuronal cells a binding site for βAPP-C100 that may mediate its toxic effects (Kozlowski et al., 1992). If we can define further the interaction of βAPP-C100 with its receptor we may be one step close to goal of developing a rational therapy for AD.

βAPP-C100 is Toxic Specifically to Neurons
We showed previously that PC12 cells transfected with a retroviral recombinant expressing the carboxyterminal 100 amino acids of βAPP (formerly termed AB1, Yankner et al., 1989; and then ßAPP-C104, Kozlowski et al., 1992; now termed ßAPP-C100) degenerate when induced to differentiate into neuronal cells with nerve growth factor (NGF; Yankner et al., 1989). Moreover, conditioned medium from these cells, but not from control cells transfected with recombinant βAPP-695, is toxic to neurons but not non-neuronal cells in primary rat hippocampal cultures. The neurotoxicity can be removed from the medium by immunoabsorption with an antibody to βAPP-C100 (Yankner et al., 1989), suggesting that βAPP-C100 is secreted by the transfected cells and is neurotoxic.

We extended our characterization of the mechanism by which βAPP-C100 may kill neurons by evaluating the pH dependence of the toxicity and by assessing the functional effects of site-directed *in vitro* mutagenesis of βAPP-C100 (Kozlowski et al., 1992). The data revealed that the neurotoxicity of βAPP-C100 is dependent upon pH, and is almost completely inhibited at pH 7.8 or above.

Transplantation of βAPP-C100 Transfected PC12 Cells Into The Brains of Newborn Mice Results In Neuropathology
To test our hypothesis that βAPP-C100 can cause neuropathology resembling that seen in AD, we transplanted PC12 cells transfected with the βAPP-C100 retroviral recombinant (Yankner et al., 1989), or with the retroviral vector alone, into the hippocampal-cortical region of postnatal day (PD) 1-2 or PD6 mice (Neve et al., 1992). Clusters of grafted PC12 cells were clearly evident in both the experimental (C100) and control animals (DO vector only) sacrificed 20 days following transplantation, although these clusters had largely disappeared by 2 months post-transplantation, leaving only scars to mark the locations of the transplants.

At 4 months post-transplantation, experimental animals exhibited significant cortical atrophy relative to controls; this atrophy was not evident at the earlier age of 2 months. Some of the mice that had been transplanted with βAPP-C100 transfected cells also revealed immunoreactivity with Alz-50, an antibody that detects an Alzheimer's disease related protein (Wolozin et al., 1986), in the somatodendritic domain of neurons in the cortex surrounding the transplants, and in dystrophic-appearing fibers in the same region.

In addition, abnormal organization of the neuropil in the CA2/3 region of the hippocampus ipsilateral to the transplant was revealed by immunostaining with F5, an antibody to the carboxyterminal end of the amyloid protein precursor. Adjacent Nissl stained sections did not reveal gross morphological abnormalities in the area of decreased F5 staining, suggesting that the disorganization evident in the immunostained section mainly involves neuropil at four months post-transplantation. Together, these results suggest that the carboxyterminal fragment of βAPP may cause specific neuropathology and neurodegeneration *in vivo*.

Transgenic Mice Expressing βAPP-C100 in the Brain Display Specific Neuropathology That Resembles Aspects of AD Neuropathology
The neuropathological effects resulting from transplantation of βAPP-C100 transfected cells into the mouse brain suggests that it may play a role not only in amyloidogenesis but also in the neurodegeneration of AD. To test further this hypothesis, we made several lines of transgenic mice expressing βAPP-C100 in the brain (Kammesheidt et al., 1992) under the control of the dystrophin neural promoter (Boyce et al., 1991).

Our initial studies of the βAPP-C100 transgenic mice entailed histological and immunocytochemical examination of 4-6 month old mice (Kammesheidt et al., 1992). These mice display, at 4 months of age, intraneuronal deposition of the β/A4 protein, abnormal intracellular accumulations of a carboxyterminal epitope of βAPP that is similar to that we previously described in AD brain (Benowitz et al., 1989), and thioflavin S fluorescence around blood vessels in the brain.

We used an affinity purified antibody raised against a peptide representing the 42 amino acid β/A4 fragment, to detect amyloid deposition in the transgenic mouse brains. This antibody does not recognize normal human βAPP, but distinctively immunoreacts with pathologic structures specific to AD and (to a lesser extent) normal aged brain. Both a quantitative and qualitative difference in the pattern of β/A4 immunoreactivity were exhibited in transgenic relative to control mouse brains. Intensely β/A4 immunoreactive material was seen in neuronal cells throughout the brains of all transgenic mice tested. In most cases the β/A4 immunoreactivity occurred as punctate deposits within neurons that have a rounded, compact appearance. Such staining was clearly visible in Ammon's horn of the hippocampus and in the stratum oriens. The intracellular accumulation of β/A4 was particularly prominent within the hilus, where the immunoreactivity was seen not only in the cell bodies but also in abnormal processes.

The emergence of β/A4 immunoreactivity in the neuropil may represent a later stage of amyloid deposition than that observed in the cell soma, since it was only seen in the three lines expressing highest levels of the transgene. Punctate accumulations of β/A4 immunoreactivity in dystrophic-appearing fibers were dramatically apparent in the striatum radiatum of the CA2/3 region of the hippocampus in these lines. Thioflavin S staining of the animals specifically in these lines also revealed accumulations of amyloid around blood vessels.

We had previously shown that staining of AD brains with F5, an antibody to the carboxyterminal nine amino acids of βAPP, exposed intracellular aggregates of this epitope in secondary lysosomes in pathologically afflicted regions of AD brain, such as in the CA1 neurons of Sommer's sector (Benowitz et al., 1989). Hence, we might expect to detect a similar phenomenon in the transgenic mice. *Indeed, staining of the brain sections with the antibody F5 showed a striking* change in the subcellular localization of the F5 epitope that was particularly evident in the CA2/3 region of the hippocampus in transgenic mice. Whereas control mice showed homogeneous light F5 immunoreactivity predominantly of the neuronal somata in this region, the F5 immunoreactivity in the transgenic mice presented as dark punctate accumulations in subcellular compartments that extended markedly into the neuronal processes. Adjacent Nissl stained sections did not reveal detectable gross abnormalities in the area of altered F5 staining, suggesting that the disorganization evident in the immunostained sections mainly involves the neuropil in transgenic mice of this age. In transgenic mice from the three lines expressing highest levels of the transgene, the cells in the CA2/3 region showed particularly dense reaction product in the neuropil, and the reactivity in the soma took the form of larger accumulations, as if the punctate vesicular immunoreactive material had fused or aggregated. The appearance of the F5 immunoreactivity in these cells was very similar to that we observed in AD (Benowitz et al., 1989).

A Newly Identified Molecule Located on the Surface of Nerve Cells May Mediate the Killing of These Cells by C100 and May be Responsible for the Destruction Found in the Brains of Patients with AD

The data that we have obtained implicate βAPP-C100 in the development of pathology very similar to certain features of AD pathology, and highlight the importance of deducing the mechanism by which this protein fragment kills neurons. In pursuit of this goal, we decided to test the idea that the neurotoxicity of βAPP-C100 may be mediated by its binding to a cell surface molecule. We subsequently discovered on NGF-treated PC12 cells a binding site for βAPP-C100 that may mediate its toxic effects (Kozlowski et al., 1992).

At least three pieces of data suggest strongly that this binding site mediates the toxic effects of βAPP-C100 on differentiated PC12 cells. First, the binding site is much more prevalent on PC12 cells rendered susceptible to the toxic effects of βAPP-C100 by treatment with NGF than on non-treated cells, to which the peptide is not toxic (Yankner et al., 1989). Second, a loss of binding occurs near pH 7.8, the same pH at which C100 loses its neurotoxicity. Third, a mutation that eliminates the neurotoxic efficacy of βAPP-C100 (tyrosine 687) also abolishes its ability to bind to the site identified in our study. Conditioned medium from our βAPP-C100 transfected NIH 3T3 and PC12 cells specifically competes with the binding of radiolabeled βAPP-C100 to this site, providing additional evidence that our PC12 cell transfectants secrete the recombinant βAPP-C100.

Future work is directed towards characterizing the mechanism by which βAPP-C100 kills neurons, focusing on its interaction with the neuronal cell surface receptor, with the goal of developing a potential therapy for AD.

REFERENCES

Benowitz LI, Rodriguez W, Paskevich P, Mufson EJ, Schenk D and Neve RL (1989): The amyloid precursor protein is concentrated in neuronal lysosomes in normal and Alzheimer disease subjects. *Exp Neurol* 106:237-250.

Boyce FM, Beggs AH, Feener C and Kunkel LM (1991): Dystrophin is transcribed in brain from a distant upstream promoter. *Proc Natl Acad Sci USA* 88:1276-1280.

Fukuchi K, Sopher B, Furlong CE, Smith AC, Dang NT and Martin GM (1993): Selective neurotoxicity of COOH-terminal fragments of the beta-amyloid precursor protein. *Neurosci Letters* 154:145-148.

Kammesheidt A, Boyce FM, Spanoyannis AF, Cummings BJ, Ortegon M, Cotman CW, Vaught JL and Neve RL (1992): Amyloid deposition and neuronal pathology in transgenic mice expressing the carboxyterminal fragment of the Alzheimer amyloid precursor in the brain. *Proc Natl Acad Sci USA* 89:10857-10861.

Kozlowski MR, Spanoyannis AF, Manly SP, Fidel SA and Neve RL (1992): The neurotoxic carboxyterminal fragment of the Alzheimer amyloid precursor binds specifically to a neuronal cell surface molecule: pH dependence of the neurotoxicity and the binding. *J Neurosci* 12:1679-1687.

Martin TL, Felsenstein KM and Baetge EE (1991): Cells transfected with amyloid precursor protein DNA fragment AB-1 produce medium toxic to differentiated PC12 cells. *Soc for Neurosci Abst* 17:1072.

Maruyama K, Terakado K, Usami M and Yoshikawa K (1990): Formation of amyloid-like fibrils in COS cells overexpressing part of the Alzheimer amyloid protein precursor. *Nature* 347:566-569.

Neve RL, Kammesheidt A and Hohmann CF (1992): Brain transplants of cells expressing the carboxyterminal fragment of the Alzheimer amyloid protein precursor cause specific neuropathology *in vivo*. *Proc Natl Acad Sci USA* 89:3448-3452.

Wolf D, Quon D, Wang Y and Cordell B (1990): Identification and characterization of C-terminal fragments of the β-amyloid precursor produced in cell culture. *EMBO J* 9:2079-2084.

Wolozin BL, Pruchnicki A, Dickson DW and Davies P (1986): A neuronal antigen in the brains of Alzheimer patients. *Science* 232:648-650.

Yankner BA, Dawes LR, Fisher S, Villa-Komaroff L, Oster-Granite ML and Neve RL (1989): Neurotoxicity of a fragment of the amyloid precursor associated with Alzheimer's disease. *Science* 245:417-420.

Alzheimer Disease: Therapeutic Strategies
edited by E. Giacobini and R. Becker.
© 1994 Birkhäuser Boston

NEUROFILAMENT PATHOLOGY IN ANIMAL MODELS FOR ALZHEIMER'S DISEASE

Masatoshi Takeda, Atsuo Sekiyama, Gen Kanayama, Satoshi Tanimukai, Toshihisa Tanaka and Tsuyoshi Nishimura
Department of Neuropsychiatry, Osaka University Medical School,
2-2 Yamadaoka, Suita, Osaka 565, JAPAN

INTRODUCTION

Functional defect of cytoskeletal systems in the brain is to be elucidated to clarify the pathological process of neurodegenerative disorders such as Alzheimer's disease (AD). Unlike microtubule or microfilament, tissue-specific intermediate filament exists in the central nervous system. Vimentin, glial fibrillary acidic protein (GFAP), and neurofilament proteins are localized in mesenchymal cell, astrocyte and neuron, respectively. Neurofilament is heteropolymer composed of triplet proteins; NF-L, NF-M, and NF-H, all phosphorylated proteins transported on a slow component of axonal flow. Phosphorylation of the rod domain of NF-L inhibits polymerization of neurofilament, and phosphorylation of NF-M, and NF-H regulates interaction with other cytoskeletal proteins, organellas, and membrane. Axonal neurofilaments are more phosphorylated than those in perikarya and dendrites. Phosphorylation of cytoskeletal protein should be closely related with the neurodegenerative process. In this chapter the aberration of cytoskeletal proteins in the brain of model animals for AD is discussed. Change in neurofilament was studied under different kinds of animal models which were designed to represent each specific aspect of pathogenetic process of AD. Abnormal accumulation of phosphorylated neurofilament protein is observed under various conditions of neuronal degeneration. Traumatic brain injury induces accumulation of neurofilament protein in neuronal perikarya at the impact site. Administration of cyclosporin A, calcineurin inhibitor, induces accumulation of phosphorylated neurofilament in rat hippocampal neurons. Buffy coat fraction obtained from patients with AD specifically induces neurofilament accumulation in neuronal perikarya in the brain stem nuclei in hamsters, which is very similar with those induced by aluminum intoxication in rabbit brain (Takeda et al., 1991a). It is speculated that accumulation of phosphorylated neurofilament in neuronal perikarya is the common pathological process among apparently different model animals, which should be relevant to AD pathology.

RESULTS

Fluid Percussion Rat Model

Fluid percussion experiments were performed to study the effect of repetition of subthreshold traumatic brain injury. First, the experiments were designed to titrate the minimum percussion transient. Rats were subjected to fluid percussion transient ranging from 1.0-4.3 atm and the brain tissue was neuropathologically studied. One hour and six hours after moderate (2.0 atm) or severe (4.3 atm) percussion transient, increased staining was observed with antibodies against amyloid precursor protein (APP), ubiquitin, and heat shock protein 72 (HSP72) at the impact site. One week after the injury neuronal loss was evident at the impact site, which was demonstrated by decrease in microtubule-associated protein (MAP2) immunoreactivity. Accumulation of phosphorylated NF-H was observed in neuronal perikarya surrounding the necrotic area. It was demonstrated that neuronal degeneration followed the induction of acute phase proteins under moderate or severe traumatic injury. The induction of acute phase proteins were not evident after mild injury below 1.0 atm.

The effects of repeated subthreshold traumatic brain injury were studied. Rats were subjected to seven times repetition of mild percussion transients (1.0 atm) every day, and the brain tissue was studied one week after the last injury. Decrease in MAP2 immunoreactivity and increase in NF-H immunoreactivity were demonstrated at the impact site. Accumulation of phosphorylated neurofilament was observed in perikarya and dendrites of neurons only at the impact site after repetition of mild percussion. The abnormal accumulation of neurofilament may represent axonal injury because the increased staining with antibodies against phosphorylated NF-H was observed in injured axons. Induction of APP, ubiquitin, HSP72 immunoreactivity was not evident at the impact site. It is shown that the mild traumatic brain injury which is not enough to induce acute phase proteins, could cause neurofilament accumulation in neuronal perikarya when the mild traumatic injury is repeated.

Cyclosporin A Administrated Rat Model

Over-phosphorylation of signal molecules and other cellular proteins is speculated to be relevant to pathological process of AD. Tau in paired helical filaments is over-phosphorylated and the kinase(s) responsible for this over-phosphorylation is under intensive search. Participation of protein phosphatase is, however, indicated by several experiments. Cyclosporin A, a calcineurin inhibitor, was administrated into the rat hippocampus. Seven days after drug administration, the effects of phosphatase activity suppression in the brain to changes in neuronal cytoskeletal proteins were studied. Rat brain homogenates injected with cyclosporin A showed about 30% suppression of Ca/ calmodulin-dependent phosphatase activity measured by ^{32}P release from ^{32}P-labeled histone, indicating that cyclosporin A acts as an inhibitor of calcineurin

after binding cyclophilin in the brain.   Hematoxylin-eosin staining revealed
basophilic neurons in the pyramidal layer of hippocampus, cerebellum,
thalamus, and cerebral cortex.   Immunostaining with anti NF-H showed positive
staining of neuronal perikarya of the basophilic neurons.   It is indicated that
cyclosporin A inhibits calcineurin activity in the brain, which results in increased
phosphorylation of perikaryal neurofilament (Tanaka et al., 1993).

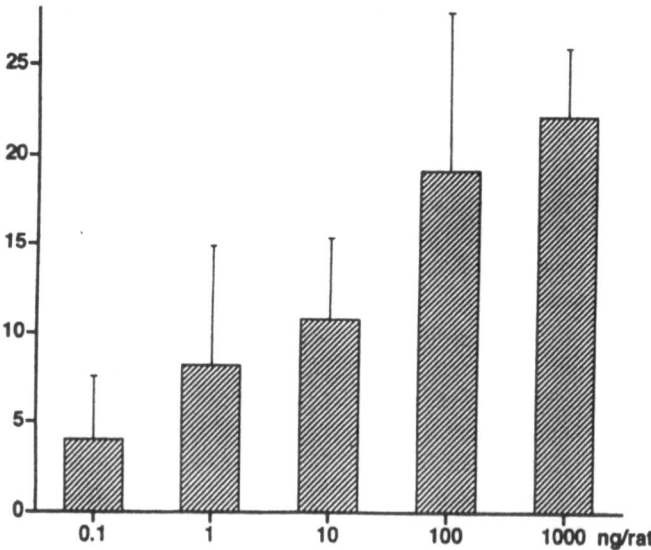

FIGURE 1. Number of immunopositive neurons in a hippocampal slice of cyclosporin A
injected rats. A hippocampal section was obtained from rat brains injects with various
concentration of cyclosporin A. The section was stained with an antibody against NF-H
and the immunopositive neurons were counted.

Alzheimer Buffy Coat Inoculation Study

We previously reported abnormal neurofilament accumulation in neuronal
perikarya in the brain stem nuclei of the hamster brain inoculated with buffy
coat obtained from members of a family with familial Alzheimer's disease
(FAD) (Takeda et al., 1991b,c). The further genetic analysis disclosed that this
family has the Hardy type mutation in APP gene. It was studied whether the
abnormal accumulation of neurofilament in the recipient hamster brain is induced
only by buffy coat with the APP mutation. Buffy coat samples were obtained
from three independent families with FAD (five patients, and seven healthy
familial members), three patients with sporadic AD, and three apparently healthy
subjects.   Seven hamsters were inoculated into the cerebral tissue with each
buffy coat sample and the brain tissue was studied by immunostaining with anti-
NF-H 18 months after inoculation. The hamster brains inoculated with the buffy
coat sample from patients with FAD and sporadic AD all produced the
characteristic neurofilament accumulation in neuronal perikarya of the lower
brain stem nuclei, while the sample from the healthy subjects did not, except the

one sample from the family with APP mutation. It is demonstrated that the buffy coat sample from patients with AD, regardless of the presence or absence of familial accumulation of the disease, induces the abnormal accumulation of neurofilament in the recipient hamster brain.

DISCUSSIONS

Head trauma is one of the risk factors for AD. Fluid percussion model can be applied to differentiate the effects of severe traumatic brain injury from those of mild injury. It was used to evaluate the effects of chronic repetition of mild traumatic brain injury, which is below the level of inducing tissue reaction of acute phase protein synthesis. After the repetition of subthreshold traumatic injury, it was demonstrated that phosphorylated neurofilament is accumulated in neuronal perikarya as well as in injured axons. It is speculated that axonal injury may trigger accumulation of neurofilament in neuronal perikarya.

Accumulation of phosphorylated neurofilament is also induced by suppression of phosphatase activity in the brain as demonstrated by the experiments of cyclosporin A administration. The abnormal accumulation of neurofilament in neuronal perikarya might be induced when the brain phosphorylation/dephosphorylation equilibrium is out of balance toward phosphorylation. Since phosphorylated neurofilament protein usually exists in axon, it is to be clarified whether phosphorylated neurofilament protein is accumulated in neuronal perikarya because *de novo* neurofilament is over-phosphorylated or axonal transport is hindered due to over-phosphorylation.

Buffy coat from patients with AD specifically induces neurofilament accumulation in neuronal perikarya of the recipient hamster 18 months after inoculation. The mechanism leading to accumulation of phosphorylated neurofilament is to be clarified, but it is to be noticed that neurofilament accumulation is observed in neuronal perikarya of the lower brain stem nuclei, which is far from the inoculation site.

Over-phosphorylation of neurofilament might be triggered by various cellular insults which cause abnormal signal transduction. Considering abnormal Ca mobilization and change in cytoskeletal proteins in Alzheimer cell (Takeda et al., 1991d) and involvement of clathrin molecule (Nakamura et al., 1994), it is speculated that phosphorylation of neurofilament protein inhibits axonal transport and eventually leads to the cytoskeletal pathology of AD.

REFERENCES

Nakamura Y, Takeda M, Yoshimi K, Hattori H, Hariguchi S, Kitajima S, Hashimoto S and Nishimura T (1994): Involvement of clathrin light chains in the pathology of Alzheimer's disease. *Acta Neuropathol* 87:23-31.

Takeda M, Tatebayashi Y, Tanimukai S, Nakamura Y, Tanaka T and Nishimura T (1991a): Immunohistochemical study of microtubule associated protein 2 and ubiquitin in chronically aluminum-intoxicated rabbit brain. *Acta Neuropathol* 82:346-352.

Takeda M, Nishimura T, Kudo T, Tanimukai S and Tada K (1991b): Buffy coat from Alzheimer's disease patients produces introcytoplasmic neurofilament accumulation in hamster brain. *Brain Res* 551:319-321.

Takeda M, Nishimura T, Tada K, Kudo T and Tanimukai S (1991c): Inoculation study of buffy coat into hamster brain. *Dementia* 2:57-63.

Takeda M, Nishimura T, Hariguchi S, Tatebayashi Y, Tanaka T, Tanimukai S and Tada K (1991d): Study of cytoskeletal proteins in fibroblasts cultured from familial Alzheimer's disease. *Acta Neurol Scand* 84:416-420.

Tanaka T, Takeda M, Niigawa H, Hariguchi S and Nishimura T (1993): Phosphorylated neurofilament accumulation in neuronal perikarya by cyclosporin A injection in rat brain. *Meth Find Exp Clin Pharmacol* 15:77-87.

Alzheimer Disease: Therapeutic Strategies
edited by E. Giacobini and R. Becker.
© 1994 Birkhäuser Boston

TRANSGENIC MICE AS A MODEL OF ALZHEIMER'S DISEASE

Linda S. Higgins and Barbara Cordell
Scios Nova Inc., 2450 Bayshore Parkway, Mountain View, CA

INTRODUCTION

A significant obstacle to determining the role of β-amyloid in Alzheimer's disease (AD) has been the lack of a manipulable small animal model. The amyloid plaque has been viewed as a major etiological factor in AD dementia and, alternatively, as an epiphenomenon. Transgenic technology provides the potential of a small animal model in which such questions might be addressed experimentally, and which would also be useful in therapeutic development.

We generated mice transgenic for the human 751 amino acid form of the β-amyloid precursor protein (β-APP), with expression controlled by the rat neuron specific enolase promoter (NSE:β-APP751) (Quon et al., 1991). β-APP751 is the major isoform which harbors a Kunitz proteinase domain, and is ubiquitously expressed. In contrast, the other major isoform, β-APP695, lacks the proteinase domain and is expressed exclusively in neurons (Ponte et al., 1988; Neve et al., 1988). In AD, neuronal levels of β-APP751 mRNA in hippocampal and cortical neurons, and this elevation correlates with plaque density (Johnson et al., 1990). Thus, NSE:β-APP751 transgenic mice mimic this imbalance of isoform expression. A pathogenic mechanism is suggested by the observation that expression of inappropriate β-APP isoforms, such as β-APP751 in neurons, leads to increased β-amyloid production (Zhong et al., 1994).

Transgenic pedigrees derived from six founder mice were established in which β-APP751 RNA expression levels were increased several- to 50-fold over endogenous murine levels. While transgene expression varied between pedigrees, it is consistent among individuals within a pedigree (Quon et al., unpublished data). In contrast to greatly elevated RNA expression, protein expression is increased 2- to 3-fold over endogenous β-APP, suggesting tight translational control (Quon et al., 1991). Mice from these six transgenic pedigrees, as well as from the wild type parental strain (WT) were characterized for potential consequences of neuronal over-expression of human β-APP751.

β-AMYLOID DEPOSITS FORM IN TRANSGENIC MOUSE BRAIN

Since β-amyloid deposition is a hallmark of AD, this feature was carefully examined in WT and transgenic mouse brain. Tissue sections were prepared and stained with a panel of β-amyloid specific antibodies. Each of these was raised to human β-amyloid synthetic peptides and produces specific immunoreactivity in human AD brain sections. Using these reagents, extracellular β-amyloid immunoreactive deposits were observed in brains of mice from all six transgenic pedigrees. Deposit morphology varied from diffuse to compact, and their size ranged from 10-50 μm. β-amyloid deposits were observed most frequently in the cortex and hippocampus, and were occasionally seen in the thalamus. The appearance of β-amyloid deposits was similar when reactivity was obtained with sera well characterized in the field, including sera 1280, 2332 and 2333, and with antibodies generated by our group (Higgins et al., 1994). One of our monoclonal antibodies, 108.1 mAb, recognizes the free COOH-terminus of β-amyloid 1-42, but not extended or truncated β-amyloid peptides (Murphy et al., 1994). Plaques and deposits in AD and Down's Syndrome (DS) brain sections react with 108.1 mAb (Murphy et al., 1994), as do deposits in NSE:β-APP751 mouse brain. Thus, at least some of the material in the transgenic mouse brain deposits is β-APP processed to β-amyloid species, as it is in human brain.

The frequency of β-amyloid immunoreactive deposits was determined using monoclonal antibody 4.1 mAb because of its low background and high sensitivity, both more critical in examining diffuse deposits than in visualizing dense core AD plaques. Since 4.1 mAb is highly selective for human over murine β-amyloid (Higgins et al., 1994), the presence of 4.1 mAb immunoreactive deposits demonstrates that at least some of the material present is transgene derived. In a survey of a large number of mice, 4.1 mAb immunoreactive deposits were detected in 27% of 122 brain sections. β-amyloid immunoreactive deposits were present in 67% of the 33 NSE:β-APP751 animals represented, including positive members of all six pedigrees (≥ 3 sections, 6 μm thick, were examined per animal). Presumably, the proportion of brains in which deposits are detected would increase if more sections were examined. In contrast to NSE:β-APP751 mouse brain, sections from WT brains and from brain of mice expressing other β-APP transgene constructs did not contain β-amyloid immunoreactive deposits are statistically significant frequencies. Only 5% (n=107) of WT and 2% (n=94) of other transgenic brain sections scored positive. Among the NSE:β-APP751 mice, there was no difference in the frequency of deposits in males and females. However, mice homozygous for the transgene had twice the frequency of β-amyloid immunoreactive deposits as hemizygous mice.

To place our understanding of the transgenic mouse brain β-amyloid immunoreactive deposits into the context of human pathology, we compared them to structures in human AD and DS brain sections. Since individuals with

DS develop AD by the fourth decade of life, the DS brain offers a view of events in the progression of AD histopathology. Only diffuse deposits are detected in young adult DS brain using 4.1 mAb immunohistochemistry, consistent with the immature AD pathology described in the young DS brain (Allsop et al., 1989; Giaccone et al., 1989). The appearance of diffuse deposits in young adult DS brain and in transgenic mouse brain was similar (Higgins et al., 1994). Staining with a number of classical histological reagents provided further evidence that deposits in NSE:β-APP751 mouse brain resembles the diffuse deposits of early AD pathology observed in young DS brain (Table I). Treatments that consistently or occasionally stain diffuse β-amyloid deposits do so in both human and mouse brain sections, whereas those specific for dense core plaques fail to detect material in young DS or in transgenic mouse brain. These data provide a profile of deposits in transgenic mouse brain that closely resembles early AD pathology such as is seen in young adult DS brain.

Stain	NSE:β-APP751 Mice[1]	Young Adult DS/Early AD[2]	Late DS/ Mature AD[2]
β-amyloid antibodies	+	+	+
Methenamine silver	+	+	+
Bielschowsky silver	±	±	+
Thioflavin S	±	±	+
Congo red	-	-	+

TABLE I. Staining characteristics of β-amyloid deposits in NSE:β-APP751 mouse brain resemble those in young adult DS brain. Staining observed: + consistently, ± occasionally, - never. [1] Higgins et al., 1994; [2] Allsop et al., 1989; Giaccone et al., 1989; Murphy et al., 1990.

TRANSGENIC MOUSE BRAIN DISPLAYS OTHER HISTOPATHOLOGICAL FEATURES

Neurofibrillary tangles containing abnormally phosphorylated tau are a second major feature of AD histopathology. An extensively documented antibody that histologically stains only abnormal tau such as is found in neurofibrillary tangles is Alz50 (Wolozin et al., 1986). Alz50 immunoreactivity was observed in NSE:β-APP751 brain sections in neural soma, processes, and fields of puncta in the neuropil. Alz50 immunoreactive neural soma were seen only in the cerebral cortex, the thalamus, and the amygdala. Immunoreactive neurites were seen in these regions as well as in the hippocampus. The aberrant subcellular localization of tau is identical to that in AD. This staining profile was not observed in brain sections of wild type mice or of mice transgenic for other β-amyloid constructs. The observed staining of neurites and soma *is* very similar to the profile obtained in young adult DS brain sections.

The histological profile of NSE:β-APP751 mice is consistent with an early AD-like phenotype. A concern in developing a transgenic model of the disease is the possibility that the murine brain is inherently incapable of producing mature AD-like pathology. It is, therefore, important that rare examples of more advanced pathology were observed in some NSE:β-APP751 mice (Higgins et al., 1994). These few brains contained large regions of dense β-amyloid immunoreactivity, often in the thalamus. The deposits were vacuolated and associated with elongated neurons of abnormal morphology, as well as with extensive gliosis, as revealed by glial acidic fibrillary protein immunoreactivity. All regions of the brain not closely affiliated with the deposits appeared normal and were well preserved. While it must be emphasized that the histopathology observed in these mice is not representative of the NSE:β-APP751 pedigree, it provides impetus for development of future rodent models.

FREQUENCY OF HISTOPATHOLOGICAL FEATURES IN TRANSGENIC MOUSE BRAIN INCREASES WITH AGE

Transgenic mice further parallel the human condition in that the frequency of early AD-like features observed in the mouse brain increases with age. The frequency of β-amyloid immunoreactive deposits and of abnormal Alz50 immunoreactive structures was determined for sections taken from twelve young (2-3 months) and twelve old (22 months) homozygous NSE:β-APP751 mice of a single pedigree. As shown in Table II the assessment, conducted by experimenters blind to the age of the mice, revealed about twice the frequency of both markers in the aged animals compared to the young mice.

Age (months)	β-amyloid immunoreactive deposits	Abnormal Alz50 immunoreactive structures
	% positive (number of sections)	
2-3	29% (35)	33% (36)
22	49% (35)	69% (36)

TABLE II. The frequency of early AD-like features increases with age in NSE:β-APP751 mouse brain.

CONCLUSIONS

The transgenic model described here typically displays features of early stage AD, including the age-related appearance of β-amyloid deposits and cytoskeletal perturbations. It is of interest that whereas a single genetic alteration was made in NSE:β-APP mice, a number of pathological events develop. It will be of interest to characterize synaptic, neurochemical, and behavioral alterations in these animals to begin to define interrelationships among purported mechanisms of pathogenesis. The observation that some mice develop mature AD-like histopathology, albeit rarely, is important since it indicates that the murine brain is capable of producing such features. These results should provide increased confidence in transgenesis as a means to test additional genetic and environmental factors which may play a role in the development of AD. Such models will be valuable in determining disease mechanisms and in assessing potential therapeutics.

ACKNOWLEDGEMENTS

This work was supported by Marion Merrell Dow, Inc. We thank our colleagues at Scios Nova who contributed to the research described.

REFERENCES

Allsop D, Haga S-I, Haga C et al. (1989): Early senile plaques in Down's syndrome brains show a close relationship with cell bodies of neurons. *Neuropath & Applied Neurobiol* 15:531.

Giaccone G, Tagliavini F, Linoli G et al. (1989): Down syndrome patients: extracellular preamyloid deposits precede neuritic degeneration and senile plaques. *Neurosci Lett* 97:232.

Higgins LS, Holtzman DM, Rabin J et al. (1994): Transgenic mouse brain histopathology resembles early Alzheimer's disease. *Ann Neurol* (In Press).

Johnson SA, McNeill T, Cordell B and Finch CE (1990): Relation of neuronal APP-751/APP695 mRNA ratio and neuritic plaque density in Alzheimer's disease. *Science* 248:854.

Murphy GM Jr, Eng LF, Ellis WG et al. (1990): Antigenic profile of plaques and neurofibrillary tangles in the amygdala in Down's syndrome: a comparison with Alzheimer's disease. *Brain Res* 537:102.

Murphy GM Jr, Forno LS, Higgins L et al. (1994): Development of a monoclonal antibody specific for the COOH-terminal of β-amyloid 1-42 and its immunohistochemical reactivity in Alzheimer's disease and related disorders. *Amer J Pathol* 244:1.

Neve RL, Finch EA and Dawes LP (1988): Expression of the Alzheimer amyloid protein gene transcript in the human brain. *Neuron* 1:669.

Ponte P, Gonzalez-DeWhitt P, Schilling J et al. (1988): A new A4 amyloid contains a domain homologous to serine protease inhibitors. *Nature* 331:525.

Quon D, Wang Y, Catalano R et al. (1991): Formation of β-amyloid protein deposits in brains of transgenic mice. *Nature* 352:239.

Wolozin BL, Pruchnicke A, Dickson DW and Davies P (1986): A neuronal antigen in the brains of Alzheimer patients. *Science* 232:647.

Zhong Z, Quon D, Higgins LS et al. (1994): Increased amyloid production from aberrant β-amyloid precursor proteins. *J Biol Chem* (In Press).

Alzheimer Disease: Therapeutic Strategies
edited by E. Giacobini and R. Becker.
© 1994 Birkhäuser Boston

AGED NON-HUMAN PRIMATES AS MODELS OF ß-AMYLOIDOSES

Lary C. Walker
Department of Pathology and Neuropathology Laboratory, The Johns
Hopkins University School of Medicine, Baltimore, MD, USA

INTRODUCTION

Because of the biological proximity of nonhuman primates and humans, monkeys are useful in the study of significant features of Alzheimer's disease (AD) (Price et al., 1994). Rhesus monkeys (*Macaca mulatta*; life span 35-40 years) are the best available laboratory model of senile plaque formation, and squirrel monkeys (*Saimiri sciureus*; life span 25-30 years) are excellent models of cerebrovascular amyloidosis (Walker et al., 1988a,b; Price et al., 1994). Aged rhesus monkeys also show mild, but statistically significant, cognitive decline (Bachevalier et al., 1991; Rapp and Amaral, 1991; Voytko, 1993), neocortical atrophy (Brizzee et al., 1980), and regional cytological and neurochemical changes in brain (Wisniewski and Terry, 1973; Brizzee et al., 1980; Goldman-Rakic and Brown, 1981; Uemura, 1980; Beal et al., 1991; Wenk et al., 1991; Stroessner-Johnson et al., 1992; Arnsten, 1993; Wagster, 1993). Other age-associated changes that closely mimic those in humans include degenerative changes in the musculoskeletal system (DeRousseau, 1986) and menopause in females (Walker, 1994). Even so, no aged monkey has yet been shown to develop AD, i.e., neither "dementia" nor neurofibrillary tangles have been demonstrated unequivocally in a nonhuman primate. However, ß-amyloid (Aß) is abundant in aged monkeys. Thus, primates are an advantageous model for studying the pathogenesis of senile plaques and cerebrovascular amyloid and for testing strategies for the diagnosis and treatment of ß-amyloidoses.

Aß IN AGED PRIMATES

The ß-amyloid precursor protein (ßPP) is conserved evolutionarily (Johnstone et al., 1991); in cynomolgus monkeys (*Macaca fascicularis*), the 695 amino acid ßPP sequence is identical to that in humans, and ßPP 751 and ßPP 770 differ by one and four amino acids, respectively (Podlisny et al., 1991). Data are accumulating on cerebral amyloid in several primate species besides rhesus monkeys and squirrel monkeys. Chimpanzees (*Pan troglodytes*) develop some cerebrovascular amyloid and senile plaques by the sixth decade of life (Cork and Walker, 1993). Senile plaques also occur in cynomolgus monkeys (Podlisny et al., 1991), cotton-topped tamarins (*Saguinus oedipus*) (Cork and Hester-Price, 1993), brown lemurs (*Lemur fulvus collaris*) (Strittmatter et al., 1993), mouse lemurs (*Microcebus murinus*) (Bons et al., 1991) and lesser bushbabies (*Galago crassicaudatus*) (Cork and Hester-Price, 1993). Tree shrews (*Tupaia belangeri*), which share a recent common ancestor with the extant primates, do not appear to manifest plaques or cerebrovascular amyloid by the age of 9 years (Walker and Fuchs, personal observations). Recently, senile plaques and cerebrovascular amyloid have been reported in marmosets (*Callithrix jacchus*) 6-7 years following the intracerebral injection of brain tissue from an AD patient (Baker et al., 1993). The injected animals were 8 years old at death; control (noninjected) marmosets ranging in age from 8 years to over 11 years had no amyloid deposits in brain.

Cerebral Aß deposits in aged monkeys also contain α1-antichymotrypsin (Abraham et al., 1989; Cork et al., 1990), apolipoprotein E (Strittmatter et al., 1993), and heparin sulfate proteoglycan (Walker and Fillit, 1993). As in humans, microglia and astrocytes are closely associated with senile plaques (Wisniewski and Terry, 1973; Walker et al., 1990), and the amyloid core is frequently surrounded by abnormal neurites from a variety of transmitter systems (Walker et al., 1988). The activity of cytochrome oxidase is elevated in senile plaques (Walker, personal observations), and this localized increase occurs in the context of a general decline in the mitochondrial enzyme in the neocortex of aged monkeys (Bowling et al., 1993). Many neurites also are immunoreactive for Cu/Zn superoxide dismutase in rhesus monkeys (Walker and Jucker, personal observations). These findings suggest that focal oxidative stress may be a significant feature of the pathogenesis of senile plaques.

Senile plaques, cerebrovascular amyloid, and diffuse parenchymal deposits all are found in aged rhesus monkeys and squirrel monkeys, but senile plaques are more common in rhesus monkeys, whereas cerebrovascular amyloid predominates in squirrel monkeys (Walker et al., 1990; Walker, 1991). This species-difference in the locus of Aß accumulation suggests that somewhat different amyloidogenic mechanisms are at play in rhesus and squirrel monkeys. Because two types of hereditary cerebrovascular amyloidosis are associated with mutations affecting amino acids at positions 22 or 21 of Aß (Levy et al., 1990; Hendriks et al., 1992), we sought a similar change in the gene encoding squirrel monkey ßPP. Preliminary data (Levy et al., in preparation) indicate that the predicted Aß sequence in squirrel monkeys is identical to that in humans and cynomolgus macaques. Thus, squirrel monkeys appear to be an appropriate model of sporadic cerebral amyloid angiopathy.

LABELING ß-AMYLOID *IN VIVO* IN PRIMATES

The development of ligands that can bind selectively to Aß in the living brain would enable the delivery of agents to Aß deposits for diagnosis and possibly for treatment of ß-amyloidoses. My colleagues and I have been studying the feasibility of labeling cerebral Aß in the simian brain *in vivo* using a sensitive murine monoclonal antibody. Because the antibody does not readily reach parenchymal or vascular amyloid from the bloodstream, we bypassed the blood-brain barrier by injecting the antibody directly into the cerebrospinal fluid of the cisterna magna (Walker et al., 1994). Using immunohistochemistry to detect bound antibody in brain sections, we found that up to 15% of cortical Aß deposits were selectively labeled *in vivo*. These findings show that it is possible to label Aß in the living brain, but it will be necessary to increase the amount of labeling, and to employ a safer mode of delivery, before *in vivo* labeling can become clinically useful. We currently are investigating other potential ligands for labeling Aß *in vivo*, such as synthetic Aß itself (Maggio et al., 1992). Circulating Aß traverses the blood-brain barrier via a saturable, specific binding mechanism in capillaries (Zlokovic et al., 1993), and thus may have ready access to Aß deposits. Radiolabeled, synthetic Aß1-40, in physiological concentrations, will bind to Aß deposits *in vitro* in aged monkeys (Walker et al., unpublished), suggesting that labeled Aß might be useful in studying the mechanisms of ß-amyloidogenesis in living primates. Such experiments might also pave the way to more effective diagnostic and therapeutic approaches to cerebral amyloidoses.

REFERENCES

Abraham CR, Selkoe DJ, Potter H, Price DL and Cork LC (1989): α_1-antichymotrypsin is present together with the ß-protein in monkey brain amyloid deposits. *Neuroscience* 32:715-720.

Arnsten AFT (1993): Catecholamine mechanisms in age-related cognitive decline. *Neurobiol Aging* 14:639-641.

Bachevalier J, Landis LS, Walker LC, Brickson M, Mishkin M, Price DL and Cork LC (1991): Aged monkeys exhibit behavioral deficits indicative of widespread cerebral dysfunction. *Neurobiol Aging* 12:99-111.

Baker HF, Ridley RM, Duchen LW, Crow TJ and Bruton CJ (1993): Evidence for the experimental transmission of cerebral ß-amyloidosis to primates. *Int J Exp Pathol* 74:441-454.

Beal MF, Walker LC, Storey E, Segar L, Price DL and Cork LC (1991): Neurotransmitters in neocortex of aged rhesus monkeys. *Neurobiol Aging* 12:407-412.

Bons N, Mestre N and Petter A (1991): Senile plaques and neurofibrillary changes in the brain of an aged lemurian primate *Microcebus murinus*. *Neurobiol Aging* 13:99-105.

Bowling AC, Mutisya EM, Walker LC, Price DL, Cork LC and Beal MF (1993): Age-dependent impairment of mitochondrial function in primate brain. *J Neurochem* 60:1964-1967.

Brizzee KR, Ordy JM and Bartus RT (1980): Localization of cellular changes within multimodal sensory regions in aged monkey brain: possible implications for age-related cognitive loss. *Neurobiol Aging* 1:45-52.

Cork LC and Hester-Price A (1993): Aging and amyloid: a phylogenetic perspective. *J Neuropathol Exp Neurol* 52:335.

Cork LC and Walker LC (1993): Age-related lesions, nervous system. In: *Monographs on Pathology of Laboratory Animals. Nonhuman Primates II.* TC Jones, U Mohr and RD Hunt, eds. Berlin, Springer-Verlag, pp. 173-183.

Cork LC, Masters C, Beyreuther K and Price DL (1990): Development of senile plaques. Relationships of neuronal abnormalities and amyloid deposits. *Am J Pathol* 137:1383-1392.

DeRousseau CJ, Bito LZ and Kaufman PL (1986): Age-dependent impairments of the rhesus monkey visual and musculoskeletal systems and apparent behavioral consequences. In: *The Cayo Santiago Macaques: History, Behavior and Biology.* RG Rawlins and MJ Kessler, eds. Albany: State University of New York Press, pp 233-251.

Goldman-Rakic PS and Brown RM (1981): Regional changes of monoamines in cerebral cortex and subcortical structures of aging rhesus monkeys. *Neuroscience* 6:177-187.

Hendriks L, van Duijn CM, Cras P, Cruts M, Van Hul W, van Harskamp F, Warren A, McInnis MG, Antonarakis SE, Martin J-J, Hofman A and Van Broeckhoven C (1992): Presenile dementia and cerebral haemorrhage linked to a mutation at codon 692 of the ß-amyloid precursor protein gene. *Nature Genetics* 1:218-221.

Johnstone EM, Chaney MO, Norris FH, Pascual R and Little SP (1991): Conservation of the sequence of the Alzheimer's disease amyloid peptide in dog, polar bear and five other mammals by cross-species polymerase chain reaction analysis. *Mol Brain Res* 10:299-305.

Levy E, Carman MD, Fernandez-Madrid IJ, Power MD, Lieberburg I, van Duinen SG, Bots GTAM, Luyendijk W and Frangione B (1990): Mutation of the Alzheimer's disease amyloid gene in hereditary cerebral hemorrhage, Dutch type. *Science* 248:1124-1126.

Maggio JE, Stimson ER, Ghilardi JR, Allen CJ, Dahl CE, Whitcomb DC, Vigna SR, Vinters HV, Labenski ME and Mantyh PW (1992): Reversible *in vitro* growth of Alzheimer disease ß-amyloid plaques by deposition of labeled amyloid peptide. *Proc Natl Acad Sci USA* 89:5462-5466.

Podlisny MB, Tolan DR and Selkoe DJ (1991): Homology of the amyloid beta protein precursor in monkey and human supports a primate model for beta amyloidosis in Alzheimer's disease. *Am J Pathol* 138:1423-1435.

Price DL, Martin LJ, Sisodia SS, Walker LC, Voytko ML, Wagster MV, Cork LC and Koliatsos VE (1994): The aged nonhuman primate. A model for the behavioral and brain abnormalities occurring in aged humans. In: *Alzheimer Disease.* RD Terry, R Katzman and KL Bick, eds. New York: Raven Press, pp. 231-245.

Rapp PR and Amaral DG (1991): Recognition memory deficits in a subpopulation of aged monkeys resemble the effects of medial temporal lobe damage. *Neurobiol Aging* 12:481-486.

Strittmatter WJ, Saunders AM, Schmechel D, Pericak-Vance M, Enghild J, Salvesen GS and Roses AD (1993): Apolipoprotein E: high-avidity binding to ß-amyloid and increased frequency of type 4 allele in late-onset familial Alzheimer disease. *Proc Natl Acad Sci USA* 90:1977-1981.

Stroessner-Johnson HM, Rapp PR and Amaral DG (1992): Cholinergic cell loss and hypertrophy in the medial septal nucleus of the behaviorally characterized aged rhesus monkey. *J Neurosci* 12:1936-1944.

Uemura E (1980): Age-related changes in neuronal RNA content in rhesus monkeys (*Macaca mulatta*). Brain Res Bull. 5:117-119.

Voytko ML (1993): Cognitive changes during normal aging in monkeys assessed with an automated test apparatus. *Neurobiol Aging* 14:643-644.

Wagster MV (1993): Changes in cholinergic receptor subtypes in behaviorally-tested aged monkeys. *Neurobiol Aging* 14:693-694.

Walker LC (1991): Animal models of cerebral amyloidosis. *Bull Clin Neurosci* 56:86-96.

Walker LC and Fillit HM (1993): Heparan sulfate proteoglycan (HSPG) core protein in senile plaques and cerebrovascular amyloid of aged monkeys. *Soc Neurosci Abstr* 19:1472.

Walker LC, Kitt CA, Cork LC, Struble RG, Dellovade TL and Price DL (1988a): Multiple transmitter systems contribute neurites to individual senile plaques. *J Neuropathol Exp Neurol* 47:138-144.

Walker LC, Kitt CA, Struble RG, Wagster MV, Price DL and Cork LC (1988b): The neural basis of memory decline in aged monkeys. *Neurobiol Aging* 9:657-666.

Walker LC, Masters C, Beyreuther K and Price DL (1990): Amyloid in the brains of aged squirrel monkeys. *Acta Neuropathol* 80:381-387.

Walker LC, Price DL, Voytko ML and Schenk DB (1994): Labeling of cerebral amyloid *in vivo* with a monoclonal antibody. *J Neuropathol Exp Neurol* (In Press).

Walker ML (1994): Menopause in female rhesus monkeys. *Am J Primatol* (In Press).

Wenk GL, Walker LC, Price DL and Cork LC (1991): Loss of NMDA, but not GABA-A, binding in the brains of aged rats and monkeys. *Neurobiol Aging* 12:93-98.

Wisniewski HM and Terry RD (1973): Morphology of the aging brain, human and animal. *Prog Brain Res* 40:167-186.

Zlokovic BV, Ghiso J, Mackie JB, McComb JG, Weiss MH and Frangione B (1993): Blood-brain barrier transport of circulating Alzheimer's amyloid ß. *Biochem Biophys Res Commun* 197:1034-1040.

Alzheimer Disease: Therapeutic Strategies
edited by E. Giacobini and R. Becker.
© 1994 Birkhäuser Boston

MODEL STUDIES OF THE ROLE OF ANTI-NEUROFILAMENT ANTIBODIES IN NEURODEGENERATION IN ALZHEIMER'S DISEASE

Lea Oron, Vladimir Dubovik, Mira Perlman,
Larisa Novitsky and Daniel M. Michaelson
Department of Biochemistry, Tel Aviv University, Ramat Aviv 69978, Israel

INTRODUCTION

Recent studies suggest that the heavy neurofilament protein (NF-H) of cholinergic neurons differs biochemically and antigenically from that of chemically heterogeneous NF-H (Faigon et al., 1991; Soussan et al., 1994) and that degeneration of brain cholinergic neurons in Alzheimer's disease (AD) and in Down Syndrome is associated with serum IgG directed specifically against *Torpedo* and mammalian cholinergic NF-H (Chapman et al., 1989; Hassin-Baer et al., 1992; Tchernakov et al., 1992). In order to examine whether the anticholinergic NF-H antibodies (Abs) associated with AD and Down Syndrome could play a role in neuronal degeneration in these diseases, we developed a rat model in which the cellular and cognitive effects of such Abs are being examined. This model is termed Experimental Autoimmune Dementia (EAD). In the following we review the evidence that the immune response of EAD rats to prolonged immunization with cholinergic NF-H induces memory and other cognitive deficits. In addition we present new EAD and *in vitro* data which suggest that these behavioral changes are due to IgG mediated damage to brain cholinergic neurons.

RESULTS AND DISCUSSION

Cognitive Dysfunction In EAD Rats
Alzheimer's disease is associated with marked changes in the spatio-temporal organization of behavior. In order to examine whether such changes occur in the EAD model, we analyzed the organization of their behavior in an open field. The experiment was performed six months after the initiation of immunization as previously described (Eilam and Golani, 1990). Analysis of the open field behavior of freely moving EAD rats revealed that the spatio-temporal organization of their behavior differs dramatically from that of either sham injected controls or of controls which were immunized with

chemically heterogenous *Torpedo* NF-H (NFHC rats). While rats of the two
control groups explored about 80 % of the open field, the EAD rats explored
only 25 % of the field. Measurements of the frequency and duration of stops
revealed that each rat of the three groups had a location where it spent most of
its stopping time and where it performed the highest frequency of the grooming
and rearing behaviors characteristic of a "home base". The EAD rats however
displayed a profound change in another behavioral measure of the home base -
the number of visits. Whereas rats of the two control groups performed
numerous round trips which started at the home base and covered most of the
open field, the EAD rats performed short sequences of stops of varying duration
and rarely returned to the home base (Eilam et al., 1993). These derangements
in the spatial organization of behavior together with the previously reported
memory deficits of the EAD rats (Chapman et al., 1991; Michaelson et al.,
1991) mimic some of the cognitive impairments of patients with AD and
dementia.

IgG Mediated Loss Of Forebrain Cholinergic Neurons In EAD
Forebrain cholinergic neurons were visualized immunohistochemically with a
mAb directed against choline acetyltransferase. This revealed that the density
of cholinergic neurons in the medial septum and vertical limb of the diagonal
band (MS+DBv) of EAD rats is lower than that of the sham injected controls
(Figs. 1A and 1C). Quantitative morphometric analysis of this effect revealed
that the density of cholinergic neurons in the MS + DBv of the EAD rats (33.2
$\pm$ 1.7 neurons/mm^2; average $\pm$ SEM; n=4) is about 20 % lower than that of
the sham injected controls (40.7 $\pm$ 4.3 neurons/mm^2; n=4) (p < 0.05). In
contrast the density of cholinergic neurons in the MS + DBv of the NFHC rats
(38.1 $\pm$ 0.9 neurons/mm^2; n=4) did not differ significantly from those of the
sham-injected controls. A similar but less pronounced effect was observed in
the horizontal limb of the diagonal band. These findings are in accordance with
a previous report in which forebrain cholinergic neurons of EAD rats were
visualized immunohistochemically utilizing a mAb to the low affinity nerve
growth factor receptor (Dubovik et al., 1993). Together these results show that
the decreased density of EAD forebrain cholinergic neurons is associated
specifically with the anticholinergic NF-H immune response of these rats.
    Immunization of EAD rats with cholinergic NF-H results in the appearance
of IgG containing neurons in the MS + DBv (43.8 $\pm$ 6.1 neurons/mm^2; n=4)
(Fig. 1D). No such neurons were detected in the MS + DBv of sham-injected
controls (Fig. 1B) whereas the levels of IgG containing neurons in the same area
of brains of NFHC rats (23.1 $\pm$ 5.4 neurons/mm^2; n=4) were about two-fold
lower than those detected in EAD rats. Specific accumulation of IgG was also
observed in neurons in the horizontal limb of the diagnonal band except that in
this area their density was lower than in the MS + DBv. Similar results were
observed when the sections were stained with either biotinylated anti-rat Fc or
with anti-rat Fab Abs, suggesting that the immunohistochemical staining is

indeed due to the presence of IgG and not to cross-reactivity with another molecule. Examination of the relationship between the levels of IgG containing neurons in the MS + DBv and the densities of cholinergic neurons in this brain area, revealed that the data is best fit by a curve which extrapolates at zero IgG containing neurons, to the average density of MS + DBv cholinergic neurons of the controls (not shown). This suggests that the MS + DBv neurons are affected by high levels of IgG but that low levels of IgG, such as those found in the NFHC rats, have no detectable effect. Examination of posterior brain areas revealed that IgG also accumulate specifically in the hippocampus and in the entorhinal cortex of EAD rats. These brain areas and the septum are connected by major pathways. Furthermore trajectories exist from the hypothalamus, where the blood brain barrier is leaky, to the entorhinal cortex (Paxinos, 1985). Additional experiments, including time course studies, are necessary for elucidating whether IgG accumulates in the brain by leakage to the cerebrospinal fluid (Michaelson et al., 1991) or via specific neuronal pathways.

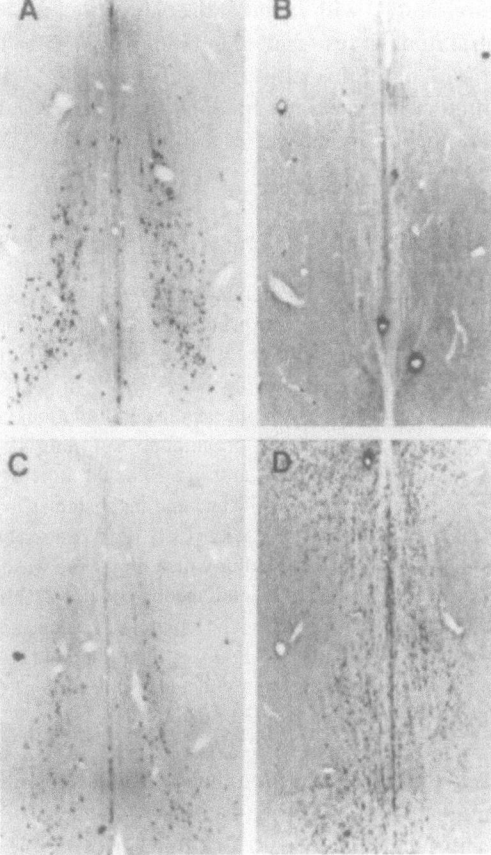

FIGURE 1. Medial septal cholinergic neruons in coronal sections (40μ) of a control rat (A,B) and an EAD rat immunized with cholinergic NF-H for six months (C,D). Sections were stained in parallel with either an anti-cholineacetyltransferase mAb (A,C) or with biotinylated anti-rat IgG (B,D). The bound Abs were visualized utilizing a Vecstatin ABC kit as previously described (Dubovik et al., 1993).

The accumulation of IgG in the MS + DBv of EAD rats and the decrease in density of cholinergic neurons in this brain area were both detectable by three to four months following the initiation of immunization and were more pronounced by six to eight months. In contrast, the short term memory deficits of the EAD rats and the disintegration of their open field behavior evolve more slowly and are significant only after more than six months of immunization with cholinergic NF-H (Chapman et al., 1989; Michaelson et al., 1991; Dubovik et al., 1993). Taken together, these data suggest that the derangement of EAD brain cholinergic neurons is due to the accumulation of anti-NF-H IgG in the forebrain, and that it plays a role in the observed behavioral deficits.

Tissue Culture Studies Of the Anti-Neuronal Effect Of Anti-NF-H Antibodies
In this section we describe results of *in vitro* studies aimed at examining whether the pathological effects observed with EAD rats can be reproduced and investigated at the cellular level. This was explored by studying the effects of anti-NF-H antisera on rat forebrain embryonic cultures enriched in cholinergic neurons. Incubation of the cultures at 4°C with rabbit antisera prepared against the NF-H protein of bovine ventral root nerves resulted in binding of IgG to the cultures (Fig. 2). The extent of binding of this antiserum was markedly higher than that of the preimmune serum. Half maximal binding was obtained at a serum dilution of 1:2000 whereas the end point was at a dilution of 1:10,000 (Fig. 2).

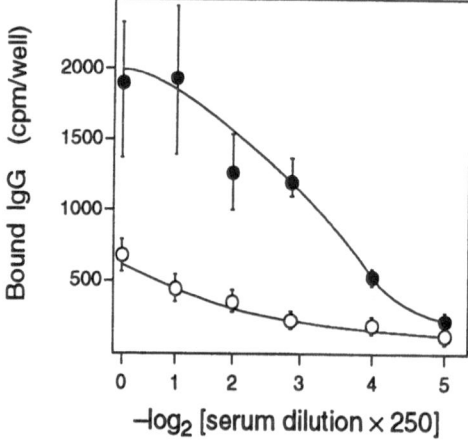

FIGURE 2. Binding of rabbit anti-NF-H antisera (●) and of preimmune sera (○) to the surface of rat primary forebrain neuronal cultures. Nine days old cultures were incubated for 1 hr at 4°C with the indicated dilutions of either preimmune or anti-NF-H rabbit antisera. The cultures were then washed and incubated (1 hr at 4°C) with [^{125}I] goat anti-rabbit IgG, after which they were washed again and incubated at 37°C for 1 hr. The bound [^{125}I] goat anti-rabbit IgG was then liberated from the neuronal outer surface (PH=2.5 at 4°C for 5 min) and counted. Omission of the first antibody abolished the binding of [^{125}I] anti-rabbit IgG to the cultures.

Conditions which disrupt antigen-antibody interactions but do not permeabilize the cells (i.e. pH 2.5 for 5 min at 4°C) (Pelchen-Matthews et al., 1989) virtually liberated all the bound anti-NF-H IgG (> 90%). Further experiments revealed that this treatment also released all the bound anti-NF-H IgG from cultures incubated at 37°C for up to 30 min. These results show that the anti-

NF-H IgG were not internalized even though the cultures were incubated at 37°C. The level of bound anti-NF-H IgG per mg protein was the same for cultures aged 9-22 days. It increased slightly at day 28, presumably due to age associated deterioration of the cultures and subsequent exposure of the intraneuronal cytoskeleton to the external medium.

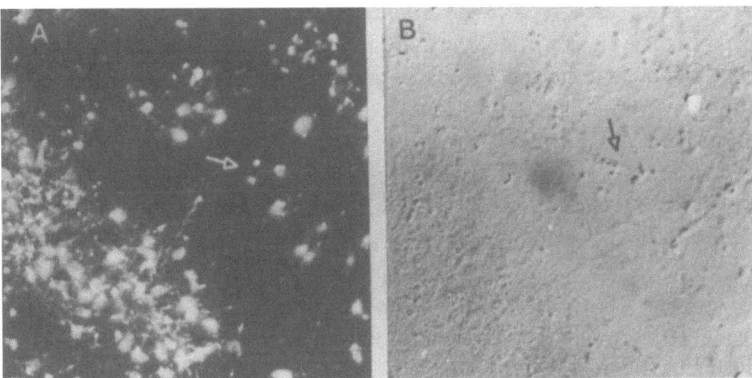

FIGURE 3. Immunofluorescence (A) and Nomarsky Optics (B) views of anti-NF-H IgG bound to a primary culture of rat forebrain neurons. Binding of anti-NF-H antisera (dilution 1:1000) was performed as described in the text utilizing a second Ab tagged with the fluorescent dye CY-3.

Immunofluorescence microscopy was employed to confirm the above binding data and to examine whether anti-NF-H IgG bind similarly to all the neurons. This was performed by incubating the cultures at 4°C with either preimmune or anti-NF-H antisera and by visualizing the bound Abs with anti-rabbit IgG second Abs tagged with the fluorescent dye CY-3. As can be seen in Fig. 3A, anti-NF-H IgG lit up both perikarya and neurites. No such staining was obtained with the preimmuned serum. Comparison of fields of fluorescently labelled neurons to those of their contours, as seen by Nomarsky optics (Figs. 3A and 3B), revealed that the labeling was selective to a subpopulation of the neurons. An example of such neurons is indicated by the arrows in Fig. 3. Further support for the assertion that anti-NF-H IgG bind to the neuronal outer surface is provided by a pilot study which suggests that incubation of the cultures with anti-NF-H antisera in the presence of complement results in marked deterioration of the neurons. Previous studies utilizing a neuroblastoma cell line have shown that an anti-NF-H mAb cross reacts with a 62-68 kD neuronal surface protein (Sadiq et al., 1991). It is tempting to suggest that rat primary cultures contain an analogous surface protein which mediates the interactions of the anti-NF-H Abs with the neuronal exterior.

CONCLUSIONS

The EAD animal model studies show that anti-NF-H IgG similar to those of AD patients induce specific neuronal and behavioral derangements. These deficits may replicate pathogenic processes in AD and support a role for such Abs in neuronal degeneration in the disease. The tissue culture experiments show that anti-NF-H Abs can interact with the neuronal outer surface. They provide a novel *in vitro* system for studying the interactions between anti-neurofilament Abs and intact neurons and for investigating the pathological consequences and specificity of these interactions.

ACKNOWLEDGEMENTS

This work was supported in part by grants to DMM from the BUPA Medical Foundation Limited and from the Simon Revah-Kabelli Fund, by grants from the Israeli Ministry of Absorption to LN and from the Branco Weiss Fund to VD. We thank Mrs. Angela Cohen for her editorial assistance.

REFERENCES

Chapman J, Bachar O, Korczyn AD, Wertman E and Michaelson DM (1989): Alzheimer's disease antibodies bind specifically to a neurofilament protein in *Torpedo* cholinergic neurons. *J Neurosci* 9:2710-2717.

Chapman J, Alroy G, Weiss Z, Faigon M, Feldon J and Michaelson DM (1991): Antineuronal antibodies similar to those found in Alzheimer's disease induce memory dysfunction in rats. *Neuroscience* 40:297-305.

Dubovik V, Faigon M, Feldon J and Michaelson DM (1993): Decreased density of forebrain cholinergic neurons in experimental autoimmune dementia. *Neuroscience* 56:75-82.

Eilam D and Golani I (1990): Home base behavior of tame wild rats *(Rattus norvegicus)* injected with amphetamine. *Behavioural Brain Research* 36:161-170.

Eilam D, Szechtman H, Faigon M, Dubovik V, Feldon J and Michaelson DM (1993): Disintegration of the spatial organization of behavior in experimental autoimmune dementia. *Neuroscience* 56:83-91.

Faigon M, Hadas E, Alroy G, Chapman J, Auerbach JM and Michaelson DM (1991): Monoclonal antibodies to the heavy neurofilament subunit (NF-H) of *Torpedo* cholinergic neurons. *J Neurosci Res* 29:490-498.

Hassin-Baer S, Wertman E, Raphael M, Stark V, Chapman J, and Michaelson DM (1992): Antibodies from Down syndrome patients bind to the same cholinergic neurofilament protein recognized by Alzheimer's disease antibodies. *Neurology* 42:551-555.

Michaelson DM, Alroy G, Soussan L, Chapman J and Feldon J (1991): Experimental autoimmune dementia (EAD): An immunological model of memory dysfunction and Alzheimer's disease. In: *Pharmacological Basis of Cholinergic Therapy in Alzheimer's Disease.* Giacobini E and Becker R, eds. Boston: Birkhauser Inc., pp. 126-133

Paxinos G (1985): The rat nervous system. New York: Academic Press.

Pelchen-Matthews A, Armes JE and Marsh M (1989): Internalization and recycling of CD4 transfected into Hela and NIH3T3 cells. *EMBO J* 8:3641-3649.

Sadiq SA, Van-den Berg LH, Thomas FP, Kilidivias K, Hays AP and Latov N (1991): Human monoclonal antineurofilament antibody cross-reacts with a neuronal surface protein. *J Neuroscience Res* 29:319-325.

Soussan L, Barzilai A and Michaelson DM (1994): Distinctly phosphorylated neurofilaments in different classes of neurons. *J Neurochem* (In Press).

Tchernakov K, Soussan L, Hassin-Baer S, Wertman E and Michaelson DM (1992): Alzheimer's disease and Down's syndrome antibodies bind to the heavy neurofilament protein of cholinergic neurons. *Research in Immunology* 6:583-588.

PART XIV

USE OF IMAGING TECHNIQUES (SPECT, MRI, PET) TO MONITOR THE EFFECT OF DRUGS IN AD TREATMENT

Alzheimer Disease: Therapeutic Strategies
edited by E. Giacobini and R. Becker.
© 1994 Birkhäuser Boston

USE OF PET TECHNIQUE TO MONITOR EFFECT OF DRUGS IN ALZHEIMER DISEASE TREATMENT

Agneta Nordberg
Department of Clinical Neuroscience and Family Medicine, Karolinska Institutet, Huddinge University Hospital, Huddinge, Sweden

INTRODUCTION

Although extensive exploration and development in the research field of Alzheimer's disease (AD) during recent years, there is still no cure of the disorder. The clinical instruments for providing an accurate premortem clinical diagnosis of AD have improved significantly. This includes various imaging techniques valuable in differentiating AD from other types of dementia. Alzheimer disease is thus no longer solely an exclusion diagnosis. Further understanding of possible genetic (Clark and Goate, 1993) and environmental (Fratiglioni, 1993) causes and their relation to the underlying pathological and neurochemical mechanisms in brain will probably provide valuable information and guidelines for design of new drug profiles in AD. Three main treatment strategies can be distinguished for treatment of cognitive impairments in AD:

1. Transmitter replacement therapy
2. Growth factors
3. Protease inhibitors

Among these strategies the possibilities to restore transmitter deficits have been extensively investigated. The cholinergic hypothesis has been in focus for many years. Up to now the cholinesterase inhibitors, eg. tacrine have shown most promising clinical effects in AD patients (Farlow et al., 1992; Knapp et al., 1994). The growth factor therapy, including nerve growth factors (NGF), has been approached in numerous animal studies and we have experience of treating two AD patients with NGF (Olson et al., 1992; and unpublished data). With increasing knowledge about the alterations in the secretory pathways which might lead to accumulation of amyloidogenic fragments in at least familiar forms of AD (Felsenstein et al., 1994) the development of protease inhibitors are of theoretical interest but have not yet been clinically tried.

This chapter will deal with the possibility to monitor by positron emission tomography (PET) the effect of cognitive drug treatment in AD. Positron emission tomography is a non-invasive technique for studies of biochemical and physiological processes in brain. It allows quantification and three dimensional imaging of distinct physiological variables. For evaluation of therapeutic effects of new AD drugs, PET offers an unique feature concerning functional aspects on brain activity which allow longitudinal PET studies in a few selected AD patients in parallel with other studies of brain functional activity such as EEG and neuropsychological performance. The pharmacological effects measured by PET can be correlated to pharmacokinetic data obtained in the same patient.

PET STUDIES OF BRAIN METABOLISM IN AD

PET studies using ^{18}F-fluorodeoxyglucose (^{18}F-FDG) have revealed abnormal reduction of glucose metabolism mainly in the parietotemporal but also frontal regions of AD brains (Rapoport, 1991). A similar pattern of changes have been observed for the cerebral blood flow (CBF) using ^{11}C-butanol or $H_2^{15}O$. Right/left assymetries in glucose metabolism are often found and the changes can be correlated to neuropsychological testings (Rapoport, 1991). Especially of interest are studies where familiar forms of AD have been investigated. In a British family with a point mutation on the amyloid precursor protein at codon 717 on chromosome 21 a symmetric parieto-temporal hypometabolism was observed in brain comparable to what is normally found in non-hereditary forms (Kennedy et al., 1993). We have also in the Swedish AD family with a double mutation at codon 670/71 on chromosome 21 (Mullan et al., 1992) found similar changes in glucose metabolism in diseased members and also in a family with mutation on chromosome 14 (Nordberg et al., in preparation). For the aspect of clinical evaluation of early therapeutic intervention in AD PET studies in family members who are carrier of a mutation will be very important in the future. This is of especially interest since longitudinal studies of functional brain activity can be initiated before the subjects have obtained the critical age for debut of memory disturbances typically for that AD family.

PET STUDIES OF TRANSMITTER ACTIVITY IN AD

Few PET studies have addressed the neurotransmitter function in AD (Nordberg, 1993). It is surprising since multiple deficits of neuroreceptors are known in AD (Nordberg, 1992). One possible explanation might be methodological difficulties in applying the PET technique. For the cholinergic transmitter system PET studies with ^{11}C-nicotine have shown a decreased uptake of the ligand to cortical regions of AD brains compared to healthy volunteers (Nordberg et al., 1990). When a two-compartment kinetic model later was applied it allowed a quantitative measurement of the ^{11}C-nicotine binding in brain revealing nicotinic receptor deficits in the temporal and frontal cortices and hippocampus of AD brains (Nordberg et al., 1994). We have used ^{11}C-benztropine for tracing muscarinic receptors in brain but since this ligand is an unspecific muscarinic antagonist more selective muscarinic antagonists are warranted. ^{18}F-6-L-dopa was used to visualize dopamine receptors which were found to be unchanged in AD compared to controls (Tyrrell et al., 1990). Losses of 5-HT$_2$ receptors were recently reported in cortical regions of AD brains using ^{18}F-setoperone and PET (Blin et al., 1993). The signal transduction system play an important role for the receptor mediated processes in synapses. The possibility to explore the function of the second messenger phosphoinositide (PI) response have so far been approached in monkey brain (Imahori et al., 1993). The PI response might be an important system to visualize by PET in AD patients treated with new selective muscarinic agonists. AD involves dysfunctional synaptic transmission and a defect coupling of the muscarinic receptors to G proteins has been observed in postmortem AD brain tissue (Warpman et al., 1993) which might be further clarified by measuring receptor-mediated PI turnover using PET.

DRUG-INDUCED CHANGES IN FUNCTIONAL BRAIN ACTIVITY IN AD

An important application of the PET technique is to examine the site of action of drugs that prove to be therapeutic in AD. This type of studies might reveal responders to a certain therapy. AD probably constitutes a whole family of diseases where only a subgroup of patient might respond to a certain therapy. PET studies can be a valuable complement to larger clinical trials especially regarding the examination site of mechanisms of action and selection of responders. We are presently in our PET studies using a multi-tracer system including tracers for glucose metabolism, CBF, nicotinic and muscarinic cholinergic receptors.

The PET technique offers unique possibility to investigate functional effect of drug treatment in AD but few studies with this design are yet available. The effect of phosphatidylserine on glucose metabolism has been studied in AD patients (Klinthammer et al., 1990) and significant enhancement in glucose metabolism during visual recognition task was reported after 6 months of treatment with phosphatidylserine (Heiss et al., 1993). Single doses of cholinesterase inhibitors such as physostigmine increase CBF with no significant effect on glucose metabolism in AD patients (Tune et al., 1991; Blin et al., 1994). Long-term treatment with tacrine for 3 months or longer improves glucose metabolism (COLOR PLATE 1) in AD patients (Nordberg et al., 1992; Nordberg, 1993). Furthermore, an increased binding of ^{11}C-nicotine can be detected in cortical brain regions after 3 weeks of tacrine treatment to AD patients (Nordberg et al., 1992). We have now longitudinally followed seven AD patients treated with tacrine 80 to 160 mg daily for 3 to 30 months. The finding is compatible with restoration of the nicotinic receptors and the PET findings are paralleled by improvement in EEG, cognitive functions and dose-related (Nordberg et al., submitted). Analysis of tacrine in CSF reveal proportionally higher concentrations when the patients have been treated with higher doses of tacrine (Johansson et al., submitted). The PET studies indicate that functional changes can be traced in brain after months of tacrine treatment in AD patients with mild dementia. Repeated PET studies performed in two AD patients receiving intraventricular infusion of NGF for 3 months have consistently shown improvements of ^{11}C-nicotine binding in cortical brain regions as well as changes in CBF and glucose metabolism (Olson et al., 1992; and unpublished observations).

COLOR PLATE 1 (located at the end of this chapter). Effect of long-term treatment with tacrine on glucose metabolism (μmol/min/100 cm^3) in an AD patient with mild dementia (MMSE 24/30). PET sections through the basal ganglia (upper panel) and cerebral cortex (lower panel) following an intravenous injection of a tracer dose of ^{18}F-fluoro-deoxy-glucose (^{18}F-FDG). The color scale illustrates Patlak images of the glucose metabolism prior and after 10 months of tacrine treatment. The patient received 80 mg tacrine daily for 9 months after which the dose was increased to 120 mg daily. Red = high; yellow = medium; blue = low metabolism.

CONCLUSION

PET studies will in the future play an important role in the evaluation of new therapeutic drug strategies and be a valuable complement to large clinical trials in AD. PET will be important for examining site of mechanism of action of a certain drug as well for evaluation of long-term treatments in AD and to select responders to a certain therapy.

ACKNOWLEDGEMENTS

The research from our laboratory reviewed was supported by the Swedish Medical Research Council, Loo and Hans Osterman's foundation, Stiftelsen för Gamla Tjänarinnor, Swedish Tobacco Research Council, KI foundations.

REFERENCES

Blin J, Baron JC, Dubois B, Crouzel C, Fiorelli M, Attar-Levy D, Pillon B, Fournier D, Vidailhet M and Agid Y (1993): Loss of brain 5-HT$_2$ receptors in Alzheimer's disease. In vivo assessment with positron emission tomography and [^{18}F]setoperone. Brain 116:497-510.

Blin J, Ray CA, Piercey MF, Bartko JJ, Mouradian MM and Chase TN (1994): Comparison of cholinergic drug effects on regional brain glucose consumption in rats and humans by means of autoradiography and positron emission tomography. Brain Res 635:196-202.

Clark RF and Goate AM (1993): Molecular genetics of Alzheimer's disease. Arch Neurol 50:1164-1172.

Farlow M, Gracon S, Hershey L and Lewis KW (1992): A controlled trial of tacrine in Alzheimer's disease. JAMA 268:2523-2529.

Felsenstein KM, Hunihan LW and Roberts SB (1994): Altered cleavage and secretion of a recombinant β-APP bearing the Swedish familial Alzheimer's disease mutation. *Nature Genetics* 6:251-256.

Fratiglioni L (1993): Epidemiology of Alzheimer's disease - issues of etiology and validity. *Acta Neurol Scand* 87(suppl 145):1-70.

Heiss WD, Kessler J, Slansky I, Mielke R, Szelies B and Herholz K (1993): Activation PET as an instrument to determine therapeutic efficacy in Alzheimer's disease. *Ann NY Acad Sci* 695:327-331.

Imahori Y, Fujii R, Ueda S, Ohmori Y, Wakita K and Matsumoto K (1993): Phosphoinositide turnover imaging linked to muscarinic cholinergic receptor in the central nervous system by positron emission tomography. *J Nucl Med* 34:1543-1551.

Kennedy AM, Newman S, McCaddon A, Ball J, Rogues P, Mullan M, Hardy J, Chartier-Harlin MC, Frackowiak RSJ, Warringon EK and Rossor M (1993): Familial Alzheimer's disease: a pedigree with a missense mutation in the amyloid precursor protein gene (APP717 valine to glycine). *Brain* 116:309-324.

Klinthammer P, Szelies B and Heiss WD (1990): Effect of phosphatidylserine on cerebral glucose metabolism in Alzheimer's disease. *Dementia* 1:197-201.

Knapp MJ, Knopman DS, Solomon PR, Pendlebury WW, Davis CS and Gracon SI (1994): A 30 week randomized controlled trial of high-dose tacrine in patients with Alzheimer's disease. *JAMA* 271:985-991.

Mullan M, Crawford F, Axelman K, Houlden H, Lillius L, Winblad B and Lannfelt L (1992): A pathogenic mutation for probable Alzheimer's disease in the APP gene at the N-terminus of β-amyloid. *Nature Genet* 1:345-347.

Nordberg A (1992): Neuroreceptor changes in Alzheimer disease. *Cerebrovasc Brain Metab Rev* 4:303-328.

Nordberg A (1993): Clinical studies in Alzheimer patients with positron emission tomography. *Behav Brain Res* 57:215-224.

Nordberg A, Hartvig P, Lilja A, Viitanen M, Amberla K, Lundqvist H, Anderson Y, Ulin J, Winblad B and Langstrom B (1990): Decreased uptake and binding of ^{11}C-nicotine in the brain of Alzheimer patients as visualized by positron emission tomography. *J Neural Transm (P-D sect)* 2:215-224.

Nordberg A, Lilja A, Lundqvist H, Hartvig P, Amberla K, Viitanen M, Warpman U, Johansson M, Hellstrom-Lindahl E, Bjurling P, Fasth KJ, Langstrom B and Winblad B (1992): Tacrine restores cholinergic nicotinic receptors and glucose metabolism in Alzheimer patients as visualized by positron emission tomography. *Neurobiol Aging* 13:747-758.

Nordberg A, Lundqvist H, Hartvig P, Lilja A and Langstrom B (1994): Kinetic analysis of regional (S)(-)[11]C-nicotine binding in normal and Alzheimer brains- in vivo assessment using positron emission tomography. *Alzheimer Dis Assoc Disord* (In Press).

Olson L, Nordberg A, von Holst H, Backman L, Ebendal T, Alafuzoff I, Amberla K, Hartvig P, Herlitz A, Lilja A, Lundqvist H, Langstrom B, Meyersson B, Persson A, Viitanen M, Winblad B and Seiger Å (1992): Nerve growth factor affects ^{11}C-nicotine binding, blood flow, EEG and verbal episodic memory in an Alzheimer patient. *J Neural Transm (P-D Sect)* 4:79-95.

Rapoport SI (1991): Positron emission tomography in Alzheimer's disease in relation to disease pathogenesis: a critical review. *Cerebrovasc Metab Rev* 3:297-335.

Tune L, Brandt J, Frost J, Harris G, Mayberg H, Steele C, Burns A, Sapp J, Folstein
    MF, Wagner HN and Pearlson GD (1991): Physostigmine in Alzheimer's disease:
    effects on cognitive functioning cerebral glucose metabolism analyzed by positron
    emission tomography and cerebral blood flow analyzed by single photon emission
    tomography. *Acad Psychiatr Scand* Suppl. 366:61-65.

Tyrrell P, Sawle G, Ibanez V, Bloomfield P, Leenders KL, Frackowiak RSJ and
    Rossor M (1990): Clinical and PET studies in the extrapyramidal syndrome of
    dementia of Alzheimer type. *Arch Neurol* 47:1318-1323.

Warpman U, Alafuzoff I and Nordberg A (1993): Coupling of muscarinic receptors to
    GTP proteins in postmortem human brain-alteration in Alzheimer's disease. *Neurosci
    Lett* 150:39-43.

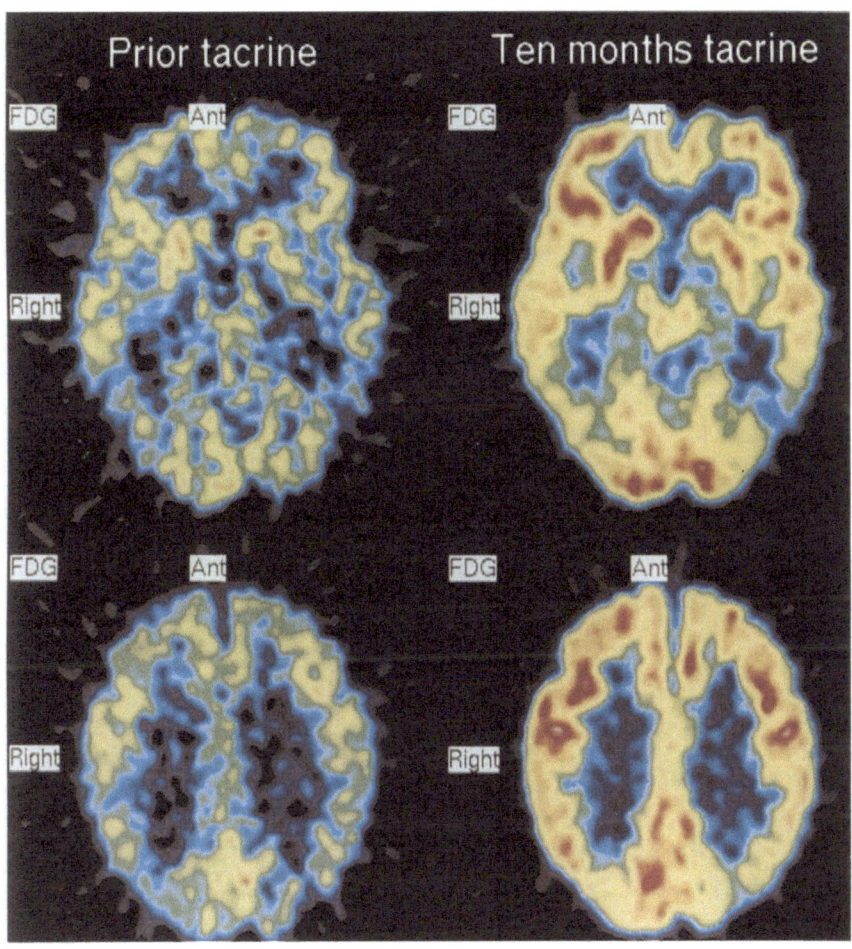

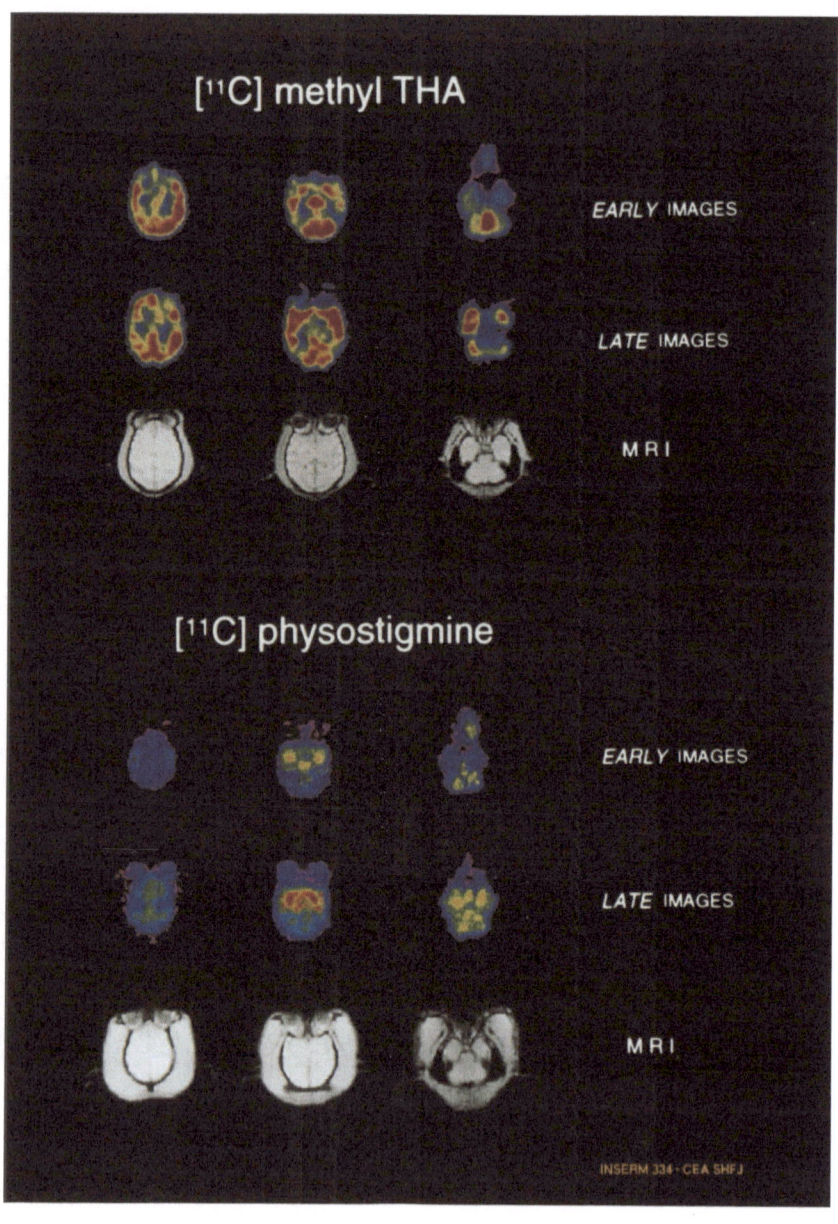

Alzheimer Disease: Therapeutic Strategies
edited by E. Giacobini and R. Becker.
© 1994 Birkhäuser Boston

POSITRON EMISSION TOMOGRAPHY WITH [11C]-METHYLTACRINE AND [11C]-PHYSOSTIGMINE

Bertrand Tavitian, Sabina Pappata, Antoinette Jobert,
Christian Crouzel and Luigi Di Giamberardino
INSERM U334, Service Hospitalier Frédéric Joliot, Direction des Sciences
du Vivant, CEA, Orsay, France

Anna M. Planas
CSIC, Barcelona, Spain

As the progressive degeneration of higher cognitive functions of Alzheimer's disease (AD) was reckoned to have an anatomical and neurochemical basis, a number of studies have used positron emission tomography (PET) to investigate the brain deficits of AD (see Foster, 1994 for a recent review). Positron emission tomography, a non invasive *in vivo* technique, can provide functional images of the brain and is thus particularly well suited to study the chemical and functional impairments found in AD.

One obvious application of PET to AD is to determine the activity of putative therapeutic agents on ligand-receptor interaction and/or brain activity. Another possible application of PET is to design new ligands capable of imaging the cholinergic deficit of AD, much in the way that dopaminergic ligands can illustrate the deficits of Parkinson's disease. However, a difficulty is that PET merely shows the distribution of tissular radioactivity concentrations after the injection of a positron-emitter-labeled compound. Only in the ideal case does this distribution correlate with the concentration of the receptor of interest.

In this paper we present data illustrating this latter approach with two new PET ligands: [11C]-methyltacrine ([11C]mTHA) is a derivative of tacrine (THA) that could be used to study the pharmacology of this drug *in vivo*; and [11C]-physostigmine ([11C]PHY) is a potent acetylcholinesterase (AChE) inhibitor whose cerebral distribution is superimposable to that of AChE.

METHODS

Both ligands were 11C-labeled (decay 20.4 min) with very high specific activity (Bonnot et al., 1991, 1993) and injected to adult anesthetized baboons. Positron emission tomography acquisition was performed either with the LETI TTV03 time-of flight camera (slice thickness 9 mm, FWHM resolution 7 mm), or the

ECAT 953B camera (slice thickness 3.375 mm, FWHM resolution 6 mm). Correct positioning was ensured by the means of a specially designed head holder (Bottlaender et al., unpublished data), and controlled by magnetic resonance imaging (MRI) in a CGR 0.5 T MRMAX. Quantitative data obtained from PET images were normalized for the radioactivity dose injected.

[¹¹C]-METHYLTACRINE

The 9N-methyl derivative of tacrine has anticholinesterasic properties similar to tacrine (Steinberg et al., 1975; Tavitian et al., 1993a) and can be readily labeled with ¹¹C (Bonnot et al., 1991). The PET images obtained early after i.v. injection of a tracer dose of [¹¹C]mTHA resemble blood-flow images and correspond essentially to the vascular passage of radioactivity. At later times, there is a preferential redistribution of radioactivity towards the cortex, notably the anterior cortex, and the basal ganglia, while the cerebellum and white matter areas have much lower concentrations. The thalamic area has an intermediate concentration. The kinetics of radioactivity washout is relatively slow: the half-time of elimination is over 4 hours in the frontal cortex; it is less than 2 hours in the cerebellum; thus regional contrast of the PET images increases with time (COLOR PLATE 2, top half). Finally, injection of a pharmacological dose of tacrine (2.5 mg/kg) 20 min after [¹¹C]mTHA displaces 50% of the radioactivity in the frontal, temporal, and parietal cortex, 40% in the occipital cortex, and 20% in the cerebellum (Tavitian et al., 1993a).

COLOR PLATE 2 (located at the beginning of this chapter). Representative [¹¹C]mTHA and [¹¹C]PHY PET scans of baboon heads. Scans were obtained in the orbito-meatal plane at different anatomical levels shown in the corresponding MRI scans: left to right, levels of the parietal cortex, basal ganglia, and cerebellum. *EARLY* IMAGES were acquired during the first minute after tracer injection. *LATE* IMAGES were acquired 100 to 120 min after [¹¹C]mTHA injection, or 20 to 25 min after [¹¹C]PHY injection, respectively. All images are color-coded with the same intensity scale, from dark blue (low radioactivity concentrations) to hot red (high activity concentrations).

Overall, the cerebral distribution of [¹¹C]mTHA is very different from that of AChE activity. This is not surprising given the number of pharmacological interactions that have been reported for tacrine aside from its inhibitory activity towards AChE (see for review Freeman and Dawson, 1991). [¹¹C]mTHA has a distribution quite similar to that of [³H]THA (McNally et al., 1989). Its' reported activity is comparable to that of tacrine (Steinberg et al., 1975), and it shows direct competition with tacrine for cerebral binding sites. Together these are strong arguments for the use of [¹¹C]mTHA to study tacrine's pharmacological properties *in vivo*. As an example, [¹¹C]mTHA's slow washout and its relatively high cortical concentration could reflect the prolonged increase in brain acetylcholine levels observed after tacrine administration (Hallak and Giacobini, 1989).

At present, the exact nature of tacrine's binding sites remains an enigma. [¹¹C]mTHA could allow to image those sites and study their fate during the course of AD, and the effect of different therapeutic strategies on them.

[¹¹C]-PHYSOSTIGMINE

Physostigmine was labeled with ¹¹C on the carboxylic carbon of its carbamic group (Bonnot et al., 1993). This is essential to ensure that radioactivity will remain on AChE after [¹¹C]PHY is injected. Physostigmine reacts rapidly with AChE and splits into eseroline and a carbamate group that links covalently to the hydroxyl group of the serine at the active site of the enzyme, and is then slowly hydrolyzed (Main and Hastings, 1966). Cerebral distribution of radioactivity after [¹¹C]PHY injection matches well with the known pharmacokinetics of physostigmine (COLOR PLATE 2, lower half). Its entry in the brain is followed by a rapid preferential redistribution to regions rich in AChE activity, essentially the caudate nucleus and the putamen. Concentrations in the cortex and cerebellum are in accordance with the moderate AChE activity in these regions, and very little radioactivity is found in the white matter. Only small differences are found between different cortical areas, although radioactivity concentrations are higher in the internal part of the inferior temporal lobe (the limbic region) than in the external part. The kinetics of radioactivity washout is in good agreement with the pharmacokinetics data of physostigmine (half-life of elimination: 38 min in striatum, 20 min in cortex, 15 min in cerebellum). Partial pre-saturation by continuous infusion of physostigmine (100 mg/kg/hr) reduces [¹¹C]PHY uptake by 50% in the striatum, 26% in the cerebellum, and 13% in the cortex (Tavitian et al., 1993b).

Concordance between AChE and [¹¹C]PHY regional distributions was further examined by autoradiographic experiments on rat brain sections. Autoradiograms from phosphor plates exposed to sections incubated with [¹¹C]PHY during 10 min, and photomicrographs of the same sections stained for AChE yield perfectly superimposable images (r > 0.9, linear regression analysis). Moreover, binding of [¹¹C]PHY to the sections is completely abolished by AChE inhibition with 10^{-5} M BW 284C51 (Planas et al., 1994).

In summary, [¹¹C]PHY is a valid PET tracer of cerebral AChE in the baboon brain. It now remains to be demonstrated whether this new tracer can document the deficit of AChE activity found in the brains of AD patients.

SUMMARY AND CONCLUSION

Two new PET ligands with potential interest for AD have been synthesized and applied to non-human primates brain imaging. (1) [¹¹C]mTHA appears to bind to the same cerebral sites as tacrine, and could thus contribute to *in vivo* pharmacological studies of this complex therapeutic agent. (2) [^{11}C]PHY shows a distribution highly compatible with that of AChE, and is promising as a tracer of AChE's active sites in pathological states in which this enzyme is implicated, such as AD (Davies, 1979; Perry, 1987; DeFeudis, 1988).

ACKNOWLEDGEMENTS

Supported in part by a grant from the MGEN. We thank F. Né for help with the phosphoimaging technology, V. Brulon and Drs. B. Bendriem and V. Frouin for PET technical support, and Dr. A. Leroy-Willig for the MRI facility.

REFERENCES

Bonnot S, Prenant C and Crouzel C (1991): Synthesis of 9-[^{11}C]Methylamino-1,2,3,4-tetrahydroacridine, a potent acetylcholine esterase inhibitor. *Appl Rad Isotopes* 42:690.

Bonnot S, Crouzel C, Prenant C and Hinnen F (1993): Carbon-11 labelling of an inhibitor of acetylcholinesterase: [^{11}C] physostigmine. *J Label Comp Radiopharm* 33(4):277-284.

Davies P (1979): Neurotransmitter-related enzymes in senile dementia of the Alzheimer type. *Brain Res* 171:319-327.

DeFeudis FV (1988): Cholinergic systems and Alzheimer's disease. *Drug Dev Res* 14:95-103.

Freeman SE and Dawson RM (1991): Tacrine: a pharmacological review. *Prog Neurobiol* 36:257-277.

Foster N (1994): PET imaging. In: *Alzheimer Disease*, Terry RD, Katzman R and Bick KL, eds. New York: Raven Press, pp. 87-103.

Hallak M and Giacobini E (1989): Physostigmine, tacrine and metrifonate: the effect of multiple doses on acetylcholine metabolism in rat brain. *Neuropharmacol* 28:199-206.

Main AR and Hastings FL (1966): Carbamylation and binding constants for the inhibition of acetylcholinesterase by physostigmine (eserine). *Science* 154:400-402.

McNally W, Roth M, Young R, Bockbrader H and Chang, T (1989): Quantitative whole-body autoradiographic determination of tacrine tissue distribution in rats following intravenous or oral dose. *Pharm Res* 6:924-930.

Perry EK (1987): Cortical neurotransmitter chemistry in Alzheimer's disease. In: *Psychopharmacology: the Third Generation of Progress*, Meltzer HY, ed. New York: Raven Press, pp. 887-895.

Planas AM, Crouzel C, Hinnen F, Jobert A, Né F, Di Giamberardino L and Tavitian B (1994): Rat brain acetylcholinesterase visualized with [^{11}C]physostigmine. *NeuroImage* (In Press).

Steinberg GM, Mednick ML, Maddox J, Rice R and Cramer J (1975): A hydrophobic binding site in acetylcholinesterase. *J Med Chem* 18:1056-1061.

Tavitian B, Pappata S, Jobert A, Crouzel C and Di Giamberardino L (1993a): Positron emission tomography study of [^{11}C]methyl-tetrahydroaminoacridine (methyl-tacrine) in baboon brain. *Eur J Pharmacol* 236:229-239.

Tavitian B, Pappata S, Planas AM, Jobert A, Bonnot-Lours S, Crouzel C and Di Giamberardino L (1993b): *In vivo* visualization of acetylcholinesterase with positron emission tomography. *NeuroReport* 4(5):535-538.

Alzheimer Disease: Therapeutic Strategies
edited by E. Giacobini and R. Becker.
© 1994 Birkhäuser Boston

USE OF SPECT IN EARLY DIAGNOSIS AND TO MONITOR THE EFFECT OF DRUGS IN ALZHEIMER DISEASE

Philippe Robert, Michel Benoit and Guy Darcourt
Memory and DAT Center, Department of Psychiatry,
University of Nice, France

Octave Migneco, Jacques Darcourt and Francoise Bussiere
Department of Biophysics and Nuclear Medicine,
University of Nice, France

Basic research to date suggests that brain imaging methods, such as Positron Emission Tomography (PET) and Single Photon Emission Tomography (SPECT) will have great success as tools to aid the clinician in the diagnosis and monitoring of a patient's clinical course. On one hand, PET techniques allow evaluation of different aspects of brain characteristics such as cerebral blood flow (CBF), metabolism or specific receptors functioning. Furthermore PET offers high sensitivity and resolution. On the other hand, the SPECT investigation field seems to be more restricted (essentially CBF); however, SPECT facilities are widely available in most hospitals since they use a much lower cost technology. Therefore, SPECT could represent an interesting tool for the clinical management of Alzheimer's disease (AD) patients. A particularly interesting point concerns the difficulty to evaluate therapeutic interventions. Activation studies consist of inducing differences in brain metabolism through manipulations of behavior or drugs. Using this technique it is possible to investigate the pattern changes of tracer uptake during a cognitive or pharmacological stress in comparison with determined basal conditions. There are at least two main practical interests to use this kind of procedure. The first one concerns the possibility to increase the accuracy of early diagnosis of dementia. In fact, pharmacological treatments developed for AD are mostly effective in the mild stages of the disease and a well chosen specific cortical "stress test" would be better suited than baseline conditions to demonstrate patterns of regional decrease in brain activity. The second one concerns the metabolic effects of these drugs and their relationship with clinical changes.

SPECT AND COGNITIVE ACTIVATION

Previous SPECT investigations mainly involved healthy subjects (George et al., 1991; Lang et al., 1988; Woods et al., 1991) or demented patients (Riddle et al., 1993; Robert et al., 1994) but were never applied to at-risk subjects when patients had only mild memory loss which are often the first signs of AD. The present study uses as a "stress test" a visuospatial memorization task and investigates the relationships between functional cortical activation and cognitive performances in patients with mild memory disorders.

Population and Neuropsychological Testing
Fifteen outpatients (mean age: 64.7 years), referred to the memory clinic for amnesic complaints, underwent two SPECTs. All had given their written informed consent. None of them had a history of cerebrovascular disease. Furthermore, the subjects were free of dementia (DSMIII-R, 1987) and of major mental disorders or drug abuse. Patients underwent a battery of behavioral and neuropsychological tests one week before the first SPECT (screening evaluation), including the COVI measure of anxiety (Covi et al., 1979), and the Mini-Mental Score Evaluation (MMSE) (Folstein et al., 1975). Memory impairment was evaluated using the Batterie d'Efficience Mnésique (BEM 84), the Signoret memory battery scale (Signoret, 1991).

Single Photon Emission Tomography
Each subject underwent two measurements of 99 mTc HMPAO brain uptake on two separate days one week apart. For each study, 740 MBq of 99 mTc HMPAO were injected via an intravenous (i.v.) line previously placed in order to avoid noxious stimuli. One SPECT (Base SPECT) was done during baseline condition, with eyes opened looking at a blank sheet. For the other SPECT (Stim SPECT) the injection of HMPAO was performed during the learning step of the Memory Efficiency Profile (MEP) test. The task consisted of memorizing drawings of familiar objects, presented in progressively abstract shapes (Rey, 1966; De Rotrou et al., 1991). These two SPECTs were performed in counterbalanced order. Eight regions of interest (ROI) for each hemisphere were drawn with a computerized method using the Talairach atlas (Talairach and Szikla, 1967) as anatomical reference (Migneco et al., 1994). The activation effect was evaluated in each ROI by the index: Stim - Base / Base x 100, where Stim and Base represent the mean counts per pixel in the ROI for the corresponding studies.

RESULTS

The mean MMSE was 27.5 (range 25-30), which was not significantly different between the COVI anxiety score assessed at the screening evaluation, before the Base SPECT and the Stim SPECT. The Spearman correlation coefficients indicated that in the right temporal, the activation effect was correlated with MEP immediate recall and BEM visual score. The right cerebellum activation was also correlated with MEP immediate recall, and with both BEM global and visual score (Fig. 1). These correlations between the neuropsychological test and HMPAO brain uptake illustrate the possibility of defining subjects with mild memory impairment according to regional cortical activation patterns provided by a SPECT technique. The follow-up of the clinical and metabolic outcome of the subjects will confirm if subjects with lower activation will have a demential evolution and therefore will highlight the potential interest to apply such a technique for the early diagnosis of dementia.

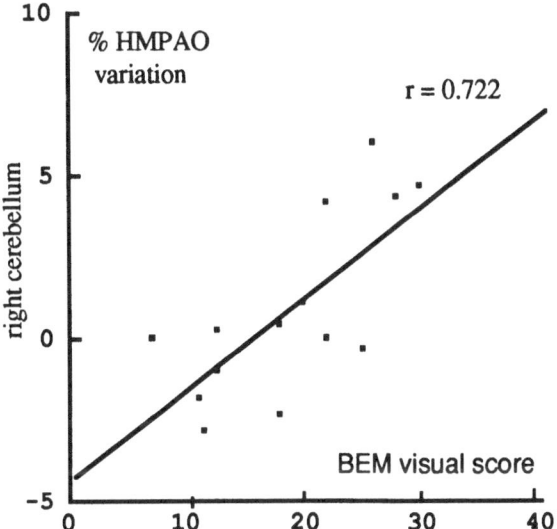

FIGURE 1. Plot of HMPAO variation [(Stim - Base) / Base] in right cerebellum by BEM visual score in 15 subjects with mild memory impairment.

SPECT AND EVALUATION OF DRUG EFFECTS

Clinical changes expected from drugs presently available or in development are either stabilization or mild improvement. Brain imaging challenges could then be useful in providing objective evidence of therapeutic results. In this field PET studies have already been used in evaluation of metabolism, CBF or neurotransmission (Heiss et al., 1989; Nordberg et al., 1992). Concerning SPECT, Table I gives an overview of the studies conducted with different tracers. The same methodology was used in all of these studies; each subject underwent 2 SPECTs, one before and the other after administration of the active agents or placebo. Four of these studies assessed the effects of single dose of cholinomimetic agents on CBF. Battistin et al. (1989), normalizing tracer uptake to the cerebellum, found that the acute administration of L-acetylcarnitine at the higher doses (1-2 mg i.v.) partially reversed the parietal CBF decline observed in the first SPECT performed after saline infusion. Using the same

Studies	SPECT tracer	Population	Type of drugs	Interval between 2 SPECT	Results: increase of tracer uptake in:
Battistin et al. (1989)	HMPAO resting condition (eyes patched)	n = 21 DAT: DSMIII mean MMSE = 12	L Acetylcarnitine	5 - 7 days	parietal, frontal and temporal ROIs
Geaney et al. (1990)	HMPAO rest condition (eyes open)	n =8 DAT DSM III-R mean MMSE = 17 n = 8 control subjects mean MMSE = 29	Intravenous saline infusion or 0.5 mg Physostigmine (blind in balanced order)	7 days	posterior parietotemporal ROI in DAT (after Physostigmine)
Hunter et al. (1991)	HMPAO rest condition (eyes closed)	n = 7 AD : NINCDS	Intravenous saline infusion or Physostigmine (0.37 to 0.5 mg)	7 days	left cortex relative to right (most significant in frontal ROI)
Agnoli et al. (1992)	HMPAO rest condition (eyes closed)	n = 10 AD: NINCDS mean MMSE = 19.6	L-deprenyl (n=5) or placebo (n=5)	60 days	L-deprenyl: no significant differences placebo:decrease in parietal ROI
Ebmeir et al. (1992)	Exametazine rest condition	n = 21 DAT:DSM III-R mean MMSE = 16.5	75 mg Velnacrine (n=11) or placebo (n=10)	2 hours	superior frontal (most in left cortex)
Minthon et al. (1993)	Xenon rest condition (eyes closed)	n = 17 DAT:DSM III-R	THA + placebo placebo + placebo	6 weeks	left posterior temporal in clinical responder during the THA period

TABLE I. Overview of the SPECT pharmacological activation studies in Alzheimer's disease.

the same type of normalization, Geaney et al. (1990) found that physostigmine produced a focal increase of CBF in the posterior parietotemporal cortex in AD patients but not in controls. Hunter et al. (1991) normalizing to white matter, found a clear increase of CBF on the left side relative to the right. Results of Ebmeir et al. (1992), normalizing tracer uptake to calcarine, agreed with this asymmetrical hypothesis. They found a relative increase of CBF in left superior frontal region after administration of 75 mg of velnacrine. In contrast, Agnoli et al. (1992) assessed CBF before and after a 60 day IMAO-B treatment or placebo. At the end of the treatment patients who received placebo showed a significant further decrease of CBF in parietal lobes while patients who received L-deprenyl showed an improvement on cognitive assessment and no changes in CBF. Minthon et al. (1993) conducted a double-blind crossover design with three types of treatments. They found that the CBF characteristics during unmedicated condition might be crucial for the effect of treatment. Clinical responder patients showed the highest mean flow values and patients who deteriorated showed the lowest. Moreover, a significant increase of rCBF was found in responders in the left temporal region after the THA treatment. In another study using both fluorodeoxyglucose (FDG), PET and iodoamphetamine SPECT, Tune et al. (1991) indicated that acute i.v. administration of physostigmine had a modest effect on both CBF and glucose metabolism. Although physostigmine enhanced CBF in most of the 6 patients, only one showed significant clinical improvement. The most straightforward interpretation of these CBF data is that, in certain brain regions of AD patients, many of the remaining neuronal structures readily respond to cholinergic agents. However the relationships between the blood flow data, the metabolic data and the cognitive effects following treatment remains unclear. Pharmacological brain imaging challenge may be useful in at least three fields; 1) the understanding of physiological effects and the localization of neurochemical targets during the development of new compounds; 2) the monitoring of the drugs effects during treatment; 3) the selection of potentially responder patients. Positron Emission Tomography seems to be more suitable for the first aim. Brain imaging could soon be useful for the two last aims. Two arguments lead to this tendency. First, the coming possibility, even with SPECT, to use receptor-specific tracers such as in Parkinson disease (Schwarz et al., 1993). This technique could allow, on a purely pharmacological basis, the possibility to distinguish responders from nonresponders. Secondly, our better knowledge of a cognitive activation paradigm that could both facilitate the early diagnosis and select patients with remaining cerebral metabolic reaction to cognitive stress test.

REFERENCES

Agnoli A, Fabbrini G, Fioravanti M and Martucci N (1992): CBF and cognitive evaluation of Alzheimer type patients before and after IMAO-B treatment: a pilot study. *Eur Neuropsychopharmacol* 2:31-35.

Battistin L, Pizzolato G, Dam M, Da Col C, Perlotto N, Saitta B, Borsato N, Calvani M and Ferlin G (1989): Single photon emission computed tomography studies with 99 mTc hexamethylpropyleneamine oxime in dementia: effects of acute administration of L-acetylcarnitine. *Eur Neurology* 29:261-265.

Covi L, Lipman R, McNair DM and Crezlinsky T (1979): Symptomatic volunteers in multicenter drug trials. *Progr Neuropsychopharmacol* 521.

De Rotrou JC, Forette F, Hervy MP, Tortrat D, Fermanian J, Boudou MR and Boller F (1991): The cognitive efficiency profile: description and validation in patients with Alzheimer's disease. *Intl J Geriat Psychiat* 6:50-509.

DSMIII-R. Diagnostic and Statistical Manual of Mental Disorders (1987): Third Edition-Revised. Washington, DC: American Psychiatric Association.

Ebmeir KP, Hunter R, Curran SM, Dougal NJ, Murray CL, Wyper DJ, Patterson J, Hanson MT, Siegfried K and Goodwin GM (1992): Effects of a single dose of the acetylcholinestrerase inhibitor velnacrine on recognition memory and regional crebral blood flow in Alzheimer's disease. *Psychopharmacol* 108:103-109.

Folstein MF, Folstein SE and McHugh PR (1975): "Mini-mental test". A practical method for grading the cognitive state of patients for the clinician. *J Psychiat Res* 12:189-198.

Geaney DP, Soper N, Shepstone BJ and Cowen PJ (1990): Effect of central cholinergic stimulation on regional cerebral blood flow in Alzheimer disease. *Lancet* 335:1484-1487.

George MS, Ring HA, Costa DC, Ell PJ, Kouris K, and Jarrit P (1991): Neuroactivation and neuroimaging with SPET. London: Springer-Verlag, p. 197.

Heiss WD, Herholz K, Pawlik G, Hebold I, Peter Kinkhammer and Szelies B (1989): Positron emission tomography findings in dementia disorders: Contributions to differential diagnosis and objectivizing of therapeutic effects. *Keio J Med* 38(2):111-135.

Hunter R, Wyper DJ, Patterson J, Hansen MT and Goodwin GM (1991): Cerebral pharmacodynamics of physostigmine in Alzheimer's disease investigated using single-photon computurized tomography. *Brit J Psychiat* 158:351-357

Lang W, Lang M, Podreka I, Steiner M, Uhl F, Suess E, Muller Ch and Deecke LDC (1988): Potential shifts and regional cerebral blood flow reveal frontal cortex involvment in human visuomotor learning. *Experimental Brain Research* 71:353-364.

Migneco O, Darcourt J, Benoliel J, Martin F, Robert Ph, Bussiere-Lapalus F and Mena I (1994): Computerized localization of brain structures in single photon emission computed tomography using a proportional anatomical stereotactic atlas. *Computerized Medical Imaging and Graphics* (In Press).

Minthon L, Gustafson L, Dalfelt G, Hagberg B, Nilsson K, Risberg J, Rosén I, Seiving B and Wendt PE (1993): Oral tetrahydroaminoacridine treatment of Alzhemer's disease evaluated clinically and by regional cerebral blood flow and EEG. *Dementia* 4:32-42.

Nordberg AA, Lilja A, Lundqvist H, Hartwig P, Amberla K, Viitanen M, Warpman U, Johansson M, Hellstrom-Lindahl E, Bjurling P, Fasth KJ, Langstrom B and Winblad B (1992): Tacrine restores cholinergic nicotinic receptors and glucose metabolism in Alzheimer patients as visualized by positron emission tomography. *Neurobiology of Aging* 13:747-758.

Rey A (1966): Les troubles de la mémoire et leur examen psychométrique. Dessart, J ed. Paris.

Riddle W, O'Carroll RE, Dougall N, Van Beck M, Murray C, Curran SM, Ebmeier KP and Goodwin GM (1993): A single photon emission computerized tomography study of regional brain function underlying verbal memory in patients with Alzheimer-type dementia. *Brit J Psychiat* 163:166-172.

Robert Ph, Migneco O, Darcourt J, Aubin V, Benoit M., Benoliel J, Bonhomme P, Giacomoni F, Bussiere F and Darcourt G (1994): Single photon emission computed tomography during cognitive stimulation: potential interest in the diagnosis of Alzheimer's disease. *Int Acad Biomed Drug Res* Vol 7, Basel: Karger (In Press).

Schwarz J, Tatsch K, Arnold G, Ott M, Trenkwalder C, Kirsch CM and Oertel WH (1993): 123I-Iodobenzamide-SPECT in 83 patients with de novo parkinsonism. *Neurology* 43(Suppl 6):S17-S20

Signoret JL (1991): Batterie d'Efficience Mnésique. Esprit and Cerveau, eds. Paris: Elsevier, p. 102.

Talairach J and Szikla G (1967): Atlas anatomique stéréotaxique du télencéphale. Paris: Masson p. 326.

Tune L, Brandt J, Frost JJ, Harris G, Mayberg H, Steel C, Burns A, Sapp J, Folstein MF, Wagner HN et al. (1991): Physostigmine in Alzheimer's disease: effects on cognitive functioning, cerebral glucose metabolism annalyzed by positron emission tomography and cerebral blood flow analyzed by single photon emission tomography. *Acta Psychiat Scandi Suppl* 366:61-65.

Woods SW, Hegeman IM, Zubal IG, Krystal JH, Koster K, Smith EO, Heninger GR and Hoffer PB (1991): Visual stimulation increase 99 mTc HMPAO distribution in human visual cortex. *J Nuclear Med* 32:210-215.

Alzheimer Disease: Therapeutic Strategies
edited by E. Giacobini and R. Becker.
© 1994 Birkhäuser Boston

NICOTINIC STIMULATION OF ANTERIOR REGIONAL CEREBRAL GLUCOSE METABOLISM IN ALZHEIMER'S DISEASE: PRELIMINARY STUDY WITH TRANSDERMAL PATCHES

Randolph W. Parks, Carter S. Young, Robert F. Rippey, Valerie Danz, Cathy Vohs, Jane R. Matthews, G. Todd Collins, Steven S. Zigler, Paul G. Urycki, Patricia Keim, Esperanza Kabatay and Robert E. Becker
Depts. Psychiatry and Psychology, Southern Illinois Univ. Sch. Med., Springfield, IL; and Depts. Nuclear Medicine and PET Imaging, Downstate Clinical Positron Emission Tomography Center, Methodist Medical Center, Peoria, IL

INTRODUCTION

We studied the effects of nicotine delivered by transdermal patch during positron emission tomography (PET) scanning while subjects performed verbal fluency as a measure of semantic memory. Since it is known that nicotine increases cognitive performance in nonclinical populations, and small but measurable improvements on selected cognitive tests in Alzheimer disease (AD) (Newhouse et al., 1988, 1990, 1993; Jones et al., 1992) we hypothesized that nicotine would increase regional cerebral glucose metabolism (rCMRglc) and verbal fluency in both AD and elderly controls.

METHODS

Alzheimer's subjects met the NINCDS-ADRDA criteria for mild AD (McKhann et al., 1984). Alzheimer disease patients were excluded if they had overlapping diseases or received on-going medications with known effects on cognition. Recruitment of normal elderly controls included a review of the medical history, a physical and neurological examination, EKG and laboratory tests. All prospective participants who were current (within past year) users of tobacco were excused from participation.

Subjects were shown a video explaining PET procedures and then asked to sign an informed consent form. Several days before PET scanning all subjects wore a nicotine patch for approximately 4 hrs. If the subject was judged clinically able to tolerate a 7 or 14 mg patch the person was enrolled and was paid a fee for participation in this study. Nicoderm® patches and placebo patches were placed on different sites of the upper right or left arm for the patch tolerance day and for each PET scan. All PET procedures were completed between 2 and 4 hrs during peak nicotine plasma levels (Physicians Desk Reference, 1994).

Monitoring of Adverse Effects During PET
The first mild AD patient was a 79 year old (MMSE=22). He smoked 3 cigarettes a day for 3 months and has not smoked in 44 years. He received the Nicoderm® (7 mg) patch and felt nausea for 15 min after wearing it for 3 hrs and 45 min just after PET scanning. The second AD patient was 81 years old with mild AD (MMSE=21) and had never smoked. He received the Nicoderm® (14 mg) patch and had no side effects. Both non-smoker elderly controls were 71 years old and had no side effects on the Nicoderm® (14 mg) patch.

PET Scanning Procedures
The sequence, administration of treatments and PET scan analysis were conducted under double-blind conditions. Each subject received two PET scans. Each PET scan was separated by at least 48 hrs. For all PET scans, subjects fasted for at least 5 hrs before the examination. The Siemens Metabtool software combined the data taken from the blood samples obtained during scanning with the radioactivity counts to produce measures of metabolic activity based on a three compartmental model. The Siemens 951 PET scanner produces 31 slices (3.37 mm between each brain slice) and has a transaxial resolution of 4.6 mm (FWHM). Ten millicuries of F-18 fluorodeoxyglucose (FDG) was injected into each subject during each PET session.

In order to reduce intra-individual variability in rCMRglc, a cognitive challenge test was performed during both the placebo and nicotine conditions (Duara, 1990). Verbal fluency, a word generation task of semantic memory, was selected for the challenge task as outlined in the Parks et al. (1988) study. Subjects remained supine with eyes blind-folded and ears unplugged. The effects of novelty due to the cognitive task was minimized by having each subject practice an alternate version of verbal fluency on another day prior to PET scanning. The scanning occurred for 30 min after the FDG half-hour uptake period.

PET Scan Analysis
Reading of PET scans was conducted as follows: 2.3 mm circles (5 circles for each unilateral ROI) were constructed for each subject (560 per subject). The regions of interest (ROI) were on slice planes parallel to the canthomeatal line corresponding to the atlas for computer tomography of transaxial scan sections (Aquilonius and Eckernas, 1980). The ROI's were first traced directly from the *subject's* MRI (5 mm slices) and overlaid at the same transaxial plane as the in

plane PET scanner slice using the same head-holder. The ROI's ran across the following number of transaxial slices: 2 (occipital and parietal), 3 (anterior and posterior temporal), 1 (anterior cingulate), 5 (inferior frontal), 6 (middle and superior frontal). The 2.3 mm circles were averaged within slice and then across slices in order to obtain the final values.

RESULTS

Brain Metabolism

Nicotine had a dramatic effect on the whole brain metabolism in both AD subjects (29.3% and 48.2%). Subject A's metabolism was 5.66 mg/min/100 g per pixel per second at baseline and 7.32 units on nicotine. Subject B's metabolism was 5.10 units at baseline and 7.56 units on nicotine. Only marginal increases were evident in both normal controls (8.2% and 6.5%). Subject C's metabolism was 4.60 units at baseline and 5.01 units on nicotine. Similarly, Subject D was 6.61 at baseline and 7.04 on nicotine. The metabolic rates for AD patients were slightly lower than those of the normals in all areas noted. The interaction between drug and disease condition was also significant. The effect of nicotine was greatest on the AD patients and negligible for normals. The drug effect range was from 19% for the anterior temporal lobe to 26.5 for the inferior frontal lobe. There was little difference in activity between sides. The increase in whole brain metabolism of AD subjects was associated with cognitive improvement in verbal fluency test performance (11% increase with 7 mg and 24% increase with 14 mg nicotine). In controls, verbal fluency test performance increased 14% with 14 mg in one subject but not in the other (20% decrease with 14 mg). This amounts to an average decrease of 6% for controls which was not statistically significant.

DISCUSSION

The increases in whole brain metabolism were greater on nicotine in both AD subjects than in elderly controls. This was surprising since the one AD subject received a nicotine dose one-half that of the others. Regional cerebral glucose metabolism increased in all frontal and temporal areas in AD subjects, and in 14 out of 16 ROI's in controls. Verbal fluency performance in AD improved with nicotine, but the effects of nicotine on verbal fluency performance in normal elderly controls was not significant.

A possible interpretation of the nicotine effects in whole brain metabolism and cognitive test performance findings in AD subjects may be that the physiological effects of nicotinic receptors in AD (Giacobini, 1990; Smith and Giacobini, 1992) were ameliorated with the administration of nicotine which increased both brain metabolism and cognitive test performance. This is in agreement with a recent PET study that found improved neuropsychological test performance and increases in both ^{11}C-nicotine uptake and glucose metabolism during Tacrine treatment with AD patients (Nordberg et al., 1992).

REFERENCES

Aquilonius S-M and Eckernas S-A (1980): *A Colour Atlas of the Human Brain Adapted to Computed Tomography*. Stockholm: Esselte Studium, pp. 1-15.

Duara R (1990): *Positron Emission Tomography in Dementia*. New York: Wiley.

Giacobini E (1990): Cholinergic receptors in human brain: effects of aging and Alzheimer disease. *J Neurosci Res* 27:548-560.

Jones G, Sahakian B, Levy R, Warburton D and Gray J (1992): Effects of acute subcutaneous nicotine on attention, information processing and short-term memory in Alzheimer's disease. *Psychopharmacology* 108:485-494.

McKhann F, Drachman D, Folstein M, Katzman R, Price D and Stadlan EM (1984): Clinical diagnosis of Alzheimer's disease: report of the NINCDS-ADRDA work group under the auspices of the Department of Health and Human Services Task Force on Alzheimer's Disease. *Neurology* 34:934-944.

Newhouse P, Sunderland T, Tariot P, Blumhardt C, Weingartner H, Mellow A and Murphy D (1988): Intravenous nicotine in Alzheimer's disease: A pilot study. *Psychopharmacology* 95:171-175.

Newhouse P, Sunderland T, Narang P, Mellow A, Fertig J, Lawlor B and Murphy DL (1990): Neuroendocrine, physiologic, and behavioral responses following intravenous nicotine in non-smoking healthy volunteers and patients with Alzheimer's disease. *Psychoneuroendocrinology* 15:471-484.

Newhouse P, Potter A and Lenox R (1993): The effects of nicotinic agents on human cognition: Possible therapeutic applications in Alzheimer's and Parkinson's Diseases. *Medical Chemistry Research* 2:628-642.

Nordberg A, Lilja A, Lundqvist H, Hartvig P, Amberla K, Viitanen M, Warpman U, Johansson M, Hellstrom-Lindahl E, Bjurling P, Fasth K-J, Langstrom B and Winblad B (1992): Tacrine restores cholinergic nicotinic receptors and glucose metabolism in Alzheimer patients as visualized by positron emission tomography. *Neurobiol Aging* 13:747-758.

Parks R, Lowenstein D, Dodrill K, Barker W, Yoshi F, Chang J, Emran A, Apicella A, Sherematta W and Duara R (1988): Cerebral metabolic effects of a verbal fluency test: A PET scan study. *J Clin Exptl Neuropsychology* 10:565-575.

Physicians' Desk Reference (1994): New Jersey: Medical Economics Company.

Smith CJ and Giacobini E (1992): Nicotine, Parkinson's and Alzheimer's disease. *Reviews in the Neurosciences* 3(1):25-43.

PART XV

CLINICAL TESTING OF EFFICACY OF NEW DRUGS IN AD

Alzheimer Disease: Therapeutic Strategies
edited by E. Giacobini and R. Becker.
© 1994 Birkhäuser Boston

MINIMAL EFFICACY CRITERIA FOR MEDICATIONS IN ALZHEIMER DISEASE

Serge Gauthier
McGill Centre for Studies in Aging, St-Mary's Hospital, Montreal, Quebec, Canada

Howard Feldman
Division of Neurology, University of British Columbia, Vancouver, BC, Canada

Erich Mohr
Institute of Mental Health Research, Royal Ottawa Hospital/University of Ottawa, Ottawa, Ontario, Canada

for the Consortium of Canadian Centres for Clinical Cognitive Research (C5R)

INTRODUCTION

There is an acute interest world-wide in developing safe and effective drugs to alleviate symptoms of Alzheimer disease (AD) in its multiple domains (mood, cognition, functional autonomy and behavior). Most of the agents under development for such symptomatic therapy are targeted to one or more neurotransmitter systems (primarily cholinergic, noradrenergic or serotoninergic). There is also hope to achieve stabilization of disease progression using drugs targeted against primary or secondary pathophysiological events (amyloid deposition, immune activation, excitatory aminoacids, free radical formation, aluminum deposition).

Since lecithin was first tried in the late 70's, a large body of experience has been gained in terms of study design and outcome variables best suited for AD. The development of tacrine since 1986 has accelerated the pace of clinical trials in AD and guidelines for minimal efficacy criteria (MEC) have been proposed in the US (Leber, 1990), Europe (CPMP working party, 1992) and Canada (Mohr et al., submitted). This review article will summarize the Canadian investigators' perspective. Discussions on this topic were initiated during a symposium organized by the C5R and held at the Institute of Mental Health

Research, Ottawa, Canada, on May 5th, 1993, in collaboration with the Health Protection Branch of the Canadian federal government.

DIAGNOSIS

Earlier and more accurate diagnosis of dementia is now possible considering public and physicians awareness of AD, as well as readily available tertiary referral sites such as the C5R network in Canada and the various AD Research Centres in the USA. Experience and consensus meetings have confirmed the essential role of history obtained from key informants and structured mental status questionnaires with a lesser emphasis on laboratory investigation in favor of selective tests based on individual patients' health profiles (Organizing committee, CCCAD, 1991). Diagnostic research criteria such as those of the DSMIIIR for dementia and the NINCDS-ADRDA for AD, supplemented by traditional inclusion and exclusion criteria, allow multicentre studies with relatively greater diagnostic homogeneity although the classification of AD "probable" versus "possible" still shows lesser reliability (Farrer et al., 1994): should we continue to exclude AD "possible" in drug trials? The importance of genotypes such as ApoE4/4 as biological markers of high risk of developing AD and of age associated memory impairment as a diagnostic borderline area remain to be established.

TRIAL DESIGNS

Experience has clearly shown the need for randomized placebo-controlled parallel groups with fixed doses, rather than cross-over after titration to "best dose" or "maximum tolerated dose" (Gauthier et al., 1991). Although the principle of "enrichment" makes intuitive sense considering the relative heterogeneity of AD in terms of neurotransmitter deficits and patterns of cognitive loss, the applicability of such efficacy studies to the population of AD patients at large may be difficult. The duration of studies aimed at symptomatic treatment is currently three to six months, whereas the minimum duration of studies aimed at stabilization treatment is currently one year. Both are generally followed by open label extension of six to twelve months, in order to allow all patients to be exposed to active medication and obtain further safety and tolerability data. The need for shorter stabilization trials in order to reduce costs and allow individual patients the opportunity to try more than one experimental drug is real but limited by the variance in rate of decline (Ritchie and Touchon, 1992). An index or sum of clinical and biological parameters (which could include functional MRI and quantitative EEG) may be usable as end point in shorter stabilization studies if patients show homogeneity of disease severity at onset of a trial (Kraemer et al., 1994).

OUTCOME VARIABLES

Efficacy is currently determined by outcome variables encompassing 1) clinical interview based impression of change (CIBIC, Leber, 1990, discussed by Rockwood, 1994), 2) structured global staging scales such as the Clinical Dementia Rating Scale (CDR, Berg, 1988) or the Functional Rating Scale (FRS, Crockett et al., 1989), 3) performance-based objective tests of cognition such as the AD Assessment Scale (ADAS, Mohs et al., 1983) or the Repeatable Battery for the Assessment of Dementia (RBAD, Randolph, 1994), 4) functional scales such as the Disability Assessment in Dementia Scale (DAD, Gauthier et al., 1993), and 5) behavioral scales such as the Behave AD (Reisberg et al., 1987). We suggest that the primary outcome variables should differ between symptomatic therapy in early AD (1, 3 and 4), symptomatic therapy in late AD (1, 4 and 5) and in stabilization therapy (1 and 2). Furthermore, MEC for symptomatic effects should be a measurable change in one domain (3, 4 and 5) without requiring a significant effect on global staging scores, whereas MEC for stabilization would require the opposite (Mohr et al., submitted). The distinction between long-term symptomatic effects and stabilization remains to be clarified.

DRUG DEVELOPMENT PROGRAMS

In addition to traditional pharmacokinetic and tolerability data, phase I studies could include functional neuroimaging using PET or SPECT to assess CNS penetration in humans, dosing and effect/type. Patients with AD may have to be included at that early stage because of potential lower tolerance to a given compound relative to healthy elderly (Cutler et al., 1992). Phase II studies aim at establishing dose-dependent efficacy in patients with "probable" AD and otherwise in good general health. We contend that phase III studies should involve patients with "possible" as well "probable" AD to be more representative of the targeted population. Conditional approval for marketing could be given pending phase IV studies which will determine long term clinical benefit, including delay or reduction of service utilization at home, need for nursing care and institution, and improved health of caregivers.

ETHICS OF RESEARCH INVOLVING PATIENTS WITH AD

Because of the declining course of competence to make choices in AD, new guidelines need to be issued to facilitate the work of Institutional Review Boards and physicians investigators, while protecting the patients' best interest, which is often the very right to participate in therapeutic drug trials, whether living at home or in institutions. Direct benefits should clearly be present for patients asked to participate in studies where more than minor increment over minimal risk is involved.

PHARMACO-ECONOMIC CONSIDERATIONS

The use of clinically-meaningful endpoints in the study of neurodegenerative diseases such as Parkinson's has allowed the introduction of pharmaco-economic considerations in phase III designs: the need for L-Dopa and risk of losing employment were primary outcome variables in the DATATOP study (The PSG, 1993). Endpoints such as loss of autonomy and institutionalization are primary outcome variables in an ongoing study of the value of selegiline in AD by the AD Cooperative Study Unit. It is even conceivable that very early interventions studies in symptomatic patients with AD identified by neuropsychological tests, quantitative electroencephalography and metabolic brain imaging, or in presymptomatic patients AD identified by genotypes such as apoE4, could use endpoints such as loss of employability.

CONCLUSION

To optimize the development of antidementia treatment harmonization of criteria for approval of drugs in AD is urgently required and we hope that this discussion of MEC will prove useful. We congratulate the regulatory agencies for their efforts at developing guidelines for MEC and we look forward to more harmonization between different countries that are actively pursuing symptomatic and stabilization therapies for AD.

ACKNOWLEDGEMENTS

The authors' research is supported by NIA, MRC, FRSQ, NHRDP, AD Society of Canada. We thank Mrs. Lyne Jean-Morrison and Miss Christina Kyriakou for expert secretarial assistance.

REFERENCES

Berg L (1988): Clinical Dementia Rating (CDR). *Psychopharmacol Bull* 24:637-639.

Crockett D, Tuokko H and Koch W (1989): The assessment of everyday functioning using the present functioning questionnaire and the Functional Rating Scale in elderly sample. *Clin Gerontol* 8:3-23.

Cutler NR, Sramek JJ, Murphy MF and Nash RJ (1992): Alzheimer's patients should be included in phase I clinical trials to evaluate compounds for Alzheimer's disease. *J Geriatr Psychiatry Neurol* 5:192-194.

CPMP working party on efficacy of medicinal products (1992): Antidementia medicinal products. Brussels, November:1-12.

Farrer LA, Cupples LA, Blackburn S, Kiely DK, Auerbach S, Growdon JH, Connor-Lacke L, Karlinsy H, Thibert A, Burke JR, Utley C, Chui H, Ireland A, Duara R, Lopez-Alberola R, Larson EB, O'Connell S and Kukull WA (1994): Interrater agreement for diagnosis of Alzheimer's disease: the MIRAGE study. *Neurology* 44:652-656.

Gauthier S, Gauthier L, Bouchard R, Quirion R and Sulta S (1991):   Treatment of Alzheimer's disease: Hopes and Reality. *Can J Neurol Sci* 18:439-441.

Gauthier L, Gauthier S, Gelinas I, McIntyre M and Wood-Dauphinee S (1993): Assessment of functioning and ADL. Abstract book of the *Sixth Congress of the International Psychogeriatic Association*, September, Berlin, Germany, 9.

Kraemer HC, Tinklenberg J and Yesavage JA (1994): "How far" versus "how fast" in Alzheimer's disease. The question revisited. *Arch Neurol* 51:275-279.

Leber P (1990):   Guidelines for the clinical evaluation of antidementia drugs. Washington, DC: Food and Drug administration, November:4.4.4.4.

Mohs RC, Rosen WG and Davis KL (1983): The Alzheimer Disease Assessment Scale: An instrument of assessing treatment efficacy. *Psychopharmacol Bull* 19:448-450.

Organizing Committee, Canadian Consensus Conference on the Assessment of Dementia (1991): Assessing dementia: The Canadian Consensus. *Can Med Assoc J* 144:851-853.

The Parkinson Study Group (1993):   Effects of tocopherol and deprenyl on the progression of disability in early Parkinson's disease. *New Engl J Med* 328:176-183.

Randolph C (1994):   *Repeatable Battery for the Assessment of Dementia (RBAD)*. New York: Psychological Corporation (In Press).

Reisberg B, Borenstein J and Franssen E (1987): Behave-AD: A clinical rating scale for the assessment of pharmacologically remediable behavioral symptomatology in AD. In: *Alzheimer's Disease: Problems, Prospects and Perspectives*, Altman MJ, ed. New York: Plenum Press.

Ritchie K and Touchon J (1992): Heterogeneity in senile dementia of the Alzheimer type: individual differences, progressive deterioration or clinical sub-types? *J Clin Epidemiol* 45:1391-1398.

Rockwood K (1994): Use of global assessment measures in dementia drug trials. *J Clin Epidemiol* 47:101-103.

Alzheimer Disease: Therapeutic Strategies
edited by E. Giacobini and R. Becker.
© 1994 Birkhäuser Boston

CLINICAL TESTING OF NEW DRUGS FOR EFFICACY IN ALZHEIMER'S DISEASE

Leon J. Thal
Dept. of Neurosciences, University of California at San Diego, La Jolla, CA

INTRODUCTION

Successful treatment of Alzheimer's disease (AD) remains a major goal. It has assumed major important public health proportions because of the almost 4 million individuals afflicted with this progressive disorder (Evans et al., 1989). Major research into the neurobiology and neurochemistry of this disorder has made it possible to design new therapeutic strategies to potentially intervene at multiple different stages in the disease process.

CLINICAL DRUG TRIALS: DESIGN ISSUES

Problems Inherent in the Conduct of Clinical Trials

There are a number of problems associated with the conduct of trials for patients with AD. First, there is no biological marker for the disease during life. Thus, diagnosis is never certain. Most contemporary series report diagnostic accuracy of approximately 85% (Galasko et al., 1994). More recently, it has been recognized that approximately one-third of AD patients develop extrapyramidal features. Pathological examination of these brains reveal the presence of both cortical and subcortical Lewy bodies, as well as sufficient senile plaques to meet diagnostic criteria for AD. We have termed this combination of patients who present with cognitive deficit, the "Lewy body variant of AD" (Hansen et al., 1990). Whether or not this important subset of patients responds to treatment in the same fashion as other patients with only plaques and tangles, but without Lewy bodies, remains to be determined.

Subjects entering into clinical trials vary greatly in terms of the clinical presentation. While all have impairment of memory, there are also varying combinations of language disturbance, visuospatial disturbance, personality change, and psychiatric features. Cognitive dysfunction may respond differentially to treatment, depending on the presence of related symptomatology.

The rate of cognitive change varies dramatically across subjects. One year rates of change on some of the most commonly used Global Cognitive Rating

Scales (GCRS), the Blessed Information-Memory-Concentration (BIMC) test, Mini-Mental State Examination (MMSE), Dementia Rating Scale of Mattis (DRSM) and the Alzheimer Disease Assessment Scale (ADAS), are approximately equal to the standard deviation for that rate of change, regardless of the instrument chosen (Galasko et al., 1991). The rate of change is reasonably constant during the middle stages of dementia, but is slower in very early and late stages of the illness. While the rate of change is predictable for groups, it is highly variable for individual patients. Most importantly, knowledge of the rate of change allows for the accurate computation of sample size for studies designed to slow decline in AD. Rates of change on noncognitive instruments have been less well studied, but have been defined for the Blessed Functional Rating Scale (BFRS), Clinical Dementia Rating Scale (CDRS) and for several activity of daily living scales.

Outcome Measures
During the past decade, the conduct of phase III studies has been improved due to several factors. First, instruments for measuring cognitive change have improved. Second, most current trials use only a few key prespecified endpoints. Finally, a set of guidelines for the conduct of clinical trials in AD was developed by the Food and Drug Administration with the support of academia. A summary of the discussion of the concepts underlying these guidelines has been published (Thal, 1991). These guidelines suggest that approval of drugs for an antidementia claim require the demonstration of cognitive improvement on a standardized instrument that captures the key features of cognitive dysfunction as well as clinically rated overall improvement on a global instrument. Improvement and/or enhancement of activities of daily living supports approval, but is not required. Although not officially released, the dissemination of these guidelines in the academic community and pharmaceutical industry has resulted in their widespread adoption for the design of contemporary AD clinical trials focused on cognition.

Design Considerations - Short-term Studies
For short-term trials designed to demonstrate improvement in cognition, three-trial designs have been commonly used. These include crossover trials, parallel trials, and enrichment designs. The use of crossover trials presents a number of problems, including the assumption that there are no carryover or periodic effects, and that the treatment response is the same in both periods. A major advantage of this design is in the economy of subjects, since each subjects acts as his/her own control. Parallel design studies have a multiplicity of advantages, including: the control population is uncontaminated by drug exposure, the absence of periodic effects, and the ability to estimate adverse events in a population free of drug. The main disadvantage of this design is that it requires more subjects to answer the question. The third approach is an enrichment *design. In this design, all patients are exposed to drug, possibly at several doses*

and placebo in order to find the optimal dose. Patients failing to demonstrate improvement on any dose are discarded from the trial. Individuals who improve during the initial dose titration phase are withdrawn from drug, washed out, then rerandomized to drug or placebo in a new double-blind, parallel phase. Thus, the population entering the double-blind efficacy portion of the trial is "enriched" by eliminating nonresponders after the dose titration phase. This design has many advantages, including: individual dose titration, enrichment of the sample population, and the ability to confirm an initial response during the dose titration phase in a second randomized, placebo-controlled, parallel phase. The major disadvantages of this design are: all subjects are exposed to drug allowing for possible carryover effects, possible failure to return to baseline during the washout phase, and difficulty in estimating the true incidence of adverse events.

Long-term Studies - Survival Analysis
While most studies designed to alter the rate of decline have utilized slope analysis, other types of analyses are possible. The technique of survival analysis, widely used in cancer studies, has rarely been applied to treatment trials of neurologic disease and has not yet been applied to treatment of AD. Nevertheless, there are a number of inherent advantages to survival analysis in AD. First, endpoints can be real life events rather than changes of slope on a psychometric test. Some important real life events for AD patients include death, institutionalization, loss of basic activities of daily living, and loss of instrumental activities of daily living. Use of these endpoints also allows for pharmaco-economic evaluation of the compound. Second, survival analysis can be carried out for multiple endpoints. Third, individuals who drop out of the study are likely to do so because an endpoint has been reached. If this occurs, the data remains informative and the statistical difficulty of handling missing data points becomes less problematic. Fourth, survival analysis allows for comparison of the entire group, despite varying length os follow-up. Fifth, patients who are doing poorly can exit study and seek alternative treatments.

Potential disadvantages to survival analysis are that the time to reach endpoints, such as death and institutionalization, are likely to be more variable than change in slope on psychometric testing. Endpoints may also be affected by social support systems and nursing care. If large numbers of subjects drop out before reaching an endpoint, the validity of the data becomes questionable. Nevertheless, the inherent advantages in survival analysis, which include the use of endpoints with face validity far outweigh the disadvantages.

SIZE OF CLINICAL TRIALS

The number of subjects needed to demonstrate drug efficacy depends on the relationship between the effect size and the standard deviation of the outcome measure (Friedman et al., 1985). With rates of change where the standard deviation is approximately equivalent to the decline over one year, a typical study using 80% power and two-sided significance with an alpha of 0.05 would require the following number of subjects per group comparing drug to placebo for significance.

Reduction in rate of decline (%)	No. Subjects per group (N)	Total Sample Size (n)
25	251	502
50	63	126
75	28	56

These sample size calculations were based on the BIMC, assuming an annual change of approximately 4 ± 4 points per year. Most contemporary phase III studies designed to examine slowing of decline in AD utilize 300 to 500 subjects to detect rates of decline between the drug- and placebo-treated group of 25-50%.

EXAMPLES OF NOVEL CLINICAL TRIAL DESIGNS

The first U.S. multicenter trial of tacrine used the enrichment design previously described. In this trial, 632 subjects with probable AD were enrolled. Of these, 215 met putative beneficial response criteria during a six-week, double-blind, dose titration phase and were randomized to receive placebo or their best-dose of tacrine (40 or 80 mg daily) in a subsequent six-week, double-blind, parallel group study. On average, treated patients showed a 2.4 point lesser decline on the ADAS-Cog than those taking placebo (Davis et al., 1992). This is equivalent to the amount of decline that untreated patients would undergo during 4-5 months. The second primary outcome measure in this study was a clinical global impression of change. The modest difference in cognitive decline observed in this study was insufficient to allow a skilled clinician to successfully identify the treated cohort. Additionally, there was a significant carryover effect at the end of the dose titration phase, such that patients on tacrine failed to return to baseline during the two-week washout phase. Two additional enrichment design trials have been carried out using controlled-release physostigmine, and in these trials, patients almost completely washed out, as expected, after drug withdrawal for two weeks. Firm conclusions regarding the utility of the enrichment design cannot be reached yet because insufficient trials have been carried out using this methodology. To use this trial design successfully, however, clearly requires the knowledge that individuals will washout and return to baseline following discontinuation of treatment.

A few trials have been designed to slow the rate of decline in AD. These include published trials studying desferrioxamine and acetyl-L-carnitine in AD. Both utilized an analysis of rates of decline on a variety of instruments as primary outcome measures. Several other trials are currently underway examining changes in the rate of decline, including a trial using a monoamine oxidase B inhibitor.

In addition, one trial is currently underway utilizing survival analysis to examine the ability of deprenyl, a monoamine oxidase inhibitor, and vitamin E, an antioxidant, to slow the rate of cognitive and behavioral decline in AD. This multicenter trials has chosen death, institutionalization, loss of basic activities of daily living and progression from moderate to severe dementia as the primary endpoints. The study will continue for two years, much longer than most previously conducted AD trials.

FUTURE RESEARCH

A whole new host of interventions will be carried out over the next decade. These will include molecules designed to: present the deposition of beta amyloid, stabilize neurofilaments, enhance synaptic regeneration, and ameliorate behavioral symptoms. Trial designs and considerations will be different for each agent tested. As molecules designed to slow the rate of decline are developed, it will be incumbent to identify subjects earlier in the course of their disease process. For some agents, administration of drugs or modification of genes could best be carried out in preclinical individuals if such individuals can be identified. The involvement of very early patients or preclinical individuals will require the development of new tools for diagnosis and evaluation. Undoubtedly such studies will only occur with agents having low toxicity, since the duration of exposure is likely to be lengthy. While clinical trials of the past were often measured in weeks or months, clinical trials in the future are likely to be measured in years.

ACKNOWLEDGEMENTS

This research was supported from grants AGO 10483 and AGO 5131.

REFERENCES

Davis K, Thal L, Gamzu E et al. (1992): A double-blind, placebo-controlled multicenter study of tacrine for Alzheimer's disease. *New Engl J Med* 327:1253-1259.

Evans DA, Funkenstein HH, Albert MS et al. (1989): Prevalence of Alzheimer's disease in a community population of older persons. *JAMA* 262:2551-2556.

Friedman LM, Furberg CD and MeMets DL (1985): *Fundamentals of Clinical Trials.* Littleton: PSG Publishing Co. Inc.

Galasko D, Corey-Bloom J and Thal LJ (1991): Monitoring progression in Alzheimer's disease. *J Am Geriatr Soc* 39:932-941.

Galasko D, Hansen L, Katzman R, Wiederholt W, Masliah E, Terry R, Hill LR, Lessin P and Thal LJ (1994): Clinical-neuropathological correlations in Alzheimer's disease and related dementias. *Arch Neurol* (In Press).

Hansen L, Salmon D, Galasko D et al. (1990): The Lewy body variant of Alzheimer's disease: a clinical and pathological entity. *Neurology* 40:1-8.

Thal LJ (1991): A Meeting Report: Antidementia Drug Assessment Symposium. *Neurobiol Aging* 12:379-382.

Alzheimer Disease: Therapeutic Strategies
edited by E. Giacobini and R. Becker.
© 1994 Birkhäuser Boston

INSTRUMENTS FOR MEASURING THE EFFICACY OF TREATMENTS FOR ALZHEIMER'S DISEASE

Richard C. Mohs, Deborah B. Marin, Cynthia R. Green and Kenneth L. Davis
Psychiatry Service (116A), Veterans Affairs Medical Center,
Bronx, New York, and Department of Psychiatry, Mount Sinai School of
Medicine, New York, New York

INTRODUCTION

Drug treatments could be developed to diminish or prevent any of the many symptoms of Alzheimer's disease (AD). Most recent efforts have been devoted to the development of treatments for the cognitive impairments associated with AD, including memory loss, dysphasia, dyspraxia and impairment of judgment. Drugs designed to treat these core cognitive manifestations of AD are called antidementia drugs. Only one drug, tetrahydroaminoacridine (THA or Cognex®) has been approved as an antidementia agent in the U.S. following completion of several large clinical trials (Davis et al., 1992; Farlow et al., 1992; Knapp et al., 1994). A variety of available psychotropic agents are currently used to help manage other noncognitive manifestations of AD including depression, agitation, anxiety and psychosis. No drugs have been developed specifically to treat these noncognitive symptoms in AD patients.

Efficacy of both antidementia drugs and drugs for the noncognitive symptoms of AD is currently determined by measuring their effects on behavior.` This paper briefly presents data on some of the instruments that are used to assess the efficacy of antidementia and other drugs for the treatment of AD. Emphasis is placed on what longitudinal data obtained from AD patients can tell us about the utility of various assessment approaches.

METHODS

The longitudinal data on AD from our center were obtained from a group of 111 patients who met NINCDS/ADRDA criteria for probable AD and who were followed with semiannual evaluations for periods of 12 to 90 months. A comparison group of 72 nondemented elderly persons was given similar semiannual evaluations for periods of 12 to 90 months. Further details about these groups are presented in Stern et al. (1994).

The assessment battery included a variety of cognitive and behavioral measures including the Alzheimer's Disease Assessment Scale (ADAS) (Rosen et al., 1984), the Blessed Test of Information, Memory and Concentration (BIMC) (Blessed et al., 1968), and the Physical and Self-Maintenance Scale (PSMS) and the Instrumental Activities of Daily Living Scale (IADLS) of Lawton and Brodie (1969).

RESULTS

Both the BIMC and the cognitive part of the ADAS (ADAS-Cog) are measures of the severity of the core cognitive symptoms of AD, i.e. the targets of antidementia drugs. Both the BIMC and the ADAS-Cog gave reliable measures of cognitive decline in AD patients followed longitudinally. The mean annual change scores were 4.1 points (SD = 4.1) on the BIMC (Stern et al., 1992) and 9.6 (SD = 8.21) on the ADAS-Cog (Stern et al., 1994). The ADAS-Cog was more sensitive to change both in mild dementia and normal aging and in severe dementia than was the BIMC (Stern et al., 1994). For neither measure was there a significant relationship of rate of decline with gender, age of onset or family history of dementia. For the ADAS-Cog there was a strong curvilinear relationship of annual change with baseline severity such that change was smaller for mildly demented and severely demented patients than for moderately demented patients. Using the ADAS cognitive and noncognitive data we found that earlier age of onset was significantly associated with greater language and praxis impairment at the initial assessment and with more depression and agitation during longitudinal follow-up (Lawlor et al., 1994).

Some of the items on the IADLS were difficult to score reliably, primarily because of gender specificity but reliability was high for all of the PSMS items (Green et al., 1993). Scores on the PSMS, which measures impairment in activities such as eating, dressing and toileting did not change until patients were at least moderately demented; scores on the IADLS, which measures impairment in activities such as handling money and using the telephone, did change much sooner but reached a ceiling in most severely demented patients (Green et al., 1993).

DISCUSSION

Broad based cognitive performance measures such as the ADAS-Cog provide reliable measures of cognitive change over a broad range of AD severity and thus are useful measures of the cognitive effects of antidementia drugs in most patients. Differences in symptom presentation related to age of onset and differences in rate of progression related to baseline severity will have to be taken into account in most clinical trials. Many of the relationships found with the ADAS-Cog have also been found using the neuropsychological battery of the

Consortium to Establish a Registry for Alzheimer's Disease (CERAD) (Morris et al., 1994).

Valid measurement of drug effects on performance of activities outside the clinical setting is somewhat more problematic. Items such as those on the PSMS clearly measure behaviors of great importance for patients and their caregivers, but these behaviors are often not impaired in patients suitable for drug treatment trials. Items such as those on the IADLS are more appropriate for the mild to moderately demented patients included in drug treatment trials but are more likely to be affected by demographic factors such as gender, type of living environment, and previous occupation. Longitudinal data on noncognitive aspects of AD will be of use in planning clinical trials of drugs for the treatment of agitation, depression, psychosis and anxiety.

REFERENCES

Blessed G, Tomlinson BE and Roth M (1968): The association between quantitative measures of dementia and of senile change in the cerebral grey matter of elderly subjects. *Brit J Psychiat* 114:797-811.

Davis KL, Thal LJ, Gamzu ER et al. (1992): A double-blind, placebo-controlled multicenter study of Tacrine for Alzheimer's disease. *New Engl J Med* 327:1253-1259.

Farlow M, Gracon SI, Hershey LA et al. (1992): A controlled trial of Tacrine in Alzheimer's disease. *J Am Med Assoc* 268:2523-2529.

Green CR, Mohs RC, Schmeidler J, Aryan M and Davis KL (1993): Functional decline in Alzheimer's disease: A longitudinal study. *J Am Geriatr Soc* 41:654-661.

Knapp MJ, Knopmen DS, Solomon PR et al. (1994): A 30-week randomized controlled trial of high-dose Tacrine in patients with Alzheimer's disease. *J Am Med Assoc* 271:985-991.

Lawlor BA, Ryan TM, Schmeidler J et al. (1994): Clinical symptoms associated with age of onset in Alzheimer's disease. *Am J Psychiat* (In Press).

Lawton MP and Brodie EM (1969): Assessment of older people: Self-maintaining and instrumental activities of daily living. *Gerontologist* 9:179-186.

Morris JC, Edland S, Clark C et al. (1994): The Consortium to Establish a Registry for Alzheimer's Disease (CERAD). Part IV. Rates of cognitive change in the longitudinal assessment of probable Alzheimer's disease. *Neurology* 43:2457-2465.

Rosen WG, Mohs RC and Davis KL (1984): A new rating scale for Alzheimer's disease. *Am J Psychiat* 141:1356-1364.

Stern RG, Mohs RC, Bierer LM et al. (1992): Deterioration on the Blessed Test in Alzheimer's disease: Longitudinal data and their implications for clinical trials and identification of subtypes. *Psychiatr Res* 42:101-110.

Stern RG, Mohs RC, Davidson M et al. (1994): A longitudinal study of Alzheimer's disease: Measurement, rate and predictors of cognitive deterioration. *Am J Psychiat* 151:390-396.

Alzheimer Disease: Therapeutic Strategies
edited by E. Giacobini and R. Becker.
© 1994 Birkhäuser Boston

PSYCHOMETRIC STRENGTHS AND WEAKNESSES OF THE ALZHEIMER DISEASE ASSESSMENT SCALE IN CLINICAL TESTING: RECOMMENDATIONS FOR IMPROVEMENTS

Ronald F. Zec, Edward S. Landreth, Eden Bird, Rosemary B. Harris, Randall Robbs, Stephen J. Markwell, and Dennis Q. McManus
Southern Illinois University School of Medicine, P.O. Box 19230, Springfield, IL 62794-9230 USA

INTRODUCTION

The Alzheimer Disease Assessment Scale (ADAS) is a brief screening test that measures a variety of cognitive functions that are typically impaired in patients with Alzheimer dementia (AD) and provides an index of overall severity of dementia. The ADAS is sensitive to the progressive decline in functioning over time in patients with dementia of the Alzheimer type (DAT) (Rosen et al., 1984) and is being used with increasing frequency as an efficacy measure in drug therapy studies.

We have previously shown that the ADAS also has utility in both early detection and staging of AD and that it is considerably more sensitive to the early detection of AD than the Folstein Mini Mental Status Exam (Zec et al., 1992a). There is, however, a "ceiling effect" on the ADAS for very early AD patients who make only a few errors on this test (Zec et al., 1992a). The low error score in very early AD patients leaves little room for this efficacy measure to detect improvement in cognitive functioning as a result of treatment interventions. This is a major concern because it is generally assumed that it is early in the course of the disorder, before too much structural damage to the brain has occurred, that treatment interventions are likely to have their maximal benefit. Furthermore, Stern et al. (1994) has recently reported that the very mild AD patients with low error scores display on average only a very modest decline on the total ADAS Cognitive score over a period of 24 months.

In this paper, we will discuss the psychometric strengths and weaknesses of the ADAS as a treatment outcome measure. We will also discuss some additions we have made to the ADAS to increase its ability to detect early AD and to increase its ability to detect improvements in cognitive functioning in early AD patients as a result of treatment interventions.

A SUBTEST ANALYSIS AND RECOMMENDED IMPROVEMENTS

Zec et al. (1992b) compared the performance of patients with mild, moderate, and severe AD and elderly controls on the ADAS. The total ADAS score was found to have the necessary psychometric properties to detect relatively small overall changes in cognitive functioning in AD patients, but the majority of the cognitive subscales were found to have limitations in detecting changes at certain severity levels. Furthermore, the ADAS does not measure several basic aspects of cognition that are known to decline very early in the course of the disease.

The following observations were made regarding the sensitivity of the various ADAS subtest scores to disease progression (Zec et al., 1992b). Word Recall and Word Recognition were maximally sensitive in the earlier stages, Remembering Test Instructions and the three rating items for spontaneous speech were sensitive in the early and middle stages, and Commands was sensitive in the middle and later stages. Orientation and the total Cognitive ADAS score were sensitive throughout the course of AD. It follows that the ADAS would not be adequately sensitive to specifically detect improvements in naming and constructional praxis during drug trials if patients with mild to moderate dementia are studied, even though these two functions are known to decline early in the course of the disorder. To improve the ability of the ADAS to detect changes in very early AD, we have added seven subtests that measure delayed memory, clock drawing, word generation, timed psychomotor performance, and verbal abstraction and have added items to the naming and constructional praxis subtests (see Table I).

The ADAS could be improved by the addition of a Delayed Recall and a Delayed Recognition test for the words on the Word Recall test. Our delayed recognition memory task for Word Recall consists of ten target words that are embedded in a paragraph. These delayed memory measures are administered after Naming Objects and Fingers (approximately a 5-minute delay). These measures of forgetting are a valuable addition to the ADAS because rapid forgetting is a cardinal feature of AD (Zec, 1993).

Another modification of the ADAS that we recommend is adding the following high, medium, and low frequency objects to Naming Objects and Fingers: toothbrush, domino, and funnel. The ADAS Naming subtest is not as sensitive to differences between normal elderly and mild dementia as would be expected from studies using more extended tests of confrontational naming, e.g., the Boston Naming Test (Zec, 1993). The additional items may improve the psychometric properties of this subtest while only adding a minute to the administration time. We also recommend that in the scoring of the extended ADAS, that the raw score (20 possible error points) for Naming Objects and Fingers be used rather than the rating score. The reason for this modification is the naming raw score for the very mild AD group (MMSE > 24) was statistically different from the elderly controls (p < .0001), whereas the rating score was not.

Seven Added Subtests		
SUBTESTS	FUNCTIONAL DOMAIN	ADDED TIME (minutes)
Delayed Recall	Delayed Memory	1
Delayed Recognition	Delayed Memory	3
Clock to Command	Conceptualization and Construction	3
Delayed True/False Word Recognition	Delayed Memory	2
Word Generation	Semantic Word Fluency	1
Letter Digit	Timed Psychomotor Performance	1.5
Similarities	Verbal Abstraction	4
Two Modified Subtests		
SUBTESTS	FUNCTIONAL DOMAIN	ADDED TIME (minutes)
Three objects added to Naming Objects	Confrontational Naming	1
Three drawings added to Constructional Praxis	Constructional Praxis	3

TABLE I. Additions to the ADAS to Form the Extended ADAS

The Constructional Praxis subscale on the ADAS is also less sensitive to early dementia than has been reported for other more complex tests of graphomotor praxis, e.g., the Rey-Osterreith Complex Figure (Zec, 1993). We recommend adding overlapping pentagons from the Folstein MMSE, the Greek cross from the Aphasia Screening Test of the Halstead-Reitan Battery, and a copy of a clock. Before copying a drawing of a clock the subject is asked to "draw a clock and set the hands at ten after eleven." These items have proven utility in the detection of constructional dyspraxia and would only add another 2 minutes to the administration time. The pentagons, cross, and copy of the clock are each scored as a maximum of one error point. The drawing of the clock to command is scored on the basis of four possible error points (i.e., for errors in making the outline of the clock face, errors in numbering, an error due to not having an hour and minute hand, and in not setting the time correctly). Drawing the clock to command has both constructional and conceptual components.

We also recommend the addition of three other subtests: Letter-Digit Test, Word Generation, and Similarities. These tests should be administered after the completion of the ADAS Cognitive subscale, so that they do not affect the performance on the original ADAS items. The Letter-Digit Test is a test of timed psychomotor performance and is similar to the Smith Symbol Digit Modalities test except that letters of the alphabet are paired with numbers rather than symbols. This subtest was added because timed psychomotor tasks can be sensitive to early AD (Zec, 1993). We recommend using the Word Generation of things that you can buy in a supermarket from the Mattis Dementia Rating Scale (Mattis, 1975). Word generation for items belonging to a specific category (i.e., semantic word fluency) is sensitive to early DAT (Zec, 1993). Finally, we recommend that a Delayed True-False Word Recognition Test be administrated several minutes after the Word Generation subtest after the ADAS Word Recognition so that forgetting over a brief delay (5-10 minutes) can be measured. Thus, Letter Digit and Word Generation are administered between the Word Recognition and Delayed Word Recognition subtests.

We also recommend that half of the WAIS-R Similarities subtest be used: items 1, 4, 5, 7, 9, 12, and 14. We recommend adding this subtest because the ADAS contains no items that measure conceptualization, a function known to be impaired in patients with DAT.

The original ADAS cognitive scale has a total possible 70 error points, whereas the extended ADAS has a total of 170 error points. The Delayed Recall and Delayed Recognition for the Word Recall Test are worth 10 points each for a total of 20 points. The Naming of Objects and Fingers are worth 20 points rather than five because of the addition of three more items and the use of the raw score are worth 20 points rather than five. Seven error points were added to the constructional praxis test. The Word Generation Test is worth a total of 24 points. The Letter Digit test is worth a maximum of 15 error points (0.5 points per item). Delayed True-False Recognition for the Word Recognition Test is worth a total of 12 error points. The half-form of the WAIS-R Similarities test is worth a total possible seven error points (one error point per item). These recommendations for an improved ADAS that would add about 20 minutes to the administration time.

RELIABILITY AND SENSITIVITY OF THE EXTENDED ADAS

In the present study, we administered the extended ADAS to 32 probable AD patients on two occasions 3-4 weeks apart. The Spearman correlation coefficients were calculated for each of the scores on the original and extended ADAS. Very high test-retest correlations were found for the total extended ADAS score ($r = 0.93$) and the total original ADAS score ($r = 0.89$). Among the seven subtests added to the extended ADAS, four were found to have high test-retest correlations [the Letter Digit (0.85), the Delayed Recall (0.83), Word Generation (0.73), and Delayed True-False Word Recognition (0.73)]. The other three subtests which were added to the extended ADAS produced correlations in the moderately range: Delayed Word Recognition (0.67), Clock to Command (0.64), and Similarities (0.62). The two subscales from the original ADAS which were modified by adding items, both were found to have high test-retest reliabilities [Naming (extended) $r= 0.83$ and Constructional Praxis (extended) $r= 0.77$, respectively].

We divided the AD group into three groups based on their total ADAS score including a mild dementia group consisting of the 12 patients with the lowest total ADAS error scores. Six of the 12 subtests which were statistically poorer in the mild group compared with the control group were subtests that were added or modified on the extended ADAS, including Naming (extended), Delayed Recall, Delayed Recognition, Clock to Command, Word Generation, and Delayed True-False Word Recognition. Only 3 of 9 subtests that were added or modified on the extended ADAS did not statistically discriminate the mild dementia group from the control group, i.e., Constructional Praxis (extended), Letter Digit, and Similarities. The 6 subtests from the original ADAS which significantly discriminated the mild dementia group and the control group included Word Recall, Orientation, Word Recognition, Language Expression, Comprehension, and Word Finding Difficulty. Three of these subtests, however, were the three subjective language rating items. Effect sizes were calculated by subtracting the mean of the mild dementia group from the mean of the control group and dividing by the standard deviation of the control group. The largest effect sizes were found for Delayed True-False Word Recognition (2.37), Orientation (2.35), Word Recall (1.72), Language Expression (1.61), Word Generation (1.65), and Delayed Recall (1.58).

CONCLUSION

The original ADAS has been shown to be useful in the early detection and staging of AD and also in measuring progression (Zec, 1993). Nonetheless, it is not as sensitive to early AD as a more extensive neuropsychological test battery. Consequently there is a "ceiling effect" on the ADAS making it difficult for this test to detect improved cognitive functioning in very mild AD patients who have low error scores. Furthermore, the ADAS has been shown to have difficulty in measuring decline over a 2-year period in very early patients (Stern et al., 1994). We added several subtests to improve the ability of the ADAS to detect early AD. We found high test-retest reliability for the total extended ADAS score and generally high test-retest reliabilities for the subtests which we added. We also demonstrated that the subtests added to the extended ADAS have enhanced the ability of this test to measure cognitive deficits in early AD patients. The considerably greater total error score on the extended ADAS raises the ceiling for the mild patients making it possible to detect cognitive improvements in these patients.   Future research should investigate whether the extended ADAS total score is more useful in measuring decline over a 24-month period in mild AD patients than has been shown for the original ADAS total score.

REFERENCES

Mattis S (1975):   Mental Status Examination for organic mental syndrome in elderly patients. In: *Geriatric Psychiatry*, Bellack R and Karasu B, eds. New York: Grune and Stratton, pp. 77-121.

Rosen WG, Mohs RC and Davis KL (1984):   A new rating scale for Alzheimer disease. *Am J Psychiatry* 141:1356-1364.

Stern RG, Mohs RC, Davidson M, Schmeidler J, Silverman J, Kramer-Ginsberg E, Searcey T, Bierer L and Davis KL (1994):   A longitudinal study of Alzheimer disease: Measurement, rate, and predictors of cognitive deterioration.   *Am J Psychiatry* 151:390-396.

Zec RF, Landreth ES, Vicari SK, Feldman E, Belman J, Adrise A, Robbs R, Kumar V and Becker R (1992a):   Alzheimer disease assessment scale: Useful for both early detection and staging of dementia of the Alzheimer type.   *Alz Dis Rel Disord -- Int J* 6:89-102.

Zec RF, Landreth ES, Vicari SK, Belman J, Feldman E, Adrise A, Robbs R, Becker R and Kumar V (1992b):   Alzheimer disease assessment scale: A subtest analysis.   *Alz Dis Rel Disord -- Int J* 6:89-102.

Zec, RF (1993):   Neuropsychological functioning in Alzheimer's disease.   In: *Neuropsychology of Alzheimer Disease and Other Dementias*.   Parks RW, Zec RF and Wilson RS, eds. New York: Oxford Press, pp. 3-80.

Alzheimer Disease: Therapeutic Strategies
edited by E. Giacobini and R. Becker.
© 1994 Birkhäuser Boston

VALIDATION OF INFORMANT-BASED COGNITIVE ASSESSMENT FOR USE IN AUTOPSY

Dennis Q. McManus, Rosemary B. Harris and Larry F. Hughes
Department of Neurology, Southern Illinois University School of Medicine, Springfield, IL 62794-9230 USA

INTRODUCTION

Currently, there are no proven animal models of Alzheimer disease (AD) (Karczmar, 1991). Human tissue must be used for studies that require fresh or optimally fixed tissue. Moreover, if an animal model were proposed, it would require validation with human tissue.

Troubling aspects of the use of human tissue include 1) storage for prolonged periods until enough samples are obtained for analysis (Faull et al., 1988; Perry and Perry, 1983; Whitehouse et al., 1984); 2) limited availability of cognitively-tested, neuropathologically verified controls; and 3) very limited numbers of individuals who come to autopsy in the early stages of AD (Davis et al., 1991). One way to ameliorate these difficulties is to retrospectively assess the cognitive functioning of individuals coming to autopsy or donating their body to science. However, the validity of retrospectively (i.e. post-mortem) applied tests is problematic. Not nearly enough research has been done to determine the feasibility of obtaining information in this manner.

Retrospective evaluation is easily performed at a standard time after death. Antemortem diagnosis of AD usually requires an informant. After death these informants are usually available. Drop out bias is not an issue and education and cultural bias are easier to control. Utilization of routine autopsy and body donor cases combined with retrospective evaluation could substantially increase the availability of clinically characterized brains for research. Finally, if a retrospective instrument can be developed that has good agreement with a standard clinical scale, then control brains can be used in ongoing prospective autopsy studies utilizing the same standard clinical scale (Morris et al., 1991).

One instrument, the Retrospective Collateral Dementia Interview (RCDI) (Davis et al., 1991), has had preliminary evaluation with a standard clinical assessment for dementia, the Washington University (WU) Clinical Dementia Rating (CDR)

(Berg et al., 1982). The RCDI had a sensitivity of 88% and specificity of 80% for detecting probable AD. However, the RCDI had only a 70% agreement with the WU CDR in differentiating the less severe stages of probable AD (normal, very mild and mild AD). It is unknown if the RCDI can reliably identify normal controls from mild AD cases that come to autopsy, because of the small study size (n=6 for controls). Further, the RCDI has not been validated with the more widely used Consortium to Establish a Registry for Alzheimer Disease (CERAD) Clinical Dementia Rating (CDR) (Morris et al., 1989). However, even given these problems, further validation of the RCDI may be able to overcome these difficulties.

Another instrument potentially useful for retrospective assessment of autopsy patients is the Informant Questionnaire on Cognitive Decline in the Elderly (IQCODE) (Jorm and Jacomb, 1989). This is a rapid instrument usually requiring about 15 min to administer. The IQCODE is resistant to education bias and was standardized with a large sample population (n=613). There was minimal overlap between dementia subjects and the normal population. However, the IQCODE has not been evaluated as a retrospective interview of autopsy cases.

PATIENTS AND METHODS

Two informant-based interviews were used; 1) RCDI (Davis et al., 1991) and 2) IQCODE (Jorm and Jacomb, 1989). Clinical evaluations were performed in an outpatient clinic utilizing CERAD CDR scale (Morris et al., 1989). A total of 70 subjects were entered in the study. Fifty-two subjects were evaluated as patients at a memory disorders clinic and 18 subjects recruited from a psychometric study of normal aging. Informed consent was obtained from all informants and the 18 subjects recruited from outside of the clinic. Informants were either a relative (spouse or child) or a close friend familiar with the daily activities of the subjects. The RCDI and IQCODE were administered by a clinical associate (Rosemary Harris) within two days of the clinical evaluation by a neurologist (Dennis Q. McManus) utilizing the CERAD CDR. The clinical associate and neurologist were kept blind about each others ratings. Once the RCDI, IQCODE and CERAD CDR were completed on a subject, disagreements were reviewed by both raters to improve agreement on the next subject assessment. Demographic characteristics of the subjects are presented in Table I.

CERAD CDR

The CERAD CDR is based upon a set criteria for diagnosing dementia and distinguishing between the common causes of dementia including dementia of the Alzheimer type, Parkinson dementia and vascular dementia (Morris et al., 1989). Information is obtained from both the subject and informant, usually a relative or close friend. The informant is asked questions about the past medical history including usage of prescribed drugs, socio-demographic information, use of alcohol and tobacco, personality changes and family history of dementia. Onset and course of cognitive changes in the areas of memory, orientation, language, judgement, home and hobby, community affairs and personal hygiene are detailed. Dementia severity is scored using the CDR which assesses six areas of cognitive function; memory, orientation, judgment and problem-solving, community affairs, home and hobbies, and personal care. Utilizing a standard set of rules the CDR is scored as follows: CDR 0, normal; CDR 0.5, questionable (or very mild); CDR 1, mild; CDR 2, moderate; CDR 3, severe dementia. Dementia was considered detected when a subject had a CDR score ≥ 0.5 (questionable dementia or more severe). This stringent criteria was used to determine if the RCDI could reliably identify CERAD normal subjects for use as neuropathologic controls.

	Controls (n=12)	Patients (n=58)
Age (years)	66.6 ± 7.3	75.8 ± 7.5
Education (years)	16.0 ± 2.8	11.7 ± 3.5
Gender	Male, 4	Male, 16
	Female, 8	Female, 42

TABLE I. Demographics. (Information was missing in 9 cases)

RCDI
Information is obtained about the subject's medical history including prescribed drugs, socio-demographic information, use of alcohol and tobacco, type and onset date and course of the terminal illness, personality problems, hearing and vision disorders, and family history of memory disorders (Davis et al., 1991). The relationship of the informant and subject prior to death is established. Onset and course of cognitive changes in the areas of memory, orientation, language are detailed as the CERAD CDR. Dementia is scored as the CERAD CDR utilizing the CERAD standard set of rules (Morris et al., 1989). The test takes approximately one hour to administer and score.

IQCODE
This instrument is an informant-based questionnaire to assess dementia in living subjects (Jorm and Jacomb, 1989). This is a 26 item interview in which an informant is asked to rate the degree of cognitive change over the last ten years. The informant rates the subject on everyday cognitive tasks as: "much better" (score of 1), "a bit better" (score of 2), "not much change" (score of 3), "a bit worse" (score of 4), and "much worse" (score of 5). Scores for each of the

26 items are averaged to give an overall IQCODE score between 1 and 5. This interview takes less than 15 min to complete. For 613 subjects from the general population the average score was 3.37 ± 51 (mean $\pm$ S.D.) and for 362 demented subjects the average score was 4.67 ± 39 (mean $\pm$ S.D.). There was minimal overlap between the two groups at a cutoff point of 4. Dementia was considered detected when a subject had an IQCODE $\geq$ 4.

Data are summarized as mean $\pm$ S.D. Contingency tables were generated for detection of dementia for the IQCODE and RCDI compared to the CERAD CDR. Only the contingency table of RCDI compared to CERAD dementia severity was generated. This was because no discrete cutoff points for the IQCODE have been defined for the degree of dementia. Degree of association of the RCDI and IQCODE compared to CERAD dementia severity rating was expressed by their respective Kendall tau-B coefficients. For the detection of dementia we utilized the Phi coefficient. All statistics were calculated using SYSTAT 5.02 for Windows.

RESULTS

The frequency of clinical diagnoses based on the CERAD assessment are listed in Table II. The detection of dementia for the IQCODE compared to CERAD is found in contingency Table III. The hit rate was 34/58 (59%). The miss rate was 24/58 (41%). Correct rejection rate was 12/12 (100%). The false alarm rate was 0/12 (0%). The Phi coefficient was 0.44 ($p < 0.01$). The detection of dementia for the RCDI compared to CERAD is found in contingency Table IV. The hit rate was 56/58 (97%). The miss rate was 2/58 (3%). Correct rejection rate was 6/12 (50%). The false alarm rate was 6/12 (50%). The Phi coefficient was 0.55 ($p < 0.01$).

Probable AD	23
Possible AD	20
Questionable	14
No Dementia	12
Other Dementia	1

TABLE II. Diagnosis frequency.

Dementia severity ratings of the RCDI compared to the CERAD is found in contingency Table V. The Kendall tau-B coefficient was 0.73 ($p < 0.01$). The IQCODE score compared to CERAD dementia rating had a Kendall tau-B coefficient of 0.54 ($p < 0.01$). A contingency table of IQCODE compared to

CERAD was not presented since cutoffs for degree of dementia severity have not been defined for the IQCODE.

	IQCODE: normal	IQCODE: demented
CERAD: normal	12	0
CERAD: demented	24	34

TABLE III. Comparison of CERAD and IQCODE frequency of dementia detection (n=70). Phi coefficient = 0.44 (p < 0.01).

	RCDI: normal	RCDI: demented
CERAD: normal	6	6
CERAD: demented	2	56

TABLE IV. Comparison of CERAD and RCDI frequency of dementia detection (n=70). Phi coefficient = 0.55 (p < 0.01).

	RCDI: CDR=0	RCDI: CDR=0.5	RCDI: CDR=1	RCDI: CDR=2	RCDI: CDR=3
CERAD: CDR=0	6	6	-	-	-
CERAD: CDR=0.5	-	9	6	-	-
CERAD: CDR=1	1	2	8	6	-
CERAD: CDR=2	1	-	4	15	-
CERAD: CDR=3	-	-	-	4	2

TABLE V. Comparison of the CERAD and RCDI dementia severity ratings (n=70). Kendall tau-B = 0.73 (p < 0.01).

DISCUSSION

Overall the RCDI is better than the IQCODE at excluding and determining the degree of dementia. This at the expense of identifying half of the cognitively normal subjects as questionably demented (false alarm rate of 50%). In contrast, the IQCODE correctly identifies all the clinically normal subjects; but at the expense of labeling almost half of the clinically demented subjects as normal (miss rate of 41%). These data suggest that the RCDI may be effective in screening neuropathological controls for clinical evidence of dementia. Further study is required to determine if the IQCODE can be useful for screening of neuropathological controls.

REFERENCES

Berg L, Hughes CP, Coben LA, Danziger WL, Martin RL and Knesevich J (1982): Mild senile dementia of Alzheimer type: research diagnostic criteria, recruitment, and description of a study population. *J Neuro Neurosurg Psych* 45:962-96.

Davis PB, White H, Price JL, McKeel D and Robins LN (1991): Retrospective postmortem dementia assessment: Validation of a new clinical interview to assist neuropathologic study. *Arch Neurol* 48:613-617.

Faull KF, Bowersox SS, Zellar-DeAmicis L, Maddaluno JF, Ciaranello RD and Dement WC (1988): Influence of freezer storage time on cerebral biogenic amine and metabolite concentrations and receptor ligand binding characteristics. *Brain Res* 450:225-230.

Jorm AF and Jacomb PA (1989): The informant questionnaire on cognitive decline in the elderly (IQCODE): socio-demographic correlates, reliability, validity and some norms. *Psychological Medicine* 19:1015-1022.

Karczmar AG (1991): SDAT models and their dynamics. In: *Cholinergic Basis for Alzheimer Therapy*, Becker R and Giacobini E, eds. Boston: Birkhauser, pp. 141-152.

Morris JC, Heyman A, Mohs RC et al. (1989): The consortium to establish a registry for Alzheimer's disease (CERAD). Part I. Clinical and neuropsychological assessment of Alzheimer's disease. *Neurology* 39:1159-1165.

Morris JC, McKeel DW, Storandt M et al. (1991): Very mild Alzheimer's disease: Informant-based clinical, psychometric, and pathologic distinction from normal aging. *Neurology* 41:469-478.

Perry EK and Perry RH (1983): Human brain neurochemistry: some postmortem problems. *Life Sci* 33:1733-1743.

Whitehouse PJ, Lynch D and Kuhar MJ (1984): Effects of postmortem delay and temperature on neurotransmitter receptor binding in a rat model of the human autopsy process. *J Neurochem* 43:553-559.

PART XVI

SOCIO-ECONOMIC ASPECTS IN THE TREATMENT OF ALZHEIMER'S DISEASE

Alzheimer Disease: Therapeutic Strategies
edited by E. Giacobini and R. Becker.
© 1994 Birkhäuser Boston

SOCIO-ECONOMIC ASPECTS OF ALZHEIMER'S DISEASE TREATMENT

Marco Trabucchi, Stefano Govoni and Angelo Bianchetti
Alzheimer Care Unit, "S. Cuore Fatebenefratelli" Hospital, Brescia, Italy

DIMENSIONS OF THE PROBLEM

Recognizing Alzheimer's dementia (AD) as a disease carries important consequences as it affects the share of expenses between health and social services for both private and public health insurance programs (NIA, 1993). Moreover, it affects the amount of resources allocated for research, the identification of risk factors and design of prevention programs.

Presently, the resources are still somewhat scattered; there is not a defined itinerary to help to pose the diagnosis or to provide care for the affected person. Families and general practitioners are not aware of the resources available and of the various structures which today take care of AD patients. In Italy, a patient waits an average of 1.5 years after the first symptoms appear before seeing a physician. Then they are evaluated by various specialists before the diagnosis of AD, which in general is made by a neurologist. This process is distressing and expensive for the families. Since resources are going to become ever more limited, models should be designed to make easier the diagnostic procedure and to organize the care system for the patient. The benefit/cost ratio analysis of each intervention will be mandatory, additionally stressing the importance of assessing the costs of AD.

In Italy, AD is prevalent in 2.6% of the population for over 60 years of age; the prevalence of the disease increases with age and is higher in women (3.4% versus 1.5% in men) (Rocca et al., 1993). A calculation based on the resident population in Italy in 1991 leads to a total of a 283,000 people affected by the disease, a number that will increase in the future if the present demographic trends and prevalence of AD do not change.

Dementia and, in particular, AD needs specific care at the diagnostic, therapeutic and rehabilitation level and the associated costs may be divided accordingly. It should be stressed that while the diagnosis involves direct medical costs almost entirely paid by the National Health Care System, therapy and rehabilitation, defined as procedures aimed to optimize at each time point of the illness the functional reserve of the patient, do include direct and indirect costs that are sometimes difficult to quantify. The costs for therapy and rehabilitation have to be further divided between hospital, nursing homes and home care. The distribution of patients among the three categories varies with the severity of illness and may differ significantly from country to country and within a country, according to services locally available. It should be stressed that in Italy the general attitude is to keep the patient at home as long as possible with a share of costs between the family, social services and the Health Care System.

COSTS OF AD IN ITALY

The data reported in Table IA are calculated considering that the diagnosis is made roughly 1.5 years after the onset of the illness and that 4-5 days are needed for the initial diagnosis, including clinical tests such as neuropsychological evaluation, biochemical examination and neuroimaging assessment. Considering that each year 40,000 new patients are diagnosed as AD, the amounts reported in Table IA lead to an annual cost of 3500 US$ per patient, an amount that can be significantly reduced in specialized centers allowing outpatient/day hospital procedures for the diagnosis. It should be stressed that expenses are partially determined by the local availability of services. If no centers specializing in the diagnosis of AD based on a day hospital assessment program are available, more likely the patient will be referred to a general hospital, increasing the costs.

Once the patient has been diagnosed as having AD, the costs will be greatly determined by the severity of the illness requiring at later stages more and more care finally leading to a totally dependent patient. As seen in Table IB, the greater burden of hospital care is due to concurrent diseases that increase dramatically the costs. In fact, it should be emphasized that AD patients require greater care than the average age-matched non-demented patient. It has been calculated that the average AD patient on each occasion of a concurrent disease will spend a period of 15-70 days in the hospital. The expenses for monitoring already diagnosed patients are calculated considering that one day every six months is needed to assess the progression of the disease. Also, behavioral disturbances represent a significant cost since they frequently require assessment and hospitalization in a psychogeriatric or mental hospital.

As dementia units in nursing homes (Table IC) are being developed today, the housing and social services will require standards higher (30%) than those for non-demented, non-self-sufficient patients, in particular for nursing personnel. The costs are roughly divided in half between medical and social services.

The annual costs of home care for AD patients greatly exceeds the other associated costs (Table ID). Costs can be divided into direct and indirect. The direct consists mostly of social and nursing services. Informal care costs are calculated as the equivalent number of hours spent for care by relatives at an hourly cost of 6 US$. The loss of resources are calculated considering that relatives lose or abandon their work and that their productivity at the working place decreases. The time that is lost from daily activities, such as taking care of children, cleaning, cooking, etc. or voluntary services in the community is also considered. Not included are costs that cannot be estimated, i.e. those linked to pain, anxiety, suffering, social distress. They are obviously of great importance but cannot be evaluated in terms of money. Costs increase in the course of the illness; i.e. medical costs increase four times from phase I to phase II (Bianchetti and Trabucchi, 1994) (annual total costs from 156 million US$ to >700 million US$) while social and indirect costs increase up to over 40 times (annual total costs from 130 million US$ to >5 billion US$).

				total	
A)	**Diagnosis**			total	**140**
	Outpatients, day hospital		31		
	Inpatients		109		
B)	**Hospital care**			total	**449**
	Monitoring [a]		56		
	Concurrent disease or complications [b]		281		
	Behavioral disturbances [c]		112		
C)	**Dementia Units in Nursing Homes** [d]			total	**1190**
	Medical costs [e]		575		
	Social services		625		
D)	**Home care**			total	**7908.5**
	Direct costs				
	Physician visits		2.8		
	Formal care (social and nursing services)		1875		
	Aids (diapers, orthopedic prothesis, etc.)		93.7		
	Indirect costs				
	Informal care		3750		
	Resources losses		2187		
E)	**Drug treatment**			total	**93.7**
	Nootropics drugs		62.5		
	Benzodiazepines and neuroleptics		18.7		
	Antidepressants		12.5		

TABLE I. Annual costs of A) diagnosis; B) hospital care; C) dementia units; D) home care; and E) drug treatment for AD patient/year (in US$). [a] geriatric or neurologic clinic; [b] acute/geriatric hospital; [c] psychogeriatric or mental hospital; [d] only for AD patients; [e] comprehensive medical exams and medications.

The expenses for drugs (Table IE) are relatively minor. For example, the money spent for aids (such as diapers) equals that spent for drugs representing less than 1% of total expenses. Twenty percent of the cost allocated for drugs is currently spent for sedatives and not for substances aimed to cure the illness. Potentially, any new drug able to slow down the progression of the disease and to improve fundamental behaviors such as incontinence and self-care could save a substantial of money, along with improving the quality of life of the patient, in terms of direct and indirect costs. Due to the high indirect social cost, such a drug would potentially represent a large benefit/cost ratio and hundreds of millions of dollars to a worldwide market (Miller, 1994; Editorial, 1993).

NEW MODELS FOR PROVIDING CARE TO AD PATIENTS IN ITALY

What type of instruments is the Health Care System developing for the future to offer sufficient and qualified support for the medical needs of demented people? Recently the local government of Lombardy (8 million inhabitants) launched a dementia care program characterized by 8 Alzheimer Regional Centers, 70 dementia units of 20 beds in nursing homes, 40 home care organizations. The goal of the System is to provide a better and less costly diagnosis and to help families to take care of the patient as long as they can and are willing to do so. It is predictable that providing help to families will allow a greater proportion of long-term hospital ward AD patients to be returned home, instead of sent to nursing homes.

STAFF (Full Time)	1,175,000
2 geriatricians; 2 neurologists; 1 psychiatrist; 1 neuropsychologist; 2 biologists; 12 professional nurses; 1 social worker; 2 rehabilitation therapists; 6 occupational and cognitive therapists; 16 blue collars	
DIAGNOSTIC PROCEDURES	
blood analysis	125,000
neuroimaging	48,750
other	15.600
FOOD AND LODGING	91,250
GENERAL FUNCTIONS	287,500
TOTAL	**1,740,000**

TABLE II. Analysis of annual costs (in US$) for a 40 bed regional center in Italy.

Table II shows an analysis of the costs of the first Italian Alzheimer Regional Center, a multidisciplinary experimental care center that provides diagnostic evaluation and treatment mainly for elderly patients with recent onset of mental impairment or long-lasting dementia. The unit is designed to provide comprehensive assessment of medical, psychological and social problems of the demented elderly and to provide therapy, rehabilitation, counseling, social, legal and ethical support to the patient and family. The Regional Center is responsible for educational programs directed to staff nurses and caregivers.

Finally, the Regional Center should also launch research programs. The involvement of the Regional Center in research should be stressed. It is our conviction that resources invested in research will bring a return in terms of awareness, new directions for diagnosis, detection of risk factors and prevention and design of new drugs. The last ten years of AD research already witness such a progress. Finally, we believe that estimating costs of AD care and benefit/cost ratio of any intervention does not reflect a selfish attitude of a society toward a disabled patient but the desire to provide the best care in spite of limited resources and coping with medical ethics and economic constrictions.

REFERENCES

Bianchetti A and Trabucchi M (1994): L'impatto economico della demenza: una ipotesi per l'Italia. *Giorn Geront* (In Press).

Editorial, US market for cholinesterase inhibitors (1993): *SCRIP* 1814:35.

Miller MW (1994): Warner-Lambert's Cognex study finds drug help 40% of Alzheimer patients. *Wall Street J* (April 6).

National Institute on Aging (1993): Progress Report on Alzheimer's Disease 1993. NIH Publication No. 93-3409.

Rocca WA, Hofman A et al. (1993): Frequency and distribution of Alzheimer's disease in Europe: a collaborative study of 1980-1990 prevalence findings. *Annals Neurol* 30(3):9.

Alzheimer Disease: Therapeutic Strategies
edited by E. Giacobini and R. Becker.
© 1994 Birkhäuser Boston

AUTONOMY IN ALZHEIMER DISEASE

George J. Agich
Departments of Medical Humanities and Psychiatry, Southern Illinois
University School of Medicine, Springfield, IL 62794-9230

Patient autonomy is a cornerstone principle of medical ethics, so much so that
bioethicists have tended uncritically to assume, and sometimes insist on, its
importance in all research and therapeutic contexts. Typically, an abstract, ideal
model of autonomy underlies and influences most treatments. This model
assumes a set of ideal capacities that the autonomous agent is supposed to
possess, namely, the ability to function as an independent, rational decision
maker, as one who knows her own desires and preferences, and whose freedom
is expressed in actions or choices that are directed at the fulfillment of her
desires and preferences. While these features represent unremittingly high
expectations for most patients, they represent an impossible ideal for Alzheimer
Disease (AD) patients. This fact alone should warn us that the standard
applications of autonomy to AD will not be without problems.

In previous work, I have argued that the standard model of autonomy involves
problems that can be best addressed not by abandoning autonomy in favor of
other ideals, but by reassessing the meaning of autonomy (Agich, 1990).
Instead of the abstract ideal of autonomy described above, I argued for a view
of *actual autonomy* that focused on the concrete phenomenological features of
human action in the everyday world (Agich, 1993). So regarded, *actual
autonomy* presents a view of the patient who has a particular developmental
history, personal beliefs, projects, and values, and who exists in a dynamic
relationship with a social world. Seen in these terms, the problem of autonomy
for AD patients becomes but one aspect of a wider problem of acknowledging
and respecting the concrete and actual experiences of individual patients. A
ready example of the importance of this perspective is in the treatment of
consent.

Consent is a necessary precondition for research or treatment, but clearly
many patients are not able to give an informed consent. Consent is usually
understood in terms of a dyadic physician patient relationship. Early AD,
however, usually involves family caregivers and later stages frequently involve
professional caregivers. For this reason, consent must be seen in a wider social
and practical context. The dynamic character of the disease process, too, must
be considered in approaching the question of consent. Although few AD

patients retain for long an ideal capacity for consent, such patients are nonetheless conscious subjects who experience an everyday world in which they prefer certain foods, certain clothes, certain persons, certain activities. Good caregivers can readily identify such preferences. In fact, good caregivers look for them and intuitively adjust their care to the elders' own idiosyncrasies. That means that the elder's comfort and sense of security in her present world, in her present identity is highly relevant as a basis for care. It is thus the AD patient's *actual* autonomy that is clinically and ethically important, and not some putative *ideal* expression of autonomous choice.

For example, it has been reported that clinical research involving early-onset AD patients who are not cognitively impaired have nonetheless utilized surrogate consent procedures before the AD patient is allowed to participate in even low-risk or low-discomfort studies (High, 1993). Naturally, when consent is understood in terms of an ideal model with high standards, AD patients who exhibit memory deficits and dysfunctions, confusion or disorientation are deemed to be not competent by definition; therefore, a surrogate must be relied on the exercise the patient's right to consent. As a result, the patient's *actual* capacity to consent can be overridden.

It has been reported that the majority of subjects participating in AD research were classified as *probable* AD, an operationally standardized classification category among clinicians and researchers (High, 1993; McKhann et al., 1984; Katzman and Jackson, 1991). An overwhelming percentage of these individuals were reported to be in excellent or good health and few were diagnostically shown to have severe or moderately severe cognitive impairment; in addition, the subjects are not reported to be severely compromised in their capacity to understand information or to ask questions. Yet, it seems that because they were diagnosed as *probable* AD, they were seen to be in the process of losing those specific human capacities of cognition and decision-making, that are thought to be necessary to provide informed consent. As a result, they have been treated as a special class of subjects who require special protections. This suggests that AD researchers are exercising extreme caution in recruiting AD patients into research, a caution that seems to be without a firm ethical foundation and one that may itself reflect social stereotypes about AD. Additional evidence for the hypothesis that social stereotyping is occurring is that IRBs are apparently approving these kind of restrictive consent procedures, procedures that assume that the AD subject is not competent to give an informed consent. A significant number of studies involving AD patients report that proxy consent was used for all of the participants. In other instances, consent is sought from a family and *assent* alone was sought from the patients themselves, much like the procedure used with children. A satisfactory ethical justification for this so-called *double consent* process, especially under these low risk/low discomfort protocols has not been made. One might thus conclude that the reported use of proxy consents and double consent represents less an attitude *of protection of the rights of* AD patients than an infantilization of the AD patient even though criticism of the infantilization of elders, especially elders requiring long term care, has been sounded in the geriatric and gerontological literature for several decades.

Confusion about the operational meaning of autonomy is also reflected in the variability of tests and procedures used to assess competence to consent to research. It has been reported, for example, that 80% of research projects employed more than one test or battery of tests to ascertain the degree of cognitive impairment and/or dementia. Other projects used a single test such as the Mini-Mental State Examination (MMSE), Clinical Dementia Rating Scale, the Blessed Scale, the Boston Naming Test, the Mattis Dementia Rating Scale, and Wechsler Memory Scale (High, 1993). There is no clear ethical basis for permitting or barring subjects from participating in research on the basis of this testing.

Consent in treatment relationships also reveal problems in the way that the autonomy of AD patients is conceptualized. Ideal physician patient relationships focus on medical or clinical decisions. And informed consent is designed to protect patients and subjects from their own ignorance of particular interventions, available alternatives, and risks/benefits to the patient or subject. Only on the basis of such information can the subject or patient make an ethically sound decision to accept or reject the proposed intervention. Disclosure clearly focuses on the technical aspects of the interaction. The concern is primarily with the nature of the intervention, any available alternatives to the proposed intervention, and an accurate and fair assessment of its risks and benefits. In AD patients, however, particularly during early stages, the focus of the relationship is less likely to be medical than about everyday actions and choices, such as should the patient be allowed to leave the house alone. For an AD patient exhibiting confusion and disorientation, this is no small issue. The emotional need and desire of a family caregiver to protect the patient complexly interplays with the patient's sometimes stubborn refusal and insistence that he or she knows his way around the neighborhood. These and other worries about maintaining physical safety for the AD patient involve choices that are not at all matters of informed consent as classically understood. To be sure, patient autonomy is at stake in these everyday cases even though the standard focus on *informed consent* seems woefully inadequate.

AD patients suffering from memory impairment and cognitive dysfunction will have difficulty in making at least some decisions. But even here we must be careful about our assumptions. Even if we focus on straightforward cases of decision making, AD patients manifest difficulties. They might, for example, misunderstand information provided to them that is relevant to carrying out an action autonomously. Or, they may be unable to use the information and relate it to a retained history and set of values. They may not be able to articulate or explain a decision made. Or they may not be able to enact a decision, because the synthetic and seamless linkage between decision and action that characterizes autonomy does not exist. As a result, AD patients may appear as if they do not know what is best for themselves and they can communicate choices that conflict not only their previous values and beliefs, but that contradict their very actions in the present.

We must remember that capacity for decision making and autonomy are dynamic; thus it is critically important that respecting the AD patient's autonomy be a regular and routine concern of caregivers, not a concern confined to isolated moments of consent to treatment or research (Sachs and Cassel, 1989). The issue of *informed consent* is not likely to be a pressing concern during most interactions with the AD patient. Because AD patients decline gradually over time, clinical encounters are likely to focus on a series of relatively insignificant concerns and problems. They will lack the conflict, emotional intensity, and drama associated with the standard model of ethical decision making. For this reason, it is easy for the physician to bypass problems associated with respecting the AD patient's autonomy. The failure to address these present and future concerns, for example, by discussing patient's beliefs and preferences for nursing home placement or end of life treatment early and recurrently, only serves to exacerbate what are otherwise difficult decisions.

Issues associated with the AD patient's actual autonomy arise in many everyday settings that are brought to the attention of the physician by caregivers. Many of these settings are not in themselves medical. For example, there is frequently conflict between the caregiver and the AD patient involving driving a car, money management, home care arrangements, and nursing home placement. These conflicts regularly come to the attention of the physician to whom family caregivers look to for authoritative advice, even though it is not clear that medical expertise is relevant to these matters. Failing to anticipate these problems well in advance of their occurrence means that the physician loses the opportunity to help support the dwindling autonomy of the AD patient. It is the neglect of these emotional and value aspects of the care of AD patients that frequently contributes to the conflict the health professional is expected to resolve, for example, between patient and family caregivers.

There is good reason to believe that the identity of a person precedes and grounds any defensible concept of autonomy. The precedence of who a person actually is over the person's own abstract capacity to choose is critical to seeing why standard views of autonomy are problematic for AD. Who a patient truly is involves the experiences, memories, habits, beliefs, and values with which that individual identifies. Should a drastic personality alteration occur such that a patient no longer identifies with her past values, but rather assumes a new set of beliefs and preferences, develops new behaviors and habits, then there are grounds to suggest that a different person is present. An AD patient who no longer recognizes family or friends, who does not know where she is, and who recalls only isolated fragments from her past is, in a very important sense, a different person than she was previously. Surrogate decision makers unfortunately seem to want to maintain the preferences or values of the patient *prior to* AD, values which the patient might not even be able to remember much less to identify with in the present. The conflicts that arise in the care of AD patients are sometimes less about the wishes or values of the patient herself than about who the patient truly is and what kinds of evidence count as expressions of the patient's own autonomy.

The deep problem that makes these cases so difficult is the age-old philosophical problem of personal identity. This problem has significant practical ethical implications that are only partly acknowledged in the bioethics literature. For example, bioethics has defended the use of advance directives as a way to insure that an ideal of patient autonomy is respected. The question that has not been adequately discussed is whether the past beliefs and values or expressed wishes of an elder carry (or should carry) more moral weight in the present than the current beliefs and values of the patient when they apply to a person who has undergone substantial behavioral and personality change. For example, an AD patient who indicated that she did not want to live in a nursing home, that she would rather die than leave her own home, might now not even recognize the home as her own, indeed, might experience it as a place of fear and dread. Should that individual's previous wishes obligate caregivers in the present to maintain her in surroundings that are alien and foreboding to her *present* self? The standard answer is to say that a patient's expressed wishes must be honored, but what counts as an expressed wish is itself not at all clear. In very few cases is there explicit and compelling evidence of a patient's actual wishes. But even when such an expression of a patient's past preferences is incontrovertible, its practical ethical use still requires justification. If the elder is a significantly different person, one who autonomously expresses preferences in her everyday actions and interactions in her life world, then why should a former self impose previous choices on a present self? While bioethicists are only now beginning to address these questions, these are everyday problems in the care of AD patients.

Physicians caring for AD patients thus need to pay close attention to the patient's own identifications and value preferences as they are manifest in the patient's own everyday life space. What is needed is not some new *technique* designed to accomplish this end, but a common sense communication about who the patient truly is. In individual cases, of course, sufficiently detailed descriptions and experiences of a particular patient are readily available, but their systematic use is frustrated by a theoretical framework that is still dependent on an outmoded model of autonomy. Substituting a model of *actual autonomy* based on the reality of patient's present and occurrent behavior and experience, for the outmoded model of ideal autonomy, is a long-overdue development.

REFERENCES

Agich GJ (1990): Reassessing autonomy in long-term care. *Hastings Center Report* 20 (6): 12-17.

Agich GJ (1993): *Autonomy and Long-Term Care.* New York and Oxford, Oxford University Press.

High DM (1993): Advancing research with Alzheimer disease subjects: investigators' perceptions and ethical issues. *Alzheimer Disease and Associated Disorders* 7(3):165-78.

Katzman R and Jackson JE (1991): Alzheimer's disease: basic and clinical advances. *J Am Geriatr Soc* 39:516-25.

McKhann G, Drachman D, Folstein M, Katzman R, Price D and Emanuel MS (1984): Clinical diagnosis of Alzheimer's disease: report of the NINCDS-ADRDA work group under the auspices of the Department of Health and Human Services task force on Alzheimer's disease. *Neurology* 34:939-44.

Sachs GA and Cassel CK (1989): Ethical aspects of dementia. *Neurologic Clinics* 7(4):845-58.

Alzheimer Disease: Therapeutic Strategies
edited by E. Giacobini and R. Becker.
© 1994 Birkhäuser Boston

ECONOMIC ANALYSIS OF ALZHEIMER'S DISEASE IN OUTPATIENTS: IMPACT OF SYMPTOM SEVERITY

E.J. Souêtre, W. Qing, I. Vigoureux and H. Lozet
Benefit Research Group, 2 rue Louis Armand, 92660 Asnieres, France

J.F. Dartigues
University Hospital of Bordeaux, France

L. Lacomblez and C. Derousené
University Hospital Pitié-Salpêtrière, Paris, France

INTRODUCTION

Alzheimer's disease (AD) is an irreversible neurological disorder of unknown etiology that affects 10% of the population 75 years of age and older (Evans et al., 1989). This prevalence rate has been shown to increase dramatically with age (Mortimer and Hutton, 1985). As the disease progresses, the patient ordinarily becomes unable to care for himself/herself and must depend on others to manage daily activities (Zarit et al., 1980). Economic consequences of AD such as direct medical costs, non-medical costs and the amount of time spent by third parties in caring for patients have been found to be substantial. Two retrospective studies carried out in the American environment have reported total costs ranging from $13.6 billion for direct health-care to $43.2 billion for indirect costs (Hay and Ernst, 1987; Huang et al., 1988). A cross-sectional study using a small sample of patients has shown that costs per patient were ranging from $11,735-$22,458 annually depending on the type of care (family care versus nursing home) (Hu et al., 1986). These findings have been supported by a recent analysis on the impact of aging on health care costs (Schneider and Guralnik, 1990); dementia was identified along with hip fracture as inducing a major share of health care cost in elderly people.

The purpose of this pilot study was to evaluate the economic impact of disease severity on the cost structure of caring for AD outpatients.

METHODS

The analytic framework of this study consisted of a cost of illness prevalence survey (Rice et al., 1985; Hodgson and Meiners, 1982). The basic design was cross-sectional, each patient being observed at a single time point. The study sample consisted of 51 outpatients 60 years of age and older and meeting the NINCDS-ADRDA (McKhann et al., 1984) criteria for probable AD. Patients excluded from the study were those that were institutionalized at the time of observation, patients with a medical history of chronic psychiatric (other than dementia) or organic disorder, patients with a history of cognitive deficits related to head injury or other neurologic organic disorder. Patients were recruited at two sites by trained neurologists who collected demographic, clinical and economic data (health-care utilization over the past three months) using a specific formatted questionnaire. In addition, economic data related to the caregiver were directly collected from the caregiver using face-to-face semi-structured interviews. The caregiver was defined as the family member that was actually spending time in relation to the patient's care. The severity of the symptoms of dementia was assessed by the neurologist using the Mini-Mental State examination (MMS) (Folstein et al., 1975) with scores ranging from 0 to 25 (maximum score is 30). In addition, the Clinical Dementia Rating (CDR) (Hughes et al., 1982) and the Geriatric Evaluation by Relatives Rating Instrument (GERRI) (Schwartz, 1983) were used as secondary clinical variables. The psychological impact of AD on the caregivers was assessed using the Hospital Anxiety Depression scale (HAD).

The costs of illness related to AD include direct expenditures for medical and non-medical care and indirect costs (Rice et al., 1985). In this study, direct expenditures for medical care included charges for the following: hospitalization, physicians' consultations, medications, laboratory tests and other diagnostic procedures, rehabilitation and specific therapies. Direct non-medical expenditures included charges for non-medical personnel such as housekeepers and purchase of specific equipment. Caregivers' medical expenditures were also collected but were not included in the cost of illness analysis *per se*. Indirect costs are represented by the value of time spent by the caregiver to care for the patient. However, indirect costs related to patients' time were not directly assessed in our study because of obvious methodological difficulties related to cognitive function impairment.

The cost evaluation was based on the societal perspective (Hodgson and Meiners, 1982; Rice et al., 1985) for the cumulative costs incurred during the three months prior to observation (Eisenberg, 1989). Hospitalization expenditures were estimated by multiplying the number of days of hospitalization by the adjusted expenses per inpatient per day (average "per diem") as reported by hospital accounting systems. Visits to physicians' offices were estimated by multiplying the number of visits of each patient by the mean fee in 1991 for an office visit according to physician's specialty obtained from the Ministry of Health official tariff (Blais, 1991). Medication expenditures were estimated by multiplying the total number of days of use (for each medication) by the public daily price (Dictionnaire Vidal, 1991) according to the daily dose actually delivered. Rehabilitation and specific therapy (psychotherapy, speech therapy) expenditures were calculated from the number of visits or sessions multiplied by the respective mean fee according to the Ministry of Health official tariff (Blais, 1991). Indirect costs, i.e. time spent, were estimated by multiplying the average number of hours spent by the caregiver by the Gross National Product per capita value for 1991.

After patients have been classified according to the severity level (MMS median score = 15), the primary comparative analysis of demographic and clinical data was based on unpaired t-test for quantitative variables and Chi-2 test for qualitative variables. The 5% level of significance was used. In addition, Spearman correlation coefficients were estimated to explore the relationship between each type of cost and the symptoms severity (MMS).

RESULTS

Fifty-one demented patients were included in the study over a three-month period. Patients' and caregivers' demographic profile is presented in Table I. Most of the patients were over 65 years of age with a larger relative number of females in the severe group (MMS ≤ 15). About 60% of the patients were retired at the time of observation and almost all the others were housewives. Income level did not differ between groups. The health insurance coverage was significantly different between the most severe patient group [72.7% of patients fully covered by French national insurance (Social Security)] and the mild cases (complementary insurance for 53.5%) (p < 0.03). The CDR mean scores were also found to differ significantly between the two groups (p < 0.01). The average age of the caregiver did not differ significantly from that of the patients, indicating the high prevalence of spouses among the caregivers. However, there were less female caregivers in the severe group. Patients were distributed over a large range of MMS scores: 28% with MMS score lower than 10; 27% with MMS scores of 11 and 15; 27% with MMS scores of 15 and 20; and the remaining 18% with MMS scores between 21-25.

In terms of cost structure (Table II), direct medical costs and direct non-medical costs represented 34% and 30% of total costs, respectively. Physician's visits represented 5%, medications 8%, diagnostic procedures 6%, hospitalization 2% and rehabilitation 13% of these total costs. Indirect costs represented 36% of the overall total cost. Among the direct costs, most of the expenses were incurred by the national health insurance (46%), whereas patients and caregivers

	MMS $\leq$ 15	MMS > 15	p
	28	23	
PATIENTS			
Age (mean $\pm$ SD)	68.0 $\pm$ 8.3	71.9 $\pm$ 9.1	ns
Sex (% female)	67.9 (n=19)	47.8 (n=11)	ns
Living situation (% with spouse)	92.9 (n=26)	91.3 (n=21)	ns
Education (% undergraduate)	57.1 (n=16)	47.8 (n=11)	ns
Professional status			ns
Retired (%)	53.6 (n=15)	65.2 (n=15)	
Housewives (%)	39.3 (n=11)	26.1 (n=6)	
Source of income			ns
Retirement allowances (%)	53.6 (n=15)	69.6 (n=16)	
Family support (5)	32.1 (n=9)	21.8 (n=5)	
Average annual household income $\pm$ SD (S)	36,663 $\pm$ 14,473	30,748 $\pm$ 9,639	ns
Health Insurance	**		
Social security full coverage (%)	71.4 (n=20)	34.8 (n=8)	
Social security + complementary insurance (%)	21.5 (n=6)	52.1 (n=12)	
CDR score (mean $\pm$ SD)	2.0 $\pm$ 0.7	1.2 $\pm$ 0.7	***
GERRI social score (mean $\pm$ SD)	2.92 $\pm$ 0.45	2.75 $\pm$ 0.51	ns
MMS (mean $\pm$ SD)	9 $\pm$ 5	20 $\pm$ 3	***
CAREGIVERS			
Age (mean $\pm$ SD)	66.9 $\pm$ 10.9	67.4 $\pm$ 8.4	ns
Sex (% female)	35.7 (n=10)	60.9 (n=14)	*
Education (% undergraduate)	35.7 (n=10)	56.5 n=13)	ns
Professional status (% retired)	64.3 (n=18)	56.5 (n=13)	ns
HAD score (mean $\pm$ SD)	14.4 $\pm$ 6.8	15.2 $\pm$ 5.7	ns

TABLE I. Socio-demographic characteristics of patients and caregivers. * $p < 0.05$; ** $p < 0.03$; *** $p < 0.01$

took over 48% in charge, the remaining being covered by the complementary
health insurance. The cost of laboratory and diagnosis tests were found to be
lower (p < 0.03) whereas drug (p < 0.05) and rehabilitation costs (p < 0.01)
were significantly higher in the most severe patient group. We found a nonsignificant trend of higher indirect costs in the group of severe patients. Total
costs were significantly higher in this group (p < 0.03).

	MMS ≤ 15 US$	MMS > 15 US$	Total Costs %	p
PATIENTS				
Direct medical costs				
Physician fees	83	104	5	ns
Drug costs	157	100	8	*
Nootropics, anti-ischemics ...	48	34		
Other psychotropics	38	17		
Other drugs	70	49		
Laboratory and diagnostic tests	42	191	6	**
Hospitalizations	70	0	2	ns
Rehabilitation, specific therapies	371	38	13	***
Direct non-medical costs				
Personnel costs	652	322	29	ns
Specific equipment purchase	33	7	1	ns
Indirect costs				
Time spent / caregiver (hours/day)	4.5 hr	3.8 hr		
Cost of time spent / caregiver	692	527	36	ns
TOTAL COST	2100	1289	100	**
CAREGIVERS				
Direct medical costs	455	213		ns

TABLE II. Total costs for three months. * p < 0.05; ** p < 0.03; *** p < 0.01.

Direct medical costs were significantly correlated with symptom severity (MMS scores) (r=0.28, p < 0.05). Direct non-medical costs were also positively correlated with symptom severity (r=0.30, p < 0.05). However, indirect costs were not significantly associated with MMS scores.

DISCUSSION

Our findings indicate that indirect costs represented the major part of total costs of AD. We also pointed out that the major share of actual expenditures associated with AD are directly incurred by the patient or his/her family. More importantly, we demonstrated that most of the costs were positively associated with AD are directly incurred by the patient or his/her family. More importantly, we demonstrated that most of the costs were positively associated with disease severity as assessed by MMS and CDR scores. A couple of limitations inherent to our study design must be taken into consideration. First, very little data exists in regard to the cost estimates of AD by severity level in the outpatient setting. Thus, it was not possible to estimate appropriate sample sizes to detect statistically significant differences between severity groups. For this reason the number of patients included in this pilot study is relatively limited and should be expanded in future studies. Second, our findings are based on the observation of outpatients; this strategy is consistent with recent studies showing that around 70% of the AD patients were actually living at home with family support (Hing, 1987; Jouan-Flahaut and Colvez, 1985; Michel et al., 1982).

The prevalence approach to cost of illness was used in this study. This strategy may underestimate indirect cost due to missing information concerning the cost of premature death and the cost of loss of productivity of the patient. Although these costs were taken into consideration in the preliminary paper of Hay et al. (1987), recent epidemiological data indicate that life expectancy may not differ in patients with AD and general population (Sayetta, 1986). In addition, the cognitive impairment associated with AD constitutes an experimental limitation to the direct assessment by the patient of the amount of time actually lost due to the disease. However, we attempted to address this issue using the disability scores derived from the GERRI scale and found the time potentially lost by the patient due to the disease ranging from 10.2 hours/day to 12.3 hours/day according to symptom severity. Similarly, research and training costs are not taken into account by this prevalence approach. However, these costs may represent less than 0.1% of total costs of AD (Hay and Ernst, 1987) and may then be dropped out of this analysis.

These potential limitations must be balanced with potential advantages of our approach; firstly our findings are available for a European setting based on a National Health Insurance System. In addition, compared to the use of databases, the cross-sectional design provided us with objective and individual data including economic and clinical parameters. Our study also included costs incurred to the caregivers that represent a major economic factor in the care of AD patients.

Our findings concerning the cost structure are consistent with those reported in earlier studies (Hay and Ernst, 1987; Huang et al., 1988). However, absolute values of costs, indirect costs in particular, differ from those published in the literature (Hu et al., 1986). The difference of setting (USA versus Europe) including different medical practice and different health care services may explain these discrepancies. Our finding concerning the relationship between symptom severity and cost is consistent with an earlier report in a smaller number of patients (Hu et al., 1986). Our findings are based on the MMS as a surrogate measure for severity. Mini-Mental State examination has been used as a major endpoint in numerous clinical studies (Yesavage et al., 1988). In addition, our findings indicate significant correlations between MMS scores and a number of relevant clinical measures such as the estimated duration of the disease ($r=0.27$, $p < 0.05$) and the CDR ($r=0.69$, $p < 0.001$). Physicians' and hospitalization costs were the only expenditures that were not associated with MMS scores. This finding may be interpreted by the active part taken by physicians to the early diagnosis of AD. Similarly, the dramatic increase in rehabilitation and support therapies with disease severity may be related to an increased need for functional and psychological support of the patient and his/her family. This is further supported by the increase in direct health care costs of the caregiver in relation to patient's disease severity. This finding is in line with previous reports on the psychological burden of caring for these patients (Hillier-Parks and Pilisuk, 1990; Morrisey et al., 1990; Quayhagen, 1989; Zarit et al., 1980). Our data concerning indirect costs may be underestimated. The time evaluation was based on the Gross National Product per capita approach. Instead, other studies have used a wage cost or an opportunity cost (e.g. cost of nursing personnel) (Hay and Ernst, 1987; Huang et al., 1988; Hu et al., 1986; Rice et al., 1991; Knapp and Beecham, 1990).

Our economic findings support some preliminary studies that pointed out the dramatic economic burden of mental disorders (Knapp and Beecham, 1990; Rice et al., 1991). These findings may be of great interest to decision-makers in the field of research and health-care policy. The relationship between AD severity and cost indicates that potentially active therapeutic interventions may be associated with a positive economic impact on both society and health insurance expenditures.

ACKNOWLEDGEMENTS

This study was made possible by a grant from Bayer Pharma and from Specia Rhone Poulenc Rorer laboratories. We wish to thank Mrs. C. Taillardat,

Dr. F. Parpeix, Dr. B. Stehle, Dr. S. Goni and Dr. P. Demol for their active participation in this study.

REFERENCES

Blais J (1991): *UCANSS: Union des Caisses Nationales de Sécuritié Sociale.* Fabrégue SA, Paris.

Dictionnaire Vidal (1991): Malesherbes, France, OVP 67ᵉ edition.

Eisenberg JM (1989): Clinical economics. A guide to the economic analysis of clinical practices. *J Amer Med Assoc* 262(20):2879-2886.

Evans DA, Funkenstein HH, Albert MS et al. (1989): Prevalence of Alzheimer's disease in a community population of older persons: higher than previously reported. *J Amer Med Assoc* 261:2551-2556.

Folstein MF, Folstein SE and McHugh PR (1975): Mini-Mental State: a practical method for grading the cognitive state of patients for the clinician. *J Psych Res* 12:189-198.

Hay JW and Ernst RL (1987): The economic costs of Alzheimer's disease. *Amer J Public Health* 77:1169-1175.

Hillier-Parks S and Pilisuk M (1990): Caregiver burden: gender and the psychological costs of caregiving. *Amer J Orthopsychiatry* 61(4):501-509.

Hing E (1987): Use of nursing homes by the elderly; preliminary data from the 1985 National Nursing Home Survey, Hyattsville, MD; US Public Health and Human Services Publication (PHS); 1250. *Advance Data from Vital and Health Statistics*, #135.

Hodgson TA and Meiners MR (1982): Cost of illness methodology: a guide to current practices and procedures. *Health and Society* 60(3):429-462.

Hu TW, Huang LF and Cartwright WS (1986): Evaluation of the costs of caring for the senile demented elderly: a pilot study. *The Gerontologist* 26:158-163.

Huang LF, Cartwright WS and Hu TW (1988): The economic cost of senile dementia in the United States. *Public Health Report* 103:13-17.

Hughes CP, Berg L, Danziger WL et al. (1982): A new clinical scale for the staging of dementia. *Brit J Psychiatry* 140:566-572.

Jouan-Flahaut C and Colvez A (1985): Etude épidémiologique de la détérioration mentale dans la population agée de haute Normandie. *Les cahiers de l'enquête Haute-Normandie*, INSEM.

Knapp M and Beecham J (1990): Costing mental health services. *Psychology Medicine* 20:893-908.

McKhann G, Drachman D, Folstein M, Katzman R, Price D and Stadlan E (1984): Clinical diagnosis of Alzheimer's disease: report on the NINCDS-ADRDA Work Group under the auspices of Department of Health and Human Services Task Force on Alzheimer's disease. *Neurology* 34:939-944.

Michel B et al. (1982): Epidémiologie de la démence sénile dans la région marseillaise. *Psychology Medicine* 14:625-629.

Morrisey E, Becker J and Rubert MP (1990): Coping resources and depression in the caregiving spouses of Alzheimer patients. *J Medical Psychology* 63:161-171.

Mortimer JA and Hutton JT (1985): Epidemiology and etiology of Alzheimer's disease. In: *Senile Dementia of the Alzheimer Type*, Hutton JT and Kenny AD, eds. New York: Alan R. Liss Inc, pp. 177-196.

Quayhagen MP (1989): Differential effects of family-based strategies on Alzheimer's disease. *Gerontologist* 29:150-155.

Rice DP, Hodgson TA and Kopstein AN (1985): The economic costs of illness; a replication and update. *Health Care Financing Review* 7:61-80.

Rice DP, Kelman S and Miller LS (1991): Estimates of economic costs of alcohol and drug abuse and mental illness, 1985 and 1988. *Public Health Reports* 106(3):280-292.

Sayetta RB (1986): Rates of senile dementia Alzheimer type in the Baltimore longitudinal study. *J Chronic Disease* 39:271-286.

Schneider EL and Guralnik JM (1990): The aging of America, impact on health care costs. *J Amer Med Assoc* 263:2335-2340.

Schwartz GE (1983): Development and validation of the Geriatric Evaluation by Relative's Rating Instrument (GERRI). *Psychological Reports* 53:479-488.

Yesavage JA, Poulsen SL, Sheikh AB and Tanke E (1988): Rates of change of common measures of impairment in senile dementia of the Alzheimer type. *Psychopharmacol Bulletin* 24:531-534.

Zarit SH, Reever KE and Bach-Peterson J (1980): Relatives of the impaired elderly: correlates of feelings of burden. *The Gerontologist* 20:649-655.

PART XVII

ALZHEIMER DISEASE TREATMENT: THE FUTURE

Alzheimer Disease: Therapeutic Strategies
edited by E. Giacobini and R. Becker.
© 1994 Birkhäuser Boston

AD TREATMENT: THE FUTURE

Peter J. Whitehouse
Alzheimer Center, University Hospitals of Cleveland,
Case Western Reserve University, Cleveland, OH

INTRODUCTION

The development of more effective medications for treatment of Alzheimer's disease (AD) and related disorders depends primarily on the basic and clinical research enterprise discovering and demonstrating the effects of medications to improve the quality of life of affected individuals. The social and political contexts in which this research is being conducted are changing; other forces are affecting our ability to find new treatments for these conditions. In this paper we will briefly review short-, intermediate-, and long-term approaches to the development of effective therapies but then focus our attention on three critical issues that will affect our ability to implement these approaches. We will discuss the need for more international harmonization in drug development, review concerns about pharmacoeconomics, and, finally, discuss ethical issues that we face in doing research in patients with dementia.

BIOLOGICAL APPROACHES

If we look back over the last 10 or 15 years, we can see that tremendous progress has been made in developing approaches to the therapy of AD. Short-term approaches are leading to the development of medications to treat the symptoms of AD. Most focus has been on cognitive symptoms and there we have seen progress in the development of drugs to treat the cognitive impairment by enhancing cholinergic function. We have seen many cholinesterase inhibitors (ChEIs) in trials and one approved in the United States (Cognex®), as well as the development of selective muscarinic and nicotinic compounds which are also in the clinic. In the intermediate term we are working to intervene to slow the progression of the disease by preventing cell death. Once again these therapies are now in the beginning stages of a clinical trial, including drugs that act on mitochondrial metabolism (acetyl carnitine), calcium metabolism (nimodipine), free radicals (deprenyl), and, finally, neuronal viability (nerve growth factor). We also know that the long-term development of more effective treatments to *cure or even prevent the* disease depends on an understanding of pathogenesis.

In the last 10 or 15 years we have made major advances in understanding molecular and cellular features of neurofibrillary tangles and amyloid. Moreover, we have identified a new genetic susceptibility condition for AD, namely apolipoprotein E (apoE) status.

INTERNATIONAL HARMONIZATION

The Third International Springfield Symposium on Advances in Alzheimer Therapy illustrates the success we have made in harmonizing our work across national boundaries. However, more work needs to be done, particularly as we focus on guidelines for drug development. It does not make sense for industry to develop drugs to treat these conditions using vastly different procedures in different countries. The International Committee for Harmonization has met twice to develop consensus about general preclinical and clinical issues, but has not been focusing on specific diseases. Performing basic research across national boundaries is relatively easy. However, clinical research is more complex, although we are making progress largely through work in epidemiology and clinical trials.

Guidelines for antidementia drugs are being developed through the Food and Drug Administration, the European Community, and Canada. In Japan there are guidelines for vascular disease which have been used to approve drugs for the treatment of vascular dementia.

One of the primary areas of focus on harmonization should be to identify the target diseases. We have actually had success in harmonizing inclusion and exclusion criteria for trials with AD so that either DSM-IV or NIH criteria will be used. This success at agreeing on diagnostic criteria has helped us avoid discussing vague entities such as chronic organic brain syndrome. However, there are many other dementias besides AD that may respond to some of the same strategies that we are developing for this condition. Vascular dementia is thought to be the second most common cause of dementia, but much vascular dementia overlaps with AD. Moreover, there are vascular aspects to the pathogenesis of AD. Parkinson's disease (PD) is also commonly associated with dementia, yet very few trials are ongoing to treat either the dementia of stroke or PD. Similarly, alcohol dementia may respond to some of the same agents that we are testing in AD. We must also keep an open mind about treatment for such phenomena as Aging Associated Cognitive Decline (AACD), which is in the process of being operationally defined. This condition is a successor to Aging Associated Memory Impairment (AAMI) and can be found listed in DSM-IV.

One illustration of a therapeutic strategy that might work in all these conditions is drugs that act on cholinergic mechanisms. Alterations in cholinergic mechanisms are important in all these conditions and either ChEIs or muscarinic or nicotinic receptor agonists may be effective. The fact that nicotine enhances cognition not only in AD but perhaps also in normal individuals allows us to at least consider the possibility that some of our therapies may be effective in normal elderly individuals or perhaps even younger cognitively intact individuals.

We also need to establish agreement about assessing the outcomes of trials. We have achieved some consensus that symptomatic therapies need to be assessed by a combination of objective and subjective instruments. In the cognitive area several objective psychometric scales are available but more work needs to be done in understanding how to assess clinicians' global impression measures and activities of daily living scales. Moreover, not enough attention has been paid to the treatment of the non-cognitive or behavioral symptoms such as agitation, depression, and psychosis. We need to be more serious about the manner in which we design studies to demonstrate slowing progression of the disease. Similar efforts are ongoing in the study of amyotrophic lateral sclerosis (ALS) and PD. Those of us interested in the treatment of degenerative dementias can benefit from these related efforts. Finally, when it comes to the development of guidelines for trials we must also consider the design of trials in different phases of the drug development. We need to involve more patients with the target condition, namely dementia, and more efficacy studies earlier in phase II studies. Moreover, we must consider the possibility that phase IV studies will become more important, particularly when we make claims about slowing progression of disease which may take some time to demonstrate successfully. Perhaps drugs can be given temporary approval, pending further demonstration in phase IV of efficacy.

PHARMACOECONOMICS

Another major international issue is the economics of developing drugs to treat AD. In Italy, more drugs are being classified as Type C which will not be reimbursed by government. In Germany, physicians are at risk for their own personal incomes if they prescribe beyond certain limits. In Japan, there have been no approvals for antidementia drugs in some time. In the United States, HMO's may exclude drugs from their formulary, or health care boards may price "breakthrough" drugs too low to recoup research costs. In whatever country, we are facing economic restrictions on drug research and development.

As the costs of research increase in both academics and industry, the products of our research are being scrutinized in terms of their impact on society. We will need to add to efficacy measures in drug studies assessments of the effectiveness of our products as well.

In the United States and United Kingdom, and I suspect in other countries, academic research institutions are faced with reductions in support from all sources including federal and state grants, industry support, and health care dollars. Health care reform is having a great impact on our entire health care system including academic centers which in some countries are particularly vulnerable.

What will be needed in the future to address at a social level the impact of drugs will be more information about the health of patients and families. Novel studies with new measurements will be needed to demonstrate that products have a significant impact on both the quality of life of patients and families and on the financial state of organizations responsible for paying for medical care. Perhaps we will be doing studies in organizations such as social health organizations which provide comprehensive care to patients with dementia. In such organizations we would be able to track the health care dollars spent by patients and caregivers not only in acute care and doctors' offices but also in community day care and in long-term care facilities.

ETHICS

Growing ethical issues face researchers in AD. A position paper is being prepared by the National Institute on Aging Alzheimer's Disease Research Centers [High DM, Whitehouse PJ, Post SG and Berg L: Guidelines for addressing ethical and legal issues in Alzheimer's disease research: A position paper (in preparation)]. The numerous ethical issues begin with the fact that we are dealing with subjects of reduced intellectual capacity. Thus their competence to make decisions about research is called into question and the role of the family becomes more important. The whole process of ensuring informed consent is more complex, and new trends in ethics, such as discourse or communicative ethics, will focus more on the process by which ethical issues are discussed rather than the conceptual framework. Too much emphasis on theoretical principles such as autonomy, justice, and beneficence (the traditional ethical categories in which to frame ethical discussions), may exclude the need to be equitable in subject recruitment, to allow appropriate opportunities for women and ethnic minorities to participate in the research.

Finally, there are issues of an international nature resulting from concerns about conflict of interest in drug trials. In the United States the Department of Health and Human Services shortly will be promulgating new guidelines that will require academic institutions that receive federal funding to set up new mechanisms for ensuring that inappropriate conflicts of interest do not diminish the trust that the public has in the information created by scientific research.

CONCLUSION

The Springfield Conference can be celebrated as illustrative of the kinds of approaches that need to be highlighted as we approach the future of drug development in AD. We can celebrate working together as an international community, working towards harmonization of our research efforts. The conference program directed us to be aware of the pharmacoeconomic considerations. Finally, the spirit of respect for each other and our patients manifested in this conference illustrates the ethical principle that we need to maintain in order to ensure that the future of AD treatment is bright.

Alzheimer Disease: Therapeutic Strategies
edited by E. Giacobini and R. Becker.
© 1994 Birkhäuser Boston

THERAPEUTIC STRATEGIES IN ALZHEIMER'S DISEASE

Lars-Olof Wahlund, Richard F. Cowburn,
Bengt Winblad and Lars Lannfelt
Karolinska Institute, Alzheimer's Disease Research Centre,
Department of Geriatric Medicine, Huddinge University Hospital,
S-141 86 Huddinge, Sweden.

INTRODUCTION

Alzheimer's disease (AD) represents an increasing financial and health care burden to society. Alzheimer's disease dementia is characterized clinically by a progressive loss of memory, intellect and personality. The neuropathological hallmarks of the disease include the accumulation of large numbers of senile plaques and neurofibrillary tangles, as well as cortical atrophy and neuronal and synaptic fallout. Despite increasing knowledge of the pathological processes underlying AD, there are at present no effective treatments to slow down the progression of the disease or to substantially ameliorate the clinical symptomatology of dementia. In this chapter, two therapeutic strategies, namely, the use of trophic factors and reducing ß-amyloid accumulation and deposition are discussed.

THE USE OF TROPHIC FACTORS

The degeneration of cholinergic innervation of the cortex is a prominent feature of the neurochemical pathology of AD. Given the relative lack of success of acetylcholine neurotransmitter replacement strategies for the disorder, emphasis has recently been placed on maintaining the survival and function of remaining cholinergic neurons in the AD brain. This approach is based on strong experimental animal data showing that exogenous administration of the neurotrophin nerve growth factor (NGF) can rescue cholinergic neurons and improve memory function following nucleus basalis of Meynert (NBM) lesions (Whittemore and Seiger, 1987). This, together with postmortem studies showing that those cholinergic neurons remaining in the NBM in AD express NGF receptor mRNA and protein (Goedert et al., 1989), has provided the rationale for NGF treatment of the disorder (Seiger et al., 1993).

The first case report of an AD patient receiving NGF treatment has recently been published (Seiger et al., 1993; Olson et al., 1992). The case in question was a 69 year old woman who had a steady deterioration of cognitive function over an eight year period. Positron emission tomography (PET) on the patient showed reduced uptake of [^{11}C]nicotine, suggestive of cholinergic dysfunction. The patient also showed decreased rates of cerebral blood flow and glucose utilization, as determined by the uptake of [^{11}C]butanol and [^{18}F]fluorodeoxyglucose, respectively (Seiger et al., 1993; Olson et al., 1992).

The patient received a 3-month intracranial infusion of a highly purified preparation of mouse submandibular gland NGF at a concentration sufficient to saturate remaining low-affinity NGF receptors. Positron emission tomography studies on the patient conducted at the end of the 3-month NGF infusion showed a marked increase in [^{11}C]nicotine uptake, compared to pre-infusion rates. This effect was seen in a number of cortical areas and was attributed to an effect on cholinergic transmission involving either an increased number of cholinergic terminals or an increased number of nicotine binding sites per existing terminal (Seiger et al., 1993; Olson et al., 1992). Unfortunately, the NGF-induced increase in [^{11}C]nicotine uptake returned to pre-treatment levels 3 months after the cessation of NGF.

Nerve growth factor treatment of this patient also gave a marked increase in cerebral blood flow, as shown by the uptake of [^{11}C]butanol. This effect was most apparent in the frontal and temporal cortices and was maintained for 3 months after the cessation of treatment when [^{11}C]nicotine uptake was back to pre-infusion levels. This more long-term effect of NGF on cerebral blood flow was suggested to result from actions on the cholinergic innervation of the cerebral vasculature resulting in vasodilatation or from increases in the sympathetic adrenergic innervation of extracerebral blood vessels (Seiger et al., 1993). Other effects of NGF in this patient included a decrease of slow wave EEG activity that was maintained for up to a year following treatment. In addition, NGF gave a transient improvement in verbal episodic memory, whereas other tasks of cognitive function, as determined using the Mini-Mental State Examination (MMSE), continued to deteriorate (Seiger et al., 1993; Olson et al., 1992).

Taken together, the reported effects of NGF on the single AD case studied to date have provided some optimism for a trophic factor based strategy for the disorder (Seiger et al., 1993; Olson et al., 1992). In order to fully evaluate the potential of this approach it will be necessary to study NGF effects in a larger patient group, preferably using improved methods for the administration of NGF in a form that will cross the blood brain barrier. Future studies should also focus on determining the involvement of other trophic factors in AD (Phillips et al., 1991), such as the NGF family members, brain derived neuronotrophic factor (BDNF) and neurotrophin 3 (NT-3). Furthermore, the importance of NGF effects on the differential splicing and release of the amyloid precursor protein (Refolo et al., 1989) will need to be evaluated when developing a trophic factor based therapy for the disease.

REDUCING ß-AMYLOID ACCUMULATION AND AGGREGATION

In recent years considerable progress has been made in understanding the underlying etiology of AD and in particular the importance of the ß-amyloid peptide.

The Amyloid Hypothesis of AD

ß-amyloid is a 39-43 amino acid peptide that forms the major component of neuritic plaques and cerebrovascular amyloid, and which is derived from the larger amyloid precursor protein (APP), localized on chromosome 21 (Glenner and Wong, 1985). In 1991, an AD family where affected members showed a pathogenic point mutation in exon 17 of the APP gene, was described (Goate et al., 1991). The discovery of this mutation, which resulted in an amino acid substitution at codon 717, C-terminal of the ß-amyloid fragment (Goate et al., 1991) was followed by the identification of other AD pathogenic point mutations at codon 717 (Chartier-Harlin et al., 1991) and at codon 670/671 (Mullan et al., 1992) of the APP gene. Of these, the so-called Swedish APP 670/671 mutation (Mullan et al., 1992) has been shown to result in a greatly enhanced production and release of ß-amyloid when transfected into cell culture systems (Cai et al., 1993). These pathogenic mutations have firmly placed APP metabolism and ß-amyloid protein deposition as central to the pathogenesis of AD and have significantly strengthened the so-called "amyloid cascade hypothesis" of AD (Hardy and Allsop, 1991; Hardy and Higgins, 1992). This hypothesis predicts that the pathological changes associated with AD are triggered by an alteration in APP processing to initiate ß-amyloid over-accumulation and subsequent plaque formation. A cascade of events including plaque maturation, neurofibrillary tangle formation and neuronal degeneration is then initiated, leading to AD pathology and the clinical symptoms of dementia (Hardy and Allsop, 1991; Hardy and Higgins, 1992).

A simplified form of the "amyloid cascade hypothesis" of AD is described below. In brief, APP is metabolized along two major pathways. The secretory pathway involves APP cleavage at amino-acid 16 of the ß-amyloid peptide, just outside the APP transmembrane domain (Anderson et al., 1991) by an as yet unidentified enzyme, termed "α-secretase". This pathway precludes ß-amyloid production, and thus plaque formation. The ß-amyloid pathway occurs parallel to the α-secretase pathway and involves cleavage of APP at the cytoplasmic N-terminus of ß-amyloid, by an enzyme termed ß-secretase. This results in the release of secreted APP extracellularly and the proposed internalization of the APP C-terminal fragment. The C-terminal fragment is then thought to undergo further intracellular processing in an acidic early endosomal or lysosomal compartment, resulting in release of soluble ß-amyloid (Haass et al.,

1992, 1993; Seubert et al., 1993). Released ß-amyloid is then thought to aggregate resulting in plaque formation and the other features of AD pathology.

Although it has become increasingly clear how APP is processed to give ß-amyloid, it should be emphasized that much about the ß-amyloid-induced cascade of events remains speculative. In particular, the proposed link between ß-amyloid deposition and neurofibrillary tangle accumulation remains to be proven. Furthermore, much debate still surrounds whether ß-amyloid is neurotoxic. *In vitro* studies have shown ß-amyloid to be neurotrophic at low concentrations and neurotoxic at higher concentrations (Yankner et al., 1990; Kowall et al., 1991), whereas groups investigating the *in vivo* neurotoxicity of ß-amyloid have produced contradictory results (Games et al., 1992). Alternatively, recent evidence suggests that the ß-amyloid peptide may not be overtly neurotoxic but instead acts to make neurons more vulnerable to degeneration caused by other factors such as glucose deprivation and/or excitatory amino acids (Copani et al., 1991).

Strategies Directed Towards the Amyloid Cascade

Despite speculation about the order of events occurring in the amyloid cascade, the hypothesis does present a number of avenues for potential intervention strategies aimed at slowing the course of the disease. For example, it is hoped that understanding the biochemical properties of the α- and ß-secretase enzymes and the factors that affect the proportion of APP committed to the alternative processing pathways will provide for attempts to slow the production of ß-amyloid. In this respect, it has been shown that APP processing can be modulated by protein kinase C (Buxbaum et al., 1990; Gandy and Greengard, 1992). Recent studies have shown that protein kinase C activation favors APP processing by the secretory pathway (Gillespie et al., 1992) to reduce the production of ß-amyloid (Hung et al., 1993). In view of the reduced levels and activity of protein kinase C in the AD brain it would appear that agents that stimulate protein kinase C would present good opportunities for therapeutic intervention.

An increased understanding of factors that influence ß-amyloid aggregation may also provide other strategies for intervention. In this respect, it has recently been suggested that the e 4 allele of apolipoprotein E (apoE), a protein involved in lipid transport, can act as a molecular chaperone for ß-amyloid making the peptide more likely to precipitate and form plaques. Thus, apoE is found as a component of AD plaques (Namba et al., 1991) and the *e4* isoform has been shown to bind ß-amyloid with greater avidity than other allelic forms of the protein (Strittmatter et al., 1993b). Moreover, allelic associations were recently demonstrated between the apoE *e4* allele and both late-onset familial AD (Strittmatter et al., 1993a) and sporadic AD (Poirier et al., 1993), whereas brains from sporadic late-onset AD patients homozygous for the *e4* allele have been shown to have a higher amyloid burden than brains from *e3* homozygotes (Schmechel et al., 1993). The identification of such important risk factors for

AD as apoE *e*4, should also provide for exciting new therapeutic strategies to slow the course of the disease, especially in those individuals that can be shown to be at high-risk.

Another major consideration for therapeutic strategies aimed at the amyloid cascade concerns the normal biological functions of APP. Amyloid precursor protein expression has been shown to be upregulated in response to cell injury or stress (Abe et al., 1991; Kawarabayashi et al., 1991), as well as to factors involved in tissue damage and recovery, such as interleukin-1 (Goldgaber et al., 1989) and the epidermal and NGF (Refolo et al., 1989). Similarly, cell culture studies have shown that APP is involved in regulation of cell growth, adhesion and neuritic outgrowth (Saitoh et al., 1989; Ninomiya et al., 1993). These effects are consistent with a role for APP in promoting cell regeneration and growth and would imply that increased synthesis of APP with the preclusion of ß-amyloid production may represent another beneficial approach for the therapy of AD.

CONCLUSIONS

Traditional therapeutic strategies for AD have focussed on ameliorating the clinical symptoms of the disease by enhancing cholinergic neurotransmission. Whereas improvement has been shown in some sub-populations of patients, it is clear that this approach is limited since it does not address the underlying cause of the disease. For the future, considerable optimism has been placed on slowing the progression of AD using approaches directed towards the amyloid cascade. In this respect, it is hoped that cell lines and transgenic animals (Lannfelt et al., 1993) that over-produce ß-amyloid will provide useful model systems for testing drugs of potential therapeutic importance for the disease.

REFERENCES

Abe K, St George-Hyslop PH, Tanzi RE and Kogure K (1991): Induction of amyloid precursor protein mRNA after heat shock in cultured human lymphoblastoid cells. *Neurosci Lett* 125:169-171.

Anderson JP, Esch FS, Keim PS, Sambamurti K, Lieberburg I and Robakis NK (1991): Exact cleavage site of Alzheimer amyloid precursor in neuronal PC-12 cells. *Neurosci Lett* 128:126-128.

Buxbaum JD, Gandy SE, Cicchetti P, Ehrlich ME, Czernik AJ, Fracasso RP, Ramabhadran TV, Unterbeck AJ and Greengard P (1990): Processing of Alzheimer ß/A4 amyloid precursor protein: modulation by agents that regulate protein phosphorylation. *Proc Natl Acad Sci (USA)* 87:6003-6006.

Cai X-D, Golde TE and Younkin SM (1993): Release of excess amyloid ß protein from a mutant amyloid ß protein precursor. *Science* 259:514-516.

Chartier-Harlin M-C, Crawford F, Houlden H, Warren A, Hughes D, Fidani L, Goate A, Rossor M, Roques P, Hardy J and Mullan M (1991): Early-onset Alzheimer's disease caused by mutations at codon 717 of the ß-amyloid precursor protein gene. *Nature* 353:844-846.

Copani A, Koh J-Y and Cotman CW (1991): ß-amyloid increases neuronal susceptibility to injury by glucose deprivation. *Neuroreport* 2:763-765.

Games D, Khan KM, Soriano FG, Keim PS, Davis DL, Bryant K and Lieberburg I (1992): Lack of Alzheimer pathology after ß-amyloid protein injections in rat brain. *Neurobiol Aging* 13:569-576.

Gandy S and Greengard P (1992): Amyloidsogenesis in Alzheimer's disease: some possible therapeutic opportunities. *TIPS* 13:108-133.

Gillespie SL, Golde TE and Younkin SG (1992): Secretory processing of the Alzheimer amyloid ß/A4 protein precursor is increased by protein phosphorylation. *Biochem Biophys Res Comm* 187:1285-1290.

Glenner GG and Wong CW (1985): Alzheimer's disease: Initial report of the purification and characterization of a novel cerebrovascular amyloid protein. *Biochem Biophys Res Comm* 120:885-890.

Goate A, Chartier-Harlin M-C, Mullan M, Brown J, Crawford F, Fidani L, Giuffra L, Haynes A, Irving N, James L, Mant R, Newton P, Rooke K, Roques P, Talbot C, Pericak-Vance M, Roses A, Williamson R, Rossor M, Owen M and Hardy J (1991): Segregation of a missense mutation in the amyloid precursor protein gene with familial Alzheimer's disease. *Nature* 349:704-706.

Goedert M, Fine A, Dawbarn D, Wilcock GK and Chao MV (1989): Nerve growth factor receptor mRNA distribution in human brain: normal levels in basal forebrain in Alzheimer's disease. *Mol Brain Res* 5:1-7.

Goldgaber D, Harris HW, Hla T, Maciag T, Donnelly RJ, Jacobsen JS, Vitek MP and Gajdusek DC (1989): Interleukin 1 regulates synthesis of amyloid ß-protein precursor mRNA in human endothelial cells. *Proc Natl Acad Sci (USA)* 86:7606-7610.

Haass C, Hung A, Schlossmacher MG, Teplow DB and Selkoe D (1993): ß-Amyloid peptide and a 3-kDa fragment are derived by distinct cellular mechanisms. *J Biol Chem* 268:3021-3024.

Haass C, Schlossmacher MG, Hung AY, Vigo-Pelfrey C, Mellon A, Ostaszewski BL, Lieberburg L, Koo EH, Schenk D, Teplow D and Selkoe D (1992): Amyloid ß-peptide is produced by cultured cells during normal metabolism. *Nature* 359:322-325.

Hardy J and Allsop D (1991): Amyloid deposition as the central event in the etiology of Alzheimer's disease. *TIPS* 12:383-388.

Hardy JA and Higgins GA (1992): Alzheimer's disease: the amyloid cascade hypothesis. *Science* 256:184-185.

Hung AY, Haass C, Nitsch R, Qiu WQ, Citron M, Wurtman RJ, Growdon JH and Selkoe DJ (1993): Activation of protein kinase C inhibits cellular production of the amyloid ß-protein. *J Biol Chem* 268:22959-22962.

Kawarabayashi T, Shoji M, Harigaya Y, Yamaguchi H and Hirai S (1991): Expression of APP in the early stage of brain damage. *Brain Res* 563:334-338.

Kowall NW, Beal MF, Busciglio J, Duffy LK and Yankner BA (1991): An *in vivo* model for the neurodegenerative effects of ß amyloid and protection by substance P. *Proc Natl Acad Sci (USA)*. 88:7247-7251.

Lannfelt L, Folkesson R, Mohammed AH, Winblad B, Hellgren D, Duff K and Hardy J (1993): Alzheimer's disease: molecular genetics and transgenic animal models. *Behav Brain Res* 57:207-213.

Mullan M, Crawford F, Axelman K, Houlden H, Lilius L, Winblad B, Lannfelt L (1992): A pathogenic mutation for probable Alzheimer's disease in the APP gene at the N-terminus of ß-amyloid. *Nature Genetics* 1:345-347.

Namba Y, Tomonaga M, Kawasaki H, Otomo E and Ikeda K (1991): Apolipoprotein E immunoreactivity in cerebral amyloid deposits and neurofibrillary tangles in Alzheimer's disease and kuru plaque amyloid in Creutzfeldt-Jacob disease. *Brain Res* 541:163-166.

Ninomiya H, Roch J-M, Sundsmo MP, Otero DAC and Saitoh T (1993): Amino acid sequence RERMS represents the active domain of amyloid ß/A4 protein precursor that promotes fibroblast growth. *J Cell Biol* 121:879-886.

Olson L, Nordberg A, von Holst H, Bäckman L, Ebendal T, Alafuzoff I, Amberla I, Hartwig P, Herlitz A, Lilja A, Lundqvist H, Langström B, Meyerson B, Persson A, Viitanen M, Winblad B and Seiger Å (1992): Nerve growth factor affects [^{11}C]nicotine binding, blood flow, EEG and verbal episodic memory in an Alzheimer patient (case report). *J Neural Transm* 4:79-95.

Phillips HS, Hains JM, Armanini M, Laramee GR, Johnson SA and Winslow, JW (1991): BDNF mRNA is decreased in the hippocampus of individuals with Alzheimer's disease. *Neurone* 7:695-702.

Poirier J, Davignon J, Bouthillier D, Kogan S, Bertrand P and Gauthier S (1993): Apolipoprotein E polymorphism and Alzheimer's disease. *Lancet* 342:697-699.

Refolo CM, Balton SRJ, Anderson JP, Mehta P and Robakis NK (1989): Nerve and epidermal growth factors induce the release of the Alzheimer amyloid precursor from PC12 cell cultures. *Biochem Biophys Res Comm* 164:664-670.

Saitoh T, Sundsmo M, Roch J-M, Kimura N, Cole G, Schubert D, Oltersdorf T and Schenk DB (1989): Secreted form of amyloid ß protein precursor is involved in the growth regulation of fibroblasts. *Cell* 58:615-622.

Schmechel DE, Saunders AM, Strittmatter WJ, Crain BJ, Hulette CM, Joo SH, Pericak-Vance MA, Goldgaber D and Roses AD (1993): Increased amyloid ß-peptide deposition as a consequence of apolipoprotein E genotype in late-onset Alzheimer disease. *Proc Natl Acad Sci (USA)* 90:9649-9653.

Seiger, Å, Nordberg A, Von Holst H, Bäckman L, Ebendal T, Alafuzoff I, Amberla K, Hartvig P, Herlitz A, Lilja A, Lundqvist H, Långström B, Meyerson B, Persson A, Viitanen M, Winblad B and Olson L (1993): Intracranial infusion of purified nerve growth factor to an Alzheimer patient: the first attempt of a possible future strategy. *Behav Brain Res* 57:255-261.

Seubert P, Oltersdorf T, Lee MG, Barbour R, Blomquist C, Davis DL, Bryant K, Fritz LC, Galasko D, Thal LJ, Lieberburg I and Schenk DB (1993): Secretion of ß-amyloid precursor protein cleaved at the amino terminus of the ß-amyloid peptide. *Nature* 361:260-263.

Strittmatter WJ, Saunders AM, Schmeckel D, Pericak-Vance M, Enghild J, Salvesen GS and Roses AD (1993a): Apolipoprotein E: High-avidity binding to ß-amyloid and increased frequency of type 4 allele in late-onset familial Alzheimer disease. *Proc Natl Acad Sci (USA)* 90:1977-1981.

Strittmatter WJ, Weisgraber KH, Huang D, Dong L-M, Salvesen GS, Pericak-Vance M, Schmechel D, Saunders AM, Goldgaber D and Roses AD (1993b): Binding of human apolipoprotein E to ßA4 peptide: Isoform-specific effects and implications for late-onset Alzheimer disease. *Proc Natl Acad Sci (USA)* 90:8098-8102.

Whittemore SR and Seiger Å (1987):   The expression, localization and functional significance of ß-nerve growth factor in the central nervous system. *Brain Res Rev* 12:439-464.

Yankner BA, Duffy LK and Kirschner DA (1990): Neurotrophic and neurotoxic effects of amyloid ß protein: Reversal by tachykinin neuropeptides. *Science* 250:279-282.

Alzheimer Disease: Therapeutic Strategies
edited by E. Giacobini and R. Becker.
© 1994 Birkhäuser Boston

NEW STRATEGIES FOR ALZHEIMER'S DISEASE TREATMENT: PLEIOTROPIC DRUGS AND MULTIFACTORIAL INTERVENTION

Ramón Cacabelos
Institute for CNS Disorders, Basic and Clinical Neurosciences Research Center, La Coruña; Neurogerontology Unit, Complutense University Medical School, Madrid, Spain

INTRODUCTION

The neuropathological hallmarks of Alzheimer's disease (AD) are senile (neuritic) plaques, neurofibrillary tangles (NFT), amyloid deposition in neural tissues and vessels, synaptic loss, and subsequent neuronal death. ß-Amyloid deposition, NFT formation and synaptic loss appear to be at the basis of AD pathogenesis (Wisniewski and Weigel, 1992; Terry et al., 1991; Hardy and Allsop, 1991). However, other neurochemical mechanisms may also account for cell death and neurodegeneration in AD, including apoptosis, neuroimmune dysfunction, excitotoxic phenomena, and alterations in neurotrophic factors and brain calcium homeostasis (Cacabelos, 1991). Family history of dementia is the major risk factor, and genetic defects in genes mapped on chromosomes 21, 14, and 19 may account for 50-80% of AD cases (Mullan and Crawford, 1993).

Potential therapeutic strategies in AD include palliative, substitutive and etiopathogenic treatments. At present, multifactorial strategies and compounds with pleiotropic activity are yielding promising results (Cacabelos et al., 1994b).

THERAPEUTIC STRATEGIES

For the past two decades many conventional drugs have been used to ameliorate cognitive deterioration and behavioral disorders in AD (Cacabelos, 1991), and more than 200 new compounds were tested in experimental animals to improve memory and learning, but less than 50 of these substances could overcome preclinical scrutiny. The success of future clinical trials with new drugs for AD will depend on: (a) a precise definition of diagnostic criteria for AD (DSM-IV; ICD-10; NINCDS-ADRDA), including biological and genetic markers; (b) a better understanding of the etiopathogenesis and the cause(s) of the disease; (c) regulatory changes affecting drug clinical trials; (d) ethical guidelines for conducting research with elderly subjects; (e) government regulations for drug administration in AD patients; (f) a rapid approach to molecular neuropharmacology; and (g) to develop more specific tools for the assessment of cognitive function, memory changes, and learning improvement. Therapeutic strategies in AD can be divided into five groups.

1. Palliative treatment. This group of drugs includes the following compounds: (a) neurometabolic enhancers, mainly represented by nootropic agents; (b) neurovascular regulators, including vasoactive agents and calcium channel blockers for improvement of brain perfusion and for optimization of cerebrovascular function; (c) drugs with potential neuroprotective effects: free radical scavengers, natural antioxidants, and phosphomonoesters involved in membrane repair; (d) psychotropic drugs for the control of depressive symptoms (antidepressants), anxiety and irritability (anxiolytics, benzodiazepines) and psychotic symptoms (neuroleptics); and (e) circadian rhythm regulators, a group of compounds with hypnotic activity devoid of benzodiazepine-like side effects, and melatonin-like compounds that act on the suprachiasmatic nucleus of the hypothalamus to regulate endogenous biorhythms. Most of these drugs are symptomatic, lacking specificity or proper anti-dementia effects. Some of them can even increase mental deterioration (i.e., neuroleptics, benzodiazepines), and most of them are currently used in the daily clinical setting (Cacabelos, 1991).

2. Substitutive treatment. Drugs included in this group are given to replace deficient neurotransmitters. They are classified into four main categories: (a) cholinergic enhancers for increasing acetylcholine transmission by providing precursors of synthesis, activating muscarinic and/or nicotinic receptors at the post-synaptic level, or inhibiting acetylcholinesterase to increase the availability of acetylcholine at the synaptic cleft. (b) Monoaminergic enhancers: the compounds belonging to this group tend to potentiate noradrenergic and dopaminergic transmission, though its use is very limited in AD, except in the case of some MAO-B inhibitors. (c) Neuropeptidergic enhancers: in the past decade several trials with neuropeptides (somatostatin, GRF, LHRH, vasopressin, ACTH, TRH, and analogs) have proved to be of limited value, due to their pharmacokinetic and pharmacodynamic properties. (d) Aminoacidergic regulators: the two modalities currently under study are GABAergic modulators with ß-carboline-like activity, and NMDA-receptor agonists or antagonists.

Replacement therapy with substitutive drugs is a supportive strategy of very modest value from a curative point of view, but it can help to relent the progression of the disease, above all in combination with non-psychotropic palliative drugs such as nootropics, calcium channel blockers, free radical scavengers, and phospholipids.

3. Etiopathogenic treatment. This strategy consists of using the present knowledge on the etiopathogenesis of AD to attempt a reduction in ßAP deposition, NFT formation, synaptic loss, and neuroimmune/inflammatory-driven cell death (Cacabelos et al., 1992, 1993, 1994a; McGeer and Rogers, 1992). For this purpose the following strategies might be used: (a) cDNA technology for regulating the expression of genes potentially involved in AD etiopathogenesis; (b) enzymatic treatments to regulate APP processing through a non-amyloidogenic pathway; (c) neurotrophic therapy for enhancing neuronal survival in vulnerable areas (neocortex, hippocampus); (d) neuroimmune intervention to regulate the immune cascade leading to neurodegeneration, abnormal astrogliosis, and cell death; and (e) anti-apoptosis and gerontogene-related intervention to regulate at the genetic and/or post-transcriptional level still unknown processes potentially directed to accelerate cell death.

The use of knockout (homologous recombination) and knockdown (antisense inhibition) are two tentative genetic interventions for therapeutic purposes. In particular, antisense oligonucleotide strategies represent an attractive approach in neuropharmacology (Wahlestedt, 1994). New DNA analogs are already in use, including 2'-modified oligodeoxynucleotides, oligodeoxynucleotides with 5'-cholesteryl moieties, and peptide nucleic acids.

In order to regulate APP processing, several strategies have been proposed including APP degradation inhibitors, phosphorylation inhibitors, APP-secretase regulators, inhibitors of amino- and carboxy-terminal ßAP-peptides (N-ßAP-peptidase), protein kinase C dephosphorylators, APP kinase modulators, APP phosphatase modulators, Ca^{2+}/calmodulin-dependent protein kinase II modulators, anti-proteolytic agents (phosphoprotein inhibitors), lysosomotropic agents, and calpain inhibitors (Cacabelos, 1991; Cacabelos et al., 1994b; Gandy and Greengard, 1992; Royston et al., 1992).

4. Pleiotropic treatments. Since it is unlikely that a single drug can preclude AD neuropathology and cognitive decline in AD, it would be wise to search into pleiotropic strategies with compounds displaying multifactorial effects. Some of these pleiotropic drugs might be found in animal, vegetal and marine extracts.

5. Neural transplantation. New developments in transplant technology and grafting, as well as genetic manipulation of pluripotential cells in culture might help to improve experimental results in neuronal transplantation with potential clinical use in the future.

From a chronological perspective we can preview for the coming years three complementary generations of anti-dementia drugs (Cacabelos et al., 1994b), beginning in 1993 with the approval of tacrine by the FDA.

CONVENTIONAL MULTIFACTORIAL TREATMENT

The therapeutic nihilism in AD prevalent for many years is at present unjustified. The administration of conventional drugs combined in a multifactorial fashion can delay the natural progression of AD for more than two years notably improving the quality of life of patients and relatives. For the past two years we were giving CDP-choline (1000 mg/day, p.o.), a choline donor involved in brain phospholipid metabolism, together with piracetam (4 g/day, p.o., t.i.d.) plus nimodipine (60-90 mg/day, p.o., t.i.d.) to a group of AD patients (N=14). Basal MMSE score was 24.5 ± 5.44 (MMSE Spanish version max. score = 35). MMSE score increased to 26.68 ± 5.12 at 3 months, 27.75

± 5.47 at 6 months, and 26.07 ± 6.69 after 12 months of daily treatment. With this supportive therapy, after one-year follow-up, 10 patients (71.43%) improved, 1 patient (7.14%) did not change, and 3 patients (21.43%) deteriorated with respect to basal mental performance. After 18 months of treatment the cognitive decline appeared again with a progression about 40-50% slower than that of patients with other therapeutic strategies or without any supportive treatment (Cacabelos et al., in preparation).

PRECLINICAL STUDIES

We are also investigating novel compounds and natural extracts with pleiotropic activities (neurotrophic, immunomodulatory, cognitive, and anti-degenerative effects) in the CNS. Two of these substances are anapsos/PL and S 9977-2.

Anapsos/PL is a purified extract of the fern *Polipodium leucotomos* with antitumor and immunomodulatory effects that improves memory and learning in rats with neurotoxic lesions in the nucleus basalis of Meynert (nbM), decreasing interleukin-1ß (IL-1ß) levels in the hippocampus and cortex of lesioned animals. In addition, anapsos/PL increases the concentration of tumor necrosis factor (TNF) in hippocampal-cortical regions, and reduces brain histamine (HA) levels (Alvarez et al., 1992). Since, IL-1ß, TNF and HA directly influence neuroinflammatory processes and neurodegeneration in AD (Cacabelos et al., 1994a), it seems plausible that PL exerts a neuroprotective effect in damaged areas.

S 9977-2 (1,3,7-trimethyl 8-[3-(4-diethylamino-carbonyl-1-piperazinyl)1-propyl]-3,7-dihydro(1H)2,6-purinedione hydrochloride) is a new trimethyl-xanthine derivative with antiamnesic and promnesic effects, enhancing brain cholinergic function, glucose utilization, and cerebral blood flow. In rats with lesions in the nbM, S 9977-2 reverses hyperactivity and memory dysfunctions, and also reduces IL-1ß in hypothalamus, hippocampus, and frontoparietal cortex (Alvarez et al., 1993).

CLINICAL STUDIES

We have also studied the therapeutic efficacy of two different compounds in AD, such as CDP-choline (cytidine-5-diphosphate-choline) and S 12024-2 (R,S 1-methyl 8(2-morpholinylmethoxy)-1,2,3,4,tetrahydroquinoleine methane sulphonate).

CDP-choline (1000 mg/day, p.o. x 3 months) significantly improved cognitive function, reducing delta and theta activity in frontal, parietal, and temporal regions as measured by brain mapping, and also improved hemodynamic parameters in the cerebral arteries studied by transcranial Doppler ultrasonography in early- and late-onset AD (N=20) (Cacabelos et al., 1992, 1993; Caamaño et al., 1994).

In phase IIa studies (double-blind, placebo-controlled protocol CL2-12024-005) with doses of 100 and 300 mg/day, p.o. for 28 days, S 12024-2 induced a moderate improvement in ADAS-Cog, MMSE and Trail Making Test in more than 75% of patients receiving 100 mg (N=11). In the same group, mild changes in brain bioelectrical activity (decrease in delta/theta, increase in alpha/beta activity) were observed. Brain hemodynamic parameters were also modified by S 12024-2, with a significant increase in diastolic velocity and a decrease in both pulsatile index and resistance index (Cacabelos et al., in preparation).

REFERENCES

Alvarez XA, Franco A, Fernández L and Cacabelos R (1992): Effects of anapsos on behavior and brain cytokines in rats. *Ann Psychiat* 3:329-341.

Alvarez XA, Franco A, Fernández-Novoa L and Cacabelos R (1993): Effects of S9977-2 on psychomotor activity, learning and brain interleukin-1ß in rats. *Meth Find Exp Clin Pharmacol* 15:587-595.

Cacabelos R (1991): Alzheimer's disease. *Barcelona: J.R. Prous.*

Cacabelos R, Alvarez XA, Franco A, Fernández-Novoa L, Caamaño J and Valle-Inclán F (1992): Therapeutic effects of CDP-choline in Alzheimer's disease and multi-infarct dementia: psychometric assessment and immune function. *Ann Psychiat* 3:233-245.

Cacabelos R, Alvarez XA, Franco-Maside A, Fernández-Novoa L and Caamaño J (1993): Effect of CDP-choline on cognition and immune function in Alzheimer's disease and multi-infarct dementia. *Ann New York Acad Sci* 695:321-328.

Cacabelos R, Alvarez XA, Fernández-Novoa L, Franco A, Mangues R and Pellicer A Nishimura T (1994a): Brain interleukin-1ß in Alzheimer's disease and vascular dementia. *Meth Find Exp Clin Pharmacol* 16:141-151.

Cacabelos R, Nordberg A, Caamaño J, Franco-Maside A, Fernández-Novoa L, Alvarez A, Takeda M, Prous J, Nishimura T and Winblad B (1994b): Molecular strategies for the first generations of anti-dementia drugs (I). Tacrine and related compounds. *Meth Find Exp Clin Pharmacol* (In Press).

Caamaño J, Gómez MJ, Franco A and Cacabelos R (1994): Effects of CDP- choline on cognition and cerebral hemodynamics in patients with Alzheimer's disease. *Meth Find Exp Clin Pharmacol* 13:211-218.

Gandy S and Greengard P (1992): Amyloidogenesis in Alzheimer's disease: some possible therapeutic opportunities. *Trends Pharmacol Sci* 13:108-113.

Hardy J and Allsop D (1991): Amyloid deposition as the central event in the aetiology of Alzheimer's disease. *Trends Pharmacol Sci* 12:383-388.

McGeer PL and Rogers J (1992): Anti-inflammatory agents as a therapeutic approach to Alzheimer's disease. *Neurology* 42:447-449.

Mullan M and Crawford F (1993): Genetic and molecular advances in Alzheimer's disease. *Trends Neurosci* 16:398-403.

Royston MC, Rothwell NJ and Roberts GW (1992): Alzheimer's disease: pathology to potential treatments? *Trends Pharmacol Sci* 13:131-133.

Terry RD, Masliah E, Salmon DP, Butters N, De Teresa R, Hill R, Hansen LA and
Katzman R (1991): Physical basis of cognitive alterations in Alzheimer's disease:
Synapse loss is the major correlate of cognitive impairment. *Ann Neurol* 30:572-580.

Wahlestedt C (1994): Antisense oligonucleotides strategies in neuropharmacology.
Trends Pharmacol Sci 15:42-46.

Wisniewski HM and Weigel J (1992): Alzheimer's disease neuropathology. *Ann New
York Acad Sci* 673:270-28.

AUTHOR INDEX

SUBJECT INDEX

Page numbers refer to the beginning of the chapter in which the entry is located.